Cancer Registry Management

Principles and Practices
for Hospitals and Central Registries

Third Edition

Editors

Herman R. Menck ▪ Donna M. Gress
Ann Griffin ▪ Linda Mulvihill ▪ Jim Hofferkamp
Carol Hahn Johnson ▪ Melissa Pearson

National Cancer Registrars Association, Inc.
Alexandria, VA

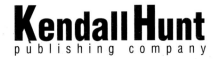
Kendall Hunt
p u b l i s h i n g   c o m p a n y

On the Cover:
The graphic illustrates the interconnection between the entities in the circles, with the focus of all activities being the patient. The process starts and ends with the patient. The hospital registry collects data on the patient. These data are submitted to the central, national, and international registries. The information is used by clinicians and researchers, and plays a major role in cancer education. The objective of these processes is to improve treatment, survival, and quality of life. All of these endeavors have a single purpose and ultimate goal: a cure for the cancer patient.

Kendall Hunt
publishing company

www.kendallhunt.com
Send all inquiries to:
4050 Westmark Drive
Dubuque, IA 52004-1840

To people whose lives have been touched by cancer:

to our colleagues, past, present, and future, who are committed to cancer data management;

to the physicians, researchers, epidemiologists, and administrators who use our data to understand disease process, improve cancer treatment, increase survival, and improve long-term quality of life for cancer patients;

to all the patients we serve;

we dedicate this book.

contents

vi

This Preface is an updated version by earlier writers and editors. Some sections of the earlier writing have been paraphrased herein. Previous editions of this book were published as two separate volumes: one primarily targeted for hospital cancer registries and the other for central or population-based cancer registries. The two separate books were considered companion volumes. This third edition brings the two companion volumes together. The first editions of these companion books were written in the early 1990s; since then, many advances have been made in cancer data collection and reporting. Previous editions were well received throughout the field and seemingly fulfilled its overall objective to provide technical and management issues defined in a comprehensive textbook. This volume, and all except one of the previous editions, is sponsored by the National Cancer Registrars Association (NCRA). This textbook is largely the result of a collaborative effort of a volunteer team of registry professionals who represent various organizations from the cancer surveillance community in North America. The editors and contributors have received no payment or honoraria.

Cancer registration is an important and fundamental tool in cancer control. A cancer registry has been defined as a system for the collection, storage, analysis, and interpretation of data on persons with cancer, within a healthcare facility or group of healthcare facilities. A population-based cancer registry collects the data from many healthcare facilities in a defined geographic area and can serve to show incidence trends for cancer of different sites over time or between population subdivisions. It can provide data to assess the effects of different types of treatments over time and to evaluate the effects of early detection programs, such as mammography or colorectal screening.

Cancer registry data can be used for epidemiologic studies, to direct resources for screening programs, and for education. Data from cancer registries can be helpful in assessing the need for new hospital construction, equipment, and staff. The medical community and the public may use registry data to pinpoint locations of facilities for cancer care.

Readers of this edition will recognize several topics and subjects that were covered in previous editions. These topics have been revisited with intent to update, enhance, and enrich the original pretext of those subjects, as new material has been discovered and technologies improved. In all cases throughout this book, new axioms and approaches are delineated in the interest of providing the reader with the most effective strategies available in the essential responsibilities of a cancer registrar.

This edition is composed of 42 chapters, which are organized into 6 sections:

- Planning and Design of Registries
- Informatics
- Operations
- Uses of Registry Data
- Standard Setters and Professional Organizations
- Central and Other Registries

Appendices include a glossary of registry terms and an index.

A Review Guide on a compact disc accompanies the book and includes a set of questions with answers for each chapter. Educators may use the questions for discussion and to help the reader focus on important points within the text. The Review Guide should be used by all readers to check their understanding of each chapter.

More than 50 authors have brought many years of experience with cancer registration to this project. Most importantly, they have brought together a comprehensive text that covers the two main types of cancer registries in North America: the hospital and population-based registries. This book will be a valuable resource for anyone intent on understanding and learning about cancer registration.

EDITORS

Donna M. Gress, RHIT, CTR

Ann Griffin, PhD, CTR

Jim Hofferkamp, BA, CTR

Carol Hahn Johnson, BS, CTR

Herman R. Menck, BS, MBA, CPhil, FACE

Linda Mulvihill, RHIT, CTR

Melissa Pearson, BS, CTR

CONTRIBUTORS

Judy H. Andrews, CTR

Lillian Antonelli-Twal, MS, CTR

Frank P. Boscoe, PhD

Connie Bura

Elizabeth Butts, MPH, CTR, CPC

M. Asa Carter, CTR

Gayle Greer Clutter, RT, CTR

Elaine Collins, RHIA, CTR

Linda Coyle, BS

Kathleen A. Cronin, PhD

Dan Curran, MS, CTR

Lois Dickie, CTR

Raye-Ann Dorn, MPH, CTR

Lynda Douglas, CTR

Eric B. Durbin, MS

Brenda K. Edwards, PhD

Nancy Etzold, CTR

Thom H. Faris, Esq., JD, CQA, CQM

Amy M. Fremgen, PhD, CTR (Retired)

April Fritz, RHIT, CTR

Laurel Gray, CTR

Donna M. Gress, RHIT, CTR

Ann Griffin, PhD, CTR

Lilly Grossman, BA

Jennifer Hafterson, BA, CTR

Elaine Hamlyn, CTR

Nadia Howlader, MS

Annette A. Hurlbut, RHIT, CTR

Sonja Jennings, CTR

Mildred N. Jones, BA, CTR

Linda L. Jund, BS, CTR

Mary Jane King, MPH, CTR

Betsy A. Kohler, MPH, CTR

Carol L. Kosary, MA

Sharon Labbate, CTR

Wendy J. Langeberg, PhD, MPH

Maureen MacIntyre, BSN, MHSA

Ruth Maranda, LPN, CTR

Colleen C. McLaughlin, PhD, CTR

Herman R. Menck, BS, MBA, CPhil, FACE

Fran Michaud, CTR

Linda Mulvihill, RHIT, CTR

Jaclyn K. Nee, MPH

David K. O'Brien, PhD, GISP

Steven Peace, BS, CTR

Melissa Pearson, BS, CTR

Jerri Linn Phillips, MA, CTR

Karen Pollitt

Wai Poon, CTR

Mary Potts, RHIA, CPA, CTR

Bonnie Quiñónez, BSB/M, RHIT, CTR

Therese Richardson, RHIA, CTR

Lynn Ries, MS

Kathleen M. Rogers, CTR

Louise Schuman, MA, CTR

Nicola Schussler, BS

Andrew K. Stewart, MA

Judith Swan, MHS

Kathleen K. Thoburn, CTR

Cindy L. Tillman, RHIT, CTR

John W. Tillman, BA, CTR

Judy Tryon, CTR

Tom C. Tucker, PhD, MPH

Judy Jacobs Williams, RHIT, CTR

Dianna Wilson, RHIA, CTR

Reda Wilson, MPH, RHIT, CTR

acknowledgments

We wish to thank the many contributing authors to this third edition. Thank you to all those who authored chapters and shared your information and ideas to advance the cancer registry profession. This includes individuals as well as staff members from the following organizations:

> National Cancer Registrars Association (NCRA)
> Commission on Cancer (CoC) of the American College of Surgeons (ACoS)
> American Joint Committee on Cancer (AJCC)
> Surveillance, Epidemiology, and End Results Program (SEER)
> National Program of Cancer Registrars (NPCR)
> North American Association of Central Registries (NAACCR)
> Department of Defense (DOD) and other Federal Registries, and the
> Canadian registry community

We thank the members and Board of Directors of the NCRA for your understanding and support during the writing of this textbook. We know you are proud of this finished product.

The quality of this book is due to the many skillful reviewers who read the manuscripts for accuracy, consistency, and completeness. We thank you for your advice and wisdom.

We would like to thank all of the authors and editors who provided and managed content for the previous editions of this textbook. This new compiled edition would not have been possible without your initial commitment to develop and prepare that original text as the original text still remains as a baseline in several areas of this new edition. Thank you for your commitment.

Finally, we thank our families, friends, and colleagues, who endured our temperaments during this enormous undertaking. We believe that it has been well worth the effort.

Herman R. Menck
Donna M. Gress
Ann Griffin
Linda Mulvihill
Jim Hofferkamp
Carol Hahn Johnson
Melissa Pearson

Planning and Design of Registries

Donna M. Gress
Section Editor—Textbook

Carol Hahn Johnson
Section Editor—Review Guide

chapter 1

Introduction to Cancer Registries

Gayle Greer Clutter, RT, CTR

Introduction

The word *cancer* is actually a catch-phrase for many diseases with a wide variety of causes. It can result from genetic predisposition, lifestyle choices, environmental factors, or a combination of these factors, and many causes are as yet unknown. Cancer in its many forms represents a major public health issue, as well as a significant challenge for individuals and the healthcare industry.

There is recorded evidence that humans throughout history have had cancer. It has been found as fossilized bone tumors, in human mummies in ancient Egypt, and in ancient manuscripts. Mummies have been found to have growths suggestive of bone cancer, or osteosarcoma, and bony skull destruction suggestive of cancer of the head and neck.[1]

Our oldest description of cancer (although the term *cancer* was not used) was discovered in Egypt and dates back to approximately 1600 B.C. Seven papyri relating the earliest known descriptions of cancer were discovered and deciphered late in the nineteenth century. These provided the first direct knowledge of Egyptian medical practice. Two of them, known as the Edwin Smith and George Ebers papyri, contain descriptions of cancer and were written about 1600 B.C. but are believed to date from sources as early as 2500 B.C. The Smith papyrus describes surgery relating eight cases of tumors or ulcers of the breast that were treated by cauterization, with a tool called "the fire drill." The writing says about the disease, "There is no treatment." The Ebers papyrus outlines pharmacologic, mechanical, and magical treatments.[1,2]

The origin of the word *cancer,* however, is credited to the Greek physician Hippocrates around 460 to 370 B.C., who used the terms *carcinos* and *carcinoma* to describe non-ulcer-forming and ulcer-forming tumors. In Greek, these words refer to a crab, most likely applied to the disease because the finger-like spreading projections from a cancer called to mind the shape of a crab.[1]

Cancer was first recorded as a cause of death in 1629 in England in the Bills of Mortality, and the first systemized collection of information on cancer was in 1728 in London. In 1839, death registration was implemented in the United States.[3,4] In 1842, an Italian physician surveyed the entire population of his hometown, Verona, to determine the prevalence of certain diseases, including cancer. Based on his surveys, he reported notable differences in the rates of certain types of cancer in nuns and married women.[5]

Cancer remains a major health concern in the United States and throughout the world with the estimated 1,479,350 new cancer cases in 2009 in the United States. The estimated number of cancer deaths for that same year is 562,340.[6] Each year, 10.9 million people worldwide are diagnosed with cancer, and there are 6.7 million deaths from the disease. It is estimated that there are 24.6 million people alive who have received a diagnosis of cancer in the last 5 years.[7]

In the United States, long-term cancer mortality data exist for all states since 1933, whereas long-term incidence data are available since 1975 only from the original registries included in the National Cancer Institute's (NCI's) Surveillance, Epidemiology, and End Results (SEER) Program, covering about 10% of the population.[8]

However, there is good news. The *Annual Report to the Nation on the Status of Cancer, 1975–2005* reported that both incidence and death rates from all cancers combined continue to decrease in men and women overall and in most racial and ethnic populations. Cancer death rates for both sexes combined declined about 1.8% per year from 2002 through 2005, almost double the 1.1% per year decrease seen from 1993 through 2002. Also, for the first time in the 10-year history of this report, incidence rates for all cancers combined decreased, falling by 0.8% per year from 1999 to 2005. This continuing decline in mortality rates is evidence of real progress made against cancer, reflecting real gains in prevention, early detection, and treatment.[9]

The statistics in this report are made possible through the marked progress made in cancer registration in the United States. Cancer surveillance is entering an exciting era where the scope of its activities will be expanded and the amount, quality, and depth of information on cancer will be richer and more readily available to practitioners, decision makers, and the public. This future is being built on a solid history of accomplishment that has placed cancer foremost among all chronic diseases in the organization and implementation of a systematic and integrated monitoring enterprise that is of essential value in both clinical medicine and public health.

Many cancer agencies and organizations rely on data collected by cancer registries. Based on accurate and timely cancer statistics, healthcare planners make decisions on resource allocation, such as the placement of radiotherapy facilities, proper staffing of cancer control programs, and "market share" reports for existing facilities. Statistics provided by population-based registries also make it possible for public health administrators to evaluate suspected clusters of cancer within communities or population groups. Cancer incidence data also provide cancer burden information for cancer surveillance and are used for comprehensive cancer control planning. Cancer data alert public health officials to trends within communities and potentially dangerous environmental or workplace conditions.

History of Cancer Registration

The term *surveillance* is derived from the French word meaning "to watch over." As applied to public health, it means the close monitoring of the occurrence of selected health conditions in the population. The ultimate goal of surveillance is the use of the data collected for the formulation of policies and programs to promote health and prevent disease. It involves the systematic collection of data to ensure consistent and comparable data are collected in a regular fashion. Data need to be collected in a timely way and should be of direct relevance to the health needs of a population.[10]

In the past, public health surveillance was primarily related to surveillance of infectious diseases and indicators of disease such as morbidity or mortality. The idea of recording information on all cancer cases in defined populations started in the mid-twentieth century. Originally, this consisted primarily of describing cancer patterns and trends. Later, information on other aspects of cancer occurrence and on the control of the disease developed. This resulted from the need for information on survival after identification of cancer at the population level, and later to study the effects of various aspects of services for prevention, early diagnosis, treatment, and care.

This cancer surveillance model was then applied in various areas around the world, and a steady increase in the number of cancer registries seen today attests to their value in cancer research and control. In 2008, these cancer registries covered around 21% of the world population.[11] Some registries cover the entire national populations, and in smaller countries this can be achieved with a single cancer registry. However, larger populations may have several registries covering specific populations. In most countries, one or more cancer registries provide coverage of a sample of the population, although this is by no means random.

The oldest example of a modern cancer registry is that of Hamburg, Germany, which was started with the idea that cancer control involves not only medical and scientific but public health and economic aspects (Table 1-1).

In 1926, an after-care organization for cancer patients was founded on a private basis. From 1929, it obtained official status as the follow-up patient care service of the Hamburg Public Health Department. Three nurses visited hospitals and medical practitioners in Hamburg, recorded the names of new cancer patients, and transferred data to a central index in the health department. The card index was, in turn, compared once a week with official death certificates and formed the basis of the Hamburg Cancer Registry.[12]

In the United States in 1926, the first site-specific cancer registry was established with Dr. Ernest Codman's Registry of Bone Sarcoma[13] and the Yale-New Haven Hospital Cancer Registry, a hospital-based registry, was established.[4,14]

Population-based cancer registration with an epidemiologic and ecologic objective started in the United States in 1935 when a division of cancer research was formed in the Connecticut State Department of Health "to make investigations concerning cancer, the prevention and treatment thereof and the mortality there from, and to take such action as it may deem will assist in bringing about a reduction in the mortality due thereto."[12] The Connecticut Tumor Registry began operation on a statewide basis in 1941, registering cases retrospectively back to 1935.[4,15,16] Further cancer registries were established in the United States and Canada in the early 1940s.

In 1937, the National Cancer Institute Act was passed establishing the NCI within the Public Health Service. It was directed by the Surgeon General to promote research, and it established a National Advisory Cancer Council.

The Danish Cancer Registry was founded in 1942 under the auspices of the Danish Cancer Society; it is

Table 1-1	History of Cancer Registration
2500 B.C.	Earliest known description of *cancer;* the "Edwin Smith" and "George Ebers" papyri describe surgery, pharmacology, and mechanical and magical treatments
400 B.C.	Hippocrates described a breast "cancer" as *karkinoma* (known now as carcinoma) during surgical removal of a tumor
1629 A.D.	Cancer is first mentioned as a cause of death in the Bills of Mortality in England
1728	London's "General Census of Cancer"—the first known systematic collection of information on cancer
1839	Implementation of death registration (what we now know as "death certification") in the United States
1842	Italian physician surveys the entire population Verona to determine the prevalence of certain diseases, including cancer
1926	The oldest example of a modem cancer registry is established in Hamburg. Germany A bone sarcoma registry is established by Dr. Ernest Codman at Massachusetts General Hospital, one of the earliest registries established for a specific type of cancer The first hospital-based cancer registry at Yale-New Haven Hospital was organized in New Haven, Connecticut
1933	U.S. long-term cancer mortality data exist for all states
1935	First population-based cancer registry in the United States established in Connecticut
1937	National Cancer Institute Act passed establishing the National Cancer Institute (NCI)
1942	The Danish Cancer Registry is the oldest functioning registry covering a national population
1956	In the United States, the American College of Surgeons Commission on Cancer encourages the development of hospital-based cancer registries
1971	The U.S. National Cancer Act budgets monies to the NCI for research, detection, and treatment of cancer

the oldest functioning registry covering a national population. Cases were reported by physicians on a voluntary basis with the support of the Danish Medical Association, whereas the National Board of Health assisted by giving full access to death certificates and all mortality data. The task of the registry was outlined as the collection of data serving as a basis: (1) for an individual follow-up of patients; (2) for reliable morbidity statistics with a view to an accurate estimate of therapeutic results; and (3) for an accurate evaluation of variations in incidence of malignant neoplasms, secular as well as geographical, occupational, and so forth.[4,17] From the mid-1940s, cancer registries were started in a number of other countries.

In the United States in 1956, the American College of Surgeons (ACoS), Commission on Cancer (CoC), through their Approvals Program, formally adopted a policy to encourage the development of hospital-based cancer registries. It was believed that by periodically reviewing the results of cancer treatment regimens, the hospitals and physicians might reveal weaknesses in local patterns of care and ultimately develop a better understanding of the disease and its treatment.

In 1971, the U.S. National Cancer Act declared "The War on Cancer" by budgeting monies to the NCI for research, detection, and treatment of cancer. This funding supported basic research and set up application programs such as the European Organization for Research and Treatment of Cancer and U.S. clinical trials programs. It established that the NCI Director would be Presidentially-appointed, and that the Director would prepare and submit a Bypass Budget directly to the President of the United States. It also established the President's Cancer Panel and the National Cancer Advisory Board, directed the expansion and development of a coordinated cancer research program, authorized the first cancer centers, and established the International Cancer Research Data Bank.[18,19] This act also resulted in the eventual establishment of the *SEER program* (Figure 1-1).[20]

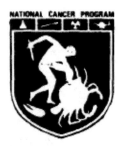

Figure 1-1. From the *1976 Seer Code Manual*, National Cancer Institute, Biometry Branch.

Types of Cancer Registries

A cancer registry is a system designed to collect information about the occurrence of cancer, the types of cancers that occur and their locations within the body, the extent of cancer at the time of diagnosis, and the kinds of treatments that patients receive. Some cancer registries also collect follow-up information regarding the patient's cancer status.

There are three main types of cancer registries: hospital based, population based, and specialty cancer registries. Depending on the operators, population-based registries can be administrative, research, or cancer control oriented. Ideally, registries of a combination of above three functions predominate because of the mission of the primary funding source. There are many different examples of specialty cancer registries.

Hospital-Based Cancer Registries

In the United States, hospital-based (or institution-based) registries are the foundation of cancer surveillance. Hospital-based cancer registries may be single hospital registries or collective (multi-institution) registries. They maintain data on all patients diagnosed and/or treated for cancer at a particular facility or facilities. The focus of the hospital-based cancer registry is on clinical care and hospital administration. The primary goal of these registries is to improve patient care by evaluation of treatment outcomes. Data collected by these registries may be used for physician education, research, and facility utilization review. Therefore, they have to collect detailed data about diagnosis and treatment, as well as recurrence and survival. Because the data collected by hospital cancer registries usually include those needed by population-based cancer registries and both use the same classifications, data are sent from a hospital cancer registry to population-based registries, thus reducing documentation efforts. CoC-approved hospital registries are required to collect active lifetime follow-up data on all patients in their registries. Most population-based registries do not collect active follow-up information.[21]

Population-Based Cancer Registries

Population-based cancer registries collect data on all cancer cases in a defined population. The main sources of information for population-based registries include: (1) information from treatment facilities, such as hospitals, cancer centers, private clinics and hospices; (2) information from diagnostic services, such as pathology laboratories; and (3) death certificate information from the vital statistics registration system. Information is collected on new cases in a defined population such as a state, country, or region for a specific disease such as cancer.[11]

State and national population-based or central cancer registries (CCRs) have an emphasis on epidemiology and public health. In contrast with hospital-based registries, they are designed to determine cancer patterns among various populations or subpopulations, to monitor cancer trends over time, to guide planning and evaluation of cancer control efforts, to help prioritize health resource allocations, and to advance clinical, epidemiologic, and health services research.

These registries also play an important role in improving patient care programs, in research into the cause of cancer, by providing data on patterns and trends, and in different types of epidemiologic study such as their ability to follow up on groups of persons exposed to a potential hazard. They comprise an essential element in the planning and monitoring of cancer control strategies and for identifying priorities in public health. Linkage for healthcare providers offers a cost-effective source of data necessary for clinical programs. These programs may include follow-up results of a mammography program, stage of diagnosis data to managed care organizations, or treatment selection data for groups monitoring clinical treatment guidelines utilization. These cancer registries may also provide services to hospital cancer programs such as shared follow-up, death clearance, and pooled data on treatment, stage, or survival.[22]

Currently, every state in the United States has a population-based state-wide CCR. The data collected by state CCRs serve a wide range of purposes. Advantages of these registries include local cancer control programs, patient care programs, administrative programs, and cancer research programs. Data from state CCRs can be used for monitoring the distribution of late-diagnosed cancer cases of those types for which early diagnosis is the strategy for control. They can also monitor distributions in communities, ethnicities, age groups, and other demographic characteristics.

Many countries have national cancer registries with varying degrees of population coverage. In 2007, 313 cancer registries replied to the invitation to participate by submitting data for volume IX of *Cancer Incidence in Five Continents.*[23] The United States has two agencies that provide national cancer data.

- The SEER Program began collecting data on cancer cases in 1973 for six states and two metropolitan areas. Over time, additional metropolitan areas and states were added to better represent the U.S. population demographics. SEER currently collects and publishes cancer incidence and survival data from population-based cancer registries covering approximately 26% of the U.S. population. The SEER Program registries routinely collect data on patient demographics, primary tumor site, tumor morphology, detailed stage at diagnosis, first course of treat-

ment, and active follow-up for cancer and vital status. From these data, SEER produces estimates of cancer incidence.

- The National Program of Cancer Registries (NPCR) Cancer Surveillance System (CSS) was authorized by the Cancer Registries Amendment Act of 1992. This law allowed the Centers for Disease Control and Prevention (CDC) to receive, evaluate, and disseminate data from participating state CCRs. In 1999, NPCR established the CSS that collects data annually from all NPCR programs. It is designed to provide cancer incidence data to meet the CDC's public health surveillance responsibilities and to help monitor progress toward NPCR goals. In 2007, these data covered 96% of the U.S. population.[24] NPCR data include the limited summary stage and treatment data, but do not include survival data.

Specialty Cancer Registries

Specialty cancer registries may be established to collect and maintain data from specific facilities, such as the ACoS CoC's National Cancer Data Base (NCDB), on a particular type of cancer site such as the Central Brain Tumor Registry of the United States (CBTRUS), or to collect data on familial cancers such as the Gilda Radner Familial Ovarian Cancer Registry. Some of these special cancer registries may also provide advocacy, educational opportunities for those who want to learn more about a particular type of cancer, and support for those who may suffer from it.

- *CoC's NCDB:* Of these special population-based registries, the NCDB is one of the oldest and largest in the United States. Begun in 1989, it is a nationwide *oncology outcomes database* for more than 1,400 CoC-approved cancer programs in the United States and Puerto Rico that includes approximately 75% of all newly diagnosed cases of cancer in the United States. Data are captured at the institutional level and reported to the NCDB. These data are used to explore trends in cancer care, to create regional and state benchmarks for participating hospitals, and to serve as the basis for quality improvement. Data collected include patient characteristics, detailed tumor staging and histology characteristics, type of first course treatment administered, and active follow-up for cancer recurrence and survival information.[25]
- *Familial and site-specific cancer registries:* The operation of this type of registry differs from the other cancer registries previously discussed. Frequently participants are voluntarily self-enrolled or enrolled by physicians. Also, in addition to maintaining a registry and doing research, they often act as patient advocates, and provide patient information and support. Some are institution based, and others are national and international cooperative groups. The following are various examples of the types of familial and site-

specific cancer registries, but they in no way represent all of them.

- *CBTRUS* was formed in 1992 to report population-based data on primary benign, borderline, and malignant central nervous system tumors. A not-for-profit corporation, it is committed to providing a resource for gathering and disseminating current epidemiologic data on all primary brain tumors for the purposes of accurately describing their incidence and survival patterns, evaluating diagnosis and treatment, facilitating etiologic studies, establishing awareness of the disease, and ultimately, for the prevention of all brain tumors. Originally, data were provided by participating state CCRs, but currently, data come from CDC's NPCR-CSS and SEER.[26]

- *The Breast Cancer Family Registry (B-CFR),* established in 1995 by the NCI, is an international coalition that includes participants from academic and research institutions and their medical affiliates in the United States, Australia, and Canada, among other countries. In addition, participants include other U.S. medical centers that run family registries, targeting a variety of malignancies including 12 primary sites, such as melanoma, pancreatic, and prostate cancer. By 2006, nearly 26,000 people had enrolled. This registry is designed for investigators interested in conducting population- and clinic-based interdisciplinary studies on the genetic and molecular epidemiology of breast cancer and its behavioral implications. The B-CFR has information and biospecimens contributed by more than 12,500 families across the spectrum of risk for these cancers and from population-based or relative control subjects.[27]

- *Gilda Radner Familial Ovarian Cancer Registry* is an international registry of families with two or more relatives with ovarian cancer. The registry is a national computer tracking system, and in addition to ovarian cancer research, the registry offers an hotline, newsletter, and ovarian cancer informational pamphlets.[28]

- *National Familial Lung Cancer Registry* was established in 1993 at Johns Hopkins Medical Institutions. If two or more people in a family have been diagnosed with lung cancer, the family is eligible to be part of the registry. Family members and patients can refer

themselves. The goals of registry are to further the understanding of the causes of lung cancer beyond smoking, and to serve as an educational resource for persons at risk for lung cancer.[29]

- The *Cancer Genetics Network (CGN)* is a research resource for investigators conducting research on the genetic basis of human cancer susceptibility, integration of this information into medical practice, and behavioral, ethical, and public health issues associated with human genetics. A core dataset is available on each participant and contains information on sociodemographic characteristics, history of cancer and/or premalignant conditions, cancer-relevant surgeries, four-generation cancer family pedigree, history of tobacco use, and expressed interest in genetic counseling. The CGN is supported through a contract from NCI's Epidemiology and Genetics Research Program to Massachusetts General Hospital in 2007.[30]

Cancer Registry Data Standardization
Why We Need Standards

One of the fundamental necessities of cancer surveillance is for users of cancer information to be assured that case definitions, coding practices, and conversions of medical terminology to useful categories is standardized. This enables compilation of case-specific information into useful and meaningful data. It also enables meaningful comparison of data across different registries. The goal is to set standards and build consensus for the collection of uniform cancer data across the world.

In the United States, cancer registries have earned the reputation as one of the most complete and highest quality public health surveillance systems (Table 1-2). This achievement may be attributable not only to current standards in case definitions and data elements, and to comprehensive case identification, but to the rigorous training and certification procedures for cancer registrars and reporters, and even to certification of registries themselves.[31]

Table 1-2	U.S. National Cancer Surveillance Programs
1973	The Surveillance, Epidemiology and End Results (SEER) Program of the National Cancer Institute (NCI) establishes the first national cancer registry program
1989	Commission on Cancer (CoC) establishes National Cancer Data Base (NCDB), a nationwide oncology outcomes database
1992	U.S. Public Law 102–515 establishes the National Program of Cancer Registries (NPCR) and is administered by the U.S. Centers for Disease Control and Prevention (CDC)
1999	NPCR establishes the Cancer Surveillance System

In the late 1980s, increased efforts to pool data collected by different cancer registries for different purposes drew attention to problems encountered as a result of insufficient data standardization. It became clear throughout the cancer registry community that the lack of standardization had a substantial cost and limited more widespread use of valuable data. Often, data were collected using different software, different data variables, different codes, and different coding rules. CCRs experienced the frustration of mapping hospital submission files into their own data systems. Software providers were frustrated at the need to prepare submissions for multiple CCRs that differed from each other and followed different models of electronic data collection. Hospital- and population-based cancer registries also report their incidence data to national organizations that aggregate and publish the data. The ways in which these data were formatted to be submitted to these organizations were determined by standards released by standard-setting organizations and often were not consistent.

Standardization of cancer registry data is now a core component of cancer registration and surveillance, and provides the foundation for developing comparable data among registries that can then be combined for the compilation of regional or national rates. These registry data must fulfill some criteria of comparability and quality control. Data standards ensure that cases are properly recorded, and that the statistical data gathered are complete and can be used to make valid comparisons. Cancer registries must conform to accepted working practices and standards so that data from different registries can be used for comparison of variations in cancer rates among different populations and across geographic boundaries.

However, case definitions and required data elements for cancer data are not federally mandated but may be established by individual state and provincial legislation. State government legislation or rules and regulation that create CCRs may define specific reporting requirements, including the specific data elements required and requirements for timely reporting. The CCR data elements and time requirements for reporting are not always the same as those for the hospital registries. Also, if a registry participates in a national program, like the NCDB, SEER, or NPCR, specific case definitions and data elements are required by each organization. In addition, each organization requires that certain electronic data edits are now run on the data to check for inaccuracies and duplicate cases before being submitted electronically. Different organizations have different standards for data reliability and completeness, and some award recognition based on the adherence to these standards.

Professional and standard-setting organizations are working together through the North American Association of Central Cancer Registries (NAACCR) to set up uniform data standards for cancer reporting for both hospital- and population-based registries. The following section describes these standard-setting organizations.

The Standard Setters
American Cancer Society

Historically, the American Cancer Society (ACS) has supported the development of standardized cancer classification systems, publishing the first code manual for the morphology of neoplasms in 1951. An example is *The Hospital Cancer Registry*, first published in 1964 (Figure 1-2). The

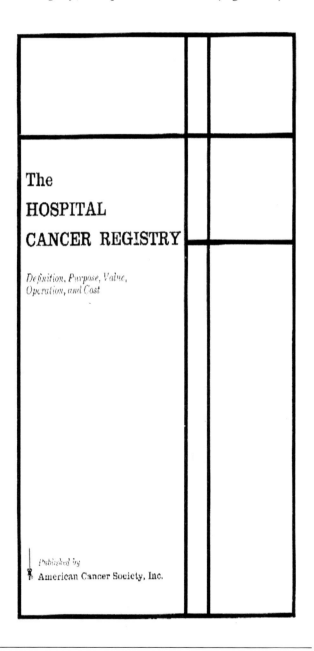

Figure 1-2. Early Manual Defining the Hospital Registry. From *The Hospital Cancer Registry: Definition, Purpose, Value, Operations, and Cost,* published by the American Cancer Society. Copyright © 1964 by American Cancer Society. This is reproduced with permission of John Wiley & Sons, Inc.

ACS has also consistently supported the standard-setting programs of ACoS, including the Fundamental Tumor Registry Operations (FTRO) Education Program, Registry Operations and Data Standards, national patient care evaluation studies, and the NCDB, as well as the efforts of the NCI, National Cancer Registrars Association (NCRA), NAACCR, National Coordinating Council for Cancer Surveillance (NCCCS), CDC, and American Joint Committee on Cancer (AJCC).[32] The ACS has been a strong supporter of NCRA, housing the first NCRA home office in 1981 in their New York City office.[33]

Commission on Cancer

In 1922, the ACoS established the multidisciplinary CoC, which was the first U.S. organization to establish standards to ensure quality, multidisciplinary, and comprehensive cancer care delivery in healthcare settings. In the 1930s, the CoC teamed up with the ACS to establish standards for cancer clinics, and in 1931, the minimum standards for cancer clinics were first published in the June edition of the CoC *Bulletin.* Since the 1950s, the CoC has diligently worked to establish guidelines for hospital-based cancer registries (Table 1-3).

The CoC has recognized the cancer registry as the focus of a hospital cancer program since 1956 with a mandatory standard that a cancer registry is required for CoC accreditation. The first manual on tumor registry operation and coding was published in 1962. An example is the *Manual for Cancer Programs,* published in 1966 (Figure 1-3). In 1974,

the CoC published the first *Cancer Registry Manual,* and in 1981, the *Cancer Program Manual* included a *Supplement for the Tumor Registry,* which described hospital-based cancer registry operations and files. With the publication of the first Data Acquisition Manual in 1988, for the first time, the coding systems for common data items required by both CoC and SEER were the same.[34] The CoC continues to provide institution-based cancer registry standards that are continually updated to meet the needs for cancer data.

In the 1980s, personal computers began to be introduced into hospital-based cancer registries requiring that most data be coded. Dr. Charles Smart of the CoC realized that this offered a great potential for sharing data electronically. He also recognized that this would require standard data item definitions and standard codes. He and his colleagues even pioneered the development of cancer registry software for personal and mini-computers with the idea of providing cost-effective registry software so that registries would all collect data using the same definitions and codes. Until that time, most registry computerization was in the larger facilities or those facilities within the SEER program, registry software was largely institution specific, and sharing of databases was difficult.

The CoC also endorsed several standards established by other organizations. Since its publication, the World Health Organization's *International Classification of Diseases for Oncology (ICD-O)* has been the standard by which primary site and morphology for neoplasms has been coded throughout the world. The AJCC published the first Manual for Staging of Cancer in 1977 utilizing the

Table 1-3	Cancer Registry Standards
1931	Commission on Cancer (CoC) published minimum standards for cancer clinics
1951	American Cancer Society (ACS) published first code manual for the morphology of neoplasms
1956	CoC requires a cancer registry as a component of an approved cancer program
1962	CoC publishes first manual on tumor registry operation and coding
1966	International Association of Cancer Registries (IACR) established
1967	First coding manual from National Cancer Institute (NCI) End Results Group
1974	CoC publishes the first *Cancer Registry Manual*
1976	World Health Organization's *International Classification of Diseases for Oncology* Surveillance, Epidemiology, and End Results (SEER) Code Manual published
1977	American Joint Committee on Cancer (AJCC) Cancer Staging Manual, First Edition SEER Summary Staging Guide SEER Extent of Disease coding
1981	CoC *Cancer Program Manual* includes a *Supplement for the Tumor Registry*
1983	National Cancer Registrars Association's (NCRA's) first certification examination
1987	North American Association of Central Cancer Registries (NAACCR) established and Uniform Data Standards Committee formed
1988	SEER Extent of Disease Codes and Coding Instructions, First Edition First CoC Data Acquisition Manual
1992	National Program of Cancer Registries (NPCR) law passed
1994	NAACCR publishes *Standards for Cancer Registries*
1997	NAACCR institutes a ceretifiction program for CCRs
2004	Collaborative Staging Manual and Coding Instructions, Version 1.0

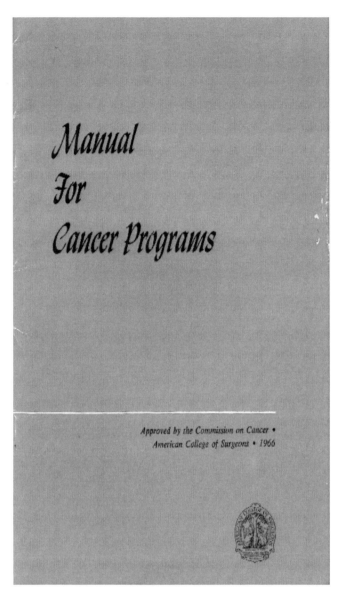

Tumor Node Metastasis (TNM) system, and CoC required the use of this staging system starting with breast cancers in 1982, adding lung and colon cancers in 1986. By 1991, AJCC staging was required for all sites.

In 1997, the AJCC in collaboration with SEER, CDC, and NAACCR established the Best Stage Task Force to address differences between staging systems, issues of clinical versus pathologic staging, and duplication of data collection. The charge to the Best Stage Task Force was to resolve these issues and define a system to use best available

information to determine a single "best stage" to meet the objectives of all surveillance organizations. Concluding in its preliminary work that defining a single "best" stage would not meet the objectives of all users, the task force determined that the cancer surveillance community would best be served by development of a uniform data collection set from which Summary Stage (SS), Extent of Disease (EOD), and TNM could be derived.[35]

This single dataset unified collection rules and standards from the various staging systems. It maintained the overall objectives of programs, resolved the differences in staging rules including timing of data collection, and allowed combining of clinical and pathologic data. The data system was based on a modified SEER EOD system and included all elements for TNM and SS. A computer algorithm would be able to derive SS and TNM. It would make use of the best available data for staging from both pathologic and clinical staging information. The system was called Collaborative Staging and was implemented throughout the United States in 2004.

The Surveillance, Epidemiology, and End Results Program

SEER is the second organization to establish standards for cancer data collection. It is a population-based cancer registry with contracted state CCRs, metropolitan areas, or rural county groupings submitting data for inclusion in the SEER database. The cancer patient data are collected from health providers such as hospitals, clinics, pathology labs, and physician offices, as well as from autopsy reports and death certificates.

The SEER Program is a continuation of at least two preceding NCI programs: the End Results Group Program and the Third National Cancer Survey. Their first coding manual was the *End Results Group 1967 Code Manual* with instructions developed to meet the specific requirements of the End Results Evaluation Program. The definitions and codes contained in this manual were not proposed as national standards but were based on more than 10 years of experience in a collaborative program that had collected information on more than 500,000 cancer patients treated in more than 100 hospitals. Data items included those for patient identification, description of the tumor, description of treatment, and follow-up information.

As mentioned earlier, SEER began collecting data on cancer cases in 1973, and the first SEER Code Manual was published in 1976. This manual was described as being a limited explanation of the format and definitions of the computerized record submitted by participants to SEER for analysis of the pooled data. SEER published the Summary Staging System in 1977 that categorized the extent of disease into five categories: In Situ, Local, Regional, Distant, or Unknown. However, SEER collected the expanded code of the EOD coding system with publication of the Extent of Disease Codes and Coding Instructions, also in

1977. These codes could be electronically converted to SS 1977 and later to TNM.

There were, however, some inconsistencies of how SEER and CoC coded data, especially for treatment and staging data. There was a conflict between the desire for a consistent coding system over time to study trends by epidemiologists (SEER) and the clinical view (CoC). Clinicians needed to keep up with how changing clinical knowledge and practices affect the staging of cancers in terms of predicted outcomes. It was the collaborative efforts of CoC and the SEER Program that led to the development of surgery-specific codes in the 1980s. Some differences also existed in registry operations and required data items as the CoC standards were designed for hospital-based programs and SEER standards were designed for a population-based registry. However, many of the SEER standards, requirements, and definitions have been incorporated as standards for both hospital-based registries and CCRs.

Quality-assurance activities have also been required by both CoC and SEER registries since the inception of the programs. In addition, SEER data are subjected to rigorous data quality edits and investigations, and must meet data quality standards. Activities include routine data edits, case-finding audits, and reabstracting audits.

National Cancer Registrars Association

Since 1983, NCRA's certification process has promoted standardization in the collection and use of cancer data through examination and certification of cancer registrars and other cancer data specialists. The CTR® (Certified Tumor Registrar) examination, establishes the standard of knowledge and experience required for professional registry practice, and measures the requisite knowledge of applicants for the professional credential of Certified Tumor Registrar.[36]

North American Association of Central Cancer Registries

Founded in 1987, NAACCR's primary role is to represent and serve as a forum for the organization, operation, quality control, and statistical reporting of population-based cancer registries. When it was first organized, it focused its efforts on achieving a consensus on cancer registration standards among the many standard setters in the United States and Canada. Because the majority of the data submitted to CCRs comes from hospital-based cancer registries, there was a need to have these standards accepted also by the CoC.[37]

In 1994, NAACCR published *Standards for Cancer Registries, Data Exchange Standards and Record Description, Volume I,* which is intended for programmers and provides the record layout and specifications for standard data exchange, *Standards for Cancer Registries: Data Standards & Data*

Dictionary, Volume II, which provides detailed standards for many aspects of the operation of a population-based cancer registry, and *Standards for Completeness, Quality, Analysis, Management, Security, and Confidentiality of Data, Volume III,* which provides CCR structural requirements, process standards and outcome measures for access to source data and completeness of reporting, data quality, data analysis and reporting, and data management.

NAACCR's Uniform Data Standards (UDS) Committee provides a formal mechanism for reviewing and recommending proposed changes in data codes and/or the addition of new items submitted by NAACCR members to ensure that data remain comparable among CCRs. The work of the Uniform Data Standards Committee built on earlier joint efforts of CoC and SEER, under the auspices of NCRA, to find ways to coordinate disparate codes and datasets. Currently, nearly all CCRs throughout the United States and Canada have adopted the NAACCR consensus standards, and these standards are updated annually.

In 1997, NAACCR instituted a certification program that annually reviewed member registries for their ability to produce complete, accurate, and timely data. NAACCR state registries voluntarily submit their nonidentified data, and NAACCR evaluates the data based on predetermined registry certification criteria. Following the evaluation, the registry receives a report containing the results of the evaluation, and those achieving certification are published on the NAACCR Web site.

For 1995 data, the first data year for NAACCR certification, only 14 state registries met the certification criteria. However, in 2005, 46 states met the criteria, demonstrating a major improvement in the quality and timeliness of the data submitted by the member registries. In 2006, cancer incidence data from 73 population-based cancer registries were evaluated as part of the certification program, and 56 U.S. registries were certified. The percentage of the population that is reflected by these certified registries for 1999 to 2003 data is approximately 82%.[38]

National Program of Cancer Registries

The 1992 law authorizing the CDC to provide funds to states and territories also authorized the CDC to set standards for data completeness, timeliness, and quality. In 1994, NPCR began providing financial support and technical assistance to statewide, population-based cancer registries. Before awarding funds, NPCR established program objectives and measuring criteria that included measures of completeness, timeliness, and data quality. These were published as NPCR standards. Each year a program evaluation was completed for each funded program to measure compliance with these objectives. NPCR adopted NAACCR's standards for uniform data elements and data exchange record layout, and defined an NPCR minimal required dataset. In 2001, NPCR began receiving data annually from funded programs, and some measures were based on the data submitted.

Baseline data from 1994 showed that only 37% of the programs met uniform data standards. This improved to 100% by 1999 and has remained at that level over the years. Baseline data on completeness was at 49% and only progressed to 63% by 1999. However, by 2009, it was at 100%. The timeliness standard was only met by 20% of baseline programs. This standard seems to be the hardest for programs to achieve, with the percentage of programs meeting the goal increasing slightly over the years to reach 56% in 2009.[39] By 2005, only 8 NPCR-funded registries met all NPCR completeness, timeliness, and quality standards, but this number increased to 24 by 2007.[40]

Quality-assurance activities that are performed in NPCR-funded CCRs and monitored by NPCR include visual review of text and codes for completeness and accuracy, use of standardized computer edits for source records and for consolidated cases, feedback to reporting facilities for reconciliation, and recoding and reabstracting audits. NPCR also conducts a continuous program of data assessment through Data Completeness and Quality Audits, an assessment where programs have an independent data audit once every 5 years.

International Association of Cancer Registries

In 1966, the International Association of Cancer Registries (IACR) was formed to foster the exchange of information between cancer registries internationally and to improve the quality of data and comparability between registries. The association is a nongovernmental organization that has been in official relations with the World Health Organization since 1979.

IACR serves as a membership organization for cancer registries concerned with the collection and analysis of data on cancer incidence and with the end results of cancer treatment in defined population groups. It is a professional society dedicated to fostering the aims and activities of cancer registries worldwide. Its members are primarily population-based registries that collect information on the occurrence and outcome of cancer in defined population groups (usually the inhabitants of a city, region, or country). For each new cancer case, registries record details of the individual affected, the nature of the cancer, information on treatment, and information on follow-up, specifically with respect to survival from the disease. In 1979, IACR had 87 member registries, and by 2006, the membership had jumped to 446 CCRs.[41]

IACR rules are established by the International Agency for Research on Cancer and IACR. These rules relate to comparability, standardization, and completeness of data. Cancer registries must conform to accepted working practices and standards to ensure that cases are properly recorded, and that the statistical data gathered are complete and can be used to make valid comparisons. To aid in this process, IACR has developed classifications such as the successive editions of the *International Classification of Diseases for Oncology,* first published by the World Health Organization in 1976. IACR also provides guidelines for registry practices and standard definitions.[42]

Other Cancer Partners
National Coordinating Council for Cancer Surveillance

In 1993, the NCCCS was created to coordinate cancer surveillance activities within the United States through communication and collaboration among major national cancer organizations, ensuring that the needs of cancer patients and the communities in which they live are fully served, that scarce resources are maximally used, and that the burden of cancer in the United States is adequately measured and ultimately reduced. It provided a forum for examining the current state of cancer surveillance operations and identifying the broad issues involved, to recommend practical approaches to facilitate the work of registries, and to contribute to the goal of coordinating data collection and improving data quality across the nation.[43]

The membership of the NCCCS includes representatives from ACS, ACoS, CDC, NCI, NCRA, and NAACCR, as well as their component programs. The NCCCS enables these organizations to collaborate on cancer monitoring and registry operations. One of the initial products of the NCCCS is a white paper entitled *Cancer Surveillance in the US: Can We Have a National System,* which provides an excellent overview of the cancer registration efforts in the United States.[44]

C-Change

Established in 1998, C-Change is composed of the nation's key cancer leaders from government, business, and nonprofit sectors. Its 130 members include the heads of federal and state governmental agencies, private businesses, the motion picture industry, and nonprofit groups whose missions relate to cancer research, control, and/or patient advocacy. Other individuals with a deep concern about cancer and who have achieved prominence in the entertainment, news, and other industries or endeavors also are engaged in C-Change. Their goal is to leverage the combined expertise and resources of its members to eliminate cancer as a major public health problem at the earliest possible time. Former President George Bush and former First Lady Barbara Bush are co-chairs of C-Change.

C-Change shares information; helps identify barriers, gaps, and opportunities related to its mission; seeks agreement on critical national priorities and supportive actions; and facilitates independent and collaborative efforts to achieve common goals.

C-Change has sponsored two Cancer Surveillance and Information Summits that brought together experts from the broad field of cancer surveillance to seek ways to reduce the burden from cancer through the full application of information. Specifically, the summits sought to review the current state of the science, identify near and long-term contributions to the surveillance enterprise, identify barriers to progress and needed areas for research and development, develop strategies and plans, and recommend key initiatives, time frames, and groups that could move the field forward.[45]

National Cancer Institute Cancer Biomedical Informatics Grid

Cancer Biomedical Informatics Grid (caBIG®) is sponsored by the NCI and its activities are supervised by the NCI's Center for Bioinformatics. It is a network that enables all constituencies in the cancer community, such as researchers, physicians, and patients, to share data and knowledge. The components of caBIG® are widely applicable beyond cancer as well. The initiative operates through an open development community made up of a wide spectrum of the cancer research community. Anyone can participate in caBIG®, and there is no cost to join. The caBIG® community includes more than 50 cancer centers; numerous other NCI-supported research endeavors; 30 federal, academic, not-for-profit, and industry organizations; and more than 900 individuals. The mission of caBIG® is to develop a truly collaborative information network that accelerates the discovery of new approaches for the detection, diagnosis, treatment, and prevention of cancer, ultimately improving patient outcomes.[46]

Cancer Data Use

Within the United States, multiple national organizations and programs actively collect and report data regarding cancer incidence, morbidity, mortality, and survival (Table 1-4). These include the CDC's NPCR, the NCI's SEER program, the CoC's NCDB, and the CDC's National Center for Health Statistics' (CDC/NCHS) Vital Statistics.[47]

American Cancer Society Cancer Facts & Figures and Cancer Statistics

The ACS has published the estimated number of new cancer cases and deaths in the current year for the total United States and individual states in its annual *Cancer Facts & Figures* publication since 1952 and in *Cancer Statistics* since 1970. The ACS estimates include the number of new cancer cases and deaths for each year, and provides the most recent statistics on cancer incidence, mortality, and 5-year relative survival.[48] They also track data regarding behaviors that influence the risk for development of cancer and the use of screening tests. *Cancer Facts & Figures* includes sections on cancer risk factors such as tobacco use, physical activity, and use of cancer screening examinations. The methods used to produce these estimates have changed over the years as data incidence and statistical models improved.[7]

Commission on Cancer Patient Care Studies

Since 1976, CoC-approved registries formed a voluntary network of contributors to annual patient care studies under the aegis of the National Cancer Data Committee of the CoC. These annual studies provide timely clinical information that is widely disseminated to physicians, allied health personnel, administrators, healthcare planners, and public and private agencies.

In 1989, the NCDB was established and the patient care studies were merged with the NCDB to meet the further expanded demand and use of registry data.[49] The use of these data has grown exponentially and has been the basis for more than 90 publications.

Surveillance, Epidemiology, and End Results Cancer Statistics Review

The SEER Cancer Statistics Review (CSR) is an annual report currently published online that contains the most recent incidence, mortality, prevalence, lifetime risk, and

Table 1-4	Cancer Data Use	
Organization	**Report**
American Cancer Society (ACS)	*Cancer Facts & Figures*
Commission on Cancer (CoC)	Patient Care Evaluation Studies
North American Association of Central Cancer Registries (NAACCR)	Cancer in North America
National Program of Cancer Registries (NPCR) and Surveillance, Epidemiology, and End Results (SEER)	U.S. Cancer Statistics Cancer Control P.L.A.N.E.T
International Association of Cancer Registries (IACR)	*Cancer in Five Continents*

survival statistics. The CSR reports and summarizes the key measures of the impact of cancer on the U.S. population. Statistics are provided in tables and graphs that are grouped by cancer site and topic. It is also possible to build your own report using the search mechanism to select individual tables and charts to include in a single file. The report includes statistics from 1975 through the most recent year for which data are available. Each year SEER also publishes various monographs on specific cancer topics. In 2008, they published *An Update on Cancer in American Indians and Alaska Natives, 1999–2004.*

SEER's publications are based on data from its population-based cancer registries, which currently cover approximately 26% of the U.S. population. For many years, the SEER Program was the only source of population-based information that included stage of cancer at the time of diagnosis, treatment, and patient survival data. The mortality data reported by SEER are provided by the National Center for Health Statistics. The population data used in calculating cancer rates are obtained periodically from the U.S. Census Bureau.[50]

North American Association of Central Cancer Registries Cancer in North America

NAACCR publishes the monograph Cancer in North America (CINA) each year. Members of NAACCR participate voluntarily in an annual call for data to develop this multiregistry, aggregated data resource for cancer surveillance and research.

In 2008, NAACCR released *CINA, 2001–2005.* This publication reported cancer incidence and mortality data from 40 CCRs for the years 1990 to 1994. In addition to publication of cancer statistics for the most recent 5-year period, the *CINA* data resource is used to create an online database called *CINA+ Online* for public queries regarding cancer incidence for the most recent 5 years, and to develop a discretionary research dataset called *CINA Deluxe* that includes data from 1995 to 2005 to facilitate analytic studies conducted by epidemiologists and other qualified researchers.[51]

U.S. Cancer Statistics

In 2002, 1999 cancer incidence data were published in the first joint report from the two federal programs that support population-based cancer registries in the United States: CDC's NPCR and NCI's SEER Program. The report contained, for the first time, official federal government cancer statistics for more than 1 million invasive cancer cases diagnosed among residents of 37 states, 6 metropolitan areas, and the District of Columbia, geographic areas in which approximately 78% of the U.S. population resided.

In 2004, U.S. Cancer Statistics (USCS) included both incidence and mortality data for 2001. The 2002 data were also provided as a Web-based version. By 2007, this report contained cancer statistics for more than 1 million invasive cancer cases diagnosed during 2004 among residents of 49 states, 6 metropolitan areas, and the District of Columbia, and these geographic areas are inhabited by about 98% of the U.S. population.[52]

Cancer Control P.L.A.N.E.T.

Cancer Control P.L.A.N.E.T. is a web portal that includes USCS data and provides dynamic views of cancer statistics for use in cancer control efforts. It provides access to data and resources that can help planners, program staff, and researchers to design, implement, and evaluate evidence-based cancer control programs.[53]

International Association of Cancer Registries Cancer Incidence in Five Continents

The Cancer Incidence in Five Continents (CI5) series of monographs, published every 5 years, has become the reference source of data on the international incidence of cancer. The first volume was published in 1966. In 2007, Volume 9 provided a wider coverage than before, presenting data from around the year 2000 (ideally the period 1998–2002) not only for entire populations but for subpopulations living in the same geographic area. This volume presented incidence data from populations all over the world for which good-quality data are available. The information provided gives a clear presentation of the changing cancer patterns worldwide. With this volume, more use was made of the Web rather than continued reliance on the printed volume. All tables previously found on printed page were made available in an electronic version. *Cancer Incidence in Five Continents, Volumes I to VIII* is a CD-ROM containing cancer incidence data from around 200 population-based cancer registries worldwide, for the period 1953 to 1997, that were published in the eight volumes of the CI5 series.[54]

Cancer Registrar Education
Basic Education

In the United States, cancer registrar education has been the pervue of several organizations over the years. Starting in the 1950s, registrar education was provided in informal settings and educational materials were scarce. There were no formal education opportunities and all training was "on the job." Some registrars came to the profession with degrees in other allied health fields, but the majority had no medical background at all.

In 1961, the Training Programs for Personnel of Cancer Patient Data Systems/Tumor Registries at the University of California, San Francisco began.[55] This program was open to all persons interested in tumor registry methodology. It was a 2-week course offered three times a year in San Francisco. An additional 1-week biostatistical and epidemiologic methods course was also offered.[56]

In 1976, the USC Comprehensive Cancer Center's Regional Activities Program was funded, and a new training program for cancer registrars was established called the USC Cancer Registrar Training Program. This program was designed to prepare individuals with the basic skills necessary to be employed as cancer registrars in hospitals or CCRs. Cosponsored by Southern California Cancer Registrars Association, the USC Cancer Registrar Training Program was a 24-day program, with classes held 2 days per week for 12 consecutive weeks. This was the only structured basic training in the United States.

SEER published the first book of the Self Instructional Manuals for Tumor Registrars series in 1980, and between 1991and 1994, five additional books were published. These included books on Objectives and Functions of a Tumor Registry, Cancer Characteristics and Selection of Cases, Tumor Registrar Vocabulary, Human Anatomy as Related to Tumor Formation, and Abstracting Medical Records. Later, other volumes were added to include Statistics and Epidemiology for Cancer Registries, as well as Antineoplastic Drugs.

In 1987, the CoC FTRO Education Program was offered as a comprehensive, in-depth, 30-hour or 3-day basic education program that was presented locally throughout the United States. It was targeted to Tumor Registrars with less than 2 years of registry experience.[57] Cosponsors were sought through a competitive selection process and locations chosen to ensure a wide geographic distribution. In 1987, six FTROs were completed in response to more than 45 proposals, and an additional 4 programs were offered in 1988, with more than 500 participants in 2 years. This was eventually repackaged into self-contained learning modules that could be more easily taught.[58]

Also in the 1970s, state cancer registrar associations started appearing modeled on NCRA with their main goal as education. Many of these organizations offered basic cancer registry training courses, and since then other organizations such as SEER, CoC, and NCRA have also offered basic cancer registry training courses.

Since its founding in 1974, NCRA has made cancer registrar education its foremost goal. Over the years, NRCA has also provided ongoing educational and professional support through regional and annual educational programs.

Educational Standards and Certification

In 1978, NCRA published the *National Tumor Registrars Association Educational Standards* as a guide for training programs offered by colleges and universities, as well as for workshops sponsored by national, regional, and local organizations. The standards included six modules focused on the basic skills pertinent to the cancer registrar's specialized knowledge needed to set up and manage a hospital cancer registry or work in a CCR. Each module also listed the recommended number of hours of instruction needed in each area.[59]

In 1990, NCRA published *Essentials for the Tumor Registrar Technician and the Tumor Registrar Administrator* as a requirement to gain American Medical Association (AMA) recognition and approval as an allied health profession. Outlined curriculum for both levels were developed. This document was to be used for development of training programs.[60]

NCRA administration believed that in the absence of formal education requirements for cancer registrars, certification would mark achievement, foster professional pride, and be nationally recognized in recruitment and retention of registry personnel. After many years of work by NCRA volunteers, in 1983, the first CTR examination was offered.

Originally, the test was administered by NCRA's Credentialing Committee, but in 1995, this responsibility was turned over to an independent board, the National Board for the Certification of Registrars (NBCR), and in 2002, NCRA established a Council on Certification to oversee all certification activities. The council consists of representatives elected by people holding a CTR credential. The Council on Certification oversees developing and administrating the professional certification examination for cancer registrars and establishes eligibility criteria for examination candidates. The council also reviews proposed questions, verifies the content of upcoming examinations, and responds to questions from examination candidates regarding eligibility status.

The educational level of CTR candidates has continued to increase over the years. When the first CTR examination was taken in 1983, approximately 40% candidates listed their highest accademic level as high school, and it remained at that level until 1993 when it began to decline. In 1998, this category dropped dramatically to less than 10% and remained at about 11% until 2008, when it again dropped to 4%. An associate's degree was consistently selected by between 30% and 40% of the candidates from 1983 through 2007, but in 2008, this increased to 68%.

The changes seen in the values for 2008 reflect NCRA's first change in the elgibility criteria for the CTR examination since its inception. These changes started a move toward the requirement of a minimum of an associate's degreee to be eligible to take the examination. In 2008, two semesters of college-level courses in Human Anatomy and/or Physiology were added to the 2 years of experience required by eligibility route 1. In 2009, 12 credit hours of college-level course education that includes two semesters of Human Anatomy and/or Physiology, one semester of Medical Science/Biology, plus one semester in Medical Terminology were required. In 2010, route 1 was eliminated and all candidates are required to have a minimum of an associate's degree. The first computer-based examination was given in 2004, and to maintain their CTR credential, certified cancer registrars must complete 20 continuing education hours every 2 years.

Because NCRA is committed to ensuring that quality education in Cancer Registry Management is provided to the public, it maintains a system of accreditation for formal education programs that provide entry-level professional preparation with a major emphasis in Cancer Registry Management. The accreditation program manages both the setting and implementation of standards throughout the United States of formal education programs at the certificate and degree level leading to the eligibility to sit for the CTR Examination.

In 1985, the first NCRA-approved formal education program was started at the University of Pittsburgh. This was a 4-year integrated Health Records Administration/Tumor Registry pilot program.[61] Many other programs followed, usually in junior colleges, but a limited number of students in any one location made making these programs financially self-supporting difficult. However, the development of Web technologies has made current programs available to a much wider audience. In 2009, NCRA listed eight approved programs, most offering both associate's degrees and a certificate program, and the majority are offered as online Internet programs.

In 2005, NCRA, in a collaborative partnership with the American Health Information Management Association (AHIMA), developed the Cancer Registry Management Program. This structured online program is designed for easy access to those interested in entering the cancer registry profession regardless of their location. The program is composed of four prerequisites and six specialization courses. It is organized into groups of courses called "clusters" that are self-paced, but each course must be completed within a limited number of weeks. Anatomy and Physiology is also offered outside of the groupings. Those who complete this NCRA-approved training program and 160 hours of work experience in a CTR-staffed registry are eligible to take the CTR examination via eligibility route 2.

In 1997, NCRA published the first cancer registry textbook, *Cancer Registry Management: Principles & Practice.* Written by a team of 85 experts, this publication contains 30 chapters, appendices, a glossary, and an index. The overall objective of this publication was to provide technical and management issues defined in a comprehensive textbook. The first edition of this book was used by many new cancer registrars studying for their certification, college and university instructors teaching cancer registry classes, and hospitals starting new cancer programs.[20] This was followed by the second edition in 2004. The second edition contains 37 chapters. A third edition was published in 2010.

Cancer Registrar Opportunities

In addition to hospital and CCRs, cancer registrars have many opportunities to pursue through various exciting career paths, including working in hospital administration, software sales and support, education, and program management in government or the private sector. Many cancer registrars also enter the consulting fields, some starting their own companies, and others have gone into the fields of information technology. Many of these careers offer flexible working arrangements, including telecommuting, and some offer travel opportunities.

According to the 2004 NCRA: University of California, San Francisco Study of the Cancer Registry Workforce, more than 50% of cancer registrars worked in the hospital setting and 38% worked in the state (or regional) CCR work setting. However, another 4% worked for consulting companies, and the remaining registrars worked for vendors, education programs, private practices and/or national standard setting organizations, and this number is growing.[62]

Hospitals or central registries tend to be the entry point into the cancer registry profession and then registrars move on to the other areas. An area experiencing a lot of growth is software vendors. Registrars not only provide software consultation, they help train hospital clients on using the software and on standard changes. However, these vendors usually want a registrar who has worked in the field, with the data and with the software, because they are looking for someone who understands the job to help improve their product. The consulting company arena, the education setting, and national standard-setting organizations are also stepping stones for cancer registrars after working in a hospital or central registry, or both. These organizations usually require CTRs with several years of experience.

Ongoing Registry and Registrar Issues

The biggest challenge for cancer registrars, no matter the work setting, will continue to be data collection, coding, and reporting standards that are constantly being updated to keep up with changing data demands. In 2010, the AJCC published the *AJCC Cancer Staging Manual,* 7th edition, and the Collaborative Stage Data Collection System version 2 used by registrars was modified to match the changes. The NCI/SEER program opened the *Hematopoietic Multiple Primary and Histology database,* and NAACCR nearly tripled the size of its data exchange record layout.

Cancer surveillance is a complex system that captures longitudinal data from multiple and varying data sources using a variety of methods. The cancer surveillance infrastructure consists of a complex network of hospitals, clinics, laboratories, health departments, nongovernmental organizations, and government agencies requiring monitoring, recording, and consolidating information on people diagnosed with cancer within the national cancer surveillance infrastructure to provide accurate and complete data on cancer incidence. The process of identifying and collecting cancer data is resource intensive, time consuming, and creates a risk for errors in transcription. Within the United States, the issues of completeness, timeliness, and quality of data prove to be a continual challenge. The time gap between a diagnosis of cancer and the availability of data for analysis is a significant problem for cancer surveillance.[63] Efforts will continue to improve on these challenges using the technology that is available.

Cancer registrars are currently experiencing the revolutionary changes caused by new features of the electronic medical record (EMR). Over several decades, the hospital cancer registry has become automated and computerized, and now the transition toward EMRs brings other challenges. In an article for *For the Record*, Susan Koering, MEd, RHIA, CTR says that "The EMR will continue to impact cancer and other disease registries in the future through ongoing upgrades and the creation of new linkages to get the exact information we want from the database and adding new disease diagnostics tests as they evolve."[64]

Surveillance informatics—the systematic application of information and computer science and technology to cancer surveillance practices, research, and learning—is a growing area of development. Ongoing cancer surveillance informatics projects will evaluate aspects of the cancer business to identify better ways to use emerging technology to incorporate automated processes and electronic data exchange. The concept of capturing data once and using it to meet multiple needs will become more critical as the need for information increases across the healthcare community. Cancer surveillance informatics projects will evaluate existing data streams such as insurance claims data that may meet data requirements for cancer registries, alleviating the need to create special data streams for cancer registries. These changes are providing new opportunities for registrars to translate their knowledge and skills into the vocabulary and systems of the electronic health data environment.[65]

This information technology has changed the dynamics of cancer registry work, and registrars are increasingly utilizing electronic health information to build the cancer registry abstract. This transformation will readjust the registrars' focus to data editing and more quality-of-care issues, but CTRs who have in-depth knowledge of the oncology arena will still need to verify and reconcile the information obtained from the disparate documentation systems and code it according to a defined dataset so it can be compared, benchmarked, and trended against national quality measures and guidelines. In addition, the CTR is still required to track any treatments the patient may have received outside of the organization to provide an entire picture of what transpired in terms of therapy for that person and to follow the cancer patients annually for their entire lifetime.

Several groups and organizations are currently working toward developing standards and technologies that will continue to benefit not only cancer registry activities, cancer research, and cancer surveillance, but the health profession as a whole. Electronic reporting in the cancer registry will be a part of a larger healthcare informatics system. Ultimately, these efforts and the work to integrate these initiatives into registry operations will provide the means to improve the process by which cancer data are collected, maintained, reported, and analyzed, thus helping to meet the goal to eliminate cancer as a major public health problem at the earliest possible time.[66]

Some changes that can be expected include increased direct downloading of demographic, cancer identification, and follow-up items; some autocoding; list-oriented (synoptic) reporting of pathology reports; increased physician office reporting; and increased free-standing laboratory reporting. Other changes will include more fluid navigation within the medical record, and centralization and filtering of data such as nurses notes, images, and laboratory reports. Increased physician coding will lessen registrar guesswork. Follow-up letters will be generated through the actual chart, providing documentation to the physician about the patient.[67]

These changes require that registrars constantly train and retrain to keep up with the advances in cancer registry science. The level of detail required continues to escalate and will almost certainly continue into the future as the value of cancer registry data is recognized and new technologies are developed. Cancer registrars will need to meet these challenges with an increased level of education and skills to meet the technical requirements of the profession.

In February 2008, C-Change convened the Cancer Information and Surveillance Summit (CSIS) II, which brought together approximately 50 experts in the fields of strategic forecasting and cancer surveillance. Summit participants made the following nine recommendations and, therefore, have outlined the areas that need to be addressed in the future:

1. **Market the value of cancer surveillance.** Public awareness of cancer surveillance databases needs to be raised, the public's fear of government use of individual/personal health data must be reduced, researchers' awareness needs to be raised, and a use case among a broad base of partners needs to be developed.
2. **Transform registries.** A tangible need is to make registry information available at the point of healthcare service and to scale the information available from population-based registries to the available resources to maintain a high-quality surveillance enterprise.

3. **Improve the coordination of surveillance and clinical data needs for quality improvement.** Tangible needs are to identify necessary data and adapt to changing information needs, to identify the multiple sources and locations of data by understanding opportunities for synergies between resources and the potential for error or conflict, and to identify and address multiple efforts to collect complete, accurate, and timely treatment data.

4. **Improve the utility of existing cancer surveillance methods using advanced tools.** Tangible gaps include the fact that existing data are underutilized, and that there are polarized perspectives of the usefulness of consumer-based, research-based, or public health–based data systems.

5. **Develop a "Cancer Patients Like Me" Web site to engage patients in submitting data that can enhance registries.** One tangible need in this area is data exchange among patients, providers, and surveillance systems for mutual benefit.

6. **Create financial incentives.** The tangible gap in this area is the financial barrier to the adoption of EMRs and their linkage to public health surveillance systems.

7. **Examine the need and opportunity for legislative policy regarding privacy and security.** There is no existing legislation or regulation to protect personal privacy in the United States; thus, a tangible need for health privacy regulations exists with the emphasis that health data should be used for the benefit of patients and not against them. The data must be available to create information for the benefit of society.

8. **Focus on workforce development and recruitment.** Currently, a need exists for the cancer surveillance workforce to develop skills for future demands related to technology and infrastructure, and to attract new workers to the field.

9. **Achieve shared meanings.** Cancer incidence standards have recently been incorporated into vocabularies and standards beyond the NAACCR standards. Specific actions needed now are to support ongoing activities, ensure progress is maintained, and harmonize ontologies and value sets. Potential goals in this area are to ensure that cancer incidence data and registries are ready for interoperability with other data sources, support the existing movement with interoperability and consensus, and ensure that linkages will result in synergistic information for better decisions by researchers, surveillance experts, physicians and other providers, and policy makers.[68]

Summary

According to the CDC, cancer registrars are the intelligence officers on the front lines, collecting critical information that is used to develop the battle plan and to deliver the necessary troops to the right location at the right time to combat the enemy—cancer. Cancer registrars are the lifeblood of cancer registries and serve as the backbone of local, state, and national cancer surveillance and cancer control programs.[5]

The future of cancer surveillance will be driven not only by innovations in methods of cancer surveillance itself, but by developments in information technology and communication, and by revolutionary new tools used in the delivery of medical care. At the same time, it will be a challenge to ensure levels of privacy and confidentiality needed to maintain the public trust.

In the Cancer Surveillance and Information Summit, a 2004 conference sponsored by C-Change, experts from the field and from allied and related disciplines in both the public and private sectors met to consider the future of the cancer surveillance enterprise. The shared view is that cancer surveillance and information is essential to fulfill a vision for a future where cancer is prevented, detected early, and either cured or managed successfully as a chronic illness.[69]

References

1. American Cancer Society. "The History of Cancer." Available at: http://www.cancer.org/docroot/CRI/content/CRI_2_6x_the_history_of_cancer_72.asp?sitearea. Accessed June 2009.

2. New World Encyclopedia. "Ebers Papyrus." Available at: http://www.newworldencyclopedia.org/entry/Ebers_Papyrus. Accessed June 2009

3. Intlekofer, R. *NPCR Education & Training Series: Data Collection Standards. Data Collection Standards in Cancer Surveillance. Centers for Disease Control and Prevention, National Program for Cancer Registries, Atlanta Ga.*

4. Clive, R. "Introduction to Cancer Registries." In *Cancer Registry Management: Principles & Practice,* edited by C. L. Hutchinson, S. D. Roffers, A. G. Fritz (p. 2). Dubuque, Ia: Kendall Hunt, 1997.

5. *Quality Cancer Data: The Vital Role of Cancer Registrars in the Fight against Cancer. Centers for Disease Control and Prevention National Program for Cancer Registries, Atlanta, GA: http://www.cdc.gov/cancer/npcr/pdf/QualityData90min.pdf*

6. American Cancer Society. *Cancer Facts & Figures 2009.* Atlanta: American Cancer Society, 2009.

7. International Agency for Research on Cancer. *Cancer Mondial.* Available at: http://www-dep.iarc.fr/. Accessed June 2009.

8. Pickle, Linda W., Hao, Yongping, Jemal, Ahmedin, Zou, Zhaohui, Tiwari, Ram C., Ward, Elizabeth, Hachey, Mark, Howe, Holly L., Feuer, Eric J. "A New Method of Estimating United States and State-level Cancer Incidence Counts for the Current Calendar Year," *CA Cancer J Clin,* 2007;57:30–42.

9. Jemal, Ahmedin, Thun, Michael J., Ries, Lynn A. G., Howe, Holly L., Weir, Hannah K., Center, Melissa M., Ward, Elizabeth, Wu, Xiao-Cheng, Eheman, Christie, Anderson, Robert, Ajani, Umed A., Kohler, Betsy, Edwards, Brenda K. "Annual Report to the Nation on the Status of Cancer, 1975–2005, Featuring Trends in Lung Cancer, Tobacco Use,

and Tobacco Control," *Journal of the National Cancer Institute,* December 3, 2008, 100(no. 23):1672–1694.

10. *STEPS: A Framework for Surveillance: WHO/NMH/CCS/03.01 Noncommunicable Diseases and Mental Health.* Geneva, Switzerland: World Health Organization.

11. Parkin, D. M. "The Cancer Registry: Its Purpose and Uses; The International Network For Cancer Treatment and Research," *Newsletter Guest Message,* Vol. 8 (no. 1), Spring 2008.

12. Wagner G. "History of Cancer Registration in Cancer Epidemiology; Cancer Registration: Principles and Methods" In Cancer Registration: Principles and Methods (IARC Scientific Publication No. 95), edited by O. M. Jensen, D. M. Parkin, R. MacLennan, C. S. Muir, and R. G. Skeet. International Agency for Research on Cancer, Lyon, France, 1991.

13. Clive, R. E. "Quarter of a Century Relationship with Cancer Registries, Commission on Cancer and NCRA." Presented at the NCRA Annual Meeting, May 1999.

14. National Cancer Institute. "SEER Training Modules: Cancer Registration & Surveillance Modules: Cancer Registration." Available at: http://training.seer.cancer.gov/registration/index.html?map. Accessed June 2009.

15. Griswold, M. H., Wilder, C. S., Cutler, S. J., Pollack, E. S. "Cancer in Connecticut. 1935–1951." Monograph, Connecticut Department of Health, Hartford, CT, 1955.

16. Connelly, R. R., Campbell, P. C., Eisenberg, H. "Central registry of cancer cases in Connecticut," *Public Health Reports,* 1968;83:386–390.

17. Storm, H. H., Michelsen, E. V., Clemmensen, I. H., Pihl, J. "The Danish Cancer Registry—History, Content, Quality and Use," *Dan Med Bull,* 1997;44(5):535–539.

18. National Cancer Institute. "Milestone (1971): National Cancer Act of 1971." Available at: http://dtp.nci.nih.gov/timeline/noflash/milestones/M4_Nixon.htm. Accessed June 2009.

19. Haran, C., DeVita, V. "The view from the top," *Cancer World,* 2005(June-July):38–43.

20. Hutchinson, C. L. "Preface." In *Cancer Registry Management: Principles & Practice,* edited by C. L. Hutchinson, S. D. Roffers, A. G. Fritz (pp. xvii-xviii). Dubuque, Ia: Kendall Hunt, 1997.

21. Knight, Karen L., Pearson, Melissa, Tingle, Wendy, Landry, Nora, Lewis, Tara, Morgan, Eileen, Rimmer, Cathy. "A Unique Role in Cancer Care and Control," *NC Med J,* 2008(July/August):69(4).

22. National Cancer Institute. "SEER Teaching Modules: Cancer Registration & Surveillance Modules: Types of Registries." Available at: http://training.seer.cancer.gov/registration/types. Accessed June 2009.

23. Curado, M. P., Edwards, B., Shin, H. R., Storm, H., Ferlay, J., Heanue, M., Boyle, P., editors. *Cancer Incidence in Five Continents, Vol. IX* (IARC Scientific Publications No. 160), Lyon, France: IARC, 2007.

24. "Macro International Awarded CDC Cancer Surveillance Contract," *Business Wire,* December 15, 2008. Available at: http://www.businesswire.com/portal/site/home/permalink/?ndmViewId5news_view&newsId520081215006341&newsLang5en. Accessed June 2009.

25. Commission on Cancer. "About the COC: National Cancer Data Base (NCDB)." Available at: http://www.facs.org/cancer/ncdb/index.html. Accessed July 2009.

26. Central Brain Tumor Registry of the United States Web site: http://www.cbtrus.org/1997report/1997report1.html. Accessed July 2009.

27. The Breast Cancer Family Registry (B-CFR) Web site: http://epi.grants.cancer.gov/CFR/about_breast.html. Accessed July 2009.

28. Gilda Radner Familial Ovarian Cancer Registry Web site: http://ovariancancer.com/app/index.php. Accessed July 2009.

29. National Familial Lung Cancer Registry Web site: http://www.path.jhu.edu/nfltr.html/ Accessed July 2009.

30. The Cancer Genetics Network (CGN) Web site: http://epi.grants.cancer.gov/CGN/. Accessed July 2009.

31. "Team Building to Enhance Data Quality," edited by Holly L. Howe and Gayle G. Clutter. A Report of the National Coordinating Council for Cancer Surveillance, March 2000.

32. Hultstrom D, editor. *Standards for Cancer Registries Volume II: Data Standards and Data Dictionary,* Seventh Edition, Version 10. Springfield, IL: North American Association of Central Cancer Registries, March 2002.

33. "NCRA History Highlights," *NCRA Abstract,* 1984:11(1):5.

34. Hoyler S. "The Data Acquisition Manual: A Step Forward for Standardized Data Collection," *The Abstract,* 1988(July/Aug);14(3):9

35. Edge, S. S., Fritz, A. G., Clutter, G. G., Page, D. L., Watkins, S., Blankenship, C., Douglas, L., Fleming, I. "A Unified Cancer Stage Data Collection System: Preliminary report from the Collaborative Stage Task Force/American Joint Committee on Cancer," *Journal of Registry Management* 1999;26(2):51–55.

36. National Cancer Registrars Association's Council on Certification History Web site: http://www.ctrexam.org/about/index.htm. Accessed July 2009.

37. North American Association of Central Cancer Registries. "About NAACCR, Inc." Available at: http://www.naaccr.org/index.asp?Col_SectionKey59&Col_ContentID541. Accessed July 2009.

38. North American Association of Central Cancer Registries. "Registry Certification." Available at: http://www.naaccr.org/index.asp?Col_SectionKey511&Col_ContentID554. Accessed July 2009.

39. Wilson, Reda J. "Evaluating NPCR—Then and Now." Poster presentation NAACCR Annual Meeting, 2008.

40. Centers for Disease Control and Prevention. "Program Manual: National Program of Cancer Registries Version 1.0: 1.0 Introduction to the National Program of Cancer Registries: Highlights of NPCR Accomplishments." Available at: http://www.cdc.gov/cancer/npcr. Accessed July 2009.

41. Parkin, D. M. "The evolution of the population-based cancer registry," *Nature Reviews Cancer,* 2006;6:603–612.

42. International Agency for Research on Cancer. "IACR Standards." Available at: http://www.iarc.fr/. Accessed July 2009.

43. "Surveillance Research Implementation Plan; The National Coordinating Council for Cancer Surveillance (NCCCS)." Prepared by the Surveillance Implementation Group (SIG) National Cancer Institute; National Institutes of Health, March 1999.

44. Swan, J., Wingo, P., Clive, R., West, D., Miller, D., Hutchison, C., Sondik, E. J., Edwards, B. K. "Cancer Surveillance in the U.S.: Can we have a national system?" *Cancer,* 1998;83:1282–1291.

45. "Symposium Report: C-Change: The Cancer Surveillance and Information Summit II: From Cancer Diagnosis to Cancer Information in Real Time: Executive Summary." Pre-

sented at Marriot Biscayne Bay, Miami, FL, February 11–13, 2008. Available at: http://www.c-changetogether.org/pubs/reports/CancerSurveillanceSummit.pdf. Accessed July 2009.

46. National Institute of Health caBIG. "About caBIG." Available at: https://cabig.nci.nih.gov/overview/. Accessed July 2009.

47. Centers for Disease Control and Prevention. "National Program of Cancer Registries; Cancer Surveillance System Rationale and Approach." Available at: http://www.cdc.gov/cancer/npcr/training/css.htm. Accessed July 2009.

48. Thun, M. J., Calle, E. E., Rodriguez, C., Wingo, P. A. "Epidemiological Research at the American Cancer Society," *Cancer Epidemiology Biomarkers & Prevention,* 2000(Sept);9:861–868.

49. Clive, R. E., Zuber-Ocwieja, K. E., Karnell, L. H., Hoyler, S. S., Seiffert, J. E., Young, J. L., Henson, D. E., Winchester, D. P., Osteen, R. T., Menck, H. R., Fremgen, A. M. "A National Quality Improvement Effort: Cancer Registry Data," *Journal of Surgical Oncology,* 1995;58:155–161.

50. National Cancer Institute. "About the SEER Cancer Statistics Review." Available at: http://seer.cancer.gov/csr/1975_2006/about.html. Accessed July 2009.

51. Howe, H. L., Lake, A., Firth, R., Lehnherr, M., Bayakly, R., Copeland, G., Wu, X. C., Stroup, A., Roney, D., editors. *Cancer in North America, 2001–2005. Volume One: Combined Cancer Incidence for the United States and Canada. Executive Summary.* Springfield, IL: North American Association of Central Cancer Registries, Inc., 2008.

52. U.S. Cancer Statistics Working Group. *United States Cancer Statistics: 1999 Incidence.* Atlanta: Department of Health and Human Services, Centers for Disease Control and Prevention and National Cancer Institute, 2002.

53. Cancer Control P.L.A.N.E.T. Web site: http://cancercontrolplanet.cancer.gov/index.html. Accessed August 2009.

54. International Association of Cancer Registries. *Publications: Cancer in Five Continents, Vol I-VIII.* Available at: http://www.iacr.com.fr/statist.htm. Accessed August 2009.

55. "Tumor Registry Training Program," *The Abstract,* 1979;5(6):9.

56. Young J. "SEER's Commitment to Training and Continuing Education of Tumor Registrars," *The Abstract* 1986(July/Aug);13(1):7

57. Continuing Education and the Commission on Cancer, American College of Surgeons. *The Abstract,* 1986(April):12(4):2

58. Opalach, G. M. "The Fundamental Tumor Registry Operations (FTRO) Program," *The Abstract,* 1989(May/June);15(1):10.

59. Shambaugh E. "President Discusses Education," *The Abstract,* 1981(April);7(2):5, 8.

60. "Tumor Registry Essentials," *The Abstract,* 1990(Winter);16(3):3.

61. "Pilot Program Begins at University of Pittsburgh," *The Abstract* 1985(Dec);12(3):2.

62. "Needed: Cancer Registrars in Various Work Settings," *Advance for Health Professionals,* 16(24):16 2006.

63. Centers for Disease Control and Prevention. "NPCR-AERRO: Developing a Cancer Surveillance Informatics Structure in the New E-Health Environment." Available at: http://www.cdc.gov/cancer/npcr/npcrpdfs/npcr_aerro_overview.pdf. Accessed August 2009.

64. Gater, L. "Reshaping Cancer Registry: Connecting Data, Improving Care," *For The Record,* 2008;20(8):16.

65. Menck, Herman R. "Leap of Faith," *For The Record,* 19(8):20, 2007.

66. National Cancer Registrars Association. "Medical Informatic Basics for the Cancer Registry." Developed by the NCRA Education Foundation and the NCRA Cancer Informatics Committee, April 2008. Available at: http://x01.us/ncraedfdn/pdfs/NCRAInformaticsBrochure.pdf.

67. Menck, H. "NCRA Studies Registry Workloads," *Advance for Health Information Professionals,* 2008;17(8):14.

68. C-Change. "From Cancer Diagnosis to Cancer Information in Real Time; February 11–13, 2008. Available at: http://www.c-changetogether.org/pubs/reports/Cancer%20Surveillance%20Information%20Summit%20II.pdf. Accessed August 2009.

69. Hiatt, R. "The Future of Cancer Surveillance," *Cancer Causes and Control,* 2006(June);17(5):639–646.

chapter 2

Standardized Data Sets

Jerri Linn Phillips, MA, CTR

Registry data collected in the absence of shared standards contribute little beyond anecdotal detail toward case management or cancer control. Shared standards assure clarity of communication, protect the integrity of data when they are pooled or compared across multiple sources, and focus attention on key aspects of cancer care and cancer control.

A registry's data set choices are revealing. Those choices reflect the answers to such questions as "What do we care about most?" and "Who funds us?" How a registry selects the data items to collect shows how much the organization cares about collaboration with others, how historical continuity is handled, and whether the impact of current technologies is properly understood. Data collected by a registry should be useful on several levels. First, the cancer registry is a source of personal and medical information necessary for planning and evaluating the individual patient's case management. Second, registry data provide administrative information for facility planners, cancer committees, and practitioners. Third, government and private agencies use registry data to develop and evaluate cancer control programs after central registries consolidate individual reports into a composite case record. Fourth, registries provide a rich source of data for investigative cancer research.

Except for individual case reports, all uses of cancer registry data involve compilations of data in statistical summaries. The interpretation of compiled data requires uniformity of definitions and consistent use of codes. Consequently, even if broadly accepted standards do not exist, most registries institute local guidelines to meet their immediate needs for data consistency. Special care should be paid to codes currently prevalent in the United States and Canada when defining the data set and the individual item definitions and codes. Registries that select nonstandard codes limit the comparability of their data and ultimately sabotage the usefulness of the data they collect.

Interest in shared or uniform registry standards for data collection and management grew with the increasingly varied uses of registry data, stimulated by the implementation of computerized registry data systems. Contemporary standards for registry data and data management emphasize standardization of the data. That is, for items characteristically collected by cancer registries, the same codes and code definitions are applied and the same guidelines are followed to edit or update data. When standard rules for case inclusion or exclusion are also followed, the resulting incidence, survival, and response rates have the same meaning no matter where they were produced. Uniform standards are necessary for registry data to be optimally useful.

The use of standard data items and codes allows a registry to build on decades of item development and avoid much of the time, effort, and expense of defining and testing new items. The use of standard item definitions enables registries to adopt or adapt existing training procedures for coders, share standard editing protocols, and generate comparable analyses. The use of standard codes has facilitated development of hospital registry software capable of providing uniform data to central registries, data exchange between central registries, and the aggregated analysis of data from multiple registries. Empirical reports presented in the context of standard data items are more readily interpretable within and beyond the boundaries of cancer registration.

Definitions

A *data set* is the collection of items maintained by a registry. It may include data items coded and submitted by hospital registries or other direct sources such as pathology laboratories or physicians' offices, calculated items based on other items (e.g., time from record completion by a hospital registry to incorporation of that record in the central registry), data linked from external sources (e.g., median family income in the patient's census area), or items generated as a part of routine record processing (e.g., number of edit errors in the record at submission).

A *standard data item* is a data item whose codes, definitions, and coding instructions are shared among registry organizations. Most cancer registry items are promulgated by one or several cancer registry standard-setting organizations: the Surveillance, Epidemiology, and End Results (SEER) Program of the National Cancer Institute (NCI), Commission on Cancer (CoC) of the American College of Surgeons (ACoS), National Program of Cancer Registries (NPCR) of the Centers for Disease Control and Prevention (CDC), Statistics Canada, and the North American Association of Central Cancer Registries (NAACCR). Some items are developed by organizations outside the immediate realm of cancer registration: World Health Organization (e.g., ICD-O-3), U.S. Postal Service (e.g., U.S. ZIP codes), or the American Joint Committee on Cancer (e.g., the *AJCC Cancer Staging Manual*).

A *standard data set* in cancer registration is the collection of standard data items defined as the minimal data set required by an applicable standard-setting organization.

A *data dictionary* defines the data items in a registry data set, including coding instructions, code definitions, and the code options. A comprehensive data dictionary also includes a history of data item changes, identifies applicable edits, and provides guidelines or examples for item usage.

Basic Types of Registry Data

The general types of data items maintained by a registry are grouped as follows by NAACCR[1]:

- **Demographic** Analytic categories of patients (e.g., age, sex, race and ethnicity, residential location, occupation)
- **Cancer Identification** Anatomic point of origin and the pathologic nature of the tumor, sequence of independent primary tumors, screening information

- **Hospital Specific**   History of patient contact and case management by a specific facility, local record identification
- **Stage/Prognostic Factors**   All forms of staging, tumor markers, secondary diagnoses
- **Treatment—First Course**   First-course treatment dates and description
- **Treatment—Subsequent and Other**   Care delivered for recurrent or progressing cancer
- **Follow-up/Recurrence/Death**   Date of follow-up, recurrence date and type, status of patient, date and cause of death
- **Patient—Confidential**   Confidential patient information used to track the individual patient (e.g., patient name)
- **Hospital—Confidential**   Confidential information about specific hospitals and hospital personnel (e.g., institution referred from); collected by central registries from source registries
- **Other—Confidential**   Other confidential information (e.g., physician identifiers)
- **Text**   Narrative support for coded information

The standard NAACCR transmission file incorporates data items in each of those categories, together with administrative items and items specific to the registry sending or receiving the transmission.

- **Record Identification**   Items used to identify the layout and content of the record being transmitted; the recipient registry may maintain information in these fields in its own data set
- **Edit Overrides/Conversion History/System Administration**   Code systems used to record and transmit data, edit overrides, record processing trail, historic codes

The information in these fields is entered at the sending registry for use by the receiving registry to interpret submitted data.

- **State/Requestor Items**   Registry-specific or other special-use items, not in the standard NAACCR data dictionary but maintained by the receiving registry

Evolution of Current National Standards for Cancer Registry Data Sets

Movement toward standardization is incomplete, ongoing, and ultimately always will be in flux as registries respond to advances in cancer diagnosis and treatment, registry operation, and data storage and transmission technologies.

Most data set items in current use had their origins in the CoC or the SEER Program. The CoC first added cancer registry operation as an approval requirement for hospital cancer programs in 1956 and published a recommended data set in 1981.[2,3] CoC refined its data set with the publication of *Data Acquisition Manual* in 1986 and added specific coding requirements with publication of *Cancer Registry Operations and Data Manual (ROADS)* in 1996, with further revisions published in 1998.[4-6] The current manual is *Facility Oncology Registry Data Standards (FORDS: Revised for 2010).*[7] The SEER Program, which evolved out of the 10 Cities Survey, later called the Third National Cancer Survey, likewise developed its central registry data set over several decades. The latest version of the SEER Coding Manual was published in 2010.[8]

Most central cancer registry data originate in the hospital. In the 1970s, concern arose over disparities among hospital data sets, and between hospital data sets and the data sets needed by central registries.[9] A joint committee representing the CoC and SEER was begun in 1983 to promote increased standardization between the two programs. The group was broadened and was formalized in 1987 as the Uniform Data Standards Committee (UDSC) of NAACCR.[10] Although CoC and SEER each retain some unique items, a significant number of items are used by both organizations. For these common items, a single standard coding schema was agreed on and is maintained through the auspices of NAACCR. The NPCR, created in 1992 and administered by the CDC, became the third major standard setter for cancer registry data, in accordance with the federal legislation that provided funding support to developing state central registries. Statistics Canada is also taking an increasing role as the fourth standard-setting organization. Finally, some items necessary for central registry operation and data exchange are defined by NAACCR.

With the computerization of laboratories, it has become possible for pathology laboratories to send reportable data to cancer registries electronically. NAACCR developed guidelines for electronic transmission of pathology reports to cancer registries using Health Level 7 (HL7) and to update existing pathology laboratory electronic reporting documentation, which can be found in the *NAACCR Data Standards for Cancer Registries, Vol. V: Pathology Laboratory Electronic Reporting.*[11] Pathology laboratory reports often contain insufficient information to complete an abstract and usually require follow-back to the treating physician or facility for additional information.

The second decade of the twenty-first century is characterized by increasing adoption of electronic medical records (EMRs) by hospitals and movement toward "interoperable" electronic data transmission for central registries. Interoperability refers to the consistency in which varied organizations and software systems handle the transmission of similar information. These two trends involve changes in the way some data items are transmitted from formats that were unique to cancer registries to formats widely used beyond those bounds. For example, through 2009, registries transmitted dates in MMDDCCYY form and allowed 00000000, 88888888, and 99999999 to designate special conditions. Beginning in 2010, registry transmission of dates shifted to CCYYMMDD form, where unknown, less significant portions of the date are transmitted as blank spaces. When the date is missing, an associated flag indicates the special reason the date is missing. That logic, and the codes used for the flags, are based on HL7 coding practices. Additional similar changes are anticipated for electronic consistency with other medical data–gathering organizations.

Guidelines for Choosing Data Set Items

Data item selection starts with consideration of the goals and objectives of the registry and the intended uses of the data collected. The data set should include items required by funding sources such as SEER or NPCR or local benefactors, expected by parent agencies such as a state health department or a university medical school, of special interest to local audiences, needed to provide support to contributing hospitals and other facilities, and needed to support and monitor the activities of the registry itself. The registry may choose to collect some items for only limited primary sites or from only certain types of contributing sources.

As a general rule, if a standard item definition already exists for a concept to be measured, use of the standard definition and codes is preferable to creating a new item. However, the particular needs of the registry may require collection of information lacking a widely accepted standard definition. Any time new codes are defined, whether by an individual registry or a major standard setter, the following factors need to be kept in mind.

Availability of the Information in the Patient Record

Otherwise promising data items are of little use if the information is infrequently recorded in the patient record. One example is usual occupation, an item required to be collected by the law that established formation of the NPCR. The concept is potentially useful for surveillance, but the information is often absent from the patient record. Standard setters should establish in advance whether an item is available in a sufficient proportion of cases to make its collection useful. Conversely, if a standard setter requires an item that is not systematically recorded in the patient record, the registrar can take some actions to have it placed there. Depending on the item, it may be necessary to have it added to the hospital's admission sheet, or it may be sufficient that the clinicians responsible for the patient's care know that the item needs to be recorded. A supportive physician, the cancer committee, or another administrative authority can be approached to assist in implementing the addition.

Accuracy and Consistency (Reliability) of Information and Coding

Reliability refers to how likely different people are to arrive at the same data code, given the same information. Reliability requires unambiguous code categories, clear and consistent rules for assigning codes, good documentation, and good training. An item that describes a medical condition, such as laboratory measures, must be collected under consistent circumstances so that the results always have the same meaning. New data items should always be pretested, ideally under field conditions and with more than one person coding the same information for the same cases. Items such as stage or extent of disease are inherently complex and require continual attention to assure reliable coding. Some items may be unreliable if they are collected for purposes other than cancer registration. In the example of usual occupation just mentioned, the information will be unreliable if what is recorded is sometimes dominant lifetime occupation, sometimes current or most recent occupation, and sometimes the patient's former occupation most likely to have contributed to the disease. In this example, the *rules* for coding are inconsistently applied, although the code scheme is the same.

Continuity over Time

When possible, data items should be defined so the categories will be adequate for describing the intended concept under changing conditions. However, changes in medicine, cancer registry use, and technology necessitate item and code revisions over time. The test of continuity is invoked whenever a data item must be modified to meet new needs or improve reliability. If the transition from old to new codes is not carefully managed, use of the item may be seriously limited. The most useful new item is one whose new codes can be mapped completely to the old ones for analysis of time trends or to combine data collected over several years in a single study.

Especially if unambiguous mapping between the old and new coding scheme cannot be obtained, it is necessary to define clearly which coding scheme was applied in an individual case or the item becomes unreliable. By agreement of major registry standard setters, new codes are implemented to begin in a specified diagnosis year. This practice requires complete consistency in handling of data from all sources and detailed records for maintaining the "institutional memory" of schema in use at any given time. Data sources and coding schema used by central registries are complex. Including some administrative data items in the data set that define the coding scheme in use when the case was abstracted and coded and the current scheme (which may be the product of conversion) is an efficient method of guiding data analysis. Central registries may want to retain both sets of items as submitted by source facilities, letting the "current" scheme represent "as submitted" and defining an additional set of coding scheme items, which will be updated if the central registry subsequently converts an item.

Changes in medical technology over time may affect the data statistically. Widespread adoption of screening techniques that lead to earlier diagnosis of a disease can lead to the erroneous conclusion that survival has improved from the time of diagnosis. "Lead time" error occurs when there is a passage of time between the time the cancer was actually diagnosed and the time it would have been diagnosed using the older techniques. A comparable shift may occur if a diagnostic technique for identifying cancer spread is more sensitive than in the past, resulting in an apparently improved prognosis for a given stage of disease. Identifying effects such as these requires familiarity with the shifts in medical techniques that may affect analyses.

Compatibility with National and International Standards

An important criterion for evaluating new items is how well they fit with existing standards that reach beyond the registry. If a standard setter or a registry needs to collect information not already in its data set, the first resource should be to determine whether a measure for that item is already adopted by one or more standard setters, beginning with the standard setters having the most direct effect on or the most in common with the individual registry.

It is important not to alter existing standard items to fit local needs, because doing so removes the value of the standard item. Some standard items appear to have more response categories than may be useful within any single registry. For example, many categories in the standard race items are fully represented only in limited regions of the country. The registry can collapse some categories in such an item for data analysis, but it is important that all categories be available for coding if they apply so the information is retained for data exchange, aggregate data analysis, and other data uses. The registry software in use where the information is originally coded can provide simple procedures, such as drop-down menus, that enable the registrar to code information to rare categories without additional labor.

Relevance to Cancer Registration

Perhaps it is obvious that a new item in a data set should be of probable relevance to tracking or interpreting cancer rates, treatment quality, or survival, or to the management of the data system. It is important also to reevaluate the data set items periodically to determine whether the items are used at all and whether they are useful for understanding or controlling cancer. A registry may choose to drop an item because it is no longer considered medically relevant, the purposes of the registry have changed, or the item is not producing the quality of information that was desired. Some items have been eliminated from the large data set defined in the NAACCR standard data set over the years for exactly those reasons, and the major standard setters also eliminate required items when their usefulness can no longer be demonstrated.

The relevance of an item is increased if the item categories are well designed to fit the intended use of the item by the registry. For example, the standard definitions of race and Hispanic ethnicity are designed to match the usual categories used in census publications so cancer rates can be calculated with numerators and denominators measured in similar terms. Although problems with these items persist because of differences in the way individuals provide the information for the census and at hospital admission, the form of the item categories does not introduce an additional barrier to their use.

NAACCR Hispanic/Latino Identification Algorithm: An Example of the Creation of a Standard Item

Development of the NAACCR Hispanic/Latino Identification Algorithm (NHIA) measure by NAACCR illustrates some of the complexities involved in creating a new data item. NAACCR convened an expert panel in 2001 to develop a best practices approach to Hispanic/Latino identification. Representatives were selected from registries that serve regions of the largest numbers of Hispanic or Latino populations in the United States. The purpose of this activity was to evaluate the various methods and to determine whether a recommendation for a single measure based on patient surname was feasible for the various central cancer registries, considering the variety of Hispanic or Latino populations in the different geographic areas.

The development and testing of NHIA was based on the experience of the U.S. states with the largest Latino populations. When it was applied to states with smaller Latino populations, several issues emerged related to over-identification and the positive predictive values of indirect identification using surname alone in areas with a low frequency of Latino populations. Based on some state-specific analyses, several registries made suggestions to improve the accuracy of the surname-matching portion of the algorithm. These suggestions were then reviewed and evaluated by the Latino Research Work Group, a group that evolved from the original expert panel on Hispanic identification.[12]

Registry-Specific Items

Any hospital or central registry can create additional data items for its own use and for maximal efficiency and consistency; that procedure should always be used rather than instituting local changes in standard item definition. For example, sometimes neurologists request the hospital registrar to record the location of meningiomas in terms of the brain lobe covered by the affected meninges. The ICD-O-3 site code for meninges does not convey that level of detail. A registry-specific item can be developed for local use with meningioma cases that will document the detail requested. It is not appropriate to use ICD-O-3 brain site codes as a proxy for that information or to attempt to add nonstandard codes to the ICD-O-3 item.

Why Data Sets Change

The reasons data sets change have already been suggested. Some changes are due to changes in medicine, especially diagnostic tools and treatment modalities. The role of genetics in cancer care is expanding rapidly, and with it the codes used to describe the cancer and the laboratory approaches used for diagnosis. Newer techniques such as robotic surgery, the ability to treat in utero cancers successfully, and targeted delivery of molecular substances to tumors all required new ways to describe how cancer is treated. Other changes result from broadened computer capabilities as they affect registries, especially Internet connectivity, electronic access to medical records, and high-speed communications of all sorts. These allow accession of more information into the registry, more variety of data uses by registries, and more rapid communication among registries. With all of these advances, increased use of registry data has led to pressure for more data items, and more detail, to be collected by cancer registries. Quality of care, cancer control, genetics repositories, and hospital programmatic needs all are aided by registry data.

Adopting New Standard Items

As recognition of the value of standard items with fixed implementation dates became widespread among central registries, it became apparent that central registries, reporting facilities, and vendors were having difficulty making and implementing changes and additions to data standards annually. In 2000, the NAACCR Board of Directors established a Standards Implementation Task Force to review the timeline for changes to data standards and to recommend guidelines for a new timeline that will meet the needs of the standard-setting organizations, central cancer registries, vendors, and reporting facilities. The Standards Implementation Task Force guidelines provide for major changes to be implemented on a 3-year cycle, with all standard setters adhering to the same 3-year cycle. Minor changes may be implemented on an annual cycle. The intent is to allow the flexibility to fix errors and clarify codes or add new codes should they be necessary during the interval between scheduled major revisions and updates. See the *NAACCR Standards Implementation Guidelines* for definitions of major and minor changes and additional information.[13] The 3-year cycle introduced complications of its own, however, in the magnitude of adjustments being made at one time. Over the next few years, the registry community can expect further exploration of the best way to implement these important changes.

The Cancer Registration Steering Committee (CRSC) was established in 2005 to ensure coordination in the development and implementation of major data items, standards, and procedures related to cancer registration. Its purpose is to provide regular communication among leaders of NAACCR and its sponsoring member organizations to facilitate coordination and promote consensus. The committee members include all sponsoring member organizations; the NAACCR president, executive director, and the program manager of standards; and the chairs of the UDSC or Registry Operations Committee.

The *NAACCR Data Standards for Cancer Registries, Vol. II: Data Standards and Data Dictionary* provides detailed specifications and codes for each standard data item in the data exchange record layout for use by central registries, software providers, standard setters, and individual facilities that do their own registry programming. NAACCR members may request the addition of new data items or request a change to an existing data item by visiting the NAACCR Web site and completing a form. When a request form is completed, it is then submitted to the chair of the UDSC. Requests are reviewed and discussed by the UDSC, and may be sent back to the submitter for additional information, tabled for further discussion, approved, or denied. When a request for a change to an existing item is approved, it is then forwarded to the Volume II workgroup to include in the next version of the Standards Volume II. Requests for addition of a new item are reviewed by the UDSC and the CRSC to determine whether it is considered a major or minor change. Then, after the UDSC and the CRSC complete their reviews, the request may be sent back to the submitter for additional information, tabled for further discussion, approved, or denied. Once a request for addition of a new item is approved, it is forwarded to the Information and Technology (IT) Committee. IT then assigns the new data item a column space within the data exchange layout and a data item number. Finally, the new data item is forwarded to the Volume II workgroup for inclusion in the next version of the Standards Volume II.

Looking into the Future

Some of the most compelling changes facing cancer registration in the near future involve the technological feasibility of more rapid transmission of data from its source to cancer registries. These changes will more readily provide data from other parts of a facility to hospital cancer registries and will provide more timely transmission of information from hospital, laboratory, and other data sources to central registries.

Real-Time Reporting

A Real-Time Reporting Task Force was formed at an NAACCR leadership retreat in 2002. The participants, who included the NAACCR Board of Directors, NAACCR committee chairs, and NAACCR staff, recognized that the future success of cancer registries will rely to a great extent on the ability of registry systems to accurately and rapidly obtain information about cancer cases, and that real-time case reporting from all reporting sources would soon become a necessity. NAACCR also recognized that real-time reporting of cancer information to regional and local registries would help to completely identify all newly diagnosed cases of cancer by healthcare facilities and help increase the registry's ability to efficiently and accurately capture information related to the diagnosis, treatment, and survival of cancer patients.

The promise of real-time data collection for cancer registries is based on the availability of networked source data from the various departments of originating facilities (hospitals, pathology laboratories, etc.) in standardized, digitized form. Real-time reporting presents central cancer registries with the opportunity to improve on current cancer surveillance methods by the automated reporting of cancerous conditions to centralized cancer registries to improve both the completeness and timeliness of cancer registration efforts. For example, laboratory information systems can be configured to search automatically for reportable cancers and send final diagnostic reports in real time to the central cancer registry. Software systems, utilizing artificial intelligence technology, are showing that information may be collected and transmitted with a high degree of sensitivity and specificity. Some systems also allow the hospital cancer registry to be integrated with the central cancer registry and share both databases and software applications with a high degree of security.

Electronic Medical Records

An abundance of changes and influences needs to occur to set the stage for real-time data collection. Current progress toward a standard EMR will help to solve one of the major problems facing medical information systems today: to develop the interfaces that will enable different information systems to speak to each other. A necessary element for a real-time cancer reporting system is to have data source streams from the key departments of the facility (admissions, radiology, oncology, pathology, etc.) brought together in a single structured and standardized database or data stream that can be transmitted in real time to the facility or central cancer registry, or both.

The degree to which such data streaming is amenable for cancer reporting is dependent on thousands of system implementations in medical facilities throughout the country. These systems form the necessary baseline with which real-time cancer reporting can eventually be accomplished.

The administrative simplification section of the Health Insurance Portability and Accountability Act (HIPAA) establishes national standards for electronic healthcare transactions, which require the use of specific electronic formats developed by the American National Standards Institute (ANSI). Today, health providers and plans use a variety of different electronic formats, which often results in cumbersome or erroneous processing and transfer of information. The adoption of Transaction and Code Set standards, therefore, will improve the efficiency and effectiveness of the national healthcare system by moving systems toward the use of electronic data interchange (EDI) and uniform sets of standards. Currently, the X12 (developed to facilitate the exchange of e-commerce data, which has a broad application but is not sufficient for HIPAA) and HL7 (a messaging standard that enables different applications to exchange key sets of clinical and administrative data standards) are both used for designated electronic HIPAA compliant transactions. Although these two standards are similar in many respects, X12 is a generalized standard and HL7 was designed as a healthcare exchange standard.

Implementing New Data Items and Data Set Changes

One step toward implementing changes in data items or data sets is publication of implementation guidelines through an NAACCR-appointed committee. Those guidelines specify for central registries, facility registries, and software providers the steps and timing each must make for changes being implemented in a given year. However, before production of that document, considerable preparation has already taken place.

Standard-Setter Responsibilities

Planning for major changes in data items or data sets involves many players and may require 2 or 3 years or more of lead time. Whether the change is spearheaded by a collaboration of multiple standard setters or by one, all should be involved in early discussions to work out any potential problems and all should be kept up to date on progress of the new rules and definitions, field testing, timelines, and related matters. Beyond U.S. and Canadian national registry standard setters, registrars (through the National Cancer Registrars Association [NCRA]), software providers, state and regional central registries, and all of their constituents need to be included in early discussions, and they will need to know what the changes will mean for their own work and why the changes are important. Central registries need to begin planning at the outset what adjustments will be required in their data system: processing of incoming records, new items in the database, and conversions. In addition, changes to data dictionaries, training, coding software used in the field, data requirements, and possible supporting legislation all need to be addressed.

Beyond informing members of the registry community about the proposed changes, the standard setter(s) behind a major change should provide written documentation about it and the reasons behind it for reference by other standard setters, state and regional central registries, and others that will need to know whether and how to adopt the new or changed item for their use. In the absence of such information, some central registries may delay deciding whether to adopt a change until it has already been in use for a year. In addition, if the change involves a conversion from existing data, the standard setter(s) should provide a simple tool that makes that conversion. Often such tools convert registry records from the preconversion NAACCR transmission layout to the postconversion NAACCR layout. Providing a conversion tool helps assure that historic data are treated the same way across registries and software systems, and improves the timing and smoothness of implementation of the conversion. The conversion algorithm and any assumptions made in developing it should be thoroughly documented in text form.

Central Registry Responsibilities

Central registry timelines need to take into account the time software providers need to develop the changes, test the revised product, and place their revisions in the field; time to write and publish updates for data dictionaries and coding manuals, distribute them, and offer training; and time to make any necessary changes to the central registry software. This means that when changes are being planned, even well into the future, central registries need to begin planning proactively for those changes.

Central registries should expect to be ready to accept the new or changed data from their constituents as soon as the constituents implement the new items. By convention, the date of implementation is set at the beginning of a calendar year. That means the registry's database must be ready to accept any new items or redirect recoded items into new fields, modified edits and other quality-checking procedures must be in place, and the ability to read the new transmission layout must be set up. It is highly advisable to retain the old items in their original form and add new fields to represent converted and newly coded items when definitions are substantially changed. Because some software providers may not provide the updates promptly and some data sources may delay installation of software updates two or more months after receipt, the central registry will need to develop and publicize a procedure to deal with the delays. That may involve requiring the source to withhold submissions until the upgrade has been implemented by the source, or implementing two-track data input for a limited time to accept old and new transmission layouts.

It puts an additional burden on facility registrars and software providers if central registries require continued use of an old transmission layout with old codes after a change is scheduled to be implemented, and that practice should be avoided.

Hospital Registry Responsibilities

Hospitals provide nearly all cancer registry data. Their ability to implement new changes in a smooth and timely manner is key to the process. Hospitals need to develop routine procedures that can be implemented whenever software updates are made available to ensure the updates are ready to use on a timely basis. In particular, the procedures should avoid long delays between the time the upgrade is made available by the software provider and the time it is implemented in the registry. Data changes are designed for implementation in a new diagnosis year, so implementation of software updates is ideally timed just before the registry is ready to abstract cases diagnosed in the new diagnosis year.

Although standard setters, central registries, and software providers must provide information about coming changes and applicable education to hospital registries, it is the responsibility of hospital registrars to take full advantage of the training offered.

Staying Informed

In a world where change itself is a constant, *change* should be an anticipated component of registry operation, data set considerations, standard item definitions, and data storage and transmission processes. By planning for change, the registry can assure the continued utility of its data. Information about pending changes is transmitted through NAACCR and by the major standard setters to their constituent groups. State and regional registries have found that participation in NAACCR's committees is useful for being abreast of issues that may affect their operations.

The registry will need to retain information about *current and past* item requirements and definitions. The registry's library should include all editions of the coding manuals of the major standard-setting organizations affecting the data retained by the registry, and the relevant editions of publications of any other code manuals used by the registry. Central registries should include manuals used by their contributing sources for coding data items. This information is necessary for assuring the data are interpreted correctly and is of particular value in interpreting analysis of change over time.

The registry's data set should include all administrative items that identify the coding scheme originally used to code and the current code form for items that change over time. The registry should retain documentation of conversion algorithms applied by the registry.

The registry's programmers will need to understand how common data changes are for registries when they develop the processing system to design computer-processing procedures that facilitate annual addition of new items, changes in data definitions, and conversion of old items.

References

1. Thornton, M., O'Conner, L., editors. *Data Standards for Cancer Registries, Vol. II: Data Standards and Data Dictionary,* 14th ed. Springfield, Ill: North American Association of Central Cancer Registries, August 2009 (revised).

2. Blankenship, C., Moore, M., Opaluch, G. M., Sylvester, J. "The American College of Surgeons Commission on Cancer and the Approvals Program" (p. 17–28). In C. L. Hutchison, S. D. Roffers, A. G. Fritz, editors. *Cancer Registry Management Principles & Practice.* Dubuque, Ia: Kendall Hunt Publishing Company, 1997.

3. Commission on Cancer of the American College of Surgeons. *Cancer Program Manual: A Supplement on the Tumor Registry.* Chicago: American College of Surgeons, 1981.

4. American College of Surgeons Commission on Cancer. *Data Acquisition Manual (DAM).* Chicago: American College of Surgeons, 1986.

5. American College of Surgeons Commission on Cancer. *Standards of the Commission on Cancer, Vol. II: Registry Operations and Data Standards (ROADS).* Chicago: American College of Surgeons, 1996.

6. American College of Surgeons Commission on Cancer. *Standards of the Commission on Cancer, Vol. II: Registry Operations and Data Standards (ROADS),* rev. ed. Chicago: American College of Surgeons, 1998.

7. Commission on Cancer of the American College of Surgeons. *Facility Oncology Registry Data Standards (FORDS): Revised for 2010.* Chicago: American College of Surgeons, 2009.

8. Adamo MB, Johnson CH, Ruhl JL, (eds.). *2010 SEER Program Coding and Staging Manual.* National Cancer Institute, NIH Publication number 10-5581, Bethesda, MD.

9. Shambaugh, E. *Comparability of Cancer Data: Proceedings of Central Registry Workshop.* Chicago: American College of Surgeons, December 7–8, 1979.

10. "Historical background and status of U.S. standards." In L. Havener, D. Hultstrom, editors. *Data Standards for Cancer Registries, Vol. II: Data Standards and Data Dictionary,* 11th ed. Springfield, Ill: North American Association of Central Cancer Registries, April 2006.

11. Havener, L., editor. *Data Standards for Cancer Registries, Vol. V: Pathology Laboratory Electronic Reporting,* version 3.0. Springfield, Ill: North American Association of Central Cancer Registries; July 2009.

12. NAACCR Latino Research Work Group. *NAACCR Guideline for Enhancing Hispanic/Latino Identification: Revised NAACCR Hispanic/Latino Identification Algorithm [NHIA v2.2].* Springfield, Ill: North American Association of Central Cancer Registries, 2009.

13. Hultstrom, D., Gershman, S., Havener, L., editors. *NAACCR Standards Implementation Guidelines.* Springfield, Ill: North American Association of Central Cancer Registries, January 2003.

chapter 3

Staffing, Office Space, Equipment, and Budgets

Laurel Gray, CTR

As registries continue to expand in their ability to provide data and enhance cancer surveillance, it is important that registrars understand the overall administration of a registry to increase the efficacy of the department. Staffing needs, space and equipment, and the timing and process for budget derivation and implementation are all components of producing a registry of quality. Teamwork and knowledge are the foundation of a registry that provides consistent, reliable records. A productive registry maintains the delicate balance of providing useful, clinical data to the physicians, whereas fulfilling requirements of the state, the Centers for Disease Control/National Program of Cancer Registries, National Cancer Institute/Surveillance, Epidemiology, and End Results, or the Commission on Cancer's (CoC's) accreditation standards. The virtues of a registry can be debated, but the registry's value is ultimately based on the final product it provides.

Staffing

Most nonregistry personnel assume that staffing should be a simple mathematical equation: caseload divided by hours equals staff. But a registry has other functions besides case finding, abstracting, and follow-up. Analyzing the workload involves taking into consideration the ancillary factors that impact a registrar's time such as chart location logistics, cancer committee meetings, cancer conferences, audits, patient care studies, data requests, and other administrative responsibilities. Every procedure takes time and affects the staffing algorithm. The more aspects that can be anticipated, documented, and planned for, the more accurate the staffing algorithm will be. Determining how many staff members are needed requires taking into consideration the type of facility, who will be accessing the registry's data, and how available patient records are. Each task takes a specific amount of time and requires a certain number of staff members to complete. By determining how much time it takes to complete the tasks and all of the ancillary steps, it is possible to ascertain how many employees are needed in the registry. There are two key factors in determining time: knowing what is being asked of the registry and knowing what is required of the registry. It is important that the goals and expectations be defined so that everyone is aware of the registry's responsibilities. A discussion with the cancer committee will determine what the facility expects from the registry and what the registry can provide for the facility. The state's reporting guidelines will show what reporting is mandated. A document with the committee goals and expectations and the state mandates should be prepared. Presenting that document to the cancer committee on an annual basis approval ensures that the registry stays on track. It is also important that realistic time frames for accomplishing tasks be accurately determined. In addition to recording the time it takes for case finding, abstracting, and follow-up, other duties need to be accounted for, such as how long it takes to aggregate patient information for abstraction, prepare for cancer conferences, or perform case audits/reabstracting. Time-motion studies provide a means to document the time needed for all tasks that ultimately enter into the equation to determine the number of staff. Transferring the studies into work-flow charts and tables makes presenting the staffing needs a snap.

Facility Type/Mission

Knowing the mission of the facility is also a factor in determining staff. Take, for example, a small community hospital (SCH) and a medium-size clinic (MC). In this example, the overall number of cancer cases is the same at both facilities. However, SCH primarily diagnoses cancer and sends the patient elsewhere for treatment. MC is a full-service facility that diagnoses, treats, and also provides ongoing primary patient care. For a diagnosis-only case, SCH reports only the minimum mandated information. SCH may need the same amount of staff time as MC for case finding, but not the same amount of staff for abstracting and follow-up. Even though the overall number of cases is the same for SCHs and MCs, MCs will need more staff to gather the additional information required for abstracting and keeping the annual follow-up records up to date. In another example, research-based facilities that depend on the registry to assist the physicians with study information may require that supplementary data be gathered. These facilities may need to allot extra time for abstracting or for producing detailed study reports. Smaller CoC-accredited facilities may require the same staffing as larger facilities that are not accredited and collect only incidence cases as mandated by the state registry. The point is that the size or overall number of cancer cases does not always equate to the number of staff needed in the cancer registry. Different facility types and different goals or missions will help determine the registry's role. The cancer committee should define the registry's role and decide what information the registry will provide to the facility's clinicians beyond the mandated requirements.

Medical Records

Another consideration in staffing is the type of medical record and what it means in terms of efficiency. Facilities that keep a single patient chart in medical records may be ready to abstract in less time than facilities that have individual departmental charts and need to allot extra time to retrieve information from different locations. As program capabilities continue to be developed and hard-copy charts are rapidly being replaced by electronic medical records (EMRs), it is common for facilities to use a mix of departmental hard copies and electronic charts. This situation still poses the challenge of gathering all of the patient's information in the most efficient manner. What is of concern in this discussion is how the current medical record system affects the registry's time and staff in obtaining the records, processing the information, and sending the chart back into the system. One example might be obtaining hard-copy medical charts at our previously discussed SCH. The first task to obtain a chart from medical records is to fill out a chart request form, which is sent to the Health Information Management (HIM) department. The chart request can be done by e-mail. This process takes a 1 minute to complete. In this facility, it takes a total of 10 minutes for a registrar to go from the registry to HIM, sign out the chart(s), and come back to the registry office. At the registry office, someone needs to log in the chart. When the abstract is completed, the chart is logged out and returned to HIM, which adds 11 minutes to the time needed to obtain the medical record for abstracting. The result is a total of 22 minutes of registry staff's time required for nonabstracting duties. The total adds up to almost 2 hours every week or 2.5 weeks just to retrieve and return charts. Again, this is an example of time that needs to be factored in and not necessarily a statement of a procedure that must take place. The time it takes to complete this task is important because it impacts staffing. If an abstractor is used to retrieve and return the chart, then that time used will result in less time to abstract. Documenting the amount of time and series of actions within a process is called a "step assessment." Step assessments will produce a productivity level, an expected amount of work for a specific amount of time. For a person who only abstracts, a step assessment will provide a benchmark for the expected number of charts to be abstracted in a daily, weekly, or monthly period. Without documentation assessing the impact of processes on the registry, there is no standard by which to evaluate an employee's level of productivity. Having a reference point will enable the cancer committee to evaluate staffing needs and propose changes.

Software

The registry software also affects the registry's staffing needs. Registry software can increase productivity if it is versatile enough to meet the registry's growing needs and there is both vendor and facility technical support. Should a registry decide to transition to new software or make a software upgrade, there are several items that should be taken into consideration. It is not just the initial purchase price or the added amount of money for integration and support programs that affect the registry. Inconspicuous associated costs such as the extra time for training and the decrease in productivity during the learning curve add to the cost. Incorporating these associated time factors into the plan will assure that the budget stays in check, submission timelines are met, and there are few, if any, surprises along the way.

Newer registry software programs are able to interact with EMRs to aggregate all patient information, and some even accentuate cancer terms and/or codes for easier screening and abstracting. These additional features allow a registry to gather more information in less time, thus increasing the efficacy of the registrar. As this technology emerges, registrars must be responsive, ready to embrace the changes, and be willing to adjust registry operations accordingly.

Time

Time is commonly underestimated in a registry, and yet staffing has to be based on the actual time it takes from the beginning to the completion of a task. Some statistics indicate that an abstractor can produce one case per hour, with approximately 15 additional minutes per case given for case finding, follow-up, and administrative tasks. Therefore, if a facility accessions 2,500 cases per year, the simple mathematical equation—caseload divided by hours equals staff—would show that the registry would need only 1.5 registrars. Does the equation account for subtle time-consuming tasks? It may be better to readjust the equation to fit the specific circumstances of the facility. Every routine, task, and procedure needs to be evaluated because it influences staffing and registry function. If it takes 5 minutes for the computer to load the registry and facility programs each morning, and 5 minutes for it to backup and shutdown in the evening, those 10 minutes need to be considered. For a full-time employee who works 2,080 hours per year (excluding personal leave time, vacation time, or sick time), a simple opening and closing process takes 50 minutes per week, which adds up to more than 1 week per employee each year doing nothing but opening and shutting down the computer. Five employees would equal more than 5 weeks of time that would need to be added to the production equation.

Other items that tend to escape the staffing algorithm are training and education. Regardless of whether staff is given time for education through the facility or personnel leave time is used, production is decreased while employees are away maintaining their certification. Mentoring CTR students or training new hires will take time from the existing staff in addition to the time needed for them to become proficient in the job. Ongoing training is needed for software and registry updates. Adjustments in productivity levels must be made to account for the time in training, and that can have an overall impact on the number of staff required.

A basic technique to evaluate how each task affects the registry is to do time-motion studies. These studies show how long it takes the employees to do a particular task and how the work transitions from one task to another. They provide information necessary to create work-flow charts and establish productivity goals.

Time-Motion Studies

Work flow (how the work or information comes into the registry, is assimilated, and is disseminated) and workload (the total amount of work or tasks) determine staff and productivity levels. The work flow is based on what type of systems and processes are available at the facility. The workload is based on the overall caseload but also takes into consideration the additional responsibilities of a registry such as cancer conferences, cancer committees, studies, audits, reviews, training, and education. Vacation time, sick time, and personal leave time, although not always preplanned, need to be anticipated in terms of the effect on productivity. To establish staffing needs, it is important to understand how the work moves through the registry, how much time each task requires, and how much productivity should be expected. Both work-flow charts and time-motion studies start by picking out one task in the cancer registry, listing all of the steps needed to complete

that task, and recording the time it takes for each step. Obtaining paper charts from the medical records department is a good example. Table 3-1 shows both types of documentation were done, a time-motion study, and a list of steps needed to accomplish the tasks (step assessment). A review of the list of steps in accomplishing a task can determine whether the current procedure is the most efficient or whether there are opportunities for improvement. Once the optimum method has been established, the time to complete the task can be multiplied by the number of times this task needs to be done (daily, weekly, monthly, or yearly). After the total time in hours needed to accomplish these tasks is recorded, the tasks and hours can be matched to the category of staff to be hired (i.e., clerical, abstractor,

Table 3-1   Time-Motion Study

Name:_____ Date:_____ Position:_____

Activity	Start Time	End Time	Comment
Phone call	8:00	8:09	Dr. X study request—logged into request log
Start up computer and registry programs	8:01	8:06	
Fill out task steps for chart request	8:07	8:10	
Chart request for abstraction	8:10	8:11	Sent chart request to medical records
Sign out charts from medical records and return to office	8:11	8:21	Returned to office (no stops)
Fill out task steps for abstraction	8:22	8:35	
Chart abstraction	8:35	9:42	
Question by coworker	9:00	9:07	
Sign out chart, remove patient from suspense file, and place in cart for return (record further tasks)	9:43	9:44	
Return and log in charts to medical records	4:30	4:40	6 charts returned, no stops

Step Assessments
Task Steps for: Chart Request, Pick up and Return

Order	Individual Tasks	Comments
1	Choose chart from suspense file	
2	Indicate chart has been requested in registry program—date and initials	
3	Retrieve electronic chart request and fill out	
4	E-mail chart request	
5	Pick up chart at medical records	
6	Return to office	
7	Sign in chart at registry	
8	Sign out chart at registry	
9	Return charts to medical records	
10	Sign in charts at medical records	
11	Return to registry office	

Task Steps for: Abstraction

case finding or follow-up clerk). The total number of hours assigned to each category of staff, divided by the average number of working hours in a year (2,080 hours minus personnel leave time, vacation accrual, and sick time allotted) is the number of staff in each category that need to be hired. It is important to account for employee accrued leave time, vacation time, and at least factor in some sick time as these are part of the employee benefits, and employees are encouraged to use their time to keep them both physically and mentally healthy. If the facility also allows for additional education time, then subtract that benefited time from the total 2,080 hours as well. After the original assessment has been completed and time has been factored, then the categories can be combined or split as needed. This is a basic staffing algorithm.

A daily productivity sheet is another form of time-motion study. It tracks the overall productivity of each individual without listing the details of each specific task. Productivity sheets work well for specific tasks. The caveat to the productivity sheet is that it is designed to show what has been accomplished, not necessarily the steps it takes to complete the task. However, tracking daily productivity sheets can help in identifying tasks outside the normal day such as time for training, monthly meetings, off-site education, unusual telephone usage, or computer issues. Using time-motion studies, a daily productivity sheet, or a combination of both, and evaluating the results at regular intervals, provides updated information regarding shifting or growing staffing needs. This assures that the registry is adjusting staff work flow and workload in the best possible way.

Is it reasonable to use someone else's time-motion studies for averages? It is always a good idea to be able to compare the facility against outside benchmarks or standards to give accountability. The NCRA publication "Salary and Compensation Considerations for Cancer Registries (2007)" is one such survey that facilities can use. Matching individual studies to national averages will also show how the facility compares with these benchmarks. This assessment can be a starting point in making procedures more efficient or noting that the facility does a particular task well. Having an outside study does not negate the need for the facility to do its own studies. Only facility studies can provide actual information about the registry's specific needs based on the facility's specific systems and processes.

Type of Staff

Some registries use all certified tumor registrars (CTRs). Others include clerical staff or mentor students in the process of becoming CTRs. Unless the registry is CoC accredited, there are no hard and fast rules regarding how many CTRs are required at the facility or which tasks only a registrar can perform. However, when determining staffing, it should be made clear that CTRs are credentialed professionals who have passed a standardized test in cancer data management. Before assigning any task, the question to answer is whether it is better handled by a professional or whether it that can be performed just as well by a more cost-effective means such as using clerical staff.

Is it better to hire a contractor or permanent staff? That is a question most registries consider at some point, particularly those that are behind in submissions or those unable to hire enough qualified staff. There are pros and cons to both choices, and there is no right or wrong; it is simply a choice. Outsourcing to a contractor means not having the responsibility of providing for permanent staff in terms of salaries and benefits, although in exchange, the hourly cost may be higher. Outside contractors can often adjust quickly to a cyclical influx of cases by bringing in extra staff, whereas hiring permanent staff takes time and does not allow for temporary adjustment in cases. However, even if an outsourcing company provides additional staff, the facility may still need to provide the contractors with space, computers, and connections for the extra staff. Facilities requiring on-site training to obtain program passwords or facility compliance will have to consider the added cost of traveling and housing for contracted staff. Permanent employees provide consistency and the ability to keep up with training on an ongoing basis. With direct hiring, costs are usually within a range and consistent. Contracting prices may change, particularly with short-term contracts, and there could be associated charges for travel. Choosing to outsource all or part of the registry or to keep the registry in-house needs to be based on the individual facility and what is the best fit.

The movement to electronic medical charts has opened the opportunity for more registrars to work remotely. While remote staffing will certainly solve space issues, it has its own unique set of concerns such as patient confidentiality and computer connectivity. Also, remote abstractors may not be able to do all the work of the registry. It may be necessary to have at least one person on-site to handle items such as cancer conferences, mail, or other types of paper reports. The decision to use all remote staff, use only on-site staff, or use a combination of both, once again needs to be based on the facility's specific processes, systems, and policies.

Office Space and Equipment

A registrar actually needs very little in terms of supplies. As we move further into the electronic age, registries will no longer need the same storage space. They will no longer need to physically pick up medical charts, or receive and file reams of paperwork. Gone are the days of index cards and rows of file cabinets. Functionality of a space, rather than the location and physical size of an office, becomes the primary concern. Today's registrars are more concerned with having updated computers with better connectivity and enhanced registry software products. Nevertheless, to properly equip an office, staff still need desks, chairs, phones, access to a printer and fax machine, paper, hole punch, pens, pencils, stapler, file hangers, files folders, writing pads, highlighters, sticky notes, and a locking file cabinet for personnel records, outside correspondence, or other papers requiring privacy according to Health Insurance Portability and Accountability Act (HIPAA). Several registry manuals for reporting and abstracting are now computerized, saving some desk space; however, keeping a full set of registry manuals and reference books on hand is always a good idea for the unexpected computer disconnects. A well-organized, prepared, work-directed office contributes to the productivity of registrars and has a favorable impact on the overall efficiency of the registry.

Although necessities may be few in regard to material supplies and equipment as compared with other departments, improper placement of equipment and furniture can turn into chronic medical issues and result in loss of time at the job. Working all day on a computer can cause excessive fatigue, eye strain, neck pain, and back pain. The U.S. Department of Labor Occupational Safety and Health Administration (OSHA) provides the following information to maintain a proper, healthy work environment. Per OSHA, simple preparation of the task area each day can prevent most of these side effects and keep a productive environment.

- Computer monitors should be placed directly in front and at least 20 inches away with the top line of the screen at or below eye level.
- Monitors should be perpendicular to windows and at right angles to light sources. Arrange the office to minimize glare from overhead lights, desk lamps, and windows. Rows of ceiling lights should face the same way (parallel) as the line of site.
- Remove the middle bulb of four-bulb fluorescent light fixtures to reduce the brightness of the light levels and make them more compatible with computer tasks.
- Bright light sources behind the display screen can create contrast problems. Use blinds or draperies on windows to eliminate bright light. Per OSHA, vertical blinds work best for East/West-facing windows and horizontal blinds for North/South-facing windows.

Maintain appropriate air circulation and avoid sitting directly under air conditioning vents that "dump" air right on top of the work area. Dry air can dry the eyes, and poor air circulation can result in stuffy or stagnant conditions. Temperatures above or below the standard comfort level can affect productivity. To avoid these issues:

- Keep relative humidity between 30% and 60%. Use a simple humidity gauge and request a humidifier or dehumidifier as needed.
- Maintain ambient indoor temperatures in the recommended range between 68° F and 74° F during

heating season and between 73° F and 78° F during the cooling season.
- Always maintain proper ventilation to ensure that there is an adequate supply of fresh air.

Good working positions will reduce the risk for development of musculoskeletal disorders. Maintain a neutral body position. A neutral body position is one in which joints are naturally aligned. To accomplish this:

- Keep the head level or bent slightly forward, forward facing, and balanced (in-line with the torso). Shoulders should be relaxed and upper arms hang normally at the side of the body. Thighs and hips should be supported by a well-padded seat and generally parallel to the floor.
- Keep hands, wrists, and forearms straight, in-line, and roughly parallel to the floor.
- Elbows should stay in close to the body and bent between 90 and 120 degrees.
- The back needs to be fully supported with appropriate lumbar support when sitting up straight or leaning back slightly.
- Knees should be about the same height as the hips with the feet slightly forward. Feet should be fully supported by the floor or a footrest.

Working in the same position or sitting still for prolonged periods is not healthy. Change working position frequently throughout the day. Even when the design of the workstations is correct, and environmental factors are at their best, users can face other risk factors, such as repetition. Avoid some of these risk factors by providing variation in prolonged tasks, such as computer data entry, so that there is time to recover from the effects of the activity.

- Utilize adjustable chairs to easily change posture to allow different muscle groups to provide support while others rest.
- Substitute keystrokes instead of using the mouse all of the time.
- Take small breaks and stand, walk, or stretch.
- Try alternating tasks by mixing noncomputer-related tasks into the workday.

There is more to office workstations than supplies and equipment. How the workstations are organized and utilizing simple strategies will keep the work area comfortable, efficient, safe, and productive. More detailed information can be found online at the OSHA Web site (www.OSHA.gov).

Budget

The majority of registries have a top-down budget. A top-down budget is prepared by top management, passed down to primary departments and then subdepartments. This type of budget is fairly typical in hospital registries.

Another type of budget is the bottom-up budget. Subdepartmental managers or supervisors (i.e., cancer registry coordinators or managers) submit annual budgets to management to be approved. These are then forwarded up through the chain of command where they are appended to the departmental budgets. A third budget option is a zero-based budget. This type of budget is prepared as though it is being done for the first time; it starts with a budget base of zero. This method calls for each department or subdepartment to look at all expenses and justify them at each budgeting cycle. The facility, specifically the financial/accounting department, will determine whether the budget cycle follows a fiscal or calendar year. A fiscal year is simply an accounting year. It can start at any point in the calendar year and continues for 12 months. For example, some facilities start their accounting years in July and end in June instead of using the calendar year.

Few established registries produce a budget from scratch or work with a budget that has not already been projected 5 years out by the facility. Rather, they make adjustments based on unforeseen changes to these 5-year plans and might be asked to submit a new budget for year 6. A 5-year budget, sometimes called a "strategic business plan," is essential to allow time to prepare for growth and associated costs for added personnel, departments, and facilities. It is a plan to prepare for maintenance, updates of capital assets (more long-term items rather than disposable supplies), and annual growth. Regardless of whether the registry is making adjustments or submitting a full budget for the following year, a review of expenditures and staffing needs should be presented to the appropriate leadership body that approves the budget.

Where does one start? What is documented? There are four sections to a budget: capital purchases, salaries and benefits, supplies (disposable items such as paper and ink), and fixed costs (recurring monthly items such as rent, utilities, or housekeeping). Again, registries are not revenue-producing departments. The money to support the registry is allocated from the sponsoring department's budget or by the facility. The capital budget covers such items as the cost of the furniture, computers, or any equipment that has a life expectancy of more than one year, and is usually associated with new hires or normal attrition of equipment. The operating budget includes salaries, benefits, disposable supplies, and fixed costs. The registry generally focuses on the salaries, benefits, and disposable supplies. Budgets should be reviewed annually to determine whether the registry stayed within expected costs in all areas, whether there were unexpected but one-time-only costs, or whether the budget needs to be increased. The registrar will need to show the original budget together with the projected changes so reviewers can clearly identify the changes. Short text documentation for major budget adjustments, such as "addition of one FTE, see justification," can be added to refer the reviewers to detailed documentation.

If there is an upward adjustment in staff, there should also be a corresponding adjustment in the capital budget for the extra furniture and equipment.

Salaries are one of the largest cost items in the registry budget. How does one determine an accurate salary range for the geographical area? Human Resources has access to salary surveys performed for most positions within a facility. Many of these are conducted by the American Hospital Association or its local/state associations. Another option is the Internet. Several sites will give a salary range based on location, education or certification, and job description, though be wary of their sources and whether the salaries have been verified. Some sites use self-reporting, and it is not uncommon for people to artificially inflate their salaries. Also check the registry want ads and look for the current pay offerings. It doesn't behoove the registrar to underestimate the cost of staff. Overestimating staffing needs and pay will also harm the budget as it can be perceived as not being credible. Finding sites where actual salary ranges can be printed out will boost a budget presentation. When contacting outside facilities to get the information, note who was contacted (the person and their title), the date and time, the department, and the salary range given. The report justifying the salaries should provide specific job descriptions and task expectations along with the salary ranges. Having this type of documentation will show that the registry has done the research and prepared a well-thought-out proposal with credible numbers.

Often overlooked is accurately requesting funds for supplies and costs of meetings. Know the costs. Keep invoices for the supplies ordered. Keep track of ordering food for meetings. If the registry pays for certification, educational meetings, and associated travel, keep records. Aggregate the information and list it as an annual cost. If the registry is CoC accredited, make sure that the survey and any associated costs are accounted for.

When economic times are depressed, every expenditure of a nonrevenue-producing department, such as the cancer registry, must reflect a proven need. As diagnostics and treatment of cancer develop, there is growth in the registry. Seldom does a registry's caseload decrease unless an entire cancer program is cut. However, budgets are often reduced. Regular time-motion studies can show that the registry is using existing staff wisely and shifting tasks and personnel as needed. By demonstrating how long it takes to do each job, these studies can also predict growth and, ultimately, the need for new staff or validation for retaining staff. Having records of the small things such as disposable supplies, dues, and meeting costs will show that registry is cognizant of what it is spending. Being able to present a credible budget, staying within the current budget, and being able to accurately predict future needs will prove the registry to be a proficient and competent partner in the facility.

Conclusion

The details may differ in each registry, but the goal of better quality data collection is universal. The improvement of registry software and EMRs has and will continue to enhance the registry processes. The direction of standard-setting organizations has been toward the gathering of more detailed information as evidenced by the many changes that were implemented in 2010. Continually monitoring the registry workflow and the time various tasks require will be necessary to keep the registry efficient and responsive to ever-changing demands. Economic pressures require that the registry manage more efficiently. Being prepared with adequate documentation will position the registry to move into the future with confidence.

chapter 4

Legal and Ethical Aspects of Cancer Data

Amy M. Fremgen, PhD, CTR (Retired)
Dianna Wilson, RHIA, CTR

Importance of Legal, Ethical Aspects

The cancer patient, the physician, the facility, the cancer registrar professional, and the general public all have a stake in ensuring that the collection, maintenance, and sharing of cancer data are done in a professional, ethical, and legally defensible manner.

1. Cancer patients are most vulnerable at the time that they are, unknowingly, providing important data. Their rights, including information confidentiality, need to be protected. The cancer registrar must know the federal and state laws governing use of these data.
2. The physician and the facility's confidentiality must also be protected by the cancer registrar unless authorized to release pertinent information. The workplace may have additional rules concerning this knowledge.
3. The cancer registrar also must be protected from unknowingly performing unethical or illegal actions.
4. The general public also has a stake in this issue, as patient cancer data are the basis for cancer research, treatment development and decisions, and program funding. The cancer registrar has an ethical and legal responsibility to ensure the quality of the data collected.
5. We live in a litigious society; thus, it is important that cancer registrars protect themselves and their employers by knowing and following all the legal requirements for working with cancer patient data.
6. Legal understanding is also necessary for making appropriate decisions in the cancer registry.
7. Ethical behavior, not regulated by law, is a major component of being considered a professional.

Cancer registrars, whether working in a health facility or central registry, need to know how to perform their duties in a legal and ethical manner.

U.S. Legal System

For cancer registrars to understand the legal aspects of cancer data, they must first understand how our government and legal system are organized. The United States has a form of government structure called *federalism*. This means that power is divided between a large, central government, located in Washington, DC, and smaller, state governments. Under this system, all powers that are not specifically granted to the central, federal government are delegated to the authority of the states.

There is a hierarchal structure of legal precedence. Federal laws have precedence over state laws and state laws over city laws. However, if a city or state law is more stringent than a federal law, it can take precedence.

Laws are defined by the Merriam Webster Dictionary Web site as follows: ": a binding custom or practice of a community : a rule of conduct or action prescribed or formally recognized as binding or enforced by a controlling authority (2) : the whole **body** of such customs, practices, or rules."[1] Law is a system of rules, usually enforced through a set of institutions. It shapes politics, economics, and society in numerous ways, and serves as a primary social mediator in relations between people.

Four Categories of Law

In the United States, there are four basic categories of laws: constitutional, statutory, regulatory, and case (common) law.

Constitutional laws are embodied in the U.S. Constitution but also in the constitutions of the 50 individual states. They refer only to the relationship between citizens and their government, not to the relationship between private entities whether they are persons or businesses. In general, these laws do not pertain to the working of cancer registries and cancer data.

Laws passed by legislative bodies, such as Congress or state legislatures, are known as *statutes*. Congress and state legislatures have both enacted laws affecting cancer registries; these laws are discussed later in this chapter.

Congress or state legislatures may also empower agencies to make laws by passing "enabling legislation." When agencies make such laws they are called *regulations*. And there are agencies, also discussed later, that do impact cancer registry work.

City governments pass laws called *municipal ordinances*. They usually do not affect cancer registries.

Case or common law is made by judges when they apply previous court decisions to current cases. Thus, common law, as established from a court decision, may explain or interpret the other sources of law. Because common law evolves on a case-by-case basis, it is also called *case law*. Common law was originally established by English courts in the twelfth century and brought to America by the early colonists. The only state that does not follow common law is Louisiana, which bases its law on early French law.

Court decisions can affect cancer registries if lawsuits involving cancer registries are brought to court.

Civil versus Criminal Law

A further classification of laws is whether they are private (civil), public (criminal), or administrative. One type of civil law is called *tort*, which is a wrongful act committed against another resulting in injury to another's person, property, reputation, or the like, and for which the injured party is entitled to compensation. Invasion of privacy can be a tort.[2] Because cancer registries are very involved with health information confidentiality and patient privacy, it is possible for a cancer registry to be involved in a tort.

Legal Aspects of Confidentiality

This discussion of the specific legal aspects of working with cancer data starts with one of the most basic: ensuring the confidentiality of the patient's medical information.

Historical Basis of Medical Confidentiality

The historical basis for the confidentiality of patient information, including cancer data, is thought to have begun with an ancient (circa 400 B.C.) Greek physician, Hippocrates, known as the Father of Medicine. He vowed, "What I may see or hear in the course of treatment or even outside of the treatment in regard to the life of men . . . I will keep to myself." More than 2,000 years later, physicians still take the Hippocratic Oath as they enter the practice of medicine.

Because of this historical precedent, over time, patients grew to trust that their doctors would honor the privacy of their medical concerns. Until recently, that trust only needed to be placed in one treating physician. Now, however, a patient may be seen by many physicians and other professional health specialists in several different facilities. There are computerized record keeping and transmission of medical records. As a result, concern over patient privacy issues has increased.

Confidentiality

The American Health Information Management Association, in its 1993 position paper on disclosure, made a distinction between confidential and nonconfidential information. Researchers using medical information often distinguish between aggregate data, which are combined without patient identifiers, and confidential data. Other registries such as the National Cancer Data Base (NCDB) at the American College of Surgeons collect individual patient information, but without patient identifiers. Although the legislation and regulations under which the cancer registry operates may only define patient-specific data as confidential (e.g., name, address, and phone number), registries should also treat any information that specifically identifies a healthcare professional or an institution as confidential.

Need for Laws Protecting Confidentiality

As mentioned earlier, healthcare providers have a strong tradition of safeguarding private health information. However, in today's world, the old system of paper records in locked filing cabinets is not enough. With information broadly held and transmitted electronically, there needs to be clear standards for the protection of personal health information.

Unfortunately, when personal health information is not safeguarded, unscrupulous people can search for it and sell it, especially in the case of celebrities who find their medical records published in the tabloids. Such events are a serious breach of both legal and ethical standards.

In the spring of 2009, the medical information privacy of a woman who gave birth to 8 babies was compromised; consequently, 15 hospital workers were fired for looking at her records without permission, and 8 others were disciplined. At that time, hospital officials did not think that any information had been given to the media.[3] Remember no one is allowed to look at anyone's medical records unless there is a valid reason for doing so. This means no one can look up the records of a neighbor, friend, or even a family member. To help prevent unauthorized viewing of medical records, almost all facilities now have a tracking system that keeps a record of who has accessed a medical record.

Cancer data are highly confidential, and one of the most important responsibilities of cancer registry professionals is to safeguard the confidentiality of cancer patient information. Improper disclosure of these data could result in emotional, psychological, and financial harm to the patients and their families. The standard of confidentiality maintained by cancer registries is similar to that of the doctor–patient relationship, and it extends indefinitely, even after the patient is deceased. Although patient confidentiality is of paramount importance, it is also critical that cancer registries implement policies to protect the privacy of physicians and healthcare facilities. The terms *confidentiality* and *privacy* are often used interchangeably in reference to medical information.

Federal Laws That Impact Cancer Data

Because of the changing methods of record keeping, laws had to be enacted to protect patient privacy beyond that generally accepted under the concept of patient–doctor confidentiality.

Privacy Act of 1974

One of the first federal laws to protect patient privacy was the Privacy Act of 1974. It was enacted to safeguard individual privacy from the misuse of federal records, to provide that individuals be granted access to records concerning them that are maintained by federal agencies, and to establish a Privacy Protection Study Commission.[4]

Thus, individuals were given the following rights:

- To find out what information is collected about them by the government

- To see and have a copy of that information
- To correct or amend their information
- To exercise control over disclosure of that information

However, it is sometimes necessary for confidential information to be shared without the knowledge or consent of the person. Thus, this law also permits federal agencies to collect, maintain, use, or disseminate any record of identifiable personal information but only in a manner that assures the following:

- Such action is for a necessary and lawful purpose
- The information is current and accurate for its intended use
- Adequate safeguards are provided to prevent misuse of such information
- Only in those cases where there is an important public policy need as has been determined by specific statutory authority

Enactment of HIPAA

In April 2001, an important federal law was enacted that impacts every cancer registry: The Health Insurance Portability and Accountability Act of 1996 (HIPAA).[5] Although the name does not seem relevant to the cancer registry, the act contains a pertinent section. Part 164 of HIPAA is considered its security and privacy portion. Its provisions safeguard patients' important confidential health data identified as protected health information (PHI) and these patients' rights to protect their privacy. As cancer registrars deal with patients' PHI, they must be aware of the pertinent legal restrictions and procedures detailed in this part of the act.

Part of what HIPAA seeks to do is set minimum standards for confidentiality of patient health information. States may enact stricter standards. (See earlier discussion of the U.S. legal system.) The cancer registry must follow whichever provisions are stricter. There is also a process for changing the provisions of the act, if necessary. Thus, cancer registry professionals must be alert to amendments to HIPAA.

Need for HIPAA Privacy Rule

In enacting HIPAA, Congress mandated the establishment of federal standards for the privacy of individually identifiable health information. When it comes to personal information that moves across hospitals, doctors' offices, insurers or third-party payers, and state lines, our country has relied on a patchwork of federal and state laws.

Under the patchwork of laws existing before adoption of HIPAA and the Privacy Rule, personal health information could be distributed—without either notice or authorization—for reasons that had nothing to do with a patient's medical treatment or healthcare reimbursement. For example, unless otherwise forbidden by state or local law, without the Privacy Rule, patient information held by a health plan could, without the patient's permission, be passed on to a lender who could then deny the patient's application for a home mortgage or a credit card, or to an employer who could use it in personnel decisions. The Privacy Rule establishes a federal floor of safeguards to protect the confidentiality of medical information. State laws that provide stronger privacy protections will continue to apply over and above the new federal privacy standards.

In the 1990s, during Congressional hearings concerning HIPAA, an egregious misuse of patient data came to light. A lay member of a state health commission had access to the state's cancer database. He used that access to search for cancer patients who had loans with his bank and then called in their loans. Although the original purpose of the act was to ensure workers' continuation of health insurance, it quickly spread to include the issue of confidentiality to prevent such abuse that is now covered in Part 164 of the act.

Understanding HIPAA

It is important for cancer registrars to be aware of the provisions in HIPAA that directly affect their work and know how to access future changes in the provisions. For example, how does HIPAA affect:

- The exchange of data within the reporting facility?
- The exchange of data within and outside of the state?
- Patient follow-up operations?
- Obtaining patient health information from external physicians?

Although the laws pertaining to cancer registries and patient information are designed to protect patient privacy, they also are designed to allow data to be used for important research and surveillance activities. Thus, the cancer registrar must also be aware of the specific requirements of state and federal laws for the content and use of the collected data.

Many cancer registry functions are carried out under the "Operations" umbrella of HIPAA regulations known as "consent for uses and disclosures to carry out treatment, payment or healthcare operations . . ." Operations include "quality assessment and improvement activities" and "population-based activities relating to improving health or reducing health care costs." This allows hospitals and physicians to disclose PHI, including first course of treatment and follow-up, to each other for specified healthcare operations, provided that both covered entities (CEs)—that is, those facilities that are covered by HIPAA rules—have a relationship with the patient. However, patient follow-up many years after treatment (or encounter) remains an area that needs further clarification in future modifications. Cancer registrars are responsible for knowing of any changes in section 164 that will impact their work.

It may be of interest to note that a precursor to HIPAA was the Medical Patients Rights Act (MPRA), which is no longer in effect as it was superseded by HIPAA. MPRA stressed that medical records needed to be handled with confidentiality, especially the disclosure of patient information without the patient's written consent. This included whether the patient was a patient. However, the act did not cover the electronic transfer of medical records, which was hardly being used when it was enacted, and it did not carry strong penalties for violations. But it was a start in getting healthcare workers to pay more attention to the important issue of confidentiality. HIPAA *does* carry strong penalties for violations of its provisions. State laws can also carry penalties for violation of privacy rules.

In spring 2009, a southern California hospital was fined $250,000 because several employees had illegally accessed the medical records of a mother who had had multiple births. The California Department of Health (CDOH) imposed the maximum fine, even though the hospital had fired the implicated employees, notified the state of the situation, and none of the information appeared in the media. The CDOH found that the facility had not done enough to stop the privacy breach, and there was a possibility of individuals facing fines as the result of further investigation.[6]

"Stimulus Bill" and Privacy

It may be surprising to learn that the American Recovery and Reinvestment Act of 2009 (ARRA), which has been called the *economic stimulus bill*, includes 21 pages pertaining to health information privacy.[7] It establishes the first federal requirements for reporting and notification of breaches of personal health data. Although many states have their own data breach notification laws, CEs will now need to review the requirements of both the ARRA and their own state. ARRA, just like HIPAA, does not overrule state requirements that are stricter than the federal provisions.

One of ARRA's disclosure provisions that may be pertinent to cancer registries requires CEs using electronic health record systems to account for all disclosures when the patient so requests. This includes disclosures that HIPAA exempts, such as for treatment, payment, and operations. ARRA also seeks to improve enforcement of HIPAA and its own regulations. It further stipulates that individuals, and not just the CEs, will be subject to penalties. This means that under the new law, individual cancer registrars could also be subject to penalties as specified.[8]

Significance of Accurate Records

In addition to confidentiality requirements, accurate record keeping is important both for legal and ethical reasons. An important provision of HIPAA is a patient's right to know to whom his or her PHI has been disclosed without his or her consent. To meet this HIPAA requirement, a facility must maintain an "accounting of disclosure," which is essentially a record (kept for the most recent 6 years of disclosures) of "what, where, when, to whom and for what purpose" any PHI was disclosed without patient consent. This includes data submissions to state and central cancer registries that are covered under law and to researchers conducting special studies.

Ordinarily, medical records cannot be sent to anyone without consent in writing from the patient and with the physician's approval. One exception to this is cancer registrars needing to send data to state cancer registries or to provide patient follow-up information. See earlier comments regarding the "Operations" umbrella of HIPAA.

Responding to a Legal Subpoena

Another exception to not providing medical information is when a court orders that a record be subpoenaed. It is highly unlikely that a cancer registrar will ever be served with a subpoena, as this would usually go through the hospital's administrative and/or Health Information Management Department (Medical Records) and legal offices. However, it is good to know that if a medical record is subpoenaed, *only the parts requested* should be copied and provided to the requesting attorney. The entire medical record of a patient is usually not necessary, unless requested, to fulfill a subpoena request. Also, if the original record is not requested, a certified photocopy may be provided. If the original is requested, a photocopy of it is placed in the file with the receipt for the subpoenaed record. The patient should also be notified by certified mail that the record has been subpoenaed. *Note:* The cancer registry abstract is usually considered a work product and not an official legal document, and thus is not usually subject to subpoena.

Important Regulatory Agencies

The process of Congress granting regulatory powers to agencies is discussed in an earlier section. Two such federal administrative agencies of significance to cancer registries are the National Cancer Institute (NCI) and the Centers for Disease Control and Prevention (CDC). They are both agencies of the U.S. Department of Health and Human Services.

SEER Program

The NCI oversees a national system of population-based registries established in 1971 when Congress passed the National Cancer Act. This act mandated the collection, analysis, and dissemination of data for use in the prevention, diagnosis, and treatment of cancer. This resulted in the establishment of the Surveillance, Epidemiology, and End Results (SEER) Program, an ongoing project of the NCI. The SEER Program operates 17 population-based cancer registries in various geographic areas of the country covering approximately 26% of the U.S. population (see Chapter 33).

National Program of Cancer Registries

The CDC implements the National Program of Cancer Registries (NPCR), which was developed as a result of Congress enacting the Cancer Registries Amendment Act in October 1992.[9] Through this legislation, the CDC was given authority to:

- Provide funds to states and territories to enhance existing population-based cancer registries
- Plan and implement registries where they do not exist
- Develop model legislation and regulations for states to enhance viability of registry operations
- Set standards for completeness, timeliness, and quality
- Provide training

Presently, there are now 48 population-based registries in 48 states/territories: 45 states, Pacific Island Jurisdictions, District of Columbia, and Puerto Rico (see Chapter 34).

Amending Existing Laws

Over time, it may become necessary to change or amend laws that have already been enacted. For example, in 2002, Congress determined that the population-based registries of NPCR needed to include benign brain-related tumors in their data collection. Thus, they enacted the Benign Brain Tumor Cancer Registries Amendment Act[10] based on testimony that supported the importance of this data item. Cancer Registrars, in addition to being aware of new laws that may affect their work, also need to keep informed about any pertinent changes to existing laws.

Commission on Cancer Standards

Both NCI and CDC work closely with the Commission on Cancer (CoC) of the American College of Surgeons. Although not a federal agency, the CoC has operated a voluntary system of accreditation for hospital cancer programs since 1932 (formerly called *approved cancer programs*). To become accredited, such programs must meet established standards, which include a requirement for maintaining a hospital cancer registry with at least one Certified Tumor Registrar (CTR). Other standards include policy state-

ments about protecting patient confidentiality and release of patient information.

State Laws and Institutional Requirements

State Laws

State laws regarding confidentiality vary; some are very specific, and others are worded in a more general manner. As mentioned earlier, the more stringent law, whether federal or state, usually takes precedent. Central cancer registries can also obtain valuable information from the North American Association of Central Cancer Registries (NAACCR) (see Chapter 28). It publishes standards for confidentiality and disclosure of data, and for what legislation and regulations should specify when setting up a mandated central cancer registry. The CDC has used NAACCR's standards in the implementation of the NPCR. Copies of the appropriate law governing the registry's area of coverage can be obtained by contacting legal counsel or the population-based registry serving the geographic area of interest.

Institutional Requirements

Institutions may have their own specific rules and regulations governing confidentiality and release of information. Institutional review boards or other committees established to review confidentiality and ethics can set up policies and procedures that need to be followed. These policies can extend from the health facility to the central cancer registry that receives its reported cancer patient data. Thus, in addition to knowing and abiding by state and federal laws, cancer registrars need to be aware of institutional regulations.

The cancer registry professional has an important role in ensuring that legal requirements are met by all those involved in the collection, maintenance, and use of cancer information. This responsibility includes being up to date on the legal requirements and the institutional policies and procedures regarding patient data, and ensuring that this knowledge is communicated to, understood, and followed by all those involved with the data.

Personnel Policies and Procedures

All cancer registry staff must be responsible for the confidentiality of all patient information encountered during the collection, maintenance, and dissemination of cancer data. NAACCR standards state that registry employees and cancer data users should at least annually sign a Personal Security Compliance Form documenting participation in the Security Awareness Program, a program that addresses the security education needs of all employees, contractors, and users as appropriate.[11] Some registries require staff to sign a confidentiality agreement annually as a reminder of the importance of this issue. A sample confidentiality pledge is shown in Figure 4-1. These agreements should be signed before the employee receives any passwords or other sign-on codes granting access to patient information.

Registry staff training should include a comprehensive session concerning the confidentiality of the data. Fictitious names or anonymous datasets should be used in training and demonstrations of the computer system used in registry operations. Nonregistry staff who request access to registry data should also sign confidentiality agreements. Nonregistry staff must agree to adhere to the same confidentiality policies as practiced by registry staff.

An example of a facility's zero tolerance policy on confidentiality was demonstrated in August 2007. A Minnesota health clinic suspended more than 100 employees for violating federal laws on patient privacy. They were suspended without pay for 3 days. Most had looked into a relative's records, and in one case, the employee altered his/her own record.[12]

In March 2008, a well-known actor was forced into announcing his diagnosis of pancreatic cancer before he had planned to do so. Unethical and possibly illegal disclosure of his medical records to the media resulted in pressuring him to quickly inform his family and friends of his disease so he could make his announcement at a very stressful press conference.[13] It is unconscionable that a cancer patient should be treated in such a way by the healthcare professionals he had relied on when he entered his healthcare facility.

Cancer Data Protection

Release of Cancer Registry Data

As the late Charles R. Smart, MD, FACS, founder of the Utah Cancer Registry and past Executive Director of the CoC of the American College of Surgeons, once said, "The purpose of the cancer registry is not just to collect the data but to use the data." The authorized use of registry data is fundamental to the success of the registry. Release of cancer data for clinical purposes, research, and administrative planning is central to the utility of the registry. However, as noted earlier, confidentiality of the patient's information and privacy of the healthcare provider and facility are protected both legally and ethically.

To ensure that information is only disclosed to authorized parties, policies and procedures for release of cancer registry data must be developed and implemented. Confidential information about cancer patients, care providers, and healthcare facilities must not be released for purposes other than those specified by the cancer registry unless

---

Confidentiality Pledge

I understand and accept the legal and moral responsibilities of maintaining the confidentiality of all data and information collected and processed by the (facility name) cancer registry. I agree not to divulge, publish, or otherwise make known to unauthorized persons or the public any information that could lead to identification of such persons receiving services, or to the identification of their health care providers. I also understand my role in ensuring the right to privacy of persons and institutions cooperating with the cancer registry data collection activities. Furthermore, I understand that the (facility name) has policies that protect the patient's right to every consideration of their privacy regarding their medical information. I understand that I must not reveal any confidential information to anyone except those individuals authorized to receive such information. I also understand that failure to adhere to this policy may result in disciplinary action up to and including automatic dismissal without further notice. I recognize that unauthorized release of confidential information may subject me to civil liability under the provisions of state or federal law.

I have read and understand (facility name)'s confidentiality policy and procedures and pledge to act in accordance with these policies and procedures.

Signature _____ Date_____

Supervisor_____ Date_____

Figure 4-1. Sample Confidentiality Pledge

all parties concerned provide written authorization and agree in writing to adhere to all confidentiality policies.

Confidential cancer registry data should never be made available for uses such as marketing products to cancer patients, healthcare institutions recruiting new patients, or insurance companies or employers trying to determine the medical status of a patient. Under no circumstances should confidential information be published or made available to the general public. Media inquiries should be referred to an administrator or another staff member who has the authority to respond.

Information should not be given to individual patients about themselves, except when required by law. Requests from patients for specific registry information should be referred to the attending physician; and the physician notified of the patient's request and the registry staff's response.

Under the Operations section of HIPAA, the cancer registry may permit the release of confidential data to other treating hospitals in their own state or other states for the purpose of patient follow-up. However, if appropriate, policies and procedures should be instituted that include a case-sharing agreement among multiple facilities and a central registry. These policies and procedures should also be approved by the institution and the hospital cancer committee.

Data Security

The physical security of confidential data stored on paper, microfilm, microfiche, and electronic media must be ensured to fulfill the legal and ethical requirements for maintaining patient confidentiality. Suitable locks and alarm systems should be installed to control access to the registry itself. Fireproof, lockable file cabinets should protect hard-copy abstracts, computer printouts, and other reports.

Employees accessing patient information on a computer screen should be careful that the screens are shielded from passersby. They also may be required to log off the computer system when not using it to prevent unauthorized access. Paper files should also be placed so as to prevent unauthorized viewing.

Personnel may not take home confidential patient information without proper authorization; they also may not remove procedure or other important registry manuals.

HIPPA security requirements include administrative provisions, physical safeguards, technical safeguards, and network and communications safeguards. Computers used for cancer registry data must be controlled by electronic and physical measures to enhance the security of the data. Electronic or technical controls include use of passwords (access controls), automatic logging of all attempts to enter a computer system (audit controls), and different levels of data access, such as read-only files.

Automatic backup systems should be in place in case of computer failure. Most facilities also have policies for off-site storage of computer files in case of on-site disasters.

The cancer registrar's manual provided by the employer should have a policy and procedures section with information concerning the security of the cancer patients' data. This material should be covered when training new registry employees.

Data Transmission

Confidential data must not be transmitted by any means—mail or other types of paper delivery system, verbal via telephone or in person, or electronic—without explicit authorization from administration. Authorization may be granted for use in follow-up activities, for the transfer of data to a central registry, and for other appropriate activities. When authorized, cancer registries should consider the use of registered mail, overnight mail, or courier service for delivering confidential data. Procedures to help ensure confidentiality include separating patients' names from other data for transmission. Another procedure is to use two envelopes with confidential data placed in a separate envelope stamped or marked confidential and that envelope inserted in a second mailing envelope.

If envelopes need to be sent to patients, for whatever reason, such as containing materials or requests for information, the envelope's return address should not use the words *Cancer Registry* or other similar term.

Confidential material should generally not be transmitted by fax. However, if it must be done, the sending registrar needs to be reassured that the receiving machine is in a restricted area where only authorized people have access. A fax is not acceptable when an original document is requested.

Encryption of data is necessary when transmitting confidential information electronically. Encryption is a process of encoding textual material and converting it to scrambled data that must be decoded to be understood. This process is especially necessary when data are transmitted over public networks or communication systems.

Another method is used by the NCDB. Data from reporting facilities are submitted through a secure, password-protected site. All CoC passwords are person specific and are linked to the individual's roles in one or more facility. Only people identified by NCDB as hospital registrars in CoC-accredited programs (or programs pending accreditation) can submit cases, except the registrar can give permission for a specific registry software provider to make the submission. The NCDB validation system checks that the registrar who submitted the data is a registrar affiliated with the program whose data are submitted in the file, and files are not processed if there is not a match.

The growing use of off-site notebook computers and remote data access by physicians and registrars has led to the need for additional security measures. Each affected facility will need to develop specific policies and procedures for maintaining database security and restricting unauthorized access to its data.

Policies should also be developed and implemented for the disposal of confidential data. The use of shredders or incinerators is common in hospitals. Paper abstracts, computer printouts, copies of pathology reports, and other materials should all be stored or disposed of properly. Care must be taken not to leave these documents lying where unauthorized persons may have an opportunity to read them.

Other Legal Issues

Although the confidentiality and quality of cancer data are the primary legal and ethical responsibilities of cancer registrars, they may need to be aware of other legal areas. For example, in interviewing a potential employee, there are certain questions that may not be asked, such as "How many children do you have?" If seeking to discharge an employee, one should be aware that the provisions in an employee handbook may be considered "implied contracts" and should not be violated. Obviously, any charge of harassment could also come under legal scrutiny. A facility's personnel office should have more specific information concerning these issues.

Ethical Aspects

Ethics can be defined as "the discipline dealing with what is good and bad and with moral duty and obligation" or "a set of moral principles."[14] For some, ethics means following the "letter of the law," whereas others may regard ethics as a statement of acceptable behavior found in a code of conduct or regulations developed by a professional organization. Professional ethics concerns "the principles of conduct governing an individual or a group".[15] To ensure the integrity of cancer data and the cancer registry profession, the National Cancer Registrars Association adopted a *Professional Practice Code of Ethics,* most recently updated in 2008, that outlines the principles of professional conduct and provides members of the association with definitive and binding guidelines of conduct (see the Appendix C). This code of ethics addresses the issues listed in Table 4-1.

In general, the cancer registrar shall maintain high standards of conduct, integrity, and fairness in all professional actions and decisions to establish and sustain an irreproachable, professional reputation, as well as bringing honor to oneself, the cancer registry profession, and the association.

The comprehensiveness of the guidelines covered in the NCRA *Professional Practice Code of Ethics* demonstrates the importance of ethical concerns. The NCRA publication was used as a guide for the rest of this section.

Cancer Registrar Practice and Standards of Conduct

Cancer registrar practice and standards of conduct address professional actions and decisions to establish and sustain an irreproachable, professional reputation. These guidelines address conducting business on behalf of employers honestly and ethically, declining favors that will influence any decisions, and avoiding commercialization of one's position. Undue pressure should not be exerted in obtaining employment/clients, and honesty and integrity in the promotion and delivery of services including an honest representation of qualifications should be followed. Professional titles and degrees must be used as earned and consistent with the dignity of the profession. Use of the CTR is reserved for those individuals who have been awarded this credential. It is unethical to use this credential if it has not been awarded or if it has been revoked. A breach of ethics by one registry

Table 4-1	Guidelines Addressed in the National Cancer Registrars Association *Professional Practice Code of Ethics*

- Cancer registrar practice and standards of conduct
- Confidentiality and privacy
- Cooperation with other professions and organizations
- Discharge of entrusted professional duties and responsibilities
- Preservation and security of cancer registry records and information
- Preservation of confidential professional determinations by official committees
- Disclosure of sensitive information during employment or contracted services
- Compensation for professional services
- Professionalism
- Increasing the profession's body of systematic knowledge and individual competency
- Participation in developing and strengthening the professional workforce
- Honorable discharge of the association's responsibilities
- Upholding the standards of the profession

professional may have a negative impact on the entire profession. Registry professionals also have an ethical obligation to recognize, encourage, and support other members of the profession. The contributions of fellow members and coworkers should be recognized appropriately to advance cancer registry practice. Publications should give credit where due to one's peers.

Confidentiality and Privacy

Confidentiality and privacy have already been addressed in this chapter, but an example provided in the NCRA *Professional Practice Code of Ethics* is reiterated here. The patient has a right to feel confident that all identifiable information about such patient possessed by the cancer registry will be kept confidential unless the privilege is waived, or release of the information is compelled by statute, regulations, or other legal means. Use and release of identifiable and nonidentifiable information shall be according to established institutional policies. With regard to the release of confidential information, it is unethical to "provide lists of patients' names for marketing research or other commercial use." Such practice is not a proper function of a health institution, and these lists should not be released by a cancer registry professional without the proper authorization. Every effort must be made to ensure that the computerization of cancer registry data is accomplished in a manner that protects the confidentiality and security of patient information.

Cooperation with Other Health Professions and Organizations

Cooperation with other health professions and organizations to promote quality of healthcare programs and the advancement of medical care is an essential factor in the cancer registry profession's greater aim of improving health services and supporting research relevant to cancer patients. All states and the District of Columbia have laws, regulations, or statutes requiring healthcare facilities and providers to report cancer data to either state or SEER registries that, in turn, report the data on a national level. In addition, many state laws have provisions authorizing the exchange of cancer registry data with registries in other states. Respecting, cooperating, and working with other health professionals will foster good relationships that will benefit both professions and, ultimately, the cancer patient.

Discharge of Entrusted Professional Duties and Responsibilities

Discharge of entrusted professional duties and responsibilities is the ethical conduct expected of the cancer registry professional. It is unethical to accept a position or contract for services for which one is inadequately pre-

pared. The cancer registry professional should seek out the special knowledge, skills, or experience of fellow professionals for referral, counsel, guidance, or consultation when requiring additional expertise to adequately perform duties for an employer. It is also unethical to vacate a position without adequate notice or to fail to complete an assignment without ensuring that the work that is entrusted will be completed in a satisfactory manner. It is incumbent on the cancer registry professional to render a truthful accounting of the status of the work for which he or she is responsible.

Preservation and Security of Cancer Registry Records and Information

The cancer registry professional should strive consistently to uphold professional standards for producing complete, accurate, and timely information to meet the health and related needs of the cancer patient. In addition, it would be unethical to participate in any improper preparation, alteration, or suppression of medical or health records, including official minutes and related documentation maintained as part of the healthcare facility's operation.

It is the responsibility of the cancer registry professional, whether a consultant, supervisor, employee, advisor, or other, to advise the employer or client if, in the registrar's professional judgment, there is the danger of making errors of commission or omission.

Cancer registrars performing remote abstracting and working from home offices must be diligent to follow the same confidentiality and privacy guidelines as they would when working in an employer's office. This would include as examples, storing patient records in a secure location where they cannot be read by unauthorized persons, not leaving patient data on unattended computer screens, and properly disposing of paperwork with patient information, that is, shredding or returning to an employer.

Preservation of Confidential Professional Determinations by Official Committees

Preserving the confidential nature of professional determinations made by official committees of health and health-service organizations is the ethical responsibility of the cancer registry professional. Cancer registry professionals shall abstain from discussing observations, comments, or findings concerning the practice of individuals that result from committee activities (such as medical audit findings, individual patient care, professional standards review recommendations, or information obtained from any other source) with anyone except the appropriate institutional authority.

Disclosure of Sensitive Information during Employment or Contracted Services

Discretion shall be exercised when releasing or discussing sensitive information acquired during employment or fulfillment of contracted services that concerns the administrative conduct or professional practices within the healthcare facility. Examples include disclosing only to the proper authorities concerning the conduct or practices believed to be violating the institution's internal policies and rules, or disclosing to proper regulatory or law enforcement agencies the conduct or practices believed to be illegal only when, after informing the healthcare facility, no corrective action has been enacted.

Compensation for Professional Services

Compensation for professional services should be accepted only in accordance with services actually performed. It is unethical for the cancer registry professional to place material gain ahead of service. Primary importance should be placed on providing a high standard of professional service; financial considerations are secondary to this objective.

The cancer registry professional should endeavor to avoid a conflict of interest by providing full disclosure to the employer, client, or professional organization of any interest in any provider of services or products.

Professionalism

Professionalism requires the cancer registry professional to represent truthfully and accurately professional credentials, education, and experience in official transaction or notice, including any other positions held and any possible conflict of interest. Misrepresentation of one's professional qualifications or experience is unethical. A statement of any other positions of possible duality of interest in the health or health-related fields, either remunerative or nonremunerative in nature, should be made available on request of the employer. Examples of possible duality of interest are outside consultation services, committee appointments, advisory positions, elected offices, business enterprises interests, and the like.

Increasing the Profession's Body of Systemic Knowledge and Individual Competency

Increasing the profession's body of systematic knowledge and individual professional competency through continued self-improvement and application of current advancements to the conduct of cancer registry practice is an ethical goal. The attainment and preservation of professional status are accomplished through the mastery and competent handling of cancer registry activities and the continual development of new knowledge and skills. This may be accomplished by reading pertinent literature; attending workshops, institutes, and other continuing education programs; and examining scrutinizing functions performed as a cancer registrar for the purpose of self-evaluation in carrying out professional duties. Advancements in the knowledge and practice of cancer registry administration are attained by participating in studies and projects related to the principles and practices underlying such practices. Examples include promoting and/or participating in advancing the development, maintenance, use, and preservation of cancer registry practices or foreseeing subjects necessary in current and future training of cancer registrars.

Dissemination of new developments or changes in methods or procedures should be shared with other cancer registry professionals in a timely manner for the purpose of increasing the knowledge and skills of the profession. Care should be taken to distinguish the sharing of such information from the promotion of products or services of the employer or favorite commercial firm.

The cancer registrar professional should provide for professional growth and development of those under the professional's supervision.

Participation in Developing and Strengthening the Professional Workforce

Participation in the development and strengthening of the professional workforce is the responsibility of all cancer registry professionals. The future of the profession is dependent on the affirmative and responsible endeavors of professionals to recruit and train other cancer registry specialists. Providing training and clinical experience to students, participating in career fairs, and writing for professional publications are all ethical undertakings that meet these objectives.

Honorable Discharge of the Association's Responsibilities

Honorable discharge of association responsibilities is expected of every cancer registry professional who accepts an appointed or elected position. Examples include the execution of one's obligation to the profession with integrity, discretion, and conscientious performance of the duties and responsibilities of the office or assignment accepted. Preserving the confidentiality of privileged information obtained through this association is one's ethical duty.

Upholding the Standards of the Profession

Breaches of ethical conduct are very serious. Any charges of unethical behavior or alleged violations are investigated by the NCRA Ethics Committee and, if necessary, brought before the Board of Directors for possible punitive action. The complaint procedure can be obtained from the chairperson of the NCRA Ethics Committee. Judgments of unethical behavior and recommendations for sanctions are the responsibility of the Ethics Committee rather than of individuals. If found guilty of a violation of the *Professional Practice Code of Ethics,* a cancer registry professional shall be subject to one or more of the following penalties: (1) rendered ineligible to be nominated for or elected to an office in the association, (2) suspension of NCRA membership, (3) revocation of NCRA membership, or (4) revocation of the CTR credential.

The most serious consequence of a finding of guilt of a violation is revocation of the CTR credential. NCRA's Council on Certification, which confers the designation of CTR on persons meeting the eligibility requirements and passing the CTR examination, is also highly concerned with the ethical behavior of CTRs. The Council on Certification Examination Handbook states, "Certification will be revoked for falsification of an application, violation of examination procedure, or violation of NCRA's Code of Ethics."[16] An appeals mechanism exists for challenging revocation of certification. In addition, the examination application requires candidates to sign the following statement: "I have read the Handbook for Candidates and NCRA's Code of Ethics and understand that I am responsible for knowing their contents. I certify that the information given in this application is in accordance with the Handbook instructions and is accurate, correct, and complete. I understand NCRA may verify my provided experience and education."[16]

References

1. Merriam Webster Dictionary. Available at: http://www.merriam-webster.com/dictionary/law Accessed March 30, 2010.
2. Fremgen, Bonnie F. *Medical Law and Ethics,* 3rd ed. (p. 33). Upper Saddle River, NJ: Pearson Prentice Hall, 2009.
3. "California Briefing/Bellflower: Workers who saw Suleman file fired." *Los Angeles Times,* March 30, 2009, p A9.
4. Electronic Privacy Information Center. "Privacy Act of 1974 and Amendments." Last updated February 2008. Available at: http://epic.org/privacy/laws/privacy_act.html. Accessed April 01, 2009.
5. U.S. Department of Health and Human Services. "The Health Insurance Portability and Accountability Act of 1996 (HIPAA) Privacy and Security Rules." Available at: http://www.hhs.gov/ocr/privacy/index.html. Accessed July 19, 2009.
6. Ornstein, Charles. "Breaches in privacy cost Kaiser; The Bellflower facility is fined $250,000 after unauthorized workers viewed the records of Nadya Suleman." *Los Angeles Times,* May 15, 2009, p A3.
7. U.S. Government Printing Office. "Public Law 111–5—Feb. 17, 2009." Available at: http://frwebgate.access.gpo.gov/cgi-bin/getdoc.cgi?dbname=111_cong_public_laws&docid=f:publ005.111.pdf. Accessed July 19, 2009.
8. Rode, D. "Recovery and Privacy," *Journal of AHIMA,* 2009;80(5):42–44.
9. Library of Congress. "Improvement of the National Program of Cancer Registries Act (Introduced in Senate)." Available at: http://thomas.loc.gov/cgi-bin/query/z?c111:S.792:. Accessed July 19, 2009.
10. The actual law itself may be found at http://frwebgate.access.gpo.gov/cgi-bin/getdoc.cgi?dbname=107_cong_public_laws&docid=f:publ260.107. Accessed April 7, 2010.
11. Hofferkamp, J., editor. *Standards for Cancer Registries, Volume III: Standards for Completeness, Quality, Analysis, Management, Security and Confidentiality of Data.* Springfield, IL: North American Association of Central Cancer Registries, August 2008.
12. "Clinic cracks down on snooping," *Advance,* August 13, 2007, p. 33.
13. "Patrick Swayze weeks to live." *National Enquirer.* Available at: http://www.nationalenquirer.com/patrick_swayze_cancer_weeks_live/celebrity/64581. Accessed July 2, 2009.
14. Merriam-Webster Online Dictionary. "Ethic." Available at: http://www.merriam-webster.com/dictionary/ethics. Accessed June 14, 2009.
15. Merriam-Webster Online Dictionary. "Ethic." Available at http://www.merriam-webster.com/dictionary/ethics. Accessed April 18, 2010.
16. National Cancer Registrars Association Council on Certification 2010 CTR Exam Handbook & Application. Available at http://ctrexam.org/pdfs/Handbook2010.pdf. Accessed January 1, 2010.

chapter 5

The Registrar and Professionalism: Networking, Mentoring, and Volunteerism

Linda Mulvihill, RHIT, CTR
Ann Griffin, PhD, CTR

People recognize the word *professional* to mean those with a professional degree, such as doctors and lawyers. However, the term *professional* is also used to describe a person with a high level of competence in a particular activity. Although cancer registrars may be considered professionals based on either definition, skilled registrars can certainly be described as having a high level of competency in cancer registration.

Cancer registration is a quantifiable, organized process by which data are systematically collected. By combining data on many patients with similar characteristics, information is provided for both medical and public health communities.

The ultimate goal of the analysis of cancer data is to prevent and control cancer, including the improvement of cancer patient care.[1] Surveillance data should be used to identify research and service needs, which, in turn, help to define training needs.[2] Cancer registrars are the professionals who provide the data for cancer surveillance. Registrars are, by definition, "official recorders or keepers of records."[3] Cancer registrars specialize in recording cancer data in a wide variety of settings (mostly hospital and central registries), thereby providing high-quality records of the cancer diagnosis and treatment experience for each cancer patient within the population. The fundamental data set includes: (1) cancer incidence; (2) cancer type (site, morphology, behavior); (3) extent of cancer progression at the time of diagnosis (stage); (4) treatment (first course and subsequent); and (5) outcomes of treatment (survival).[4] The cancer registrar of today is charged with developing the knowledge base required to collect high-quality records to meet these specifications of various standard-setting organizations.

Technological advances in cancer diagnosis and management, in addition to the technological advances in the software used to process registry data, necessitate continual education and professional development. The data collected have become progressively more complex, and consequently, more time will be required for professional development and education to stay abreast of change. The registrar must address the additional challenges of implementing new data standards and data management. Registrars are expected to understand and apply all data standard changes. Employers who support professional development will attract and retain today's registrar.[5]

Professional Development

Continuing education is the cornerstone of the registrar's professional development. It is required to maintain the Certified Tumor Registrar (CTR) credential to ensure proficiency in cancer registration. As the technology involved in cancer surveillance becomes more advanced, continuing education will become more vital, not only to the profession, but also to the cancer surveillance and research community.

The registry profession, historically, reviewed paper medical records to abstract information onto a paper form. Early on (1970s), cancer registrar education was not systematic or formalized. Organizations that utilized cancer data, and later required its collection, developed more formal training in cancer registry over time (e.g., self-instruction manuals developed by the Surveillance, Epidemiology, and End Results [SEER] program). Several non-degree training programs were developed, such as the University of San Francisco's 2-week course (no longer available) and the University of Southern California, Cancer Surveillance Program's 4-week course. Education opportunities have evolved from self-instruction manuals to college degree programs in Cancer Information Management. (A complete listing of college degree programs is available online at: www.ncra-usa.org, click on Accredited College Programs.)

The registrar of today utilizes electronic health records and sophisticated registry software that will increasingly link the patient's information automatically to the registry database. The CTR's knowledge of the cancer disease process and the data standards to capture the information for each type of cancer is essential to the shift from data collection to complete data management. The major function of the registrar's job will become that of a data manager and analyst. Educational requirements for certification and recertification (education and certification requirements are available online at: www.ncra-usa.org) will most likely continue to increase in step with emerging technology, both in medicine and in database management. For the registry professional, an emphasis on cancer surveillance will be added to the current core knowledge of the cancer disease process and data standards. This will include the calculation of survival rates, cancer program information, analyzing referral patterns, the evaluation of the efficacy of treatment modalities, and compliance with cancer treatment guidelines.

Just as a commitment to continuing education for professional growth is important, the future direction of cancer surveillance may dictate advancing professional development through earning a degree or an advanced degree in addition to maintaining certification requirements. Some knowledge simply cannot be learned on the job or in continuing education classes or workshops. Continuing education cannot incorporate all of the information, and on-the-job training is time limited. As the data requirements increase and become more complex, the greater the responsibilities that are placed on the registrar, the greater the need for higher education. Educational background enables one to understand the implications of change and to position one to have the necessary knowledge to anticipate future skills. Education to prepare for a world with informatics will play a pivotal role in the future of the cancer registry profession. The transition to the electronic health record from the registry perspective will depend on the registry professionals' capability to utilize information technology. Part of the successful transition may involve some basic core competencies for anyone who uses the electronic record in his or her daily work.

Formal education offers new networking opportunities by increasing one's knowledge about the whole healthcare environment, such as a better understanding of how cancer information is integrated into the health system and a general understanding of technological issues. Education can increase job satisfaction and personal satisfaction. It offers the opportunity to learn about and understand other disciplines. This, in turn, enables one to see the larger picture and make communications more effective. Online coursework enables the full-time worker to be a part-time student at his or her convenience. Professional growth demands that we look beyond the day-to-day job activities and position ourselves for challenges in the future. Degrees that provide benefits on the job today may be mandatory in the future.

The commitment to professional development and growth is an individual commitment, but employers should be coaches for professional development and should support the registrar's efforts. Taking an active role in preparing for the future may well be the clearest sign a registrar can give management to recognize the registrar's skills and knowledge base. Individual employee professional development results in organizational professional development. It is important that management recognizes the importance of the registrar's work and the registry's contributions to the organization. The registrar should take personal responsibility for his or her own professional growth by assessing the work environment through reading, continuing education and networking. The registrar should evaluate how their job duties or position in the organization is changing: It is important to consider what skills and/or experience will be required to keep up with future changes in technology and workflow. Registrars should discuss their duties with the information technology department and ask about new changes in technology that may facilitate registry duties (e.g., electronic pathology casefinding). Registrars should be active in pursuing the right education, training or assignment opportunities at their place of employment through professional organizations, education programs, and online coursework. It is up to the registrar to find the next training opportunity!

Professionalism

Never has it been more important to maintain professionalism in the registry field. Staffing registries of various sizes can be expensive in today's economy. The choice between hiring full-time, in-house staff instead of the cheaper alternative of contracting out registry services may be facing many facilities. It is imperative that registrars step up and prove their worth as professionals who cannot easily be replaced, either by technology or impermanent staffing.

Professionals are characterized by a commitment to service, are autonomous in their work, and maintain a level of competence and good judgment that make them universally needed and respected. Professionals are bound by a code of ethics, have membership requirements (licensure, certification), adhere to standards, and support professional development outside the work environment (maintain membership in associations or professional organizations such as the National Cancer Registrars Association [NCRA] or American Health Information Management Association [AHIMA]).

Back in the early days of cancer registration, the only education required of a registrar was a high-school diploma. Registrars were commonly thought of as "clerks" or "coders." Keeping up with the registry profession today requires a lot more knowledge than a high-school diploma. Registrars can demonstrate their worth to their institution by maintaining a professional attitude throughout daily work activities. The cancer registrar can be the most valuable member of the cancer program team by taking the lead in coordinating: (1) high-quality data collection, (2) compliance with cancer program standards, (3) promotion of data analysis and dissemination of outcomes both inside and outside the institution, and (4) integration of all aspects of the cancer program.

How the registrar looks, talks, acts, and works can determine whether they are perceived as a professional or an amateur. Further, the registrar's professional conduct elevates cancer registry as a profession in the eyes of administrators, medical staff, and physicians. Professionalism can go a long way toward supporting the registrar when it comes time to budget for space, equipment, education, and more staff. Registrars who do not have experience as a "professional," or are new to the cancer registry field, should choose a mentor. The best place to find one is a current or former board member of the local, state, or national registrar's association.

Mentoring

Professional development is a lifelong process in which individuals no longer stay on one career path their entire life. They will experience transitions in choice of career because of changes in the economic climate or likely personal interest and/or aptitude. Mentoring is a learning approach that is highly suited (and valuable) to supporting a person who is undergoing either an initial or alternate career choice.

The concept of mentoring is as old as Greek mythology. A mentor promotes the passing down of knowledge, values, and/or life skills to a less experienced person (mentee). It is a reciprocal relationship, built on trust and accountability, where the mentor enjoys sharing his or her experience and serving as a role model to a mentee who benefits from the exchange.[6]

Mentoring in the cancer registry profession is essential. However, it is often difficult to develop effective mentoring relationships because of the specialization of the field, lack of formalized education (until recently), and simple lack of registrars with long-term experience having time to share. Even registrars who transition into the registry profession from other careers still need to accumulate experience through "hands-on" training. For most in the cancer registry profession who have benefited from mentoring, as a relationship, it has been mainly on an informal level. Many cancer registrars are the only staff member at a hospital working in the registry. The usual scenario involves a single registrar at a facility under the supervision of a manager of another type of department (e.g., Medical Records/Health Information Management, a clinic practice, Quality Improvement). The registrar in this position would benefit most from a mentor/mentee relationship with a registrar from a nearby (if possible) hospital facility. Rather than waiting for a formalized mentoring program, many registrars either gravitate to a more experienced registrar or a more experienced registrar informally "adopts" a less experienced registrar. This requires that, together with registry experience, registrars volunteer their time and expertise. The topic of volunteerism is addressed further later in this chapter. At any stage of professional development it does not hurt to seek out the guidance and wisdom of a registry professional who has more experience. The development of such a relationship is a benefit to the mentee and an honor and privilege to the chosen mentor.

With any career choice or transition, there is a learning curve. Mentoring helps reduce choices made by trial and error, can make transitions smoother, and supports people making decisions about their careers and defining long-term career goals. The benefit of mentoring for an employer can be shorter learning curves, fewer mistakes, smoother transitions, and happier employees. Probably the greatest benefit of mentoring a fellow registrar is the succession of mentoring by that individual of another registrar in the future, and so on.

Patient volume and data collection standards do not leave registrars with much additional time. However, each of us has the opportunity to serve as a role model at many points in our careers. In turn, each of us could benefit from the guidance of a fellow registrar. Building a support network of fellow registrars can make the difference between a feeling of isolation and overwork to a feeling of community and a shared burden. In some area of registry work where the registrar has formulated a "best practice" or succeeded with a performance improvement project like increasing the compliance with AJCC[7] staging at the facility, the sharing of that information with other registrars leads to less stress, improved quality, and camaraderie in the shared mastery of the myriad challenges registrars face every day. On the other hand, if the registrar is stumped by a problem with no solution in sight or is unsure about new data collection standards, he or she should not hesitate to reach out to fellow registrars for brainstorming potential solutions. If a registrar has generously volunteered his or her time with a peer, the peer registrar, in turn, can pass on shared knowledge or experience later on. It is the cancer patient who will ultimately benefit from registrars helping one another and working together.

Networking

Networking is about making connections with fellow registrars who can either provide information or introduce others who have information. It could be information such as a job posting, a "best practice" relative to a registry duty, or just advice on how to handle a difficult employee, coworker, or supervisor. Networking can be either formal or informal.

The best way to begin networking, if new to the registry field, is to join the state cancer registrar's association (formal networking). If a registrar has been in the registry profession for some time, then he or she should consider being of service to the state or national registrar's association, perhaps as a committee volunteer or in an elected office. Don't hesitate — a component of networking is a willingness to ask for help from a more experienced person. Within a place of work, it is important to venture out to tumor boards (cancer conferences) and meet anyone unfamiliar. When coordinating the Cancer Committee, express an interest in the performance improvement or education activities of nursing staff. Join a hospital-sponsored Relay for Life team. Remain visible to cancer program members. Sign up for newsletters or other forms of workplace communication. All of these avenues broaden a network of people, ideas, and/or services that can provide important information in the future.

NCRA has special interest groups for members. At one time, Yahoo groups served as a forum for posting questions and getting answers in these special interest groups. Today, NCRA has ventured into popular social networking outlets such as Facebook and Twitter,[8] giving members a less formal, but convenient, way of communicating. Another popular online networking opportunity is available through LinkedIn, where a registrar can join and "connect" with other members, create a résumé, and look for open positions in cancer registry.[9]

Networking creates a community of people who support each other, who provide emotional support and information that will help each other. Networking spreads the word regarding new developments in cancer registry: new tools, processes, leaders, training programs, products, and services, and is a good way to discover the solution to a problem faced at work. It is satisfying to provide a key piece of information that makes a real difference in the life of a network member. Choosing members takes some thought, but once started, networks can grow quickly. Keep an open mind in travels and interactions with colleagues. Exchange business cards. And don't hesitate to share information that may be valuable to fellow registrars.

Volunteerism

Volunteering is the practice of people working on behalf of others without financial remuneration or material gain. This does not mean that volunteerism is without benefits. Organizations benefit by meeting their goals in an economic manner while individuals receive multiple social benefits. Employers benefit from volunteerism because not only are volunteers presented with opportunities to make new friends and social contacts, but they can acquire leadership and management experience (e.g., through serving on boards, task forces, or ad hoc committees). Volunteering can enhance specific work-related skills and knowledge, and can open up future opportunities. As Margaret Mead once said, "Never doubt that a small group of thoughtful committed citizens can change the world; indeed, it is the only thing that ever has."[10]

Taking on interesting challenges in volunteer leadership helps registrars realize their potential and gain personal satisfaction. Healthcare organizations welcome candidates with good experience and leadership skills, as well as qualifications on their résumés. Volunteer positions can help fill those résumé gaps. Being a volunteer, especially as a mentor to another registrar or serving as a board member of a professional organization such as the NCRA, is highly rewarding, and far outweighs the loss of personal time or freedom that volunteerism sometimes entails. Volunteering for the American Cancer Society or community outreach efforts impacts the lives of cancer patients, and can often provide balance to a stressful career by blending direct personal interactions and "human touch" with the less personal registrar duties involving data collection.

Conclusion

Professional development can no longer be viewed as an event that occurs once a year; rather, it must be continual. Individual professional development enhances organizational development. Registrars are self-motivated, self-directed professionals in a small, unique field and may not be presented with employer direction to meet career challenges. Professional development and growth may, by necessity, be self-motivated and self-directed for registrars. The registrar's motivation and confidence will grow along with professional development. Through mentoring, volunteerism, and networking, registrars can take care of each other and promote the registry profession in keeping up with our future role as leaders in the "war on cancer."

Linda Mulvihill is a Public Health Advisor for the Centers for Disease Control and Prevention. The findings and conclusions in this report are those of the author(s) and do not necessarily represent the official position of the Centers for Disease Control and Prevention.

References

1. Clive, R. E. "Introduction to cancer registries" (pp. 3–4). In C. L. Hutchison, M. R. Menck, M. Burch, R. Gottschalk, editors. *Cancer Registry Management: Principles and Practice,* 2nd. ed. Dubuque, Ia: Kendall Hunt Publishing Company, 2004.
2. Thacker, S. B. "Historical development" (p. 7). In S. M. Teutsch, R. E. Churchill, editors. *Principles and Practice of Public Health Surveillance.* New York: Oxford University Press, 1994.
3. *Merriam-Webster Dictionary: Third New International Dictionary of the English Language.* Springfield, Mass.: Merriam-Webster, 2006.
4. Clive, R. E. *Cancer Registry Management: Principles & Practice,* 2nd ed. Dubuque, IA: Kendall Hunt, 2004.
5. Mulvihill, L. G. *Salary and Compensation Considerations for Cancer Registrars.* Alexandria, Va.: National Cancer Registrars Association, 2007.
6. Cuerrier, C. "Mentoring and professional development, document #13." Ottawa, Ontario, Canada: Canadian Career Development Foundation, 2004.
7. Greene, F. L., et al. *AJCC Cancer Staging Manual,* 6th ed. New York: Springer, 2002.
8. Hefner, L. "Social networking for registrars. *ADVANCE for Health Information Professionals,* 2009;19(10):12.
9. McEvoy, C. "The Webs We Weave." *ADVANCE for Health Information Professionals,* 2009;19(10):14.
10. Lutkehaus, N. C. *Margaret Mead: The Making of an American Icon.* Princeton, NJ: Princeton University Press, 2008.

chapter 6

Health Information Privacy and Security

Thom H. Faris, Esq., JD, CQA, CQM
Annette A. Hurlbut, RHIT, CTR

Introduction
Need to Protect Confidential Information

"Have you ever been diagnosed with a sexually transmitted disease?" "Have you ever experienced high blood pressure?" "Do you drink alcohol or use illegal drugs?" Patients peruse the waiting room, looking around to ensure that no one is looking at their answers. But what happens after the new patient information is handed over to the receptionist? Who has access to the medical records that include all of your physician's notes about your most personal conditions, feelings, traits, and problems? What do they do with the information, and who are "they" anyway? Medical records can contain the most highly personal and sensitive information about a person.

Enter the Computer Age. Handheld computers, the Internet, e-mail communication, and the use of personal computers enable people unknown to you to store nearly limitless amounts of data, perform timely searches and reports, and distribute large quantities of information to a wide audience in practically no time. The healthcare industry is now able to make patient records and image data instantaneously available at multiple locations, as well as provide summary analysis of multiple patient, facility, or regional studies with very little effort. Information is power.

Junk mail, credit card offers, e-mail spam, and telemarketing—how do they find us? Marketing firms exist in today's business world solely for the purpose of accumulating and selling information about individuals. Your name, address, and information about your spending habits, property interests, creditworthiness, political affiliation, or health conditions are routinely sold without your slightest awareness. The best information-gathering services are able to accumulate information about millions of people using highly focused research efforts. This information is of great value to those looking for someone to buy their products, creating a product to sell, or determining how to relate their advertising to their market. Information is money.

Health Information and Cancer Registry

Hospital and central cancer registries necessarily deal with significant amounts of confidential information, including patient identification information and detailed medical histories. Cancer registry personnel routinely collect, evaluate and interpret, and disclose patient health information. It is critical that registrars be very familiar with what comprises confidential health information; the regulations and laws applicable to the access, use, and disclosure of confidential information; and the processes and technologies necessary for protecting the privacy and security of this information.

Notable Incidents

The following are actual events that demonstrate the relevance of privacy and security protections in health information management:

- A hospital employee's child copied patient contact information from hospital records and "jokingly" notified the patients that they were diagnosed with HIV.
- A county health board member, who was a banker, reviewed patient information under his control to determine which of his customers were diagnosed with cancer. He recalled their mortgages for immediate payment.
- A health information Web site mistakenly posted the names, addresses, and telephone numbers of thousands of users who requested drug and alcohol addiction information.
- A pharmacy clerk's son informed a prescription holder's children that their father had AIDS.[1]
- A hospitalized patient discovered that more than 200 hospital employees had accessed her health information.
- The purchaser of a used computer discovered that it contained detailed prescription and identification records kept by the pharmacy that previously owned the computer.
- An auction bidder attempted to purchase a health practice's medical records for the purpose of, among other plans, selling the information back to the patients.[2]

Initial Legal Protection

The initial protection of confidential patient information was developed on a state-by-state basis. State statutes and regulations have been sporadically adopted spanning many decades, disciplines of applicability, and scopes of coverage. The Health Privacy Project, sponsored by the Institute for Health Care Research and Policy of Georgetown University, conducted a detailed comparative analysis of all state statutes seeking to protect the privacy of patient health information.

The project highlighted the following trends:

- State privacy legislation is predominantly enacted on an entity basis. Statutes typically regulate the activity of specific types of entities; therefore, different entities are subject to different levels and types of controls.
- Only two states have even attempted to enact comprehensive privacy law. Almost all states seek to implement privacy protections within other larger statutes, resulting in piecemeal protection based on ancillary topics.
- State statutes infer a duty to maintain confidentiality. Although penalties for specified breaches are

provided, the explicit duty to keep information confidential is, most often, conspicuously absent.

- The statutes that are in place today have not remained current with technologic advancements or healthcare industry standards.[3]

Such a piecemeal system for the protection of confidential patient health information causes many problems. Treatment, billing, and general healthcare operations may be spread across a number of states, resulting in complex law-to-be-applied questions. Patient information is subject to differing levels and types of protection, depending on where treatment was provided or healthcare operations are performed. Clearly, comprehensive federal protection is necessary to provide uniform and fair health information management privacy and security practices.

Current Drivers of Privacy and Security Protection

HIPAA

The Health Insurance Portability and Accountability Act (HIPAA) was enacted by Congress to answer the pleas of the healthcare industry to simplify and reduce the sky-rocketing costs of healthcare administration. The industry and government agreed that requiring standardized health transactions and coding standards would decrease administrative overhead. HIPAA promotes "good business" for the healthcare industry by pursuing the most effective and efficient use of modern information technology. HIPAA also calls for the implementation of commonsense privacy and security protection of the personal patient information reflected in the data to temper the risks posed by the powerful information technology. This portion of HIPAA is entitled "Administrative Simplification."

The U.S. Department of Health and Human Services (DHHS) defines the purposes of the Administrative Simplification rule thusly:

1. To protect and enhance the rights of consumers by providing them access to their health information and controlling the inappropriate use of that information
2. To improve the quality of health care in the U.S. by restoring trust in the health care system among consumers, health care professionals, and the multitude of organizations and individuals committed to the delivery of care
3. To improve the efficiency and effectiveness of health care delivery by creating a national framework for health privacy protection that builds on efforts by states, health systems, and individual organizations and individuals.[4]

The Security and Electronic Signature Standard ("Security") and the Privacy of Individually Identifiable Health Information Standard ("Privacy") comprise a team of regulations intended to protect patient health information. *Privacy* defines the permissible means of access, use, and disclosure of the applicable patient information, whereas *security* governs the operational and technical mechanisms necessary to protect this information.

Several other federal enactments have recently been implemented to protect confidential data in other areas, including the following:

- *The Gramm–Leach–Bliley Act:* protects consumers of financial institutions from unknown or deceptive use of their personal financial information and provides the opportunity to opt out of certain disclosure practices
- *The Privacy Act (of 1974):* protects the individually identifiable information held by the federal government from inappropriate use or disclosure
- *The Public Health Service Act:* protects information obtained during drug- or alcohol-related treatment at federally funded facilities from inappropriate use or disclosure

Industry Standards

Trade and professional associations consist of learned professionals who evaluate and resolve issues that affect their industry. Ethical canons are typically pledged that promote the development of "best practices" for the industry, including minimal standards of quality assurance, development and operational methodologies, and product acceptability. Association participants represent many years of experience in the field and can provide intimate insight into the values and perils associated with particular processes, technologies, and product requirements. They contend—and the federal government quite often accepts—that legitimate self-regulation by industry standards reasonably ensures adequate results for consumers, mitigates unreasonable risks and side effects, and levels the playing field for competitors.

Healthcare industry participation in the development of privacy and security standards is of the utmost importance. Existing associations have been developing applicable standards for many years. Privacy and security technology continuously advances; however, it is not usually practical or efficient to use the newest technology. Cutting-edge privacy and security devices, tools, and processes are often expensive, unwieldy, unpredictable, and prone to failure. Also, information system applications have traditionally been developed in near isolation. Privacy and security vulnerabilities are identifiable as the information travels between these information management systems, technologies, and processes. Cooperation within the industry is necessary to mitigate these identifiable gaps. Industry associations analyze these issues, based on their experience and tribulations, and identify minimal compliance standards to be satisfied by all applicable industry participants.

Duty of Care

Regardless of the existence of specific state law, a patient will be able seek legal compensation for healthcare organization security and privacy breaches on the basis of civil negligence theory. A patient will be able to legally recover damages if the healthcare organization caused unprivileged access, use, or disclosure of Protected Health Information (PHI) by failing to perform a duty to use reasonable care in the exercise of information security or privacy. This legal action is based on a party's negligence. Intentional disclosure or distribution is not necessary.

The key issue for legal consideration is whether a duty of care exists for the healthcare organization to provide adequate security and privacy. A duty of care is a socially defined standard of care for the protection of others against unreasonable risks. A standard of care arises from foreseeability of injury to a third party and a reasonable expectation that the responsible party would prevent that harm.[5] Standards of care are often based on standard business practices, providing clear indication of which actions are considered reasonable by the industry. An organization can create an unreasonable risk for harm to a person by failing to provide protections that are common to the same industry.

Furthermore, common business practice does tend to indicate that a standard of care exists, but it is not always necessary to substantiate that the standard of care exists. The famous *T. J. Hooper* case *(T.J. Hooper, et al. v. Northern Barge Corp., et al.)* provides legal precedent that a standard of care may exist even when current common business practice does not dictate that it exists.[6] The *T. J. Hooper* was a tugboat that lost its barge and cargo during a storm. The captain indicated that he would not have ventured into the storm if he knew that the storm was coming but did not have a radio receiver to notify him of the impending storm. Very few tugboats at that time were equipped with radio receivers, as it was very new technology. The court found that the owner of the tugboat had a duty of care to provide the receiver to prevent unreasonable risk to the cargo owner's property:

> *Indeed in most cases reasonable prudence is in fact common prudence; but strictly it is never its measure; a whole calling may have unduly lagged in the adoption of new and available devices. It [the industry] may never set its own tests, however persuasive be its usages. Courts must in the end say what is required; there are precautions so imperative that even their universal disregard will not excuse their omission.[7]*

The requirement for adequate information security and privacy in the healthcare industry is becoming unquestionable. Numerous standards, as well as plenty of state and federal legislation, make it clear that carefully protecting confidential information that is entrusted for healthcare purposes is prudent. Although there will be plenty of argument reserved for what levels of protection are to be considered reasonable, there is no doubt that the failure to provide reasonable privacy and security protection is actionable.

Patient Interests

Patients want nothing less than complete privacy and security applied to all of their medical information, but the complexity and reality of the modern healthcare system complicates the realization of their expectations. Many patients' rights advocacy groups and vocal patients express the concern that the patients should have full control of their medical information; however, this position is not fully compatible with the provision of quality health care.

Gone are the days in which a doctor keeps each patient's record in a single folder, hidden from all potentially prying eyes. We no longer pay with eggs or even the whole chicken if complex treatment is required. Payment is an intricate network of health insurance claims, authorizations, coordination of benefits analysis, copays, billing agencies, collection agencies, and public programs. The family doctor has become a multiphysician network with shared administrative resources. Referrals to specialists are common to diagnose and treat particular disorders. Support organizations play significant roles in accumulating, transferring, and coding health information for numerous operational purposes. Data are collected to identify disease trends, evaluate treatment effectiveness, assure the quality of healthcare operations, and improve many other healthcare aspects. Society's interest in maintaining order requires that certain suspected abuses and dangers be reported to public officials. In short, patient health information may pass through many hands as it travels the many well-beaten paths of the healthcare system.

Healthcare organizations must realize that the complexity of the healthcare system does not lessen the need to adequately protect confidential information while still providing patients with quality health care. In fact, many medical advances increase patient interest in a tighter grip on the data: the breakdown of the human genome, hereditary predictability, statistical inferences based on physical characteristics, and better early detection methods and technologies. The intended or unintended release of confidential health information can easily result in serious ramifications that irrevocably affect patients' lives.

Some patients, worried about the potential distribution of their information and the growing risk for privacy breaches, are taking impractical steps to protect their confidential information. Some patients pay cash for insurance-covered care instead of permitting their information to travel the course of medical billing. Many patients withhold, alter, or request their doctor to refrain from recording pertinent information in their records. Others refuse recommended tests or treatment altogether.[8] Current and accurate information is necessary to achieve correct diagnoses and treatment of the illnesses and diseases that afflict those seeking health care. Organizations that foster practices that discourage the intended free flow of information between doctor and patient interfere with the healing process to which the healthcare industry is committed.

Identifying Confidential Information

Although this chapter focuses on the confidentiality of *patient-related health* information, there are several distinct types and levels of confidential information associated with healthcare organizations. *Webster's II New College Dictionary* defines *confidential* as follows: "1. Communicated or effected secretly. 2. Entrusted with the confidence of another. 3. Denoting intimacy or confidence."[9]

HIPAA protects *individually identifiable health information,* which refers to any information related to the condition of the patient, treatment, or billing that reasonably identifies the patient. Information is individually identifiable if it explicitly identifies the patient by name, identifier, address, Social Security number, phone number, or similar information, or if the content provides some information that permits reasonable deduction of the patient's identity.[10] Health information legislation and regulation, such as HIPAA, typically protects information that connects patient identification with other health information. Healthcare organizations must protect the privacy and security of individually identifiable health information to comply with the law.

Health organizations also compile significant quantities of information about the organization, its employees, and its business partners that must be adequately protected. All business entities collect information regarding employees that is likely protected by federal and/or state law, such as employees' personal and salary information. The law does not require the same protection of organization planning, financial, and performance data; however, an organization will compile and maintain significant information that it would probably not intend to subject to public review. Business partners will also provide information to the organization that they would not like to place into public view. In fact, nondisclosure agreements may require an organization to take proactive steps to maintain the privacy and security of the information. The organization must identify internal organization, employee, and business partner data, and ensure that necessary privacy and security controls are implemented to adequately protect the information.

All organizations must conduct analyses of all information under their control to determine what must be considered *confidential.* Applicable standards and regulations immediately classify certain data as confidential as a matter of law. An organization must continue reviewing their information to determine what other collected, created, and maintained information must or should be protected

from unintended access, use, or disclosure based on personal, business, or proprietary interests. An organization must determine and establish sufficient and appropriate privacy and security controls to protect all of the confidential information received, maintained, or transferred by the organization.

Privacy versus Security

Perhaps the only issue in competition with the rivalry created by the famous "chicken or the egg" question is the ability to separate the concepts of information privacy and security. Together, privacy and security form a team of protections that prevent unintended access, use, and disclosure of confidential information. It is difficult to examine either of the concepts separately without overlapping the other. Privacy generally refers to the requirements of restricting access, use, and disclosure of confidential information to parties with privilege to the information; however, security's operational and technical protections are the tools that ensure implementation and maintenance of these requirements. Many protections, therefore, may be considered privacy and/or security. *Webster's II New College Dictionary* does little to clarify the distinction: Privacy comprises "seclusion or isolation from the view of, or from contact with, others," whereas security is defined as "the degree to which a program or device is safe from unauthorized use."[11] Regardless, we can consider these two information management necessities as coconcepts working in calculated unison to protect confidential information from unintended access, use, and disclosure. The descriptions below reflect the predominant role of the defined protection, admitting that the roles may often be complicated and reversible.

Privacy

Health information privacy prevents the unreasonable offense of a patient's interest in restricting unnecessary knowledge of personal information provided by the patient to assist diagnosis or treatment, or derived during medical care in furtherance of those healthcare objectives. Although it has been made clear that no absolute constitutional right to privacy exists, law is being established providing that individuals generally have the right to determine the use and disclosure of intimate or personal information. Patients provide information to medical practitioners and allow the collection of health-related information for the purpose of identifying and treating their medical afflictions. Privacy protections are aimed at meeting confidentiality expectations for data provided or accumulated to that end.

The following privacy practices define typical elements necessary to reasonably protect the privacy of confidential information. Cognizance of these elements pertains to privacy issues to be considered when handling confidential information within many different types of organizations, not limited to the healthcare industry and HIPAA. These are general considerations and may or may not be legally required in specific circumstances, depending on the type of confidential information, specific regulatory context, and type of organization.

Organizational Control of Confidential Information

The organization must take affirmative steps to ensure that the privacy of the confidential information is adequately protected from inappropriate access, use, or disclosure.

Minimum Necessary

Organizations must follow reasonable standards for using only the minimum amount of information necessary when pursuing permissible uses and disclosures of confidential information. This requirement to use only the minimum necessary to accomplish the intended objective pertains to all uses and disclosures of confidential information, regardless of who is to use or receive disclosure of the information or the intended use of the information (with the exception that the minimum necessary requirement of HIPAA does not apply to healthcare facilities for the purpose of providing treatment to patients). The minimum necessary standard is not intended to impose an overly strict standard to scrutinize all uses and disclosures of confidential information. The organization should use professional judgment, and establish applicable policies and procedures to define the minimum necessary for routine uses and disclosures.

Privileged Use

As prescribed by the actual requirements of the organization and applicable law and regulation, the organization should establish a documented system of procedures and policies that provide for all routine privileged use and disclosure of confidential information. The management system requirements should clearly demonstrate all legally and ethically acceptable uses and disclosures of confidential information within the organization, including identification of which employees may access the confidential information, the particular portions of information that may be accessed, and the specific purposes for which the information may be used. Organizational privacy management personnel must take steps to ensure that all access, use, and disclosure of information is appropriately privileged.

Privileged Disclosure

Organizations must ensure that all disclosures of confidential information to third parties are legally permissible. Disclosures necessary to support the operation of the organization, necessary to support the needs of the individual, or that the organization is legally bound to provide are typi-

cally permissible, whereas uses that are solely intended for the benefit of the organization will probably require notice and the individual's ability to opt out or authorization of the patient, if permissible at all. Applicable regulations may provide a list of permissive or mandatory disclosures that the organization may consider privileged as a matter of law. Privileged disclosures should be described in detailed written procedures for consistent application and foolproof employee decision making.

Disclosure Accounting

Depending on applicable law, some organizations must maintain records that track confidential information disclosures made by the organizations. The accounting need not typically include information regarding regular internal uses and disclosures related to providing requested services to the individual. The disclosure accounting must include the date, destination, purpose, and description of all information subject to disclosure. The disclosure tracking records must be provided to internal auditing personnel to ensure compliance with internal procedures and policies, to regulatory auditors as part of regulatory inspections, and to requesting individuals to notify them of the full distribution of their confidential information.

Current and Accurate Information

The organization must take reasonable steps to ensure that all confidential information remains sufficiently current and accurate to prevent any inappropriate detriment to the individual.

Individual Ability to Review

Many regulations, including HIPAA, provide the individual with the right to review records maintained about him or her. State cancer registries must review applicable state law to determine whether such requirements apply to them. Individuals may be irrevocably harmed by the use or distribution of false or inaccurate information about them. The ability to review provides the individuals with the ability to understand precisely what information an organization has accumulated about them and the accuracy of that information.

This right does not provide the individuals with a virtual search warrant to enter the organization's premises to demand an inspection of any information in the business records that may pertain to them. If applicable, the organization should define acceptable means for providing the contents of the applicable records to the individuals, including the means of filing the requests, reasonable timelines for supplying the information (within regulatory requirements), format for information delivery, and cost to be charged for the disclosure.

Individual Ability to Correct

Individuals must have the ability to address any believed inaccuracies in records maintained about them, especially if the records will be used in a manner that may unduly affect their well-being. State cancer registries must review applicable state law to determine whether such requirements apply to them. If applicable, an organization must establish a formal process to incorporate an individual's requested corrections without changing the source record the information was taken from; for example, changing the state registry record will not mandate a change to the original hospital medical record. The process may permit the correction of or amendment to the confidential record to clearly note the individual's contention with the maintained information. Organizations that do not agree with the request of the individual must at least document the individual's objection to the decision not to correct or amend the information. Future users of the confidential information must be made aware of the individual's contention with the record.

Culture of Confidentiality

Organizations that routinely deal with confidential information must establish a culture of confidentiality to reasonably sustain the privacy and security of the information. The consideration for confidentiality must permeate regular business activities to the extent that it is not simply a precaution to follow but is ingrained into the fabric of the organization's routine operational practices, policies, strategic objectives, and priorities.

Policies and Procedures

An organization should establish internal procedures as part of their operational management system to appropriately document intended usage of confidential information and restrict all improper access, use, and disclosure. The operational management system provides organizational management with appropriate direction for managing the organization by concisely stating particular information control requirements. Policies and procedures related to privacy and security efforts may be integrated into existing operational procedures that already govern the operation of the organization. Requirements specific to privacy protections, such as training, internal audit, document control, and other elements discussed in this chapter, can easily be integrated into existing operational procedures handling those matters. Operational policies and procedures provide a clear and consistent means of communicating specific requirements, as well as avail employees of the opportunity to reference the information at a later date.

Employees

All employees must be made aware of the importance of maintaining the privacy of confidential information. Training must be provided to all employees when they be-

gin work at the organization, stressing that all activities, responsibilities, and decisions must consider what is in the best interest of maintaining the privacy of confidential information. Employee managers must consider the effectiveness and appropriateness of their employees' efforts in maintaining privacy during employee reviews, including compliance with all applicable procedures. Internal auditing must review all required activities to ensure successful implementation. Employees must be held strictly accountable and appropriately disciplined for any breach of privacy caused by their inappropriate actions or failure to follow procedures.

Control of Associates

Organizations must take reasonable steps to protect the confidential information that they must pass to business associates and ensure that it remain reasonably protected. An organization cannot and should not control the operations of an associate to ensure that privacy breaches do not occur; however, the organization should contractually require that privacy protection equivalent to the organization's standards be applied to the confidential information. An organization must ensure that privacy breaches caused by the business associate be communicated to the organization and mitigated or cured, if possible. The organization must terminate the contract and cease doing business with the associate if the associate fails to adequately address a breach or maintains inadequate privacy protection.

Adequate Security

In clear overlap of the two information protection considerations, privacy requires an organization to establish adequate information security. The requirements listed earlier can be met only if operational, physical, and technical security measures are in place to support the privacy efforts. Attempts to keep information private are fruitless when no boundaries are in place to prevent others from freely accessing, taking possession of, or disclosing the information.

Use of De-identified Information

Although organizations may not legally commercially profit from distributing individuals' confidential information without their express permission, an organization may be permitted to remove the identifying information from the data to utilize the lessons learned, examine the case study, or draw statistical inferences by aggregating remaining information. Following are some means of ensuring adequate de-identification of data.

No Identification Captured

No privacy concern typically exists if the information does not contain individually identifiable information and cannot otherwise be used to link the information to a particular individual. An organization can use this information without further regard to privacy.

Removal of Identification

The organization that routinely handles or maintains individually identifiable information as part of its standard business practices may wish to utilize portions of the information for other commercial purposes. The privacy concern becomes moot if the organization takes steps to remove all individually identifying information and reasonable inferences from the data.

Coding/Encryption

Rather than fully removing identifying information from the data, the organization may encode or encrypt the identifying information to prevent any unintended recipients from interpreting or understanding this information. The de-identified information could then be re-identified at a later point when a legitimate and privileged business need arises.

Aggregation with De-identified Results

Another means of benefiting from the value of discreet confidential information without unnecessarily disclosing specifics is to produce summary reports from the aggregation of confidential information. An organization may aggregate individually identifiable information from many patients or healthcare provider facilities for important organizational functions, such as the purpose of quality assurance comparison of operations. The individually identifiable information may play a significant role in performing the aggregation and comparison, such as eliminating duplicate cases; however, the final reports or conclusions cannot disseminate any individually identifiable information.

Complaint Handling Process

All organizations should provide the ability for individuals to file complaints regarding alleged privacy and security breaches. Organizational representatives can be appointed to receive such complaints and ensure timely, independent, and adequate investigation of the individual's claim. The representative must have sufficient responsibility and authority to provide redress to the complainant, take reasonable steps to cure or mitigate any actual breach, improve the privacy and security system to prevent similar events in the future, and ensure necessary disciplinary action is taken against any culpable employees.

Security

Information security is a comprehensive system of overt actions taken to protect the confidentiality, integrity, and availability of an organization's electronic data, work product, information systems, and other related intellectual and physical property. The overt actions must reflect operational policies and procedures, physical safeguards, and technical security devices.

- *Confidentiality:* protection of entrusted information from unauthorized use, access, or disclosure
- *Integrity:* preservation of the specific nature, character, and content of the information
- *Availability:* ability to access, use, or disclose the information as intended in an effective and efficient time, place, and manner

The following practices and mechanisms provide a high-level overview of the typical elements necessary to reasonably protect the security of confidential information. Although the considerations are not solely applicable to the security of health information, implementation of these requirements should nonetheless be considered minimally acceptable security protection for individually identifiable health information.

Operational Policies and Procedures

Organizations must establish formal operational procedures and policies to provide security guidance and instruction to all applicable personnel and to ensure that all pertinent functions are consistently performed in accordance with the organization's security needs.

Security Management Planning

Organizational security management must evaluate the flow of confidential data throughout the organization and identify all unreasonable security vulnerabilities. This data flow analysis must consider all inputs, internal uses, data resting points, storage mechanisms, transmissions, external disclosures, and third-party access points to identify all potential security weaknesses. Security management must determine which vulnerabilities are considered unacceptable and establish appropriate security protections or mitigations to reduce the vulnerabilities to reasonable levels. The results of the security vulnerability analysis shall be formulated into a security risk management plan and translated into specific organizational requirements, as defined later. Organizations must routinely review both the vulnerability analysis and security risk management plan to ensure that they remain effective as the organization evolves.

Security Configuration Management

The security risk management plan must be translated into specific requirements for implementation and maintenance. Security management must clearly specify the entire security system, including technical requirements and data flow modeling. Procedures must be established to control all changes to the security specifications, including validation of the effectiveness of any planned changes.

Management Responsibility

Organizational management must ensure that adequate authority and responsibility are delegated to effect the implementation and maintenance of the security management plan. Management should appoint a security officer, with executive responsibility, and provide him or her with full authority and responsibility to oversee the entire security system, establish policy and procedures to provide reasonable security protection, and respond to security breach incidents and other significant issues. The security officer must routinely report on the status of the organization's security efforts to executive organization management to review the suitability and effectiveness of the security management plan. The executive managers must identify, evaluate, and resolve deficiencies in operations or the security management plan to ensure that confidential information is maintained and used in a reasonably secure environment. The organization shall ensure that adequate resources are dedicated to implement and maintain the security risk management plan.

Information Handling Procedures

Similar to and perhaps in conjunction with privacy procedures, information handling procedures shall establish appropriate controls over the handling and control of confidential information during all pertinent operations. Procedures should detail confidential information handling requirements during the entire flow of information throughout the organization. Specific designation of personnel and limited amounts of data for use must be specified, as well as any security vulnerability mitigations deemed appropriate by the security management plan. The information handling procedures must consistently secure the handling of confidential information as long as it is used or controlled by the organization.

Access Controls

Security management must create operational procedures to identify which particular employees or classes of employees may have access to defined confidential information. The procedure must define operational steps to ensure that access rights are correctly assigned and exercised.

Personal Authorization Controls

Security management must procedurally define actions to be undertaken to verify the identity and authority of employees before granting access to, use of, or disclosure of confidential information. This will include new employee rights as-

signment procedures, grant of access to particular buildings and areas, key distribution, release of information authority, and supervision of visitors and contractors. Records must be maintained of all approved grants of access.

Information Technology Use Policies

Security management must recognize the security risks inherent in the use of certain technologies and proceduralize appropriate controls. E-mail and Internet use poses substantial risks, with direct ingress and egress from the outside world into and out of an organization's network. Uncontrolled disclosures could potentially contain confidential information. Uncontrolled incoming files could contain viruses, worms, or Trojan horses. Procedures must be established to ensure appropriate controlled use of these and other similar communication technologies.

Employee Training

Employees must be aware of potential vulnerabilities and the organization's means of controlling those vulnerabilities. Employees must receive training on hiring and routinely thereafter to ensure that they can consistently fulfill all security requirements that apply to their responsibilities. Training elements must include a description of the following:

- The organization's security vulnerabilities (not those to which the employee is a potential wrongdoing party)
- The employee's responsibility for mitigating those vulnerabilities
- All security requirements that pertain to employee job functions
- Information about social engineering—a type of attack where the employee is subjected to trickery by another person and persuaded to inappropriately provide information used to breach security—and tips to recognize, avoid, and report social engineering attempts
- The identification of confidential information and the controls necessary to protect the confidentiality, integrity, and availability of that information
- Applicable laws and regulations
- Incident reporting and response procedures
- Disciplinary procedures for failure to follow established procedures and policies, and direction of the security officer

Employees must receive sufficient training to ensure their full awareness of performing their security requirements and the importance of those requirements. Security culturing efforts are also necessary to ensure that employees perform their security responsibilities with diligence. Management must demonstrate complete and consistent support for the security management plan and security management. Employees must be made aware of the priority of security and the fact that they will be held accountable for their security responsibilities.

Disciplinary Action

Security management must establish policies and procedures to appropriately discipline employees for any breach of security caused by their inappropriate actions or failure to follow procedures. Disciplinary action procedures must be clearly defined and consistently applied across the organization. Management discretion must be removed from the process to ensure that the message is very clear that the protection of security and privacy of confidential information is a top organizational priority. Disciplinary action must apply to all levels of the organization.

Employee Termination

Human Resources and Information Technology representatives must immediately terminate all access rights and abilities of employees who have left the organization, including the removal of all computerized and physical access rights and passwords, collection of keys or tokens, and return of all equipment held by the employee. An organization must take immediate steps to ensure that the terminated employee retains no ability to access confidential information or systems.

Vendor/Associate Control

Security management must ensure that third parties receiving access to confidential information adequately protect the security of that information. Organizations must ensure that partners or associates intended to receive distributions of confidential information legally agree to provide security protections at least equivalent to the organization. See the earlier "Control of Associates" section for more information.

The organization must ensure that any business partners that may have electronic or physical access to confidential information located within the organization's facilities do not pose an unreasonable security risk to the confidential information. The vulnerability analysis must consider potential third-party access, use, and disclosure when identifying security management plan requirements. Care must be taken to supervise and control the access of necessary partners and contractors, such as after-hours maintenance, network administration, vendor technical support, and temporary office personnel.

Internal Auditing

The organization must take proactive steps to evaluate the sufficiency and effectiveness of all security measures established under the security management plan. Internal audits must be performed to determine whether security-based operational procedures have been correctly and effectively established. Internal auditors must review operational records, speak with responsible employees, and observe process activities to ensure intended awareness of employees and effectiveness of security requirements. Audit results must be made available to security and executive management to determine whether additional or improved action should be taken.

Security management may also find value in having external personnel attempt to breach the organization's security system. Attempted attacks on operational systems, physical safeguards, and security technology can yield valuable improvement information about the effectiveness of security efforts and any continuing vulnerabilities.

Contingency/Disaster Recovery Planning

Security management must identify potential events that could interfere with the organization's business operations and establish a plan for continuing operations if each contingent event were to occur. A vulnerability analysis must be performed to indicate what potential disasters, failures, or other events could reasonably be expected to occur and interfere with business operations. Plans must be created that include steps to ensure that information necessary for business continuation is routinely archived and protected, and will be made available for timely restoration in case of a disaster. The organization must be able to restore the information and re-establish necessary business operations, as the plan defines necessary.

Incident Handling

Formal process must be established to report, investigate, and resolve incidents that may reflect security breaches. See the "Complaint Handling Process" section earlier in this chapter.

Compliance Certification

Business partners, regulatory authorities, and consumers require assurance that an organization is in full compliance with security requirements and is able to adequately protect the confidentiality, integrity, and availability of confidential information. The organization must employ either internal or external review authority to reliably determine and certify that adequate security is effectively implemented.

Physical Safeguards

Appropriate physical safeguards must be established to prevent unreasonable threats to an organization's buildings, equipment, and media, as deemed appropriate by the security risk management plan. The organization must consider physical threats, such as disaster, physical or electronic break-in, theft, and careless or intentional physical access to confidential information. Physical safeguards shall be implemented in layered coordination with each other and with other security requirements to protect information from identified threats. It is important to remember that these safeguards are intended to protect against both external and internal threats, as the interest to be protected is the controlled access to confidential information.

Locks

An individual cannot improperly access, use, or disclose confidential information if he or she cannot get to it. Buildings, rooms, file cabinets, and even workstations can be locked to prevent access by anyone who does not hold a key, token, or access code. The most critical areas, such as a network administration control room, shall typically have the most restrictive locking systems—possibly within a locked cage in a keypad-controlled room within a facility accessible only by pass card or key fob.

Physical Barriers

Walls, fences, doors, and shaded glass may be used to provide additional layers of security protection. For instance, the walls or shaded windows between the reception area and the administrative office prevent bored patients from incidentally eavesdropping on patient-related office conversations or viewing open medical records on the desk. Also, record casing could be used to provide fire resistance to critical business information. Physical barriers apply a layer of protection between the information and the persons or dangers to be kept away.

Monitoring

As no security is invulnerable, security management must be notified when security breaches are attempted. Intrusion alarms will directly alert security management, law enforcement personnel, or whomever the organization deems appropriate in case of break-in or unauthorized entry attempt. Alarms can trigger actions to investigate breaches or attempted breaches, make security management aware of the disclosure of accessed information, and provide a deterrent to prevent continuation of the security breach attempt. Smoke and other detectors must be installed to provide awareness of conditions that may be hazardous to equipment, personnel, or information. Well-lit areas ensure that suspicious or inappropriate activity does not escape unnoticed. Video monitoring permits the supervision of multiple areas with less attention. Also, video monitoring provides a deterrent because the attacker will fear being caught if he or she is being watched at that time and/or recorded. Security guards may be utilized to provide focused surveillance of areas requiring more intense protection. Monitoring provides organizational timely awareness of the occurrence of activities in identified areas of concern.

Visitor Control

Visitors represent potential customers, job candidates, personal friends, business partners, and salespeople—and no one wants to upset a coworker or manager by harassing their visitors. In fact, they can often wander facilities unchallenged, especially if they are dressed in formal attire or provide the impression that they know where they are going.

Visitors inherently have no access right to any of the organization's information. Security management policy must provide definite controls over the ability of visitors to have any access to any secure locations or information. In fact, visitors should be required to sign a visitor log, tagged with a name badge, escorted at all times, and confronted if they are found roaming the building unattended.

Control of Media

Information from heavily secured networks can still be copied to CDs and memory sticks, which provide few or none of the protections performed by the network. Employees can take work home or leave it in their cars and expose it to all kinds of security risks. Archive tapes that are necessary to recover systems when disasters strike can potentially permit anyone who swipes a tape to replicate an organization's stored data. An organization's vulnerability analysis must identify which uses of media, information transfer, storage requirements, and work processes represent reasonable practices. Procedures should be established to detail all media use, storage, and disposal practices.

Control of Equipment

Information technology equipment is the gateway into an organization's computer network. Network security can be defeated if an administrative access terminal is left unprotected. Employee workstations will necessarily be placed in an open work environment, so they must be subject to username and password logon and time-out after periods of inactivity.

New technology offers great advances in efficiency and effectiveness but often carries its own security quandaries. Following are some examples and security considerations:

- *Laptop computers.* Laptops are often and easily stolen. They can hold large quantities of confidential information, which is often unprotected and accessible just by turning on the computer. "Remembered" dial-ins and passwords can permit purported privileged access to a protected network with a single click.
- *Wireless devices.* A wireless device connects to a host network via a wireless transmitter and receiver. It connects into an independent access point into the network; however, other wireless devices can just as easily tap into the network's wireless connection. The lack of access controls will result in full access to

the network. Also, wireless communications can be captured and easily read if not encrypted.

- *Personal Digital Assistants (PDAs).* PDAs can be subject to all of the concerns above but typically offer less CPU processing power and storage space. Therefore, security protections that could mitigate the above vulnerabilities often interfere with the speed and efficiency of operation of the device.

An organization must carefully consider how the devices will be used in its vulnerability analysis, and define appropriate control procedures and technical protections.

Corporate Security Culturing

A fine line exists between adequate security control and going overboard. Security vulnerability mitigations can be burdensome, time consuming, and confusing. Procedures may often seem overly strict and a waste of time. Therefore, it is essential for all employees to fully understand and support an organization's security efforts. Employees must be trained not only on the security protections, but also why each protection is necessary. Whenever possible, employees should be permitted to participate in the evaluation, implementation, and maintenance of security requirements. Employee support is necessary to fully recognize vulnerabilities, and identify and report actual or potential security breaches.

An organization must not thwart employee trust by using security mechanisms to unnecessarily monitor or punish employee performance. An employer will quickly turn into "Big Brother" if network audit trails are used as employee timecards or production gauges, if area monitors are used to watch general employee activity, or employee communications are overly monitored or scrutinized. Security is intended to protect privacy, not permit its invasion.

Technical Security Mechanisms

Security technology must be implemented to protect information stored on a computer network or otherwise electronically communicated from unauthorized access, use, or distribution. An organization's security risk management plan must consider all potential points of access of electronic information, including the following four access concerns:

1. *Network.* Network access must not be permitted without valid login.
2. *Network file structure.* User and user group rights must be assigned based on the need and privilege to access information.
3. *Software applications.* Applications typically permit the assignment of either user group or function to recognize access privileges.

4. *Communications.* Communication mechanisms must not permit receipt or review of any confidential communications by any unintended parties.

Firewalls

A firewall is the front-line perimeter protection that separates a network from the world on the other end of a communication connection. There are many variations of firewalls, but they all primarily have two functions: (1) the control of the specific information that comes into the network through the firewall and (2) the control of the information that exits the network through the firewall. These controls affect the most basic access control into and out of the protected network.

Firewalls can protect the network in a number of ways. The easiest way to think of it is as a gatekeeper. Security management programs the firewall to permit or reject passage of certain types of traffic that pass through it. Typically, it is programmed to support security policies that have been enacted by the organization. The difficulty with firewall operation is that each permitted communication weakens the protection value of the firewall. The firewall is opened to permit incoming and outgoing transmission for e-mail, Internet use, authenticated interactive session logins, and many other uses. Incorrectly or loosely configured firewalls provide little protection to the network.

Intrusion Detection

Nearly all entities attached to the Internet receive some sort of malicious attack: scans to find communication openings left open in the firewall, attempts to crack or guess passwords to enter the network via an existing user account, Trojan horse programs that enter the network attached to e-mail or other validly transferred files and then open a port in the firewall from inside, or attempts to interfere with communications by hitting the site with repeated information requests. Intrusion detection applications review firewall logs or other communication data to identify suspected attack attempts. The detection system alerts security management of the attempted breach of access control protection.

Alarms

Alarms notify security management of suspicious access control activity that may represent a security breach or attempted breach in progress. Intrusion detection systems send an alarm when external breach attempts or other abnormal conditions are suspected by the application. Alarm systems also review internal access activities or attempted access activities to identify suspicious activities (e.g., repeated login failures, attempts to access multiple unauthorized network locations, repeated access of a particular record by many employees, or one employee accessing many records). The alarm provides security management an early detection notice of a breach or potential breach to allow time to apprehend the perpetrators and mitigate or prevent the damage caused by the incident.

Access Control

Access controls protect information resources by restricting access to particular users or classes of users. Firewalls are the first line of organization access controls, preventing unauthorized network access. Lower level access controls are implemented within the network and within applications that maintain and control confidential information. Access rights may be restricted on a user level or to defined user function(s). This may be implemented by network access to particular organizational groups, classifications, or levels of employees, or employees charged with defined functions.

User Authentication

Network and application administration must verify that users are who they purport to be before access is granted. Authentication may take the form of password or personal identification number (PIN) entry, biometric evaluation (e.g., fingerprint, voice recognition, or retinal scan), or electronic or physical token. Authentication information must be kept personal and confidential to remain effective, so passwords and PINs must be subject to standard protections: minimal length, complex configuration, no common words, routine change, and time-out after a number of failed attempts.

Audit Trail

Audit trails track the details of substantial user accesses, changes, and decisions related to confidential information. The audit trail provides a mechanism for the review of access activities, as well as material to be examined for suspicious access, use, or disclosure activities as part of a security audit.

Encryption

Confidential information transmitted across an open network, such as the Internet or widely accessible network, must be transmitted in a manner that cannot be intercepted and understood by unintended recipients. In short, all e-mails, electronic data interchange transmissions, and similar transfers must be subject to reasonably unbreakable encipherment or encryption, unless they are transmitted across a dedicated communications line.

Virus Protection

Viruses can be introduced into an organization's network by nearly any transmission from the outside world: e-mail, downloaded files, or media brought into the office. All files brought into the network should be scanned on incoming transmission. Also, security management must routinely perform up-to-date virus scanning of the entire network and all connected workstations. Viruses and other malicious software ("mal-ware") must be detected and neutralized before they are permitted to cause damage to information or applications stored within the organization's network. Virus incidents must also be considered within an organization's incident handling procedure.

Summary

Protecting confidential health information is everyone's job. Organizations in the healthcare industry hold some of the most personal and private information about an individual. Medical information can provide an understanding of what kind of lifestyle an individual has led, how long he or she is likely to live, and what ails and aches he or she currently suffers. We all want to retain the privacy of our confidential information; it is in the best interest of the patient, and now it is legally required.

Confronted with the need to determine what would be considered adequate privacy and security, healthcare organizations must look to numerous developing industry standards, federal and state regulations that state that "reasonable" protections must be applied, and an industry history of checkered performance. It is now within an organization's grasp to evaluate its own operations and practices to determine which privacy and security risks are reasonable and which must be mitigated. The bottom line is that "adequate protection" means "reasonable protection" based on the abilities of current technology, current industry practices, and what the organization determines to be reasonable under the circumstances.

Privacy and security standard development is not unique to the health information industry. It is affecting nearly all information-based industries. Organizations will find it in their best interest to create dynamic systems that remain current with the industry standard protections— not the state of the art, but what provides the best protection of confidential information without undue effort or cost to the organization.

References

1. Health Privacy Project. *Medical Privacy Stories* (pp. 1–7). Washington, DC: Institute for Health Care Research and Policy, Georgetown University, 2002.
2. 65 Fed. Reg. 82467 (December 28, 2000).

3. Pritts, J., Goldman, J., Hudson, Z., Berenson, A., Hadley, E. *The State of Health Privacy: An Uneven Terrain—A Comprehensive Survey of State Health Privacy Statutes* (pp. 8–9). Washington, DC: Health Privacy Project, Institute for Health Care Research and Policy, Georgetown University, 1999.

4. 65 Fed. Reg. 82463 (December 28, 2000).

5. Kenneally, E. "The Byte Stops Here: Duty and Liability for Negligent Internet Security," *Computer Security Journal,* 2000;XVI(2):3–6.

6. Salaverry, P. "From Boats to Bytes: Establishing a Y2K Standard of Care," *Texas Lawyer,* 1999;14(46):25.

7. *In re Eastern Transp. Co.; New England Coal & Coke Co. v. Northern Barge Corporation; H. N. Hartwell & Son, Inc., v. Same.* 60 F. 2d 737, 740 (2nd Cir. 1932).

8. 65 Fed. Reg. 82468 (December 28, 2000).

9. Severynse, M., editor. *Webster's II New College Dictionary* (p. 236). Boston: Houghton Mifflin Company, 1995.

10. *Privacy of Individually Identifiable Health Information.* 45 CFR 164.501.

11. Severynse, M., editor. *Webster's II New College Dictionary* (pp. 880, 998). Boston: Houghton Mifflin Company, 1995.

Informatics

Ann Griffin
Section Editor—Textbook

Jim Hofferkamp
Section Editor—Review Guide

Computer Resources

Eric B. Durbin, MS

Most of the work performed within a cancer registry relies heavily on computer resources. Cancer registries are repositories of data, and much of the work that is performed in a cancer registry involves some manipulation of that data. This simple "manipulation" of data, however, actually involves extraordinarily complex procedures and operations, and must adhere to a vast array of rules and data standards. Fortunately, we have computer resources to help us navigate these complexities. This chapter offers a synopsis of the computer resources currently required by both central and hospital cancer registries. Essential hardware, software, and interoperability resources are presented, followed by a discussion of computer resource management, protection, security, and maintenance. Although this chapter is current as of the time of publication, some technologies discussed here will be supplanted by newer technologies as computer resources continue to evolve at their rapid pace.

Hardware Resources

Local Area Networks and Wide Area Networks

At the heart of any modern office with shared computer resources is a computer network, often referred to as a Local Area Network (LAN). To utilize shared file system servers, application servers, or an Internet gateway, each desktop or laptop computer must connect directly or indirectly to the LAN.* The backbone of the LAN is typically made up of network switches or hubs that reside in a wiring closet. Network cabling usually leads from the wiring closet to individual office locations, allowing individual computers to access the network through a network card and cable. The most common network technology, called Ethernet, currently supports data transmission rates of 10, 100, or 1000 Megabits per second (MB/S).

Many LANs are also equipped with wireless access points that allow laptop and other computers to participate in the network over wireless radio frequencies. Wireless access points require particular attention to network security. Wireless technologies allow computers to communicate without being physically attached to the network. It is therefore impossible to control unauthorized computers that can potentially "see" the wireless signal. The wireless access points can be configured to limit access to specific computers identified by each computer's unique Media Access Control (MAC) address to prevent unauthorized access over wireless networks. The wireless network signal must also be encrypted so that network communications cannot be intercepted by an unauthorized third party.

---

*Individual computers may also access the Internet through a computer modem. Today, this is more common to home installations than office installations.

Some hospitals are part of a larger system with facilities located either within a small geographic area or across an entire state or the country. These facilities may also share computer resources and network communications through a Wide Area Network (WAN). Many central registries are also part of WAN within a university or state health department. The WAN connects the facility networks, whereas the computer resources within each facility are connected by the LAN.

Firewalls

Individual LANs (hardwired, wireless, and mixed) are often connected to a larger institutional WAN, an Internet gateway, or both. Because of the confidentiality requirements of cancer registries, any registry LAN that is not entirely self-contained should be isolated from the external network through a firewall. A firewall is a computer or dedicated hardware device that restricts access between a protected network and an "external" network.[1] Firewalls can be configured to allow only certain types of network traffic or even certain specific computers to reach internal network resources. A registry should allow only traffic that is deemed absolutely necessary to reach the internal network from outside. Many registries do not allow any such traffic. The firewall can also be used to restrict traffic that originates from computers on the protected LAN. For example, the firewall could be configured to prevent users from accessing a particular Web site.

A firewall can be configured to provide a safe way for outside users to access Web servers or other such resources while keeping the protected network closed. This logical network partition often referred to as the demilitarized zone (DMZ). Computers in the DMZ can be "seen" from the outside, whereas internal computers cannot. Figure 7-1 is a logical diagram of a registry network configured with a DMZ.

Remote Network Access

Many computer networks are also configured with remote access capabilities. Remote access points may be used to allow staff to work from home or off-site, or may allow information technology (IT) staff to remotely check system status and perform maintenance during evenings and weekends. Remote access may be implemented using telephone modems but is increasingly implemented over the Internet using a Virtual Private Network (VPN) connection. When remote access is provided through any publicly accessible mechanism such as the Internet, it is imperative that communications be authenticated and encrypted. Authentication requires the user to enter a correct login and password to gain access. Encryption encodes or scrambles the data stream between the network and remote user in such a way that it would be nearly impossible for an unauthorized party to intercept and decipher anything that is transmitted. VPN access utilizes software that provides

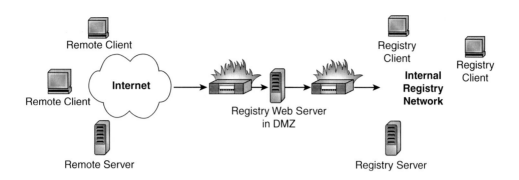

Figure 7-1. Registry Network with Demilitarized Zone

an authenticated, encrypted connection. This setup is becoming increasingly common as many hospital registrars are now working from home. It is also used when there is a shortage of hospital registrars and contractors who may even reside out of state are used to meet the staffing shortage.

Desktop Computers, Laptop Computers, and Computer Servers

To make use of the registry software systems, a registry must acquire and maintain the computers to run them. Three classes of computers are presented here. These include desktop computers, also known as workstations or personal computers (PCs), computer laptops, and computer servers. Desktop computers are installed in staff work space, laptop computers are mobile and are used by staff in and out of the office, and computer servers are usually installed in a secured computer room that is accessible only by technical staff. In terms of hardware configurations and performance, advances in computer technologies have rendered the distinctions between desktop, laptop, and server computers much less obvious.

Desktop computers are used for a variety of functions in the registry. One of their primary uses is to invoke and interact with the registry software system. Registry abstracting software is usually run on or from a desktop computer. Most desktop computers are configured with basic office software including spreadsheets, word processing, e-mail, Web browsers, and small database applications. Many other registry software applications also run on desktop computers.

Laptop computers have similar internal hardware specifications and function quite similarly to desktop computers. The primary distinguishing factor is their small physical size and portability. Because of this, laptop computers are particularly vulnerable to being lost or stolen. Extra precautions should be taken when using laptop computers to store confidential registry data. Laptop computers should require a password and login for access, and

any directories that contain confidential data should be encrypted and require password authentication for access. If properly protected, a laptop computer will not allow unauthorized access to any confidential information, even if physically accessed by an unauthorized user.

Desktop and laptop computers usually access e-mail and the Web, and are therefore vulnerable to malware such as computer viruses, worms, and spyware. Worms are unauthorized programs that propagate themselves from computer to computer.[2] Viruses are unauthorized programs that also propagate themselves and may interfere with computer operations or destroy data. With the increased utilization of the Web, spyware applications have become a growing concern. Spyware applications secretly transmit data or reports of user activities to a third party. Virus scanning applications must be installed and remain current with patches and updates from the operating system vendor to protect desktop computers from such threats. Once installed, virus scanning applications also require frequent updates to remain current with the information necessary to identify new threats.

Server hardware specifications are also similar to desktop and laptop computers. Servers, however, are frequently configured with multiple central processing units (CPUs), more random-access memory (RAM), and increased disk capacities. Registries that maintain multiple servers usually prefer rack-mounted models that make efficient use of floor space. Registries may also utilize virtual server technologies. Virtualized servers are configured with software that allows a single hardware server to support multiple simultaneous virtual servers. A computer room housing multiple physical servers may require supplemental cooling capabilities. Central registries typically maintain servers dedicated to registry operations, whereas the servers that maintain registry data in a hospital are often also utilized by other departments.

Server disk storage systems may benefit from built-in disk redundancy provided by Redundant Array of Independent Disks (RAID). RAID configurations allow one or more disk drives to fail or become corrupt while continuing to maintain the integrity of the data they are storing. With a RAID disk system, failed drives may be replaced before they lead to a loss of data. Because servers maintain important data and user files, they should always be equipped with a reliable file backup and retrieval system. Magnetic tape backup devices continue to be a highly reliable mechanism for this purpose.

Uninterruptible Power Supplies and Generators

Servers and critical desktop systems should also be equipped with an Uninterruptible Power Supply (UPS). A UPS provides a redundant backup power supply to protect computers in the event of a power surge or temporary power outage. When a computer abruptly loses power, data may be lost or corrupted and hardware may be damaged. A UPS provides protection against abrupt power loss by switching over to battery power with time to initiate an orderly shutdown of the computer systems. A UPS should be sized to provide battery power to protected computers for as much time as it takes to conduct an orderly shutdown. A registry can further accommodate longstanding power outages with an appropriately sized power generator. Hospital registries (and some central registries) may be equipped with electrical outlets connected to backup generators. It is important to discuss with the hospital IT department whether the registry can utilize these outlets for their computers.

Web Servers

A computer that provides access to Web pages is referred to as a Web "server." A Web server is actually a software application that allows data and information to be accessed from the Web. Web servers do not require specialized or dedicated hardware and can even be installed on laptop computers. Commonly used Web server software applications include the open source Apache HTTP server (The Apache Software Foundation: http://www.apache.org/) and the commercial Microsoft Internet Information Services (IIS; Microsoft Corporation: http://www.microsoft.com/) Web server. Web servers may be designed to provide browser-based access for internal users, external users, or both. Additional information about Web servers, Web sites, and central cancer registries can be found in Chapter 10.

When a Web server is made available for public access (i.e., when the Web server is accessible from the Internet), additional precautions must be taken to ensure that only authorized information be made available. It may be risky to physically store any confidential information on an Internet-accessible Web server. Internet-accessible servers should always be isolated from other registry computers by placing them in the network DMZ. As a good rule of thumb, it should be assumed that all publicly accessible computers can be broken into by an unauthorized user. Such a security breach should never automatically grant the invader access to any information beyond what is hosted on the Web server.

Software Resources

Databases

All cancer registries store the registry data in an underlying database. A database is responsible for organizing and storing the data so that it may be manipulated and retrieved efficiently. The database is actually a specialized software application that manages the storage and retrieval of data. Commercial and open source database products are widely utilized. Commercial databases include Oracle, Sybase, and Microsoft SQL Server, among others. Commercial database products usually require the purchase of a license for their use.

As an alternative to commercial databases, open-source databases such as MySQL and Postgres are also currently being used in registries. Open-source applications are freely distributed and licensed. The underlying source code used to develop the application is available for all open-source applications.[3] An advantage of having access to the source code is that the application can be modified by programmers to meet any needs beyond the scope of the distributed application. In addition, registry software developers may be able to rely on themselves to track down and correct errors or bugs in the application. Open-source software is also supported through online discussion forums where problem resolutions or helpful suggestions can often be found. Reliable use of open-source software does, of course, require sufficiently technical staff, contractors, or consultants to support it.

In addition to the organized storage of registry data, most database applications provide the ability to query the database using various criteria that may be specified by a user or by the registry application. The database products listed above all support a database computer language called the Structured Query Language (SQL). SQL supports commands to create, update, and delete data. SQL provides the ability to submit both simple and highly sophisticated requests to the database application. A SQL query to select all data for female breast cancer cases might be similar to the following:

SELECT * from PatientData, CaseData
WHERE PatientData.Sex = '2'
AND CaseData.SEERSite = '26000'
AND PatientData.Key = CaseData.Key

Databases for cancer registries are usually designed to store various data elements together in logical groupings known as *records* or *tables*. For example, it may be beneficial to store all patient demographics together in one record and case-specific information in another record. Each record consists of the individual data fields such as Social Security number, last name, accession number, case sequence number, primary site, and so on. When such a database design is implemented, the patient records must be tied to their case records using a key variable that is common to both types of records and unique to the patient record. For example, the NAACCR Patient ID NUMBER (Item #20) would be a good candidate for this purpose. Notice that the last clause in the example SQL statement uses a common "Key" in the patient data and the case data to tie or relate the two data records. A database organization using keys to link record types is known as a *relational database design*. Most database products today support relational databases, including the commercial and open-source databases previously cited. Fortunately, the details of the registry database structures are hidden from the users for most operations. Familiarity with the registry database structure may, however, be important to the user when extracting record-level data for research or other purposes.

A distinction should be made between NAACCR data exchange records and central registry database records. The various NAACCR Data Exchange Standards[4] define how data should be formatted to exchange data with another organization. NAACCR data exchange standards are essential for data exchange, but they do not determine how data should be stored in a central registry database. The underlying data stored in the central registry database can be and usually are stored in a completely different order and structure than a NAACCR exchange record. In fact, it might be meaningless to store some NAACCR fields in a registry database. For example, the NAACCR field DATE CASE REPORT EXPORTED (Item #2110) is a variable that is generated only when a NAACCR file is exported and could not be meaningful for records manually entered by staff at the registry.

Central Registry Data Management Systems

The most important software used by a cancer registry is that which manages the registry database. Data management is usually accomplished using a primary registry software application, often referred to as the Data Management System (DMS). Registries typically make use of additional software applications in conjunction with the DMS. Central and hospital DMSs share many common functions. The hospital DMS is most often is used to manage data directly entered for one or more facilities by one or more registrars. The central registry DMS, in contrast, is utilized to import, consolidate, and manage data originating primarily from external reporting sources.

Eight key central registry DMS functions are presented in the following list. Some of the central registry tasks are essential and performed at all central registries, whereas others are optional. A number of these functions are also performed at hospital registries.

1. Data import and data entry include:
   - Importing new and updated case reports from a variety of reporting sources such as hospitals, other state registries and nonhospital facilities
   - Allowing staff to enter and edit case reports from nonelectronic sources
   - Importing electronic pathology reports
2. Record consolidation includes:
   - Identifying when case reports have been submitted for the same patient
   - Identifying and consolidating multiple reports for the same primary cancer
   - Distinguishing when case reports represent multiple primaries
   - Identifying and resolving conflicting information
   - Tracking any conflict resolutions
3. Record linkage includes:
   - Supporting record linkages with external data sources for follow-up such as state death certificates, the National Death Index (NDI), the Social Security Administration (SSA), the Centers for Medicare and Medicaid Services (CMS), the Department of Motor Vehicles (DMV), voter registration files and others
   - Supporting the process of "death clearance" whereby death certificate only cases are identified and entered
4. Quality assurance includes:
   - Performing edit checks on new and existing case reports
   - Generating registry management reports
   - Generating random case samples for quality-assurance activities
   - Supporting case-finding and reabstracting audits
5. Reporting and analysis includes:
   - Generating case summary reports
   - Generating ad hoc reports and data lists
   - Performing epidemiologic analysis of data
   - Calculating crude and age-adjusted cancer incidence rates
   - Supporting publication of an annual report
6. Data exchange and export includes:
   - Selecting subsets of records for export
   - Supporting data exchange in standard formats such as the NAACCR standard record layout as defined in NAACCR's *Standards for Cancer Registries, Volume II*[5]
   - Exporting ad hoc ASCII formats for research studies
   - Reporting to national and federal agencies such as NAACCR, the Centers for Disease Control and Prevention's National Program of Cancer Registries (CDC/NPCR), and/or the National Cancer Institute's Surveillance, Epidemiology, and End Results (NCI/SEER) Program
7. Security includes:
   - Requiring password authentication to access registry data
   - Facilitating the protection of confidential information
   - Supporting various security access levels and roles such as abstractors, visual reviewers, managers, and researchers

8. Task and record management includes:
- Tracking registry staff productivity
- Providing record modification audit trails

Central registry DMS applications may be purchased or licensed from a number of vendors, or they may be developed internally by registry staff, contractors, or both. The SEER Program and NPCR now provide their own central registry DMS to interested constituents. Because of the highly complex nature of registry data and registry operations, central registry software systems are technically challenging to implement. These systems are certainly more difficult to implement than they first appear, particularly to software designers new to cancer registration.[6] After starting a new job at the Kentucky Cancer Registry, the author recalls suggesting that a registry DMS to server both hospital and central registry operations could be developed in 6 months. Now, after 20 years of continuous development and refinement of registry DMS, it is apparent that this initial assessment was a little naïve. Notably, however, a number of perfectly functional and innovative central registry software systems continue to be successfully developed by central registries.

In addition to initial development, any registry DMS must be maintained. Registry data elements, standards, and operations change over time. NAACCR policy establishes updates to the data exchange standard on an annual basis. When contemplating whether to develop a system, adopt a federal system, or license a commercial registry system, continuing maintenance and technical support are important factors to consider. Central registry software maintenance requires continuing effort that is comparable with that of the initial development.

Hospital Registry Data Management Systems

Of the key functions cited earlier for central registries, hospital registries also perform most of them except perhaps for importing and consolidating complete abstracts from external sources and conducting record linkages with data files from external agencies. In addition to the key functions in common with central registries, many hospital registries rely on the registry DMS to support active patient follow-up activities and submit data to the American College of Surgeons' (ACoS) National Cancer Database (NCDB) and Rapid Quality Reporting System (RQRS). The hospital registry DMS may also interface with the hospital's electronic medical record system to allow direct import of demographics and other abstracted data elements.

The majority of central registry cases are provided by hospital registries. Central registries, therefore, have a vested interest in the quality of the reporting hospital registry DMS. Hospital registry DMSs must follow the same national data coding standards and rules, and must support data export in standard formats such as the NAACCR

data exchange standard. Central registries operations can be severely challenged when coordinating the transition to new coding standards such as the sweeping changes that occurred in 2010. The failure to remain current by a single hospital vendor may impede the central registry's ability to convert to a new standard.

To ensure the data quality abstracted by their reporting hospitals and to control data standard transitions, some central registries have chosen to provide the registry DMS to their reporting hospitals. Just like central registry software systems, a hospital registry DMS may be developed, acquired from a federal agency, or licensed from commercial vendors. When done well, there is a distinct advantage to a central registry that receives hospital reports from a single reliable software application. Such central registries can ensure that abstracting rules and edit checks have been consistently applied, and that new data standards have been introduced in a systematic fashion. However, this approach also runs the greater risk for widespread reporting failure if the hospital software vendor is unable to perform in a reliable and timely fashion. Hospital DMS development is just as challenging as at the central registry, and providing hospital technical support can be even more challenging.

The majority of central registries receive data from a variety of commercial, federal, and institutionally developed systems. The wide acceptance of NAACCR standards for data transmissions has reduced a number of problems that central registries used to face when receiving data from various hospital software packages. More recently, coordinating the timing of updated NAACCR standards in software among a variety of vendors represents the most significant challenge for these central registries. It is always advantageous for a central registry to maintain contact with the hospital software vendors to remain informed about potential software issues and standards revision timelines.

Other Useful Software Applications

A number of other software applications are frequently used by registries. Several specific products are listed in this section. Such references do not represent an endorsement, and the omission of any product does not suggest that it should not be considered.

Performing record linkages between the central registry database and external data files is a common and important function for central registries. Probabilistic record linkage systems allow records to be linked while taking into consideration the weighted match probabilities of different data variables. According to Matthew Jaro, an early developer of record linkage software, "Probabilistic linkage technology makes it feasible and efficient to link large public health datasets in a statistically justifiable manner."[7] Probabilistic linkages offer greater flexibility than deterministic linkages that tend to rely on exact variable matches. For example, small typographical errors in names and Social Security numbers in one or more records from the same patient may still result in a valid match when using a probabilistic record linkage. CDC/NPCR recently developed a standalone probabilistic record linkage application called LinkPlus (http://www.cdc.gov/cancer/npcr/tools/registryplus/lp.htm) for this purpose. Other commercial probabilistic packages also exist. These possibilities are discussed further in Chapter 17.

Statistical analysis of registry data is an essential function of any cancer registry. Commonly utilized data analysis applications include SAS (SAS Institute: http://www.sas.com/), Stata (StataCorp: http://www.stata.com/), and SEERStat (NCI/SEER: http://seer.cancer.gov/seerstat/). SAS and Stata are commercial products, whereas SEERStat was developed for public use by the NCI/SEER Program. Some registry DMS applications support statistical analysis of the registry abstracts.

Geospatial analysis of registry data is becoming increasingly important to central cancer registries and some hospital registries. Geographic information systems (GISs) can be used to map and analyze cancer incidence and mortality rates and trends, environmental risk factors, socioeconomic data, healthcare facility data, and other data relevant to cancer control. GIS software applications include ArcView/ArcGIS from ESRI, Inc. (http://www.esri.com) and cancer-rates.info (http://www.cancer-rates.info/) developed by the Kentucky Cancer Registry. GIS systems may require the geocoding of registry data to apply GIS methods below the county level. Please also refer to Chapter 37 for further information regarding GIS systems and geocoding.

Consistent edit checking of registry data elements is essential to registry data accuracy, consistency, and reliability. CDC/NPCR developed and maintains a standalone edit checking application called NPCR-EDITS (http://www.cdc.gov/cancer/npcr/tools/edits/). The underlying EDITS engine is also supported as a software library that can be incorporated into registry DMS applications. The SEER Program also developed a standalone edits application for SEER central registries called SEEREdits (NCI/SEER: http://seer.cancer.gov/). For further information about edit checking, refer to Chapter 8.

In recent years, central registries have widely implemented software applications and infrastructure to support real-time electronic reporting of anatomic pathology reports, also known as e-path. A commercial application that supports e-path transmissions from pathology laboratories to registries are TransMed and Autocode, which were developed by Artificial Intelligence in Medicine, Inc. (AIM: http://www.aim.on.ca/). The AIM system supports simultaneous reporting to both hospital registries and central registries for hospital-based pathology laboratories. CDC has also implemented e-path support through the Public Health Information Network Messaging System (PHIN-MS: http://www.cdc.gov/phin/).

Collaborative Stage Data Collection System (CS) is a coding system for staging of cancer that brings together the principles of several staging systems.[8] CS is utilized by the hospital registry, as well as the central registry. CS was first implemented in registry software systems for 2004 diagnoses and was recently completely revised for 2010 diagnoses as Collaborative Stage Data Collection System version 2 (CSv2). To facilitate a consistent and reliable implementation of the complexities of the CS rules and processes among all registry software vendors, various CS stakeholders have worked together to produce a CS software library that could be incorporated into any registry software application. The library is supported as a Microsoft Window's Dynamic Link Library (DLL) and is available in source code for compilation into registry software on other operating system platforms such as Unix and Linux. The CS implementation and software distribution has been highly successful to date and will serve as a model for future support of complex data coding standards.

Interoperability Resources

Semantic and Syntactic Interoperability

Interoperability has become an important issue for both hospital and central cancer registries. The significance of interoperability boils down to the ease in which registries can incorporate electronic data from external sources into the registry, as well the ease in which external recipients can incorporate registry data for their use. Interoperability is often described in terms of semantic and syntactic interoperability. Semantic interoperability pertains to sharing a common "meaning" of a data representation among two or more entities, whereas syntactic pertains to using a common data representation or coding system. As an example, consider two data standards designed to represent the presence of a new fictitious biomarker called *Beta*. Beta is an important factor in the treatment strategy for a particular cancer diagnosis. Imagine that cancer registries and pathology laboratories have adopted their own standards for recording this variable. Unfortunately, the two standards are syntactically the same, yet semantically different, as illustrated in Table 7-1. Notice that the two groups have adopted a very different meaning for code "2." In this example, the two data "standards" are not interoperable, and such data from pathology laboratories could not be stored or exchanged using the registry definition.

Data Standards

The key to successful interoperability lies in adoption and adherence to widely utilized data standards. Fortunately, cancer registries have a longstanding history in both the

Table 7-1	Example of Semantically Different Codes for a Data Variable	
Registry Code Set		**Pathology Code Set**
0—Biomarker β not detected		0—Biomarker β not detected
1—Biomarker β detected		1—Biomarker β detected
2—Biomarker β test not performed		2—Biomarker β inconclusive
3—Biomarker β status unknown		3—Biomarker β status unknown

development and adoption of data standards. The most important technological advance for cancer registries in the past two decades has been the development and widespread acceptance of the NAACCR data exchange standard, currently published as *Standards for Cancer Registries, Volume II* (http://www.naaccr.org/). This standard specifies a common file layout of well-defined cancer registry data variables. As a result of the publication and adoption of this standard, cancer registries in the United States and Canada have converged on a common set of core data variables that are easily exchanged among cancer registries, federal agencies, researchers, and others. Registries can support a single software interface to export a standard NAACCR file to submit for out-of-state data exchange and annuals data calls from NCDB, SEER, CDC, and NAACCR. Likewise, only one single software interface is required to import registry data from numerous software vendors and registry DMSs. NAACCR data exchange standards have allowed the development of standalone edit checking software, NAACCR record viewers, among others.

For many years, supporting interoperability solely among the registry community was sufficient to meet registry interests. However, as other entities who provide data important to cancer registries have become more technologically advanced, and as clinicians and researchers have become more technologically sophisticated, "playing" only among ourselves is no longer acceptable. To meet increasing demands on registries for clinical relevance and an ever-expanding data set, registries must pursue efficiencies to be gained through the adoption of interoperability standards with all stakeholders. Efficiencies will be gained by adopting external data standards while we continue to promote the adoption of registry standards by others. For example, for many years, cancer registries had adopted an unusual practice for representing two variables in individual therapy date fields by using "88888888" to mean "therapy planned but not given" or "99999999" to mean "unknown if given." External users of registry data were required to deal with this anomaly to receive and store such data in their database systems. Beginning in 2010, NAACCR adopted date representation standards more commonly utilized by others, thereby adopting a more interoperable standard that makes registry data easier to use by the greater community.

An emerging and prevalent interoperability data exchange standard has been developed by the Health Level Seven (HL7) organization (http://www.hl7.org). HL7 standards have been widely implemented by the healthcare industry and their use increasingly recognized by federal agencies and standard-setting organizations such as the Healthcare Information Technology Standards Panel (HITSP: http://www.HITSP.org). NAACCR has developed and promoted an HL7 standard for the transmission of electronic pathology reports to cancer registries, known as *Standards for Cancer Registries, Volume V: Pathology Laboratory Electronic Reporting* (http://www.naaccr.org/). The HL7 standard in NAACCR Volume V has become a de facto international standard and has facilitated the rapid deployment of electronic pathology reporting systems between pathology laboratories and cancer registries.

A resource that helps the cancer research community increase utilization of registry data can be found in the National Cancer Institute's Cancer Data Standards and Registry and Repository (caDSR).[9] The caDSR attempts to solve the challenges that arise from the lack of interoperability among representations of similar or common data elements (CDEs). The caDSR incorporates registered CDEs used across cancer research domains to facilitate interoperability among research stakeholders. Data variables defined in NAACCR Volume II have been registered in the caDSR, making them more accessible to cancer researchers.

Managing, Protecting, Securing, and Maintaining Computer Resources

Technical Staff

Computer resources must be properly managed to serve the mission of the central registry. The majority of central registry operations also rely on support from technical informatics staff. It is always in the best interest of the registry to employ technical staff whose time is devoted 100% to the registry. Particularly in a central registry, the data, rules, and operations are so complex that it may take more than a year for new technical staff to develop sufficient familiarity to efficiently support them. Staff person who only spends a portion of his or her time working for the registry may not be able to deliver an acceptable level of support. Many registries must operate within the constraints of their parent organization and may not have the option of maintaining their own technical staff. When it is possible, however, dedicated technical staff for the registry should be a priority. Descriptions of the three key roles of technical staff are presented here.

Efficient and timely systems support can directly impact a registry's overall productivity. Servers usually maintain data and software utilized by many staff such that a single system failure may have a far-reaching and costly impact. The system administrator(s) are responsible for maintaining servers and communications infrastructure such as the network devices, firewalls, wireless access points, and cabling systems. System administrators are also responsible for electronic and physical security of computer systems. Another key responsibility for the system administrator is disaster recovery planning. These duties require expertise in server operating systems support. Desktop support is another important support function that is generally closely coordinated with the server administration. Desktop support requires knowledge of hardware specifications, installations, and maintenance. Malware scanning and security updates should be guaranteed by desktop support staff. Good desktop support staff must be patient and able to communicate well with nontechnical registry staff.

Registry operations require considerable technical support beyond server and desktop support. Familiarity with the registry software system and administration is vital. Registry DMS require updates and upgrades, many of which may impact the content and integrity of the data. Inability to roll back from an errant central software update could be disastrous. Day-to-day registry operations also require technical support to manipulate data. As data submissions near, technical support may be required to generate NAACCR formatted data files and perform standalone edit checks. Requests for cancer committee and research data may require the development of custom software applications to manipulate data before release. Data linkages require considerable technical support and an understanding of probabilistic linkage methods. Web-based data submission systems require additional expertise with Web-based technologies and related security concerns. All of these operations require general computer expertise and comprehension of the registry data and registry operations.

Staff who can perform software development is another requirement of most central registries. Depending on the registry, these needs range from developing small applications to manipulate data files to developing a complex registry DMS. Software development requires specific skills and the most intimate understanding of registry data, standards, and rules. Development and support of a central registry DMS requires considerable expertise in software design and development technologies. Software develop-

ment technologies evolve at an amazing pace, so software developers must balance the desire to implement newer technologies with the practical concerns of maintaining functionality of existing software. In addition to developing software, developers must be able to provide technical and end-user documentation, and be able to provide technical support to software users.

Hospital registries typically utilize the facility's IT department and are not usually large enough for dedicated staff. IT staff assigned to support hospital registry operations may have no prior knowledge of the registry and its unique needs. Therefore, it is important for the registry to maintain documentation regarding hardware, software, data, and operations to assist the IT department in serving their needs. Installation information should be documented, such as where the applications are installed, where the data are stored, and other specifics, especially in departments where there are multiple workstations accessing a single database.

Disaster Recovery Planning

Registry computer resources should always be protected by a comprehensive disaster recovery plan. In 2005, Hurricanes Rita and Katrina provided a sobering demonstration of the value of proper disaster recovery planning as experienced by the Louisiana Tumor Registry (LTR). In the aftermath of these hurricanes, the LTR offices, including all of their computers and servers, were rendered inoperable and inaccessible for months. Fortunately, LTR's data and systems had been properly backed up by their software vendor, Larry Derrick at Rocky Mountain Data Management Systems. Larry was able to restore their central registry data and system on an alternate server at a remote location and enabled staff to resume their central registry operations long before they could return to their offices and computers. A key lesson to be learned from this experience is, "The only thing more difficult than planning (response) for an emergency is having to explain why you didn't."[10]

Perhaps most important to a disaster recovery plan is the implementation of a reliable data backup and retrieval system. Central registry data by nature are highly dynamic and are updated frequently, representing significant hours of staff time. For this reason, data and registry systems should be backed up on a daily basis at minimum. A proper backup scheme should provide for the restoration of a fully functional central registry system with little loss of committed effort (i.e., no more than a single day's work effort). Although tape backup is currently the most common mechanism, remote server backup such as that used by the LTR in 2005 is an increasingly attractive option. When relying on tape backups, the tapes themselves are as vulnerable to physical disaster as the computer servers. For this reason, weekly or monthly tape backups should be stored off-site.

As part of the disaster recovery plan, the technical staff should consider and plan for all of the procedures that would be required to restore a registry from a completely failed server. To restore tape backups, one must bring up a functional server and software application needed to perform the restoration. Operating systems, applications, and data should be protected by the backup system. A backup scheme should be designed to capture the registry system when it is in a stable state. For example, a database backed up while in the process of updating records may not be recoverable. With a sound backup and recovery plan in place, it is also important to periodically test and confirm that the backup and restoration procedures actually work.

Hospital registries should discuss disaster recovery plans with the facility IT department. Most hospitals have extensive backup plans in place for the myriad of patient information it holds for all departments. It is important for the registry to understand this process and ensure that the registry data are being protected according to the same standards as other health information within the facility. The registry should coordinate periodic validation of the disaster recovery plans with the IT department.

Secure Electronic Transmissions of Registry Data

The Internet has become the most widely utilized medium to transmit electronic data between remote computers or "hosts." The architecture of the Internet has been designed in such a way that data may be transmitted between any two hosts securely, even when those transmissions occur across a publicly accessible network. This is accomplished through data encryption. A software library, called the Secure Socket Layer (SSL), has been developed that automatically manages the process of establishing secure encrypted connections between two host computers. Software applications that utilize the SSL library can exchange confidential data over the Web or Internet while maintaining security and confidentiality. Two commonly utilized SSL tools used to securely transmit data include the secure file transfer protocol (SFTP) and the secure hypertext transfer protocol (HTTPS). SFTP is used for file-based data transfers between hosts. HTTPS is a secured version of the standard Web-based communication protocol. To exchange data using SFTP or HTTPS, both host computers must have Internet connectivity and be configured with tools that use the SSL library.

E-mail remains an alternative but less practical method to securely transmit confidential data. Because most e-mail is ultimately transmitted across the Internet, special precautions must be taken when transmitting sensitive data in e-mail. Like all Internet transmissions, unintended recipients can potentially intercept e-mail messages. Attachments can be protected by encrypting the data file before attaching to the e-mail message. Typically, a password must be provided to the recipient for them to decrypt and access the file. Several software packages support file-based encryption. WinZip (http://www.winzip.com) is a relatively inexpensive product that supports the Advanced Encryption Standard (AES), an encryption standard adopted by the U.S. government. Files encrypted by products that do not support AES encryption may be more vulnerable to an attack by an unauthorized party. Sensitive data should never be included in the body of an unencrypted e-mail message.

Another means of securely transmitting data is by using traditional physical media such as diskettes, magnetic tapes, CD-ROMS, DVDs, USB flash drives, and computer hard drives. Whenever any such media are shipped, similar precautions should also be taken to protect the data in the event that the media are intercepted either by accident or by a nefarious intent. Again, data encryption is the key to securely transporting data using electronic media. A utility such as WinZip may be used to encrypt the data before writing to the media. Data on hard drives and flash drives may also be encrypted using applications provided with the flash media or by the operating system. Checkpoint, Inc. (http://www.checkpoint.com) offers a variety of products that support encryption for hard drives and media.

Infrastructure Planning and Maintenance

All registry computer resources must be maintained. It is important for cancer registries to maintain relatively current desktop and laptop computers. With the rapid advancement of CPU speeds and disk capacities, each new generation of software applications requires increased computing capacities to run them. Registries rely heavily on computer resources, and staff productivity should not be limited by slow or outdated hardware. Fortunately, the cost/performance ratio improves with each new generation of computer technology. Computer hardware in a registry should be replaced at least every 5 years and optimally every 3 years.

Servers are more expensive than desktop and laptop computers, and a central registry may not have financial resources to replace them every 3 years. When servers are utilized by multiple registry staff, a server hardware failure may be costly in terms of lost productivity during the downtime. It may be in the registry's best interest to acquire a maintenance contract that will replace the server or failed components within a relatively short turnaround time. Contract options usually range from next business day delivery of replacement parts to same-day replacement by a technician. The original hardware cost, the age of the hardware, and contract options will determine the cost. Maintenance costs must be weighed against hardware replacement because the cost of maintenance contracts over time may actually exceed the cost of replacing the hardware. For most hospital registries, server upgrades are managed by the IT department.

Conclusions

Cancer registries offer an exciting and rigorous environment for the applied use of computer resources. Current trends suggest that central registries will continue to evolve into near real-time repositories of population-based cancer surveillance data, whereas many hospital registries are already performing concurrent abstracting. Both hospital and central registries are becoming increasingly interoperable with electronic data sources such as pathology and electronic medical records. Increased interoperability will shrink the time from diagnosis to availability of analytic registry records. The registry data set will likely become more complex and richer with biomarkers, genomic, proteomic, and even diagnostic imaging data. As a result, registry data will become more clinically relevant and important to research and cancer control.

It has been suggested that technology will eventually eliminate the need for cancer registrars and other registry staff. It has been suggested the role of the hospital registrar will shift from data collection to quality review and dissemination of data that is automatically collected through computerized systems. Is it possible that future cancer registries will consist of nothing more than highly sophisticated and fully automated computer systems? While we ponder these questions, we can rest assured that registry staff have plenty of work to keep them occupied, and that computer resources will continue to play an increasingly important role in registry operations. Computer resources will continue to evolve and be leveraged to increase the efficiency, productivity, value, and capabilities of current and future cancer registries.

The author wishes to gratefully acknowledge Donna Gress for her insightful suggestions regarding computer resources for hospital registries.

References

1. Zwicky, E. D., Cooper, S., Chapman, D. B. *Building Internet Firewalls* (p. 102). Sebastopol, CA: O'Reilly & Associates, 2000.

2. Garfinkel, S., Spafford, G. *Practical Unix and Internet Security*. Sebastopol, CA: O-Reilly & Associates, 1996.

3. Open Source Initiative Web site: http://www.opensource.org/.

4. NAACCR Data Standards for Cancer Registries. Available at: http://www.naaccr.org/. Accessed on August 5, 2010.

5. *Standards for Cancer Registries, Volume II,* 15th ed., Record Layout Version 12.1. Springfield, IL: North American Association of Central Cancer Registries, June 2010.

6. Phillips, J. L., Menck, H. R. "Computerization." In H. R. Menck, C. Smart, editors: *Central Cancer Registries Design, Management and Use.* Amsterdam: Harwood Academic Publishers GmbH, 1994.

7. Jaro, M A. "Probabilistic Linkage of Large Public Health Data Files," Statistics in Medicine, 1995;14(5–7):491–498.

8. American Joint Committee on Cancer Web site: http://www.cancerstaging.org/.

9. National Cancer Institutes. "Cancer Data Standards Registry and Repository (caDSR)." Available at: https://cabig.nci.nih.gov/concepts/caDSR/

10. Chen, V. "Registry's Response to a Natural/National Disaster." CDC-NPCR Program Directors' Meeting, Atlanta, GA, March 8, 2006.

chapter 8

Data Edits

Judy Jacobs Williams, RHIT, CTR

History of Data Standardization and Edits Development

Data Standardization

In these challenging times, there are many tools to assist registrars in doing their jobs, and the most important of these is referred to as the "Edits." To understand the Edit process, it is appropriate to first learn its history. Data standardization was the key to developing the Edits. The process to automate and coordinate data editing could not begin until data collection was standardized. The earliest standard setters were the American College of Surgeons' (ACoS) Commission on Cancer (CoC) and the Surveillance, Epidemiology, and End Results Program (SEER). These two entities established the first coding rules and guidelines in the 1950s. The first data collection manual published by the CoC was the *Supplement on the Tumor Registry,* in addition to its *Cancer Program Manual 1981.* Hospital registries at that time generally used the CoC rules, whereas central registries used the SEER rules. Therein lay the primary problem: The two agencies did not agree on data fields, coding rules, and definitions. The solution was to bring the two agencies together to define one common set of data items, field lengths, and codes. In 1988, this joint effort resulted in the publication of two manuals outlining coding and staging requirements: the *Data Acquisition Manual (DAM) of the American College of Surgeons* and the *SEER Program Manual.*[1] This effort between two diverse organizations achieved the shared goal of data standardization that still exists today.

In the 1980s, the California Cancer Registry requested that SEER and the CoC establish a formal committee to pursue further data standardization to help apply standards within California.[1] In 1987, the American Association of Central Cancer Registries (AACCR) was formed and, as a result, created the Uniform Data Standards Committee (UDSC). This committee assumed the duties of the California committee. Membership in the UDSC expanded to include all of the major standard-setting organizations. In 1992, all of the participating groups agreed to use the second edition of *International Classification of Diseases for Oncology* (ICD-O) for cancers diagnosed in 1992 and later. This was a major breakthrough for data standardization, and this progress continues today under the guidance of the Volume II Workgroup of the UDSC committee. With the addition of Canadian registries in 1995, AACCR became the North American Association of Central Cancer Registries (NAACCR), as it is known today.

Edits Development

Data standardization and increasing advances in technology brought with it the need for a computerized editing program. In the late 1980s, registries were deciding their own rules for editing data. In 1990,[2] the NAACCR Data Evaluation and Publication Committee identified that the missing link in data standardization was an automated programmable editing system that could be used by all registries. The Centers for Disease Control and Prevention (CDC) and subsequently National Program of Cancer Registries (NPCR) began the task of developing EDITS software with two purposes in mind: (1) to improve the quality of data, and (2) to standardize the way data items are checked for validity. As a result of this effort, the first NAACCR standard edits were made available to the public in 1996. The EDITS software tools, consisting of EditWriter and GenEDITS Plus, are distributed free of charge through the CDC Web site (http://www.cdc.gov/cancer/npcr/tools/edits) or from the NAACCR Web site (www.naaccr.org), found under Cancer Data Standards/NAACCR Data Standards for Cancer Registries/Standard Data Edits. [0](Instructions for downloading, installing, and running GenEdits Plus with the current NCDB Metafile can be found online at: http://www.facs.org/cancer/ncdb/datasubmission.html.)

The original GenEDITS software was DOS-based. The current iteration of the software, called GenEDITS Plus, is a newer, more user-friendly Windows version.[2]

Data Changes

Even after data collection and edits were standardized, problems continued to arise because of changes being made at different times by different standard setters. To reform and regulate the changes, NAACCR recently formed a committee, the "Standards Implementation Task Force," which is charged with the yearly review of the timing of data changes. This committee was established so that major changes will be made at the same time, to make the implementation of these changes easier for both the registries and the vendors. The committee makes recommendations according to the needs of the standard-setting organizations, central cancer registries, cancer registry software vendors, and reporting facilities. As a result, all standard setters have agreed that major changes will now be implemented on a 3-year cycle. Minor changes may be implemented annually.[3]

Standardization of Data Edits

Standardization of data edits remains challenging for both hospital and central cancer registries. These challenges include:

1. Differing computer language in registry systems
2. Standard specifications may be programmed differently
3. Incomplete editing of data during data abstraction
4. Documentation of edit algorithms used are not always available for data researchers
5. Data collected and consolidated from varied reporting sources and applications are not always uniform; therefore, data analysis may be affected

6. Standard changes are difficult to synchronize across software providers
7. Registries use different software providers

Standards for Cancer Registries, Volume II: Data Standards and Data Dictionary, Thirteenth Edition provides the answer to quality data collection: "Uniform, standardized edits must be applied to all cancer registry data in order to generate data that are comparable across registries."[4]

Using edits helps to define the criteria for data quality: Standardize data collection processes and provide clean data for analysis. Standard data edits are created to test data against coding rules. It is important that the user understand where to find that rule and which standard-setting agency created the rule, so that the edits are used appropriately.

Definition of Data Edits

Data edits verify data accuracy through the use of a computer software algorithm. These algorithms check the content of data fields against an encoded set of acceptable values. Data edits enforce valid relationships between codes and data items, and apply pass/fail criteria to data. Data quality feedback is provided via the Edit Report. Mistakes are corrected and data are rerun through the EDITS program to ensure edit resolution.[5]

The *'Why, When, Where and How'* of Edits

Why: Edits help to identify incorrect data.
When: Edits are applied on State or SEER submissions, NCDB Call for Data (Hospital Registries), NAACCR or NPCR Call for Data (Central Registries).
Where: Edits are integrated into hospital or Central Registry data collection software or used as stand-alone program (GenEdits Plus).
How: Edits flag blank fields.
Edits indicate single-field edit errors.
Edits specify disagreement between multiple data fields.
Edits indicate potential errors that require manual review.

The Mechanics of Edits

The edit components work together like joining pieces of a puzzle (Figure 8-1). Without one component, the edit will not work, just as the puzzle would not be whole without all of its pieces. There are three edit components: a *Metafile*, an *Edit Set,* and individual *Edits*.

A *Metafile* (sometimes called a *Runtime Metafile*) is a set of instructions that are necessary for the GenEDITS "engine," or driver, to run. A Metafile contains everything necessary to edit the data, except the data. The Metafile is created with the EDIT Writer program from the CDC. An example of a Metafile is the NAACCRv11 Metafile. Metafiles are considered "portable" because the same edits may be used for different purposes; for example, the NAACCR v11 Metafile edits may also be used for the NCDB Call for Data Metafile.

There are seven key components of a *Metafile*: data from each standard-setting agency (SEER, the CoC, NAACCR, or a state central registry), the data dictionary, record layouts, individual edits, edit sets, error messages, and user lookup tables.[6]

1. **Standard-setting agencies** refer to organizations such as the CoC, SEER, or NAACCR, and could indicate that the edit was created by a state central registry or by software providers.
2. The **Data Dictionary** contains all data elements or fields to be edited in the *Metafile*.
3. The **Record Layout (also referred to as record format)** is a named grouping and organization of fields from the Data Dictionary into a particular file format, such as the NAACCR Data Exchange Record. Many record layouts can be defined within the *Metafile,* with each corresponding to a particular data set or file format. Examples of the use of a record layout within a metafile are: (a) the NAACCR v11 metafile requires the use of the NAACCR v11 Record Layout; and (b) state "XX" metafile requires the use of the State "XX" Record Layout.
4. **Edits are individual data checks that** contain the logic needed to edit each field. Each Edit contains a name,

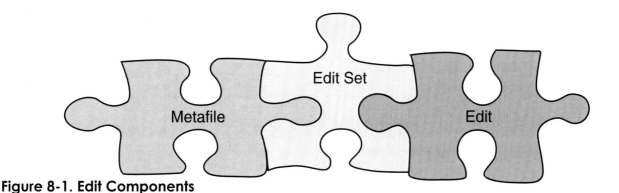

Figure 8-1. Edit Components

the standard setter requiring the edit, and a predefined error message.[6] For example:

> Edit Name: Text—Histology Title (NAACCR)
> Edit Error Message: Text—Histology Title must not be blank

5. The **Edit Sets** are groups of individual edits, combined for a purpose. Standard setters or state registries may want to use a subset of the edits. This subset is referred to as an *edit set*. Multiple edit sets can be used on the same data. For instance, the NAACCR metafile contains edit sets for hospital use, as well as central state registry use. Examples of edit sets are the NAACCR edit sets, the various SEER edit sets, the NCDB edit set, the Canadian edit set, and state-specific edit sets. Each edit set uses a specific record format or layout within the metafile as explained in the definition of "Record Layout."

6. Error messages are contained in the metafile to explain the edit. Each edit is numbered and references the standard setter requiring the edit. The error message is the key to understanding the edit.

The error messages are referred to within an Edit by their unique name and contain the information needed to make the correction to the data field. The error message may also explain why the edit was activated.

7. The **User Lookup Tables** are reference tables within the Metafile for performing lookups and for building list choices.

Types of Edits

There are three different types of Edits[7]:

- Single Field Edits or Item Edits check only one data field at a time.
  - Purpose is to verify and validate field values
  - Example: Race Codes must have only the allowable values
  - These error messages will usually begin with "xx not a valid value for…"
- Inter-field or Multi-Field Edits compare related data item codes for correctness.
  - Purpose is to identify errors
  - Example: Females cannot have prostate cancer
  - These error messages will usually begin with "Conflict among or between…"
- Inter-record or Multi-record Edits compare data on more than one like record.
  - Purpose is to identify errors common to all records
  - Example: Multiple Primaries must have the correct sequence numbers assigned in chronologic order

Consequences of Not Using Edits

Now that the mechanics of Edits are known, why use them? Or more importantly, what are the consequences of NOT using Edits?

Inconsistent data quality + Loss of data integrity = Loss of credibility in cancer registry data

Edits are the quality-control gatekeepers. The cancer registry data collection must be accurate to produce accurate data. Data presented without the use of edits may not represent the true picture of the data being presented. Incorrect data are worse than having no data at all. *Team Building to Enhance Quality Assurance* states the value of edits in this way: "Standardized edits are one of the single most important cancer registry quality assurance tools available."[8]

Resolving Edits

To resolve edits, one must know how to interpret the Edit Report (Figure 8-2). The Edit Report is the result of the edit process on a file or on one case. The Edit Report contains information for each edit error including the Edit Number, the Edit Name, and the Error Message. *The error message is the key to understanding how to correct the error.* One must also pay close attention to the error summary, which is another key feature of the Edit Report used for registry quality control. Frequently encountered errors may mean that staff education is needed.

Edit Over-rides

According to the *Standards for Cancer Registries, Volume II: Data Standards and Data Dictionary,* 14th edition: "Some computer edits identify errors. Others indicate possible errors that require manual review for resolution"[9]

The EDITS program provides a mechanism to note that questionable data are correct. Edit Over-ride Flags are an indication that case was reviewed by the managing physician or the Cancer Committee, and the *unusual* data in question were determined to be correct. Over-ride Flags can eliminate the need to review the same case multiple times. Over-ride Flags may be used for individual facility quality control and as a Central Registry quality-control method.

Examples of questionable data that will generate an over-ride flag are as follows:

Site and Age

- Patient age younger than 45 with Adenocarcinoma of Prostate
- Patient age younger than 30 with Multiple Myeloma

```
Data File - C:\Program Files\Good Registry Systems\040420.XCD
Range Processed - 1 - 2
Metafile - C:\RegPlus\GenEDITSplus\metafiles\NCDB_20_06182009.rmf
Date of Run  - 9/5/2009
Edit Set 1 - NCDB — All Edits for Call Period 20
Record Count - 2
Total Error Records - 2
Total Error Messages - 47
Total Warning Messages - 0
Legend: - Rep: = Reporting Facility
Legend: - ANH: = Accession Number—Hosp
Legend: - SNH: = Sequence Number—Hospital
Legend: - Dat: = Date of Diagnosis
Legend: - Pri: = Primary Site
Legend: - HTI: = Histologic Type ICD-O-3
Legend: - Abs: = Abstracted By
Legend: - Ven: = Vendor Name
#1 Rep: 0006999990 ANH: 200800001 SNH: 00 Dat: 01222008
Pri: C711 HTI: 9440 Abs: LEJ Ven: Good Registry Systems


Edit: Ambiguous Terminology DX, Date of DX (SEER IF157) ¨ Edit Name
E: If year of Date of Diagnosis > 2006, then Ambiguous Terminology DX cannot be blank ¨ Edit Message
Date of Diagnosis (283) [01222008] _ _ _ _ _ _ _ _ ¨ Data fields involved
Ambiguous Terminology DX (324) [<BLANK>] _


Edit: Date of 1st Crs RX—COC, Dates of RX (COC)
E: Conflict between Date of 1st Crs RX—COC and treatment dates
Date of 1st Crs RX—COC (843) [01242008] _ _ _ _ _ _ _
RX Date—Surgery (755) [01242008] _ _ _ _ _ _ _
RX Date—Radiation (779) [02152003] _ _ _ _ _ _ _ _
RX Date—Other (827) [00000000] _ _ _ _ _ _ _
RX Date—Systemic (795) [00000000] _ _ _ _ _ _ _


Edit: Date of Conclusive DX, Date of DX (SEER IF164)
E: If year of Date of Diagnosis > 2006, then Date of Conclusive DX cannot be blank
Date of Diagnosis (283) [01222008] _ _ _ _ _ _ _ _
Date of Conclusive DX (325) [<BLANK>] _ _ _ _ _ _ _
```

Figure 8-2. Example of an Edit Report

Site and Histology
- Second Primary coded to Unknown Primary with specific Histology
- Lymph Node Primary other than Lymphoma
- Ill-Defined Sites with a specific Histology
- Histology/Behavior of *in situ* not microscopically confirmed

An Over-ride Flag is indicated in the Edits by codes:

1 = Reviewed and although unusual, is correct (in the case of *in situ* behavior, this code also indicates pathologist stated behavior to be *in situ*)

2 = Reviewed and behavior is *in situ,* but is not microscopically confirmed (Override Histology only)

3 = Reviewed and conditions 1 and 2 both apply (for Override Histology only)

Blank = Not reviewed or reviewed and corrected

Edit Resolution: Resources for Registrars

Understanding terminology, definitions, and the correct coding for the fields in question is the key to deciphering edits. Registrars should refer often to the current editions of the coding manuals: *Facility Oncology Registry Data Standards Manual (FORDS),* the *SEER Program Coding Manual,* the *Collaborative Staging Manual,* the *AJCC Staging Manual,* NAACCR's *Standards for Cancer Registries, Volume II: Data Standards and Data Dictionary,* and the ICD-O-3 manual. Most of these manuals are available as electronic copies. An invaluable source of information about edits is found in another free program available from the CDC: *Registry Plus Online Help.* This program contains detailed explanations of all edits and is kept current. Both GenEDITS Plus and Registry Plus Online Help are stand-alone programs and can be installed on the desktop.

Links

GenEDITS Plus: http://www.cdc.gov/cancer/npcr/tools/edits/

RegistryPlus Online Help: http://www.cdc.gov/cancer/npcr/tools/registryplus/

The following are suggestions to assist in edit resolution:

- Learn as much as possible about GenEDITS and Metafiles.
- Check for common errors in the registry and provide education for staff.
- Record edits that are routinely troublesome.
- Look up the definitions of the fields in question.
- Find a mentor, someone with experience.
- Call the state or central registry for edit assistance.
- Use the Inquiry & Response of the ACoS or "Ask NAACCR."
- For possible software issues with edits, contact the vendor.

Cancer registrars today should consider the Edits as a vital part of the registry quality-control process. In the past, registrars had to rely on visual review to ensure error-free data for reporting. The advances in electronic data collection combined with electronic methods of editing the data provide an easy pathway to assure high-quality registry data.

References

1. *Standards for Cancer Registries, Volume II: Data Standards and Data Dictionary* (Chapter I1:15), 13th edition, edited by L. A. Havener, M. L. Thornton. Springfield, IL: North American Association of Central Cancer Registries, April 2008.
2. *Standards for Cancer Registries, Volume II: Data Standards and Data Dictionary* (Chapter IV:28), 13th edition, edited by L. A. Havener, M. L. Thornton. Springfield, IL: North American Association of Central Cancer Registries, April 2008.
3. *Standards for Cancer Registries, Volume II: Data Standards and Data Dictionary* (Chapter 2:16), 14th edition, edited by M. Thornton, L. O'Connor. Springfield, IL: North American Association of Central Cancer Registries, February 2009.
4. *Standards for Cancer Registries, Volume II: Data Standards and Data Dictionary* (Chapter IV:26), 14th edition, edited by M. Thornton, L. O'Connor. Springfield, IL: North American Association of Central Cancer Registries, February 2009.
5. *Standards for Cancer Registries, Volume II: Data Standards and Data Dictionary* (Chapter IV:25), 13th edition, edited by L. A. Havener, M. L. Thornton. Springfield, IL: North American Association of Central Cancer Registries, April 2008.
6. Centers for Disease Control and Prevention. "Key Components of a Metafile." Available at: http://www.cdc.gov/cancer/npcr/tools/edits/editmeta.htm. Last accessed 11/22/2010.
7. *Standards for Cancer Registries, Volume II: Data Standards and Data Dictionary* (Chapter IV:25), 14th edition, edited by M. Thornton, L. O'Connor. Springfield, IL: North American Association of Central Cancer Registries, February 2009.
8. Coppola, K., Bott, R., Cain-Rucker, C., Lee, L. "Quality Assessment and Continuous Quality Improvement" (p. 41). In *Team Building to Enhance Quality Assurance: A Report of the National Coordinating Council for Cancer Surveillance,* edited by H. L. Howe, G. G. Clutter. Atlanta: Centers for Disease Control and Prevention, March 2000.
9. *Standards for Cancer Registries, Volume II: Data Standards and Data Dictionary* (Chapter X:247), 14th edition, edited by M. Thornton, L. O'Connor. Springfield, IL: North American Association of Central Cancer Registries, February 2009.

chapter 9

The Electronic Health Record Environment

Herman R. Menck, BS, MBA, CPhil, FACE
Elaine Collins, RHIA, CTR

Background

Since the 1980s, the idea of developing an electronic health record (EHR) has been a topic of discussion across the healthcare community. For many, the vision became clearer with the 1991 Institute of Medicine (IOM) report, "The Computer-Based Patient Record."[1] By 2009, computerization of health information had become a part of the national news and a matter of public discourse. Potential improvements in quality of care and cost savings for patients have been frequently predicted for the EHR, which has become a cornerstone of the health policy of the United States.

Although the detailed technical aspects of the EHR can be complex, the concept is not. Recently, an American Health Information Management Association (AHIMA) columnist noted, "When my mother was diagnosed with a serious illness, the number of doctors she needed to see increased, as did the number of medications she was prescribed. For each appointment she stuffed all her prescription bottles in a plastic bag and then into her purse so that she could tell each physician which medications she was taking."[2] Many Americans are weary of clipboard completion of forms each time they visit a doctor's office, and understand the limitations of such personal and ad hoc remembrances. People have become aware that electronic technology may provide alternatives to traditional paper-based medical records, for example, allowing their information to be stored centrally and accessed by multiple providers and facilities, or to be stored and updated on small electronic devices that can be physically transported among providers.

It is useful to review the history and sequence of events in this EHR evolution to understand this marked change in the public's perceptions and attitudes, and to understand the various stakeholders and their respective roles and certain terminology. A summary follows, beginning with some definitions of terms, standards organizations, policy institutes, local and regional programs, and federal programs.

Then after this glossary of terminology, organizations and events are listed and the implications of the EHR for the Cancer Registrar are discussed, including recommended steps for future preparation.

Terminology

Electronic Health Record

The EHR refers to all types of health records, notably including the electronic medical record (EMR) and the personal health record (PHR). The EMR is an electronic record of an individual's health-related information that can be created, gathered, managed, and consulted by authorized clinicians and staff within one health care organization.

Personal Health Record

The PHR is defined as an electronic, universally accessible, layperson comprehensible, lifelong tool for managing relevant health information, promoting health maintenance, and assisting with chronic disease management via an interactive, common data set of electronic health information and e-health tools. The PHR is owned, managed, and shared by the individual or his or her legal proxy(s) and must be secure to protect the privacy and confidentiality of the health information it contains. It is not a legal record unless so defined and is subject to various legal limitations.

Interoperability and Harmonization

Interoperability refers to the ability of diverse systems to interoperate, or to work together, particularly in the exchange of information between systems, with the information carrying the same meaning through the exchange process. Harmonization refers to the adjustment of differences or inconsistencies among different measurements, standards, or systems to make them uniform or mutually compatible.

Standards Organizations

American National Standards Institute

An early participant in the EHR evolution, American National Standards Institute (ANSI), founded in 1918, is a nonprofit, voluntary collaboration for standardization activities. It is composed of government agencies, organizations, companies, academic and international bodies, and individuals. The ANSI represents the interests of more than 125,000 companies and 3.5 million professionals. ANSI is the official U.S. representative to the International Organization for Standardization facilitating voluntary consensus standards and conformity assessment systems, and safeguarding their integrity. ANSI convened a Health Information Standards Planning Panel in 1991 to coordinate the development of healthcare information standards in the United States and to participate in emerging global efforts, including the development of a framework for understanding healthcare terminology needs.

Health Level Seven

Health Level Seven (HL7) is one of several ANSI-accredited Standards Developing Organizations operating in the healthcare arena. Most Standards Developing Organizations produce standards for a particular healthcare domain such as pharmacy, medical devices, imaging, or insurance (claims processing) transactions. HL7's domain is clinical and administrative data.

HL7's mission is as follows:

To provide standards for the exchange, management and integration of data that support clinical patient care and the management, delivery and evaluation of healthcare services. Specifically, to create flexible, cost effective approaches, standards, guidelines, methodologies, and related services for interoperability between healthcare information systems.

HL7 is like most of the other Standards Developing Organizations in that it is a not-for-profit volunteer organization. Its members—providers, vendors, payers, consultants, government groups, and others who have an interest in the development and advancement of clinical and administrative standards for healthcare—develop the standards. Like all ANSI-accredited standards development organizations (SDOs), HL7 adheres to a strict and well-defined set of operating procedures that ensures consensus, openness, and balance of interest. A frequent misconception about HL7 (and presumably about the other SDOs) is that it develops software. In reality, HL7 develops specifications, the most widely used being a messaging standard that enables disparate healthcare applications to exchange keys sets of clinical and administrative data.

LOINC

The LOINC terminology database facilitates the exchange of clinical results, such as blood hemoglobin, serum potassium, or vital signs, for clinical care, outcomes management, and research. Currently, most laboratories and other diagnostic services use HL7 to send their results electronically from their reporting systems to their care systems. However, many laboratories identify tests in these messages by means of their internal and nonstandard code values.

LOINC codes are universal identifiers for laboratory and other clinical observations that solve this problem. The laboratory portion of the LOINC database contains the usual categories of chemistry, hematology, serology, microbiology (including parasitology and virology), and toxicology, as well as categories for drugs and the cell counts you would find reported on a complete blood count or a cerebrospinal fluid cell count. Antibiotic susceptibilities are a separate category. The clinical portion of the LOINC database includes entries for vital signs, hemodynamics, intake/output, electrocardiogram, obstetric ultrasound, cardiac echo, urologic imaging, gastroendoscopic procedures, pulmonary ventilator management, selected survey instruments, and other clinical observations.

SNOMED

SNOMED Clinical Terms (SNOMED CT) is administered by the International Health Terminology Standards Development Organization (IHTSDO), an international not-for-profit organization. SNOMED was developed and is maintained to advance excellence in patient care through the delivery of a dynamic and sustainable, scientifically validated terminology and infrastructure that enables clinicians, researchers, and patients to share healthcare knowledge worldwide, across clinical specialties and sites of care. The vision of SNOMED International is to be the leader in clinical terminology for encoding the medical record through the Systematized Nomenclature of Medicine, better known as SNOMED. SNOMED CT is a comprehensive and precise clinical reference terminology that healthcare providers, healthcare information technology (IT) suppliers, providers, payers, purchasers, and institutional researchers can use to improve the comparability of data. Backed by more than 40 years of pioneering research and development in the United States and United Kingdom, SNOMED CT allows for consistent capture of detailed clinical information.

College of American Pathologists Cancer Protocols

The College of American Pathologists (CAP) produces cancer protocols as a resource to pathologists in effectively delivering the information necessary to provide quality patient care. The protocols consist of cancer case summaries (checklists) accompanied by background documentation. The background documentation includes detailed outlines, explanatory notes, and references, and it is presented to you for information only. The American College of Surgeons Commission on Cancer (ACoS CoC) has recognized the value of the CAP cancer checklists in caring for cancer patients. Starting in January 1, 2004, the ACoS CoC mandated that pathologists at CoC-approved cancer programs include only the scientifically validated or regularly used data elements of the checklists in their surgical pathology reports on cancer specimens.

Other Standards Development Organizations

Many other organizations are also involved in the development of standards that define the content and format of electronic health information. Beginning in the late 1970s, their work has helped to lay the foundations for the emerging EMR. The Accredited Standards Committee X12 develops standards for electronic data interchange for billing transactions. The American College of Radiology and the National Electrical Manufacturers Association have collaborated to develop the Digital Imaging and Communications in Medicine (DICOM) standard. The American Society for Testing and Materials, one of the largest SDOs in the world, has supported a committee since 1990 to develop multiple health informatics standards, including clinical content of patient records and exchange of clinical observation messages. The Institute of Electrical and

Electronics Engineers develops standards for medical device information, including linking bedside instruments with health information systems. The National Council on Prescription Drug Programs has developed standards for prescription management and payment services.

Policy Institutes

Institute of Medicine

The IOM was chartered in 1970 by the National Academy of Sciences to examine policy matters pertaining to the health of the public. The Committee on Improving the Patient Record of the IOM published a 1991 report, "The Computer-Based Patient Record: An Essential Technology for Health Care."[1] The high demand for the original report and continued interest in computer-based patient records (CPRs) led the IOM to produce a second revised edition in 1997. The initiation of the second report corresponded with the midway point of a target set in the recommendations of the first report for achieving widespread implementation of CPRs in 10 years, approximately 2000. This date, of course, turned out to be premature.

In 2003, the IOM listed a group of eight key functions for safety, quality, and care efficiency that EMRs should support:

- Physician access to patient information, such as diagnoses, allergies, laboratory results, and medications
- Access to new and past test results among providers in multiple care settings
- Computerized provider order entry
- Computerized decision support systems to prevent drug interactions and improve compliance with best practices
- Secure electronic communication among providers and patients
- Patient access to health records, disease management tools, and health information resources
- Computerized administration processes, such as scheduling systems
- Standards-based electronic data storage and reporting for patient safety and disease surveillance efforts

Computer-Based Patient Record Institute

The Computer-Based Patient Record Institute (CPRI) was formed at the suggestion of the IOM in 1992. Three basic elements constituted the vision for CPRs, which was developed in the 1980s:

- Patient records should do a better job in their traditional role of keeping track of patient care events. They should support the creation of a longitudinal view of a patient's health history, offer greater flex-

ibility in the retrieval and display of patient data, and capture data elements essential to understanding the clinical thought process behind patient care decisions and to assessing the effectiveness of treatments.
- CPR systems should offer expanded functions that actively support clinicians in the care process and lessen the amount of time required for nonclinical tasks.
- Patient record systems should support the information needs of the full range of legitimate users (including physicians, nurses, and other caregivers; patients; administrators; third-party payers; and researchers), becoming the core of health information systems both within and beyond healthcare organizations (e.g., regional health databases or information systems).

The CPRI vision recognized key characteristics of CPR systems:

- Connectivity, data format, and data content standards must be met for systems to meet the needs of all users.
- Moreover, users must understand that the patient record is a resource for improving the effectiveness and efficiency of clinical processes and procedures. Complete and accurate data offer benefits well beyond the individual patient.
- Information management (including record keeping) is a critical component of the healthcare delivery process.

The vision of the CPRI documented in 1992 clearly illustrates the multidecade effort toward the development of the EHR; an effort that continues and is just starting to reach fruition.

Local/Regional Programs

Community Health Information Network

Community health information organizational theory, formulated in the early 1990s, supported the development of the Community Health Information Network (CHIN), the forerunner of the current Regional Health Information Organizations (RHIOs). As an example, the Oregon CHIN (OCHIN) was founded in 2000 as a collaborative project of stakeholders, safety net healthcare providers, and CareOregon. OCHIN's first charge was to design and implement a statewide data infrastructure that would offer practice management software to safety net community clinic partners. This computer software allowed OCHIN partners to achieve greater efficiency in appointment scheduling, resource utilization, and financial functions.

OCHIN's second charge was the rollout of EMR software that would greatly improve care for uninsured Oregonians by automating the collection and transmission of data needed by providers to better serve the patient.

OCHIN installed a common integrated practice management system in 14 individual clinics covering 85 sites from Seattle, Washington, to Santa Cruz, California.

Regional Health Information Organization (Also Linked with the Health Information Exchange)

A health information exchange (HIE) is a system that moves healthcare information electronically across organizations within a region, community, or hospital system according to nationally recognized standards. An HIE can also be described as the gathering of healthcare information electronically across organizations within a region or community. The HIE provides the capability to electronically move clinical information between disparate healthcare information systems while maintaining the meaning of the information being exchanged.

An RHIO brings together healthcare stakeholders within a defined geographic area and oversees the HIE among them for the purpose of improving health and care in that community. RHIOs are the building blocks of the proposed National Health Information Network (NHIN) discussed in the following section. The Inland Northwest Health Systems/Northwest RHIO (Washington) is an example, with a common EMR system in all participating hospitals and clinics, integrated systems linking urban and rural providers, and a single source for laboratory test results for inpatient and ambulatory care. The RHIO is centered in Spokane, with connections to communities across the state and more than 2,600,000 patient records in the system.

Federal Programs

National Committee on Vital and Health Statistics

The National Committee on Vital and Health Statistics (NCVHS) was originally created by the Department of Health and Human Service (HHS) in 1949. Early on, the NCVHS was concerned with improved coordination and standardization of federal health statistics. The NCVHS functioned as an early federal advisory committee on health data, statistics, and national health information policy.

Beginning in the early 1990s, the committee was regularly briefed by such groups as the CPRI and the Medical Records Institute on progress toward the CPR. In 1996, the Health Insurance Portability and Accountability Act (HIPAA) focused the attention of this committee on the striking changes in health care, health data, and information systems. Responsible for overseeing the implementation of HIPAA, the NCVHS also developed plans for a National Health Information Infrastructure (NHII). The national environment for health information systems had changed dramatically, with both information transportability and data privacy issues coming to the fore of public attention in the mid-1990s.

Health Insurance Portability and Accountability Act of 1996

HIPAA was adopted to ensure health insurance coverage after a person leaves an employer and also to provide standards for facilitating healthcare-related electronic transactions. Recognizing that advances in electronic technology could erode the privacy of health information, Congress incorporated into HIPAA provisions that mandated adoption of federal privacy protections for certain individually identifiable health information. HIPAA's Privacy Rule provides federal protections for personal health information (PHI) held by covered entities and gives patients an array of rights with respect to that information. However, balancing the protection of individual health information with the need to protect public health, the Privacy Rule expressly permits disclosures without individual authorization to public health authorities authorized by law to collect or receive the information for the purpose of preventing or controlling disease, injury, or disability, including but not limited to public health surveillance, investigation, and intervention.

National Health Information Infrastructure

NCVHS started the NHII initiative in 1997. The purpose was to form a conceptual framework around all existing, developing public and private sector health information networks in community, provider, and personal dimensions.

In 2001, the NCVHS published "Information for Health: A Strategy for Building the National Health Information Infrastructure." The strategy was designed to improve the effectiveness, efficiency, and overall quality of health and health care in the United States. The information infrastructure would be a comprehensive, knowledge-based network of interoperable systems of clinical, public health, and PHI that would improve decision making by making health information available when and where it is needed. The infrastructure would be built on the basic elements of values, practices and relationships, laws and regulations, privacy, standards, technology, and systems and applications, supporting all facets of individual health, health care, and public health.

Public Health Information Network

The Public Health Information Network (PHIN), launched by the Centers for Disease Control and Prevention (CDC) at the first annual PHIN conference in 2002, took a major step toward realizing the goals of the NHII report for the capture, storage, communication, processing, and presentation of information in the population health dimension. Through defined data and vocabulary standards, and strong collaborative relationships, the PHIN enables consistent exchange of response, health, and disease tracking data between public health partners. Ensuring the security of this information is also critical, as is the ability of the network to work reliably in times of national crisis. PHIN is composed of five key components:

- Detection and monitoring
- Data analysis
- Knowledge management
- Alerting
- Response

Multiple systems support communications for public health laboratories, the clinical community, and state and local health departments. Each has demonstrated the importance of being able to exchange health information. However, many of these systems operate in isolation, not capitalizing on the potential for a cross-fertilization of data exchange. PHIN is designed to act as a crosscutting and unifying framework that can better monitor these data streams for early detection of public health issues and emergencies, so that systems, no longer operating in isolation, can capitalize on the potential for a cross-fertilization of data exchange.

Office of the National Coordinator for Health Information Technology (2004)

On January 20, 2004, in his State of the Union Address, President George W. Bush stated, "By computerizing health records, we can avoid dangerous medical mistakes, reduce costs, and improve care." These remarks signaled the appearance of new federal initiatives to promote and standardize the development of electronic health information systems nationwide, focusing on the personal health and healthcare provider dimensions identified in the NCVHS report on the information infrastructure.

The Office of the National Coordinator for Health Information Technology (ONCHIT) was created by executive order 13335 in April 2004. The Secretary of HHS was directed to move the President's Health Information Technology (HIT) Plan forward, to develop and adopt health information standards that would be used to implement a nationwide EHR by 2014. The IT agenda was established:

- Interoperable EHR are adopted on a widespread basis within 10 years
- Medical information follows the consumer
- Clinicians have complete, computerized patient information
- Quality initiatives measure performance and drive quality-based competition
- Public health and bioterrorism surveillance are seamlessly integrated into care

The EHR would provide a way for Americans to access their healthcare information at any time and place, and patient health information would be shared among healthcare providers when authorized by the patient.

National Resource Center for Health Information Technology

As part of the HIT initiative, the Agency for Healthcare Research and Quality (AHRQ) in 2004 created the National Resource Center for Health Information Technology (the National Resource Center) to provide technical assistance to facilities in the effective use of IT resources. The AHRQ funds and manages grants to communities, hospitals, providers, and healthcare systems to build information networks, and maintains an IT Knowledge Repository including real-world experience with systems developments. The AHRQ defines its mission as helping clinicians develop higher quality, safer health care; putting the patient more squarely at the center of health care; stimulating planning and implementation of health IT, especially in rural and underserved areas; identifying the most successful approaches, as well as barriers, to implementation; and making the business case for health IT by evaluating costs and benefits.

caBIG®

The Cancer Bioinformatics Grid, or caBIG®, is a specialized health information network among the 2004 initiatives of special interest to oncology data professionals. Sponsored by the National Cancer Institute, the design for caBIG® is to harness the same technology that supports the EMR to the use of the medical research community. As described on its Web site, the mission of caBIG® is to develop a truly collaborative information network that accelerates the discovery of new approaches for the detection, diagnosis, treatment, and prevention of cancer, ultimately improving patient outcomes. The goals of caBIG® are to connect scientists and practitioners through a shareable and interoperable infrastructure; develop standard rules and a common language to more easily share information; and build or adapt tools for collecting, analyzing, integrating, and disseminating information associated with cancer research and care. caBIG® software and resources are widely distributed, interlinked, and available to everyone in the cancer research community, but institutions maintain local control over their own resources and data. caGrid (or the Grid) is the underlying network architecture and platform that provides the basis for connectivity of caBIG® software tools.

Nationwide Health Information Network

In November 2004, the ONCHIT issued a request for information regarding the development of the Nationwide Health Information Network (NHIN), a realization of the

NHII vision, through which the federal government would directly support and fund the development of a secure, nationwide, interoperable health information infrastructure. The infrastructure would allow connection between providers, consumers or patients, and other healthcare systems involved, enabling the sharing of healthcare information as a patient moves around from one clinical care setting to another. The NHIN would promote a more effective marketplace, greater competition, and increased choice through accessibility to accurate information on healthcare costs, quality, and outcomes. The ultimate goal would be fully informed clinical decision making to improve patient and national health.

The NHIN is described as a "network of networks" connecting diverse entities that need to exchange health information, such as state and regional HIEs, integrated delivery systems, health plans that provide care, personally controlled health records, federal agencies, and all related interconnected systems. Contracts were awarded to nine broad-based regional and state health networks in 2007, as trial implementations for participation in the NHIN Cooperative, a collaborative to test and demonstrate the exchange of private and secure health information among providers, patients, and other healthcare stakeholders.

American Health Information Community

The American Health Information Community (AHIC), a federal advisory committee, was formed in 2005 by the HHS. The purpose of this committee, with members from both public and private sectors, was broad in scope: to serve as an advisor to the HHS Secretary on the development of an interoperable HIT framework. Workgroups and subcommittees were formed to address specific topic areas, including EHRs, confidentiality, privacy and security, chronic care, population health, consumer empowerment, and personalized health care. Identified work on specific use cases was completed in December 2008, and the AHIC was discontinued. The work, however, represented a milestone toward the development of an interoperable healthcare system in the United States.

Health Information Technology Standards Panel

Health Information Technology Standards Panel (HITSP), established by the Office of the National Coordinator (ONC) in 2005, was a second collaborative partnership among the public and private communities. HITSP was formed to specify data items and technical standards to meet clinical and business needs for sharing information between systems, and to harmonize data and standards across different systems. HITSP worked with SDOs and also received guidance from the AHIC on specific use cases where standards harmonization was needed.

The ANSI provides a governance model for HITSP operations. Work products from HITSP include 14 Interoperability specifications, 9 Service Collaboration specifications, 10 Transaction Package specifications, 20 Transaction specifications, 28 Component specifications, and 4 Technical Notes. The specifications identify harmonized standards and provide detailed technical guidance on how the standards should be used.

The Interoperability specifications, for example, include:

IS01—Electronic Health Records Lab Results Reporting
IS02—Biosurveillance
IS03—Consumer Empowerment and Access to Clinical Info via Networks
IS04—Emergency Responder EHR
IS05—Consumer Empowerment and Access to Clinical Information via Media
IS06—Quality
IS07—Medication Management
IS08—Personalized Healthcare
IS09—Consultations and Transfers of Care
IS10—Immunizations and Response Management
IS107—EHR Centric Interoperability Specification
IS11—Public Health Case Reporting
IS12—Patient–Provider Secure Messaging
IS77—Remote Monitoring

Certification Commission for Healthcare Information Technology

After standards have been developed and harmonized, they are ready for implementation by software vendors. An automated and algorithmic certification process is needed to ensure that data and technical standards are implemented properly. Software applications must be able to receive and understand health information from other systems seamlessly.

The Certification Commission for Healthcare Information Technology (CCHIT) was formed in 2005 to certify and accredit electronic health information systems as meeting the requirements to securely and accurately share confidential health data with other approved health systems as directed. The system must be able to perform a set of required functions as described by HITSP and NHIN. This certification provides healthcare professionals with the confidence that they are making an informed decision on the purchase of an information system that will securely manage confidential data, provide intended functionality, and exchange information with other healthcare systems.

Health Information Security and Privacy Collaboration

Established in 2006 by Research Triangle Institute (RTI) International under contract with HHS, Health Information Security and Privacy Collaboration (HISPC) originally included 34 states and territories as collaborating participants. With the start of Phase 3 in April 2008, the number had expanded to 42 states and territories. HISPC addresses the privacy and security challenges presented by electronic HIE through multistate collaboration projects. Each HISPC participant maintains a steering committee and contact with a range of local stakeholders to ensure that developed solutions accurately reflect local preferences.

The third phase is composed of seven multistate collaborative privacy and security projects focused on analyzing consent data elements in state law, studying intrastate and interstate consent policies, and developing tools and strategies with the following purposes:

- Help harmonize state privacy laws, educate and engage consumers
- Develop a toolkit to educate providers
- Recommend basic security policy requirements
- Develop interorganizational agreements

Patient Safety and Quality Improvement Act

The Patient Safety and Quality Improvement Act (PSQIA) was passed in 2005, but the regulations implementing the act were published in 2008 and became effective in 2009. PSQIA establishes a voluntary reporting system to enhance the data available to assess and resolve patient safety and healthcare quality issues. To encourage the reporting and analysis of medical errors, PSQIA provides federal privilege and confidentiality protections for patient safety information called "patient safety work product." Patient safety work product includes information collected and created during the reporting and analysis of patient safety events. The confidentiality provisions are designed to improve patient safety outcomes by creating an environment where providers may report and examine patient safety events without fear of increased liability risk. This work is performed in close collaboration with the AHRQ and the Office of Civil Rights.

Nationwide Privacy and Security Framework for Electronic Exchange of Individually Identifiable Health Information

This report, released by the ONC in 2008, outlines principles that guide public and private sector entities that hold or exchange electronic individually identifiable health information and the development of any compliance and enforcement approaches, including industry self-regulation. The principles include:

- Individual access
- Correction
- Openness and transparency

- Individual choice
- Collection, use, and disclosure limitation
- Data quality and integrity
- Safeguards
- Accountability

Health Information Technology for Economic and Clinical Health Act of 2009

Starting in 2009, the Obama administration supplemented the Bush administration's initiatives, making "broad adoption of standards-based electronic health information systems, including electronic health records" a central part of the technology agenda. The Obama healthcare platform states, "Most medical records are still stored on paper, which makes them difficult to use to coordinate care, measure quality, or reduce medical errors," and implementation of the EHR will bring "improvements such as reduced hospital stays, avoidance of duplicative and unnecessary testing, more appropriate drug utilization, and other efficiencies." An "electronic medical record…will reduce error rates" and "reduce our long-term cost of health care."[3]

The American Recovery and Reinvestment Act (ARRA) of 2009, or the "Stimulus Bill," included the Health Information Technology for Economic and Clinical Health (HI-TECH) Act, which provides grants and funding for health organizations that successfully demonstrate meaningful use of a certified EHR technology for health IT adoption. The initial definition of meaningful use, published in July 2009, is a matrix of 2011 objectives and 2011/2013/2015 measures in columns, by five rows of categories:

- Improve quality, safety, and efficiency, and reduce health disparities.
- Engage patients and families.
- Improve care coordination.
- Improve population and public health.
- Ensure adequate privacy and security protections for personal health protection.

Providers must demonstrate meaningful use of EHRs, possibly certified by CCHIT, to qualify for Medicare and Medicaid incentive payments starting in 2011 under the economic stimulus law. Penalties are also assessed at some point against providers who choose not to participate in the program.

Office of National Coordinator for Health Information Technology (2009)

The ONC received legislative mandate under the HI-TECH Act. The ONC remains organizationally located within the Office of the Secretary for HHS and continues as the principal federal entity charged with coordination of nationwide efforts to implement the most advanced health IT in the collection, use, and electronic exchange of health information. The ONC's mission was restated to include development of a nationwide HIT infrastructure, with secure and protected patient health information, with the purpose of improving healthcare quality at the time and place of care, reducing healthcare costs, promoting early detection, prevention, and management of chronic diseases, and establishing governance for the NHIN. Two new Federal Advisory Committees were also created to assist the ONC.

Health Information Technology Policy Committee

The HIT Policy Committee will make recommendations to the ONC on a policy framework for the development and adoption of a nationwide health information infrastructure, including standards for the exchange of patient medical information. Any policy recommendations endorsed by the ONC can then be brought to the Standards Committee for their consideration.

Health Information Technology Standards Committee

The HIT Standards Committee will make recommendations to the ONC on standards, implementation specifications, and certification criteria for the electronic exchange and use of health information. The HIT Standards Committee will develop a schedule for the assessment of policy recommendations developed by the HIT Policy Committee. In developing, harmonizing, or recognizing standards and implementation specifications, the HIT Standards Committee will also provide for testing of standards by the National Institute for Standards and Technology. In Table 9-1 below, Federal Initiatives on IT standards are summarized.

Table 9-1	Summary of Federal Initiatives on IT Standards					
				Federal Initiatives		
Standards Organizations	Regional Initiatives	Year	Legislation	Agencies	Systems
American Society for Testing and Materials (ASTM)		1898			
ANSI		1918			
		1949		NCVHS	
American Joint Committee on Cancer (AJCC)		1959			
Institute of Electronic and Electrical Engineers (IEEE)		1963			
IOM		1970			
National Council on Prescription Drug Programs (NCPDP)		1977			
Accredited Standards Committee X12 (ASC X12)		1979			
American College of Radiology/National Electrical Manufacturers Association (ACR/NEMA) (DICOM standard)		1983			
Health Level 7—IEEE P1157 Medical Data Interchange Committee		1987			
ASTM Committee E31 on Healthcare Informatics	CHIN	1990		Agency for Health Care Policy and Research (AHCPR) AHRQ	

(Continued)

Table 9-1	Summary of Federal Initiatives on IT Standards *(continued)*

			Federal Initiatives		
Standards Organizations	**Regional Initiatives**	**Year**	**Legislation**	**Agencies**	**Systems**
IOM Committee on Improving the Patient Record—ANSI Health Information Standards Planning Panel		1991			
CPRI		1992			
LOINC—College of American Pathologists (CAP) SNOMED		1994			
		1996	HIPAA		
		1997			NCVHS NHII Æ NHIN
CAP Cancer Protocols		1998			
Certification Commission for Health Information Technology (CCHIT)	RHIO	2004		ONCHIT >ONC	CDC—PHIN
				AHRQ National Resource Center for Health Information Technology	NCI Cancer Biomedical Informatics Grid caBIG
		2005	Patient Safety and Quality Improvement Act (PSQIA)	AHIC—to 2008	
HISPC		2006		HITSP	
		2009	HITECH	ONC Health IT Policy Committee ONC Health IT Standards Committee	

Implications for the Cancer Registrar

The role of the cancer registrar will change as the EHR evolves and registry systems are integrated into the hospital and regional information infrastructure. How should registrars best prepare for the future? Most positively, the EHR changes may provide new opportunities for registrars to translate their specific knowledge and skills into building the vocabulary and systems of the electronic health data environment.

Technologic change is not new to the cancer registrar. In the last several decades, a continuing series of changes have virtually reformulated many aspects of registration, including the transition from mainframes to PCs and Web computing, the emergence of transportable registry software from vendors, data and data edit standardization, digitization of data sources, insinuation of computers into virtually all registry processes, necessary increase of IT consulting and staffing, increased security and privacy concerns, e-mail with attachments, conference calls, and cell phones.

Maintaining a professional level of awareness of the EHR evolution is a time-consuming task. Nonetheless, it is imperative that cancer registrars:

- Stay current with developments in the EHR environment, and potential impacts on their organizations and job duties.
- Adapt their roles to fit emerging EHR changes.
- Work proactively within their organizations to ensure the registry participates in and benefits from the design of new EHR systems.
- Remain aware of regional HIE and patient PHR developments.

The pace of EHR change seems to be quickening. Predictable changes directly affect registry casefinding, abstracting, and follow-up in an EMR hospital.

Electronic Casefinding

Digitized pathology reports automatically and electronically transmitted to the registry at the time of sign-off by the pathologists will automate most of casefinding. Digitized pathology reports are also increasingly being sent to central and state registries from hospital and stand-alone pathology laboratories.

Online Access/Abstracting to the Electronic Medical Record

Registrars have access from their computers to the parts of their facility records that are in electronic form, and may dispense with reference to paper records altogether depending on the pervasiveness of the facility electronic information systems. Whether the cancer registry patient abstract will become part of the medical record, will be maintained solely in the registry's standalone database, or become integrated into an oncology module of the larger system is not clear. If the cancer registry abstracts and staging forms are maintained in the EMR, then other users, including clinicians, can potentially access the abstract for quality of care purposes.

The pace of integration of disparate systems can affect registry workflow. Registries draw information from laboratory, pathology, radiology, transaction, and documentation systems. Registries may also have to compete with other units within a healthcare system for IT financial and personnel resources.

Abstracting information from an EMR has led directly to changes in working conditions:

- Flexibility in work location, with off-site access to electronic data sources
- Elimination of chart request and retrieval processes
- Use of multiple monitors to display record documents and abstracting screens
- Work processes dictated by the available EMR technology and access to software generated versus scanned documents
- Follow-up procedures dependent on the breadth of the information network

The working registrar, as well as management, must have user-friendly Internet access. Other access needs include the ability to download reference manuals and software upgrades and to participate in online training. The computer and Internet are as essential to regular work processes as the telephone.

Computer-Assisted Abstracting

Programs that identify reportable terminology, and apply site and histology codes to pathology diagnoses are available and in use. Programs that code a wider array of data items from the pathology report, either by parsing natural language or by mapping coded information from electronic pathology checklists to registry codes, are in development and testing phases. The CAP electronic checklists offer pathologists a method of recording medical information directly into an electronically coded and transmissible data stream. Data elements on the checklists map to many items in the cancer record, including cancer identification, cancer staging, surgical treatments, and some prognostic elements. The registrar may be presented with the complete text of the report, coded data fields, and flags characterizing the tightness of the relationship between coded and reported information. The checklists may eventually serve as a model for the recording of cancer information by other specialties, including radiology and medical and radiation oncology.

Potential for Timeliness

Rapid notification of patient diagnoses enhances surveillance and epidemiologic research. Patient care requires record access concurrent with and after completion of treatment regimens. As new treatments are completed, the patient record might warrant updating. Currently, the times scheduled for reporting reflect a compromise with the various needs; reporting once at diagnosis, again after first course of treatment, and then annually for follow-up. The future of immediately accessible electronic data may bring use of a more time-layered cancer record, with signal events being posted as often as they occur.

Increased Data Sources

It may become possible or necessary for the abstractor to use data sources in the future that are not now easily usable or normally considered because of current lack of requirement or precedent. These might include billing records, clinic logs, frequent use of disease index input, and medication administration records. These additional sources might be present within or without the hospital setting. Additional prognostic indicators, morbidity data, test results, and risk factors are possible examples. There may be more crosstalk or networking by registry staff with other hospital systems or clinics throughout RHIOs.

Electronic Health Record–Assisted Follow-up

Registries obtain follow-up information from facilities, physicians, and patients. As the information network for the registry expands and communication across the network is facilitated, the registry gains access to more sources of follow-up information and prospects for automating the retrieval of information. Some registries are currently using secure Web-based sites to communicate directly with patients. The PHR is another potential channel for communication, envisioning a reminder and messaging package built into a module for oncology data managed by the patient.

Secure Web-Based National Data Systems

Historically, cancer registry data systems were developed as stand-alone, facility, or vendor-designed configurations. More recently, statewide and standardized Web-based systems have been developed for direct access by multiple organizations, centralizing and focusing system design and support efforts. This development inherently establishes greater interoperability among organizations, and potentially leads to cost savings and easier data sharing between hospital, central, and state registries. Web-based systems are being opened to physician and clinic offices to support incident reporting of cancer cases to central registries.

No national Web-based system is in universal use today. However, it is possible that physician and clinic staff, hospital, central, state, and national registry personnel will ultimately utilize one unified, standardized data system for the collection of cancer data, similar to those used by banks, airlines, and other businesses.

Security

The EHR is premised on the assumption that adequate privacy and confidentiality can be achieved. Although abuses get periodic media coverage and security breaches occur, national online systems are pervasive, with the general public perceiving that the benefits outweigh any risks that may arise. The NHIN and its component parts must continue to support that perception if they are to succeed. The need for strategic backup and restore procedures, and recovery from disaster, also become critically important at every level of the system, including all registry databases.

With electronic records, registry managers need a straightforward understanding of their currently available disaster recovery plan. Backup and restore capabilities are a necessary protection against a possible loss of all registry records and files, and cessation of operations. How would the registry be reconstituted in the event of a wide-ranging fire, theft, or natural disaster? Backup/restore capabilities are sometimes provided by IT systems procedures beyond the control of the registry. This delegates future responsibility for the registry to someone unfamiliar with the functioning of the registry and whose work priorities are set elsewhere, and should be limited as much as possible and done with caution. A periodic audit of restore capabilities may become an essential requirement for registry management.

Cost Impact

Online abstracting and follow-up from the EMR are expected to achieve time savings once established. More data sources may provide a greater wealth of data, which may add review time but result in a more complete abstract. Savings based on increased data system interoperability, or possible use of a statewide or even national unified Web-based registry database would decimate total national IT development and support costs, but are less certain. Physician office reporting to state registries or RHIOs might significantly reduce costs for central registries. Strengthening security, backup, and restore procedures increases costs.

Design of vendor software will be significantly influenced by changes in the data set, need for more online documentation, interface with the EMR, increased record linkage, increased interface with regional software, and other changes. The possibility of a single national cancer registry data system also used by hospital registrars would profoundly affect vendors.

The march toward electronic technology and EMR-related changes is not without obstacles that cause delays, or worse. These include the tendency for organizations to be chronically challenged in their ability to plan and complete IT projects. Organizations must periodically renew their investments in large-scale systems as technology becomes obsolete, which may require total system redesign and conversion of legacy databases. Registry needs that require IT participation compete for resources with all the other organizational needs. This is seldom positive. Another obstacle to automation of registry efforts is the clinical reluctance to use structured forms and lists versus dictation. In addition, there can be deep-seated personal and institutional inertia and resistance to change.

Changing Role

It is possible that the cancer registrar's job will increasingly move away from coding, abstracting, and data entry from the health record toward data management: monitoring, review, editing of digitized information, with emphasis on quality control and interpretation of the abstract data. A goal will be to better understand and improve the quality of care. This shift in role may eliminate the more mundane tasks of abstracting and increase data mining.

Conversely, it is also possible that instead of becoming simpler, abstracting, staging, and managing data set changes (collaborative stage, multiple primaries and histology coding rules are past examples) will become more complex, and the CTR skill aspect of cancer registration will become more difficult. Annual educational updates may become increasingly important and intense.

If the role of the CTR is changing, then training of the appropriate job skills will need to be strengthened. More computer user knowledge will be necessary for some, including IT terminology, concepts, and methods. Some registrars may wish to learn facets of system administration, database architecture, security networks, assessment of data sources, and basic database queries, for example, SQL. Many registrars are sophisticated computer users already, and they will have a solid base from which to expand their skills.

Five Power Steps for Registrars to Prepare for the Future

The five power steps for registrars to prepare for the future are as follows:

- Keep abreast of IT and EHR changes.
- Strengthen computer skills.
- Establish a computer helper/mentor.
- Think positively about a faster pace and volume of changes.
- Develop and understand a prudent disaster recovery plan.

Previously, the question was asked: Will EHR and related computerization prove to be a labor-saving process, which also improves quality of data and care, or an unpleasant diversion that is difficult, requires a lot of learning, constant updating, fine-tuning, and continuing support? The answer in the end may be yes to both questions. The EHR will present short-term challenges and difficulties, but will also result in long-term improvements and gains for patient care.

References

1. Institute of Medicine. "The Computer-Based Patient Record: An Essential Technology for Health Care." September 1991. Washington, DC: Institute of Medicine-National Academy Press.
2. Rulan, V. "The Right Information at the Right Time," *Journal of AHIMA* 2009(Aug);80(8):10.
3. Obama-Biden 2008 Presidential Campaign Platform. "Barack Obama and Joe Biden's Plan to Lower Health Care Costs and Ensure Affordable, Accessible Health Coverage for All. Available at: http://www.barackobama.com/pdf/issues/HealthCareFullPlan.pdf. Last accessed July 1, 2010.

chapter 10

The Web and the Cancer Registry

Dan Curran, MS, CTR

Introduction

The Basics

The World Wide Web was created in 1991 and started to become popular in the mid-1990s.[1] By 2008, the Web had grown to more than *one trillion* pages, and now it is an essential tool for cancer registrars.[2] Together with the Web, Internet communication in the form of e-mail became indispensable for business communication.

This section covers an introduction to the Web and Web browsers, two important cancer registration Web sites, National Cancer Registrars Association (NCRA) and North American Association of Central Cancer Registries (NAACCR), a discussion on how to find information on the Web, the use of e-mail, collaboration tools, advanced Web topics, and the future of the Web.

Internet/Web Overview

The Web browser is the software tool that displays Web pages. There are several brands of browser such as Mozilla Firefox and Google Chrome, but they all have similar basic features. The most popular browser is Microsoft Internet Explorer, which is described in this chapter. The first browsers only displayed text and links to other pages called *hyperlinks*.

Hyperlinks

Hyperlinks are either displayed as underlined words or words that are a different color from the rest of the sentence. Clicking on the hyperlink will cause the browser to open another Web page. Images can also be hyperlinks. Hovering the mouse over text or images determines whether it is a hyperlink. Hyperlinked text or images will cause the mouse pointer, normally an arrow, to change into a hand pointing its finger.

Web Browser Basics

The Microsoft browser described in this chapter is Internet Explorer Version 7 (Figure 10-1).

The browser consists of a window that displays the Web page. A common feature of browsers are tabs; instead of launching a new browser, the user can click on an empty tab to reveal a new window. A single browser can display several tabs.

Surrounding the window are the various features that allow the user to interact with the browser. Each browser has its own set of features; however, the most common are as follows:

1. **Address Bar:** type in the Web address. The Web address or URL (Uniform Resource Locator) is a Web page's Internet address. Click on the down arrow on the right side of the Address Bar to list recently visited Web sites. Click on the listed site rather than typing it in again. An example of a URL is the one used by the NCRA: http://www.ncra-usa.org.

The components of the URL are:

- http—stands for HyperText Transfer Protocol. (https—some Web sites are secure and will have the "s" after the http. This commonly seen on e-commerce sites. Read the security information on the site before entering confidential information.)
- www—stands for World Wide Web
- ncra-usa.org—computer or "domain" name with the computer name suffixes. Some of the most common are as follows:
  .com—commercial
  .edu—educational
  .gov—government

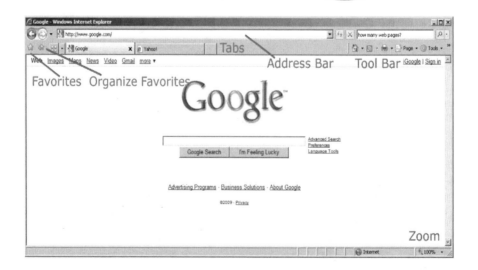

Figure 10-1. Internet Explorer 7

.mil—military
.net—networking
.org—noncommercial

It is a common practice to type in "http://www." before the domain name. However, the http:// is optional. Many sites can be reached by using the domain name alone, or the so-called naked domain. Ncra-usa.org would work as the "naked domain" for NCRA's Web site.

Why was ncra-usa.org chosen instead of ncra.org? Domain names are assigned on a first-come, first-served basis by companies called *domain registrars,* and another organization registered ncra.org first.

Typing in a new Web address in one tab will not affect the Web page displayed in another tab. In Figure 10-1, the Google home page is displayed in one Tab, whereas the Yahoo home page is hidden. Clicking on the Yahoo tab would display the Yahoo page.

2. **Zoom:** this feature is used to enlarge or reduce the window size of the Web page. Click down to zoom in or out. Select a value greater or less than 100%.

3. **Favorites:** the star icon (alone or with a plus sign in front) can be used to add and organize Web sites/pages that the user would like to visit again. Thus, the term *Favorites.* Examples of Favorites for cancer registrars would be links to NCRA, Surveillance, Epidemiology, and End Results, NAACCR, their state registry Web site, Social Security Death Index, the National Provider Identifier (NPI) site for physicians, and so on. Click on "Add to Favorites" (see Figure 10-2) to save a single Web address. Click on "Add Tab Group to Favorites" to save all open tabs. All tabs will open when chosen from Favorites.

4. **Organizing Favorites:** choose the Organize Favorites menu (Figure 10-3) to create new folders, rename existing folders and favorites, move favorites between folders, and delete folders. Think of the Favorites as files on a hard drive; it would be difficult to find files if they were not organized into folders. It is the same way with Favorites.

5. **Tool Bar:** contains icons that open various menus. Important icons include Home, which opens the home page. Print is for printing options. Tools are used to set preferences such as the following:

Setting the Home Page: The home page is the page that displays when the browser first opens. If using Internet Explorer, first browse to the desired home page. Next, click on the Tools menu and then Internet Options as seen in Figure 10-4. Click on the "Use current" button to set the home page.

6. **Other options:** Each browser brand will have its own array of options whose settings are generally adequate for most users. A couple of the more common options are as follows:

General: Besides setting the home page, the General tab also has a Delete button that will erase the browsing history, cookies, and other stored information. Cookies are small files stored on your computer that identify you to the site on your return. However, they may be used maliciously and so it is a good idea to use the Delete button after browsing if using a public computer. Regularly scanning your computer for malicious cookies is also recommended.

Security: The default security level may be changed here. Selecting less than the default or medium level is never a good idea, but increasing the security level may prevent you from using some Web site features. If only a few Web sites are blocked because of your security settings, but you trust the site, click the Sites button on this tab to add it as a trusted site.

Privacy: This tab controls how the Web browser deals with cookies. Overriding the default cookie handling may prevent you from processing Web payments or having your user name and password remembered at a Web site.

Programs: MS Internet Explorer defaults all programs such as e-mail and calendar to Microsoft products. Use this tab to select other programs.

Advanced Settings: These settings are best left alone unless you are an advanced user or directed by technical support staff. If a change in these settings ever cre-

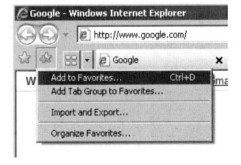

Figure 10-2. Add to Internet Explorer Favorites

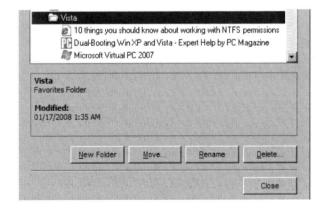

Figure 10-3. Organize Favorites

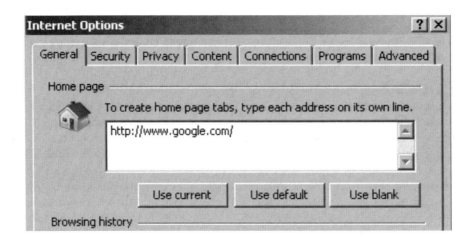

Figure 10-4. Setting the Home Page

ates a problem, you can select the "Restore advanced settings" button.

Further Information: The Expert Village Web site hosts a series of 21 free educational videos to assist learning Internet Explorer 7. The Web address is: http://www.expertvillage.com/video-series/579_using-windows-internet-explorer.htm

Use of Web Sites

The NCRA (www.ncra-usa.org) and NAACCR (www. naaccr.org) are the only two nation-wide membership organizations with Web sites for cancer registrars in the United States. These sites contain information that is useful for both members and nonmembers.

National Cancer Registrars Association

The NCRA Web site has a number of informative pages. Users can navigate the site by clicking the higher level links along the top two rows to go to major sections of the Web site, or click the links on the light blue vertical strip on the left. Some links will change color when placing the mouse over them, whereas others will show the link underlined. Links will not be revealed unless the mouse pointer is placed over them. Type in search terms in the field labeled "Search NCRA" in the upper right side of the home page.

Contents include:

- **NCRW** (National Cancer Registrars Week)—official press release, state proclamations, and celebration ideas
- **Annual conference**—online registration, link to hotel online reservations, registration brochure, and tour information
- **CTR exam**—link to www.ctrexam.org

- **CEs**—submit CEs online at the end of your 2-year cycle, application to get an educational program approved, and a list of NCRA-approved educational programs
- **Approved college programs**—list of NCRA-accredited programs that offer classes that satisfy eligibility requirements for the CTR Examination Eligibility Routes
- **Informatics brochure**—read the *Medical Informatics Basics for the Cancer Registry* brochure by the NCRA Education Foundation and the NCRA Cancer Informatics Committee
- **Job bank**—post a résumé or read job ads
- **Membership login**—access to the members-only area. Logging in to the NCRA Web site requires an NCRA ID number and a password, which is the first initial and last name, no spaces, and all lowercase.
- **Edit my profile**—update e-mail, address, phone number, and view the status of continuing education renewal and membership
- *The Connection*—read NCRA's newsletter
- **Archive**—view current and past editions of *The Connection* and *Journal of Registry Management*
- **Discussion forums**—each SIG (Special Interest Group) has its own section
- **Training**—sign up for live or archived Webinars on important topics such as CSv2
- **Other**—Membership Benefits Guide download, Membership Directory lookup, Membership Renewal

North American Association of Central Cancer Registries

Although the NAACCR organization is geared toward central registry topics, hospital registrars will benefit from the site as well. NAACCR provides the infrastructure for the standard-setting organizations to develop and harmonize data standards. The left dark blue vertical strip on the left lists links to the major sites. Placing the mouse pointer over section names will display the subsections, and then left clicking on the subsections will bring up a new Web page.

Some highlights of the site (www.naaccr.org) include:

About NAACCR

Committees: http://www.naaccr.org/MyNAACCR/public/committeelistpanel.aspx
Committees and their chairs' contact information are listed; click the committee name to link to a page with the committee's minutes, roster, and reports

Press releases: http://www.naaccr.org/About-NAACCR/PressReleases.aspx
Links to recent press releases and a link to the archived press releases

Employment opportunities: http://www.naaccr.org/Membership/JobOpportunities.aspx
Job listings

Cancer Data Standards

Data standards for cancer registries: http://www.naaccr.org/StandardsandRegistryOperations.aspx
Listing of NAACCR standards volumes that may be downloaded in .pdf format; included here is Volume V
(http://www.naaccr.org/StandardsandRegistry-Operations/VolumeV.aspx), the electronic pathology standard

Education and training:
Links to Webinars, In-Person Workshops, the Annual Meeting, and Online Training Modules

Research:
Links to research tools and data sets, such as the NAACCR CINA (Cancer in North America) Deluxe Data File; http://www.cancer-rates.info/naaccr/ is a link to the CINA+ Online Cancer in North America database

Other

The NAACCR Membership Directory, newsletter archive for *The Narrative,* and the NAACR calendar of events are available.

Just below the navigation menu is a white-colored field. Type in search terms and then the Search button below to return search results.

How to Find Information on the Web

The World Wide Web is like a giant library without a Dewey Decimal System. The sheer size and complexity of the Web, although one of its strengths, is also a source of frustration to Web users who have problems finding exactly what they want. If you have ever found too many or not enough sites, or have forgotten the site that you found last week, this section should help with several hints and tips.

Identify a Useful Links Page

Why go searching for valuable pages if your colleagues have already done the work? The NCRA links page (http://www.ncra-usa.org/i4a/pages/index.cfm?pageid=3312) has an extensive list of sites for the cancer registry professional. Your state's cancer registrar's association Web site is another good place to look.

Directories

Some companies such as Yahoo! have tried to make sense of the Web by creating a directory where the representative of the Web site chooses a category for the site. Instead of using www.yahoo.com, use http://dir.yahoo.com.

Click on the Directory link under "Select Search Category" and type in a generic search word such as cancer. Click on the Health: Diseases link, and then on Cancers when the new page comes up. Clicking on each category will reveal sites that have been organized under that category.

Advanced Search

Visitors to search engines will often type in a keyword or two and click on the Search button. A more effective strategy is to find the "Advanced Search" link and use the options presented for a more targeted search.

With www.google.com, for example, the Advanced Search options include searches that will return more results (with at least one of the words) or fewer results (all of the words, exact phrase, none of the words). Searches can also be limited to just text or links on the pages.

Bookmarks or Favorites

As mentioned earlier in this chapter, it is important to use the Bookmark (Firefox) or Favorites (Internet Explorer) menu to find valuable sites in the future.

Web Archives

It is frustrating to visit a Web site and return sometime later and realize that the content had been removed. Web archive services such as the Wayback Machine (www.archive.org/web/web.php) link to an earlier version of the desired Web site.

Management and Research Tools

It may be difficult to retrieve information from the Web with even the best organized and extensive Bookmarks or Favorites. The use of a Web research tool such as Evernote (www.evernote.com) can help. These tools make it easy to capture the information from a Web page, categorize it, and make notations about the information.

RSS Feeds

RSS (Really Simple Syndication) feeds are Web documents that can be subscribed to by using software called *newsreaders* or *aggregators*. An example of a newsreader may be found at the Google Web site (www.google.com). Click on the *more* link and then Reader to bring up the Google Reader.

Aggregators collect updated feeds and display them for the user. The feed displays like a regular Web page and usually has links back to the originating Web site. Currently, RSS is mostly implemented by Web logs and news sites, but governmental and central registry Web sites may use this technology as it becomes more commonplace. RSS's popularity with news sites suggests that RSS may be a good way for central cancer registries to distribute news press releases and other public relations materials.

To find the number of RSS feeds related to cancer, for example, go to www.google.com and type in the search criteria filetype:rss cancer.

As an example, note the RSS Feed symbol in the upper left corner of http://www2c.cdc.gov/podcasts/rss.asp. The links on the page can be used by software such as Google Reader.

Online Collaboration and Communication

The Web allows for collaboration between registry staff or cancer registry association volunteers who are not in the same office. Many options are available, but this chapter discusses only a couple software titles. However, the features mentioned are implemented in all of the major collaboration tools.

SharePoint

SharePoint is widely used in the corporate world, in part, because it is included with Windows server operating sys-

tems (OSs). There are a variety of configurations. Basically, a file can be set up for download only, or the file can be configured to allow those with sufficient permissions to "check out" the file for editing. Like a library, where a book that is checked out is not available to other patrons, the person who checks out the file in SharePoint is the only one who can edit the current version of the file. Once the file is edited and checked back in, others can now check it out.

Figure 10-5 displays a static list of files that may only be downloaded and not modified by the user. In this case, an administrator only wants to post information, and not collaborate with others. Clicking on the file name reveals a menu that allows the user to view the properties of the file, send it or download it, or set up an alert. Alerts are e-mail messages that are automatically sent to the user when a file is changed. Figure 10-6 displays the same menu, but because the permissions are set differently, the user can check out the file. The file can be saved to the local hard drive and then checked back in, as shown in Figure 10-7, or edited within the SharePoint space.

SharePoint also has a Workspace feature. It is an area designed for collaboration between members of a project team. The files can be checked out for modification. Other features include a calendar, task list, and discussion area for team members. See Figure 10-8 for an example of a SharePoint Workspace.

Google Sites

Google has a free version of file sharing called Sites. Browse to the www.google.com site. Click on the *more* link and then Sites to bring up Sites page. A Google login is required to set up a site, but members that you invite do not have to create a Google login, only a log in to the site.

As shown in Figure 10-9, the Google product can do much more than share files. Web pages can be created, different online applications called gadgets can be hosted on a page called a Dashboard, and task lists created.

Files posted to the site are tracked in a different way than SharePoint. The version number, as illustrated in Figure 10-10, is displayed in the far right column.

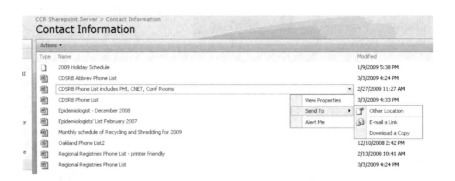

Figure 10-5. A File Directory in SharePoint Where the Files Can Only Be Downloaded and Not Checked Out or Modified

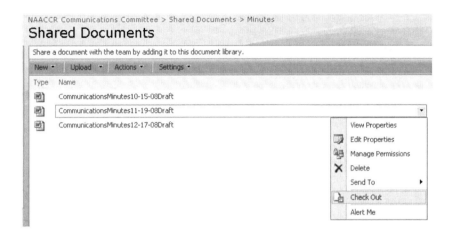

Figure 10-6. The Click Down Menu Is Being Used to Check Out a File from SharePoint

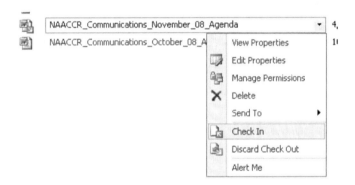

Figure 10-7. The Click Down Menu Is Being Used to Check in a File to SharePoint after It Was Modified

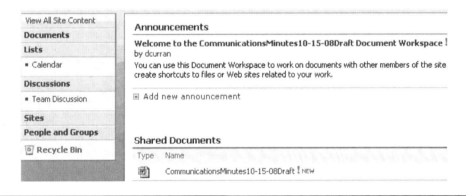

Figure 10-8. SharePoint Workspace with Files, Calendar, Task List, and Discussion Area

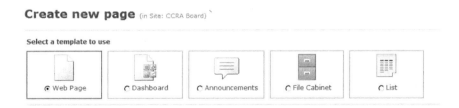

Figure 10-9. Web Page Options for Google Sites

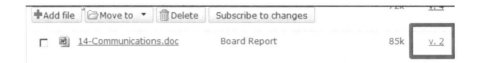

Figure 10-10. Google Sites File Folder

Version history for 14-Communications.doc

« Back to page

Version	Last edited	Edited by
Version 2 (current)	Jan 20, 2009 4:10 PM	Daniel Curran
Version 1	Jan 20, 2009 4:10 PM	Daniel Curran

Figure 10-11. Version History Example for Google Sites

Click on the version number to bring up the version history of the file, as shown in Figure 10-11. Older versions of the file are stored here.

Google Sites, like SharePoint, also allows the user to set up e-mail alerts when a file or folder is updated. Google Sites is not as feature-rich as SharePoint, but it could be used by cancer registrar associations to set up Web pages or file sharing sites for their boards or members.

Real-time Collaboration and Remote PC Control

Webex and GoToMeeting are well-known Web-based software products that allow two or more PCs to share documents or allow one person to control another's PCs.

Some common examples in the cancer registry field are:

- Sharing slides for Webinars, such as the NAACCR Webinar series
- Sharing a Microsoft Word document that is discussed over a teleconference line while one of the participants edits the document based on the discussion in real time
- A support technician gains control of the user's PC to help with a support issue regarding cancer data management software

A user who is logged in to one of these sessions is not in danger of losing control of his or her PC. A user has to request control from the other party, and once control is granted, it can be taken back by a mouse click. In Figure 10-12, windows from a brand of secure meeting software is shown. The window on the left shows options such as "Sharing," which when pressed displays the "Share Application" window on the right, and a disabled "Take Control" button, which would become active if another user joined the meeting.

Some software products have additional features. These include VOIP (Voice Over Internet Protocol) teleconferences, secure file transfer, and the ability to save the session and play it back like a movie.

A Technical Introduction to the Web

Web surfers are familiar with the .html or .htm extension of Web documents. HTML, or Hypertext Markup Language, is the common language of the World Wide Web. HTML uses a series of commands enclosed in less-than and greater-than signs that specify the appearance of the page. To see the Web page code in a Web browser, click on the Page menu and then on View Source (Internet Explorer), or View and then Page Source (Firefox).

Pure HTML code is static—the look of the page stays the same for all visitors to the Web site. However, a number of Web technologies allow Web pages to change depending on circumstances and the visitors' interaction with the site. This group of technologies is collectively known as Dynamic HTML, or DHTML.

The major technologies are listed here.

PHP: Hypertext Preprocessor

PHP stands for "PHP: Hypertext Preprocessor"—the acronym is part of the name. PHP is a script that augments the HTML code on a Web page. It is often used to interact with

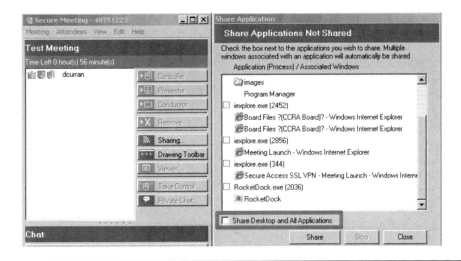

Figure 10-12. The Control Panel of Juniper, a Webex-like Software. The window on the right allows the user to select individual applications to share from his or her PC, or he or she can select the option in the red box that will share the entire desktop.

online databases, especially MySQL, a popular database use by Web developers. Both PHP and MySQL are examples of open-source software, which is developed by volunteers.

Active Server Pages

Active Server Pages (ASP) generate html pages from a server using scripts and display the pages with a .asp extension.

JavaScript and VBScript

JavaScript and VBScript are scripting languages that add dynamic and interactive features to Web sites such as navigation tools, forms, animation, and other multimedia displays.

Cascading Style Sheets

Cascading Style Sheets (CSS) are used by Web designers to apply style changes throughout a Web site by making a change to a single file. CSS may also be applied to make a dynamic navigation menu.

ColdFusion

ColdFusion is a Macromedia product that uses a language similar to HTML called ColdFusion Markup Language (CFML). ColdFusion is often used to interface with databases.

Common Gateway Interface

CGI, or Common Gateway Interface, is a standard interface for programs that are executed when called by Web pages. CGI programs are written in PERL, C, or other languages. These programs provide tools to Web sites such as bulletin boards, calendars, search engines, and guest books.

Use of Adobe Portable Document Format

Adobe Acrobat is recommended for publishing documents to the Web. Acrobat preserves the formatting of the original document, yet it is compact and can be secured. Acrobat Reader is available as a free download, so each visitor to a Web site will be able to view and print documents with the .pdf suffix. As you know, all of the national standard-setting organizations use Acrobat format.

Multimedia

There are two ways to receive video and audio from a Web site: (1) download the media file like any other file and open it in the appropriate viewer, or (2) receive it from a streaming media server.

Future Trends: Cloud Computing

When we think of software, we picture programs that have been installed from a CD, DVD, or some Internet source. The data that we enter or manage using the software are then stored on the PC hard drive or a server hard drive. But imagine software that is not installed on the PC and data that are not stored on hard drives owned by the registrar or their facility but rather by some third party. This is what cloud computing is all about.

A cloud has been used for a long time in network diagrams to represent the Internet. Cloud computing refers to the underlying infrastructure that provides computing services over the Internet.[3] Because a facility's resources are not used to provide the computing power behind the application or the data storage capacity with this computing model, the idea is that the cost of maintaining hardware and software will be less. The software and data storage are rented—software-as-a-service (commonly abbreviated as SAAS) as Google Apps (http://www.google.com/apps) calls it. Google Apps is an example of a software suite that resides completely in the cloud.

One of the components of Google Apps is Google Docs (http://docs.google.com), which is free to use and only requires registration. The document is edited within the Web browser and saved to Google's servers. It provides all of the basic word-processing functions. It may be all of the word-processing power needed for home or small business use.

If software like Google Apps was used at work, the user or IS/IT staff would never have to worry about installing the latest security update or updating to the latest version. But there could be potential pitfalls to renting software. John Dvorak, a columnist with *PC Magazine* (pcmag.com), mentions the possibilities of vendors going out of business or increasing prices.[4]

An even larger and overriding concern in cancer registration is the security of Protected Health Information. It could be that as security concerns are addressed, our hospital and central registry IT/IS departments will be willing to relinquish local control of data. However, as Dvorak also notes, computer hardware and particularly storage are extremely inexpensive right now, which would reduce some of the cost savings that would be realized from going with a third-party vendor.[5]

Major Players

Microsoft and Google are the major players in cloud computing. Microsoft has recently announced Azure, which they describe as a cloud OS.[6] Azure users will launch software that launches from Microsoft's servers rather than their own hard drive.

Microsoft touts the time savings from less maintenance and no need to install updates. PC-based OSs are still in Microsoft's future, however. The successor to Vista, Windows 7, will be a more familiar PC-based Windows OS.

Google's entry in the cloud OS is their Chrome Web browser.[7] A late 2010 release will come installed as an OS on some notebook computers. Google also has plans to integrate its online applications with Chrome. In addition, Google Gears[8] will allow developers to add more desktop-like features to their Web applications and allow for client-side databases.

Amazon Web Services (AWS; http://aws.amazon.com) is another important player. AWS is owned by the same company that owns the Amazon bookstore. It provides the infrastructure for many cloud-based companies. Years ago, a single computer or physical server would function as a single unit. Now it is possible for a single powerful physical server to host several virtual servers. Providers like AWS can increase a customer's server power on demand without having to add additional physical machines. At the same time, a customer would pay for less server power when the need decreases, thus saving the expense of paying for their own hardware that would sit idle when not needed.

Web 2.0

Cloud computing technologies have contributed to the evolution of the Web. Cloud-based software has given people the unprecedented ability to share information. Tim O'Reilly has given a brief definition of Web 2.0. He wrote, "Web 2.0 is the business revolution in the computer industry caused by the move to the internet as platform, and an attempt to understand the rules for success on that new platform. Chief among those rules is this: Build applications that harness network effects to get better the more people use them. (This is what I've elsewhere called harnessing collective intelligence.)[9]"

A classic example of a Web 2.0 application is Wikipedia.com. It is an encyclopedia where users develop and fact-check the content themselves. Myspace.com and Facebook.com are examples of social Web 2.0 sites. Linkedin.com is a professional networking site. Youtube.com is also a Web 2.0 site used to share video clips.

References

1. CERN—European Organization for Nuclear Research. "A Little History of the World Wide Web from 1960s to 1995." Available at: http://ref.web.cern.ch/ref/CERN/CNL/2001/001/www-history/. Accessed July 1, 2010.
2. The Official Google Blog. Available at: http://googleblog.blogspot.com/2008/07/we-knew-web-was-big.html. Accessed July 1, 2010.
3. Perry, G. "How Cloud & Utility Computing Are Different." Available at: http://gigaom.com/2008/02/28/how-cloud-utility-computing-are-different/. Accessed July 1, 2010.
4. Dvorak, J. "Straightening Out Cloud Computing," *PC Magazine*. Available at: http://www.pcmag.com/article2/0,2817,2329303,00.asp. Accessed July 1, 2010.
5. Dvorak, J. "Retro Computing and the Cloud." *PC Magazine*. Available at: http://www.pcmag.com/article2/0,2817,2337643,00.asp. Accessed July 1, 2010.
6. Raphael, J. "Microsoft Redefines the OS: Azure and Windows 7 Explained," *PC World Magazine*. Available at: http://www.pcworld.com/article/152899/microsoft_redefines_the_os_azure_and_windows_7_explained.html. Accessed July 1, 2010.
7. Bajarin, T. "Chrome's and OS, Not a Browser!" *PC Magazine*. Available at: http://www.pcmag.com/article2/0,2817,2330510,00.asp. Accessed July 1, 2010.
8. Hendrickson, M. "A Fresh Look at Google Gears." *Tech Crunch*. Available at: http://www.techcrunch.com/2008/10/04/googles-gears-not-just-for-offline-accessibility/. Accessed July 1, 2010.
9. O'Reilly, T. "O'Reilly Radar: Web 2.0 Compact Definition: Trying Again." Available at: http://radar.oreilly.com/archives/2006/12/web-20-compact-definition-tryi.html. Accessed July 1, 2010.

Operations

Donna M. Gress
Section Editor—Textbook

Carol Hahn Johnson
Section Editor—Review Guide

chapter 11

Casefinding

Mary Potts, RHIA, CPA, CTR
Jennifer Hafterson, BA, CTR
Wai Poon, CTR

To determine which cases are to be reported, the timeliness of and requirements for reporting abstracted data to various users, an organization needs to consider the purpose of the central registry, how the data will be used, the impact on procedures because of state, provincial, and territorial legislation, and the needs of the central registry and funding agencies. The information in this chapter is intended to help define these areas of responsibility.

Reportable Cases

Reportable List

The reportable list is the governing document for casefinding in the registry. The list should include all diagnoses that are to be reported and clarify the types of diagnoses that are not reportable. The Surveillance, Epidemiology, and End Results (SEER) Program of the National Cancer Institute (NCI) has historically established a standard for population-based registries in the United States, whereas the American College of Surgeons (ACoS) Commission on Cancer (CoC) has set the standard for hospital-based registries. The North American Association of Central Cancer Registries (NAACCR) published consensus standards in 1994.[1] These were subsequently adopted by the Centers for Disease Control and Prevention (CDC) as standards for their National Program of Cancer Registries (NPCR).

Reportable Diagnoses

Reportable cases usually include all carcinomas, sarcomas, melanomas, leukemias, and lymphomas with a behavior code of 2 or higher, and benign/borderline intracranial tumors with a behavior code of 0 or 1 as identified in the latest edition of the *International Classification of Diseases for Oncology* (ICD-O). NAACCR has adopted the third edition of ICD-O, known as ICD-O-3, as the standard effective for cases diagnosed January 1, 2001, and later.[2]

For example, the SEER Program's reportable list includes all benign/borderline intracranial tumors with a behavior code of 0 or 1 and all cases with a behavior code of 2 (in situ) or 3 (malignant) in ICD-O-3 with some exceptions.[3] The in situ and malignant diagnoses that are not reportable include the following:

- Malignant neoplasms, NOS (morphology codes 8000-8004) of nongenital skin (C44._)
- Epithelial carcinomas (8010-8045) of nongenital skin (C44._)
- Papillary and squamous cell carcinomas (8050-8082) of nongenital skin (C44._)
- Basal cell carcinomas (8090-8110) of any site except genital sites
- Cervix carcinoma in situ (any/2) and CIN III of the cervix (C53.0-C53.9) (cases diagnosed after January 1, 1996)

- Prostatic intraepithelial neoplasia, grade III (C61.9) (collection stopped effective with cases diagnosed 1/1/2001 and later)

Central registries sometimes include benign and borderline malignancies (behavior code 0 and 1) other than intracranial tumors if there is local interest in studying a particular disease. These diagnoses have been referred to as "reportable by agreement." Examples of reportable-by-agreement tumors include the following:

- Lung (C34._), bronchial adenoma, NOS (8140/1)
- Thyroid (C73.9), papillary adenoma, NOS (8260/0)
- Bladder (C67._), papilloma, NOS (8120/1)

Nonreportable Diagnoses

The central registry may also choose to maintain a list of frequently misclassified tumors; tumors submitted as reportable but on review were not. Such a list helps newer registrars properly determine reportability. A list of nonreportable diagnoses might include the following:

- In situ tumors (behavior code of 2) of the cervix (C53._)
- In situ or localized stage basal and squamous cell carcinoma of the skin (C44._)
- Papillary urothelial neoplasm of low malignant potential (PUNLMP) (C67._)

What to Report

Most central registries are population based, and as such, they are required to enter into the registry all reportable cases occurring in residents of the defined geographic reporting area, even if the patient is diagnosed and/or treated at a facility outside of the region. Although 100% registration is difficult to achieve, procedures must be in place to achieve the most complete coverage possible with the resources available. Clear and precise definitions of which cases are to be reported must be provided to all data collection sources. The definitions should address the following:

- *Reference date.* The central registry must select a reference date, usually January 1 of a year, from which its coverage begins. All cases diagnosed among area residents on or after the reference date must be included. As an example of a reporting rule, the central registry can require reporting of all hospital inpatients and outpatients who have active cancer or who are receiving cancer-directed treatment that were admitted on or after the central registry's reference date. This particular example means that a hospital treating a patient in January of the reference year must report the case to the central registry even if the patient may actually have been diagnosed earlier in December, before the central registry's reference date. Including patients with active disease who were diagnosed before the reference date will simplify future casefinding because such patients will continue to be seen frequently at health care facilities and potentially be included in the casefinding source records for several years. Because the casefinding source records are accounted for by the patient's earlier cancer record in the central registry database, no further investigation related to that primary needs to occur.

- *Diagnoses.* The central registry must develop a list of reportable diagnoses and distribute it to the reporting hospitals. An example of such a list is as follows: All diagnoses meeting the criteria of reportability of the NPCR and SEER programs, and these additional case types of local interest to researchers: adenocarcinoma of the cervix diagnosed 1/1/2006 forward and borderline ovarian cases diagnosed 1/1/2008 forward.

- *Residency.* The population-based registry must record all reportable diagnoses of residents of its defined reporting region but may also elect to register nonresidents. Collecting information on nonresidents facilitates sharing data with registries in neighboring regions (i.e., where formal agreements are in place or laws and confidentiality policies permit), simplifies death clearance processing, and allows preparation of individual hospital reports that include all of the hospital's cases. Rules should be developed to promote the consistent classification of reportability for groups whose residency status is ambiguous: snow birds, employees temporarily assigned outside the region, military personnel, college students, undocumented aliens, and prisoners. Wherever possible, rules that establish residency should be comparable with the U.S. Census Bureau rules to determine place of residence, so numerator definitions will be the same as the definitions for the population at risk when incidence rates are calculated.

- *Diagnostic confirmation.* Some central registries elect to register only pathologically confirmed cases. Most, however, also include clinically diagnosed cases. Explicit rules must be stated for each central registry.

- *Class of case.* Hospital registries are required to abstract analytic cases per CoC requirements. Patients who were diagnosed or who received any part of first course of treatment at a hospital are classified as analytic cases for that hospital. Although nonanalytic cases are not required to be abstracted by hospitals per the CoC, central registries may require a nonanalytic case from a hospital if the patient is a resident of the reporting region and the patient's cancer has not been previously reported as an analytic case by at least one facility. Examples of nonanalytic cases include the following: (1) a patient who receives non–first-course treatment for a cancer; (2) a patient pursuing a second opinion regarding first-course treatment options at a hospital, but receives the treatment at another facility; and (3) a patient with a history of cancer but who is being seen at a hospital for another condition.

Recognizing Differences in Hospital Reporting Requirements and the Impact on Central Registry Completeness

In general, all analytic cases for hospital registries for CoC accreditation are also reportable to state central registries, particularly if the state registry has data exchange agreements with other states. There are, however, additional case types required by NPCR/SEER, the two standard setters that provide the framework for minimum state reporting requirements. The reportable diagnosis list of the central registry should clearly state the case types that are additional to those required by the CoC and which hospital registrars frequently misclassify as not reportable to the central registry. Examples include:

- Autopsy-only cases
- Anal intraepithelial neoplasia (AIN III)
- Ductal intraepithelial neoplasia (DIN III)
- Lobular neoplasia and lobular intraepithelial neoplasia (LN/LIN III)
- Pancreatic intraepithelial neoplasia (PanIN III)
- Vagina intraepithelial neoplasia (VAIN III)
- Vulva intraepithelial neoplasia (VIN III)

The central registry should monitor the submission of these case types by the hospital registries and provide annual reminders that these case types are state reportable. In additional, central registries should be aware that hospital registries may collect additional case types of interest as specified by the hospital cancer committee.

Casefinding

The goal of the central registry is to identify and register all reportable cases. With an unlimited budget, the central registry could review every casefinding source available, both hospital and nonhospital sources. Funding, however, is limited for all central registries. An effective casefinding plan for the region must take into account the various characteristics of the reporting region. Examples of issues that impact casefinding include the following:

- Scope of legislative rules as to the casefinding sources the central registry can require and the clarity of legislative rules regarding the responsibility of health care providers in identifying and reporting cases to the central registry.
- Identifying and categorizing reporting entities: The casefinding plan may need to have different provisions based on the types of reporting entities.
- The types of casefinding sources available: To date, approximately 95% of cancer cases are histologically confirmed, which means that casefinding from

pathology sources is a good strategy for most cancer types. One needs to be aware, however, of which cancers may be under-reported from pathology sources and determine a plan for identifying those particular cases from other sources. In addition, as imaging technologies improve and other diagnostic tools evolve, other casefinding sources may become more important than they are today.

- Availability of electronic reporting of casefinding sources, particularly full-text pathology reports, and the ability of the central registry to process the electronic sources: Manual casefinding from hard-copy sources is labor intensive, and this may define the amount of casefinding that the central registry can perform.

Given the variation in the characteristics of reporting regions, there is no one best way in which to perform casefinding. Each central registry must determine which procedures promote the most complete reporting in the region given the current operating environment. The registry must also continually monitor the advances in the region's health care facilities and in central registry software applications to take advantage of new opportunities to improve casefinding completeness.

Legislative Rules

Although cancer is a reportable disease in all 50 states and the District of Columbia, there is variation in the legislative rules regarding the actual means of reporting cancer cases to the central registry in each state. Any strategic plan for casefinding must be supported by the reporting rules. If the rules lack the necessary clarity such that certain facilities, such as free-standing diagnostic centers, do not see themselves as being required to report casefinding sources to the central registry, then the central registry may need to go through the state's legislative rule-making process to include facilities that either diagnose or treat cancer patients. The central registry should, however, continue with its current casefinding plan within the scope of the existing reporting rules while work progresses on revising the rules to allow for an improved casefinding plan to be implemented.

The reporting rules should also have a forward view to them in terms of the mechanics of providing casefinding sources to the central registry. Although the capability of electronic reporting of casefinding sources varies greatly across health care facilities, the rules should state that health care facilities need to provide electronic sources as the capability becomes available. Legislative reporting rules are not opened for revision frequently, so it is up to the central registry to provide language that enables the registry to move toward the receipt of electronic casefinding source records even if the current casefinding procedures all involve hardcopy sources. Even if the current staff level of the central registry precludes the registry from performing 100% casefinding from all hospital and nonhospital

sources, the reporting rules, however, should still include the provision for the receipt of such sources for the central registry to perform selective casefinding on specific disease types or audits.

Types of Reporting Entities

The central registry needs to identify the various reporting entities within the geographic region and classify them. The casefinding plan for these entities will vary based on the legislative rules discussed earlier and the resources of the central registry.

- Hospitals
  - With CoC-approved cancer programs
  - Without CoC-approved cancer programs
- Free-standing pathology laboratories
  - Clients include one or more hospitals
  - Clients include physician offices or clinics
  - Clients include one or more hospitals and physician offices or clinics
- Dermatopathologists offices
- Free-standing radiation therapy centers
- Free-standing medical oncology centers
- Multispecialty clinics

Hospitals with CoC-approved cancer programs must have a hospital cancer registry with at least one certified tumor registrar (CTR).[4] The hospital registrar is the main contact person for the central registry to discuss casefinding responsibilities and audits. If the legislative rules permit, the central registry may obtain copies of the same casefinding sources, including pathology reports, which the hospital registrar receives to perform independent casefinding audits on all or some of the source records. Because some hospitals provide coding and billing services to individual physician offices, the central registry should confirm with the hospital registrar that the hospital registrar is providing to the central registry any nonhospital casefinding sources that might be beyond the scope of CoC reporting because such sources are needed by the central registry to ensure complete incidence reporting. In addition, the central registry needs to ensure that the hospital registrar's casefinding includes the identification of case types that are state reportable but not hospital reportable.

Hospitals without CoC-approved cancer programs generally do not have a hospital cancer registry, and the central registry typically must work with the Health Information Management (HIM) director to ensure that state reporting requirements for casefinding are met. The HIM department is also commonly referred to as the medical records department. The size of the hospital does not necessarily indicate whether a hospital has a CoC-approved cancer program. For example, a large health maintenance organization (HMO) system may not pursue CoC accreditation, whereas a small community hospital may be accredited. Again, legislative rules vary by state. Some states may require that all hospitals, CoC and non-CoC, of a certain size hire a CTR or contract with a healthcare staffing agency with CTRs to perform state-required casefinding and abstracting. Other states may require that non-CoC hospitals provide the casefinding sources to the central registry to perform the casefinding, and that the non-CoC hospitals are responsible for the abstracting of the specific cases identified by the central registry.

With free-standing pathology laboratories, the central registry must ensure that casefinding is occurring from the reports of all clients, both hospital and nonhospital, processed by the pathology laboratory staff. The central registry's casefinding plan should address whether central registry staff or pathology laboratory staff will perform the casefinding on the nonhospital pathology reports.

Some dermatologists are also pathologists who read their own slides and generate pathology reports. Some procedures previously requiring hospitalization are now performed in an outpatient surgery center setting, and this is true of procedures for the diagnosis and treatment of melanoma. Some state reporting rules mandate self-reporting of melanoma cases by dermatologists and dermatopathologists. Other state reporting rules mandate that the dermatologists and dermatopathologists provide their pathology reports to the central registry for casefinding, and that the physicians must provide additional information on the specific cases the central registry requests.

If there are any free-standing radiation oncology centers or medical oncology centers in the central registry's reporting region, the central registry must determine whether it will require the submission of casefinding sources from these facilities. First, do the reporting rules provide for such entities to provide casefinding sources, and second, does the central registry have the staff resources to perform all the casefinding, selected casefinding, or audits? Some central registries have the staffing resources available to perform casefinding of free-standing radiation therapy centers on a routine basis and may opt to perform selective casefinding or auditing on medical oncology centers.

The central registry's reporting region may have one or more multispecialty clinics. The size of the clinic and whether its cases can be identified from pathology reports at a free-standing pathology laboratory may determine whether a central registry pursues additional casefinding sources from the clinic if the reporting rules provide the option to obtain such casefinding sources from these facilities.

Sources of Cases

The two most important casefinding sources for both hospitals and central registries are pathology reports and the disease index. These two source types and their processing are described in greater detail in the next section. Pathology reports represent a "full-text" casefinding source document, which consists of patient identifiers (e.g., name, birth date, Social Security number, medical record number), health care provider identifiers (e.g., facility name and physician name), date of service (e.g., date specimen collected), and the full

text of the pathology report describing the specimen and the pathologist's description of the patient's reportable disease. The disease index represents a "codified" source document, which consists of patient identifiers, health care provider identifiers, date(s) of service, and one or more disease codes indicating that the patient's medical record should be reviewed for a reportable disease. A disease code, which is described in more detail in the Disease Index section later in this chapter, is not sufficient in itself to state that a patient has a reportable disease. Some of the casefinding sources listed later are full-text sources and others are codified sources.

Hospital Sources

- Pathology reports—review all surgical, autopsy, cytology, hematology, gynecologic, and cytogenetics reports. Also review all reference studies applicable to cancer diagnoses, such as immunohistochemistry, fluorescence in situ hybridization, flow cytometry, and other tests as they become available. Review the hospital and nonhospital pathology reports.
- Medical records reports—disease index and daily discharges
- Radiation oncology reports—radiation oncology log (if it is not included in the disease index) and/or treatment summaries
- Medical oncology reports—oncology therapy log (if it is not included in the disease index) and/or treatment summaries
- Outpatient records (if they are not included in the disease index)
- Other departments—surgery reports
- Diagnostic radiology reports—nuclear medicine log and reports and radiology (scan) log and reports.

Nonhospital Sources

- Pathology reports from free-standing pathology laboratories (review the same types of pathology reports as listed earlier)
- Disease index from outpatient centers such as private clinics, HMOs, and ambulatory surgery centers
- Disease index and/or full-text treatment summaries from free-standing outpatient cancer centers, such as radiation oncology centers and medical oncology centers
- Pathology reports from dermatologist offices for melanoma identification
- Disease index from hospices and nursing homes
- Death certificate file and/or hard-copy death certificates of residents with a cause of death from a reportable tumor
- Out-of-state data exchange with facilities, such as state registries, state departments of health, hospitals that serve as referral centers, and pathology laboratories in other states

Because most central registries rely on hospital registrars to identify cases from the hospital setting, central registry staff resources are often allocated to audit the casefinding of hospital registries and to perform most or all of the nonhospital casefinding. Examples of nonhospital cases include patients seen only in a physician's office or nursing home. Population-based registries must include nonhospital cases to have complete incidence statistics. With advances in cancer registry software applications, some central registries are able to perform 100% casefinding on all sources, hospital and nonhospital, if the majority of the casefinding source records are provided in an electronic format.

Pathology Reports

At a minimum, the central registry should pursue reporting from every pathology laboratory within the defined geographic coverage area because more than 95% of the cancer cases in the United States are histologically confirmed. If the state reporting rules provide for pathology laboratories to submit to both the central registry and the hospital registry, the central registry should require submissions. Some pathology laboratories provide services to physician offices in addition to their hospital clients. By obtaining 100% of the pathology reports in the region, the central registry can ensure the casefinding of histologically confirmed nonhospital cases and can perform up to 100% quality control on histologically confirmed hospital cases.

The Pathology Data Work Group of the NAACCR interoperability Ad Hoc Committee is responsible for maintaining the *Standards for Cancer Registries, Volume V: Pathology Laboratory Electronic Reporting*. Volume V[5] provides two recommended data formats for pathology laboratories to report electronically, an HL7 record format and an alternative pipe-delimited format. Selection criteria for reports to submit vary by state for central registry reporting and by hospital for their facility reporting. One method for automated report selection involves comparing the text of a pathology report against a list of words and phrases that indicate past or present existence of a reportable tumor. Additional methods, such as selecting from synoptic reporting data items, are evolving as more pathology reporting systems implement College of American Pathologists (CAP) cancer reporting protocols; however, a pathology laboratory may choose to continue to use a narrative style versus a synoptic style to meet the CAP protocols. Additional artificial intelligence is required for parsing discrete data items from narrative style. Hospital registrars should check with their state registries about the selection criteria used in their region, and they should check with their registry software vendors about the electronic pathology casefinding capabilities, current and planned, for the products used by the hospital registry.

Some hospital registrars will need to manually review their hospital's pathology reports because of the lack of an automated pathology casefinding system. Methods for this type of review vary by hospital. Some pathology laboratories provide hard copies of all anatomical pathology reports to the hospital registrar on a daily or weekly basis for the registrar to review for reportable cases. Other pathology laboratories may provide the hospital registrar with online access to newly completed pathology reports for an online review of reportability. Some central registries require that hospital registrars forward to the central registry copies (hardcopy or electronic) of the reportable pathology reports if the central registry is not already receiving these pathology reports directly from the laboratory.

Central registries may require low-volume pathology laboratories, particularly dermatopathologist offices, to submit hard-copy pathology reports if their laboratory information system lacks the capability to provide electronic files. Alternately, central registry staff may visit such laboratories on a scheduled basis to review the pathology reports onsite to identify potentially reportable cases. Such requirements vary by state and region. Although some of these facilities may offer to have their own staff perform the screening of pathology reports for the reportable diagnoses, the central registry should evaluate whether sending a staff member is feasible, both logistically and financially. Cancer registrars are specifically trained in identifying reportable cases; administrative and support staff members at pathology laboratories generally lack that training.

Disease Index

Casefinding applications for both hospital registries and central registries should include the ability to process disease index files. The hospital registrars should work with their medical records departments to obtain a monthly electronic disease index of patient encounters with one or more potentially reportable *International Classification of Diseases, 9th Revision, Clinical Modification* (ICD-9-CM) codes.[6] Central registries are responsible for providing to hospitals a list of the mandatory and optional ICD-9-CM codes that should be included for casefinding purposes per the reporting rules of the state or region. The Centers for Medicare & Medicaid Services posts the annual updates to the ICD-9-CM codes on its Web site. These updates are effective October 1st of every year and should be reviewed for new reportable codes. SEER maintains casefinding lists on its Web site of reportable ICD-9-CM codes. See Table 11-1 for the fiscal year 2009 casefinding list from SEER.

If the state reporting rules provide for hospitals to submit disease index files to both the central registry and the hospital registry, the central registry should require such submissions. This has become increasingly important because some hospitals provide coding and billing services to physicians' offices, which makes the disease index file another casefinding source for identifying and registering nonhospital cases. The disease index should include physician information so that the central registry can follow back to physician offices for these nonhospital

Table 11-1	Comprehensive ICD-9-CM^ Casefinding Code List for Reportable Tumors (Effective Date: 1/1/2009)^

ICD-9-CM Code^	Explanation of Code
140.0 – 208.9	Malignant Neoplasms
209.0 – 209.3	Neuroendocrine tumors (Effective date: 1/1/2009)
225.0 – 225.9	Benign neoplasm of brain and spinal cord neoplasm
227.3 – 227.4	Benign neoplasm of pituitary gland, pineal body, and other intracranial endocrine-related structures
227.9	Benign neoplasm; endocrine gland, site unspecified
228.02	Hemangioma; of intracranial structures
228.1	Lymphangioma, any site
230.0 – 234.9	Carcinoma in situ
236.0	Endometrial stroma, low grade (8931/1)
237.0 – 237.9	Neoplasm of uncertain behavior [borderline] of endocrine glands and nervous system
238.4	Polycythemia vera (9950/3)
238.6	Solitary plasmacytoma (9731/3)Extramedullary plasmacytoma (9734/3)
238.7	Other lymphatic and hematopoietic tissues (This code was discontinued as of 10/2006 but should be included in extract programs for quality control purposes)
238.71	Essential thrombocythemia (9962/3)
238.72	Low grade myelodysplastic syndrome lesions (includes 9980/3, 9982/3, 9985/3)
238.73	High grade myelodysplastic syndrome lesions (includes 9983/3)
238.74	Myelodysplastic syndrome with 5q deletion (9986/3)
238.75	Myelodysplastic syndrome, unspecified (9985/3)
238.76	Myelofibrosis with myeloid metaplasia (9961/3)
238.77	Post transplant lymphoproliferative disorder (9987/3)
238.79	Other lymphatic and hematopoietic tissues (includes 9960/3, 9961/3, 9970/1, 9931/3)
239.6	Neoplasms of unspecified nature, brain
239.7	Neoplasms of unspecified nature; endocrine glands and other parts of nervous system
259.2	Carcinoid Syndrome
259.8	Other specified endocrine disorders
273.2	Gamma heavy chain disease (9762/3); Franklin's disease (9762/3)
273.3	Waldenstrom macroglobulinemia (9761/3)
285.22	Anemia in neoplastic disease
288.3	Hypereosinophilic syndrome (9964/3)
289.83	Myelofibrosis (NOS) (9961/3)
289.89	Other specified diseases of blood and blood-forming
511.81	Malignant pleural effusion (code first malignant neoplasm if known)
789.51	Malignant ascites (code first malignant neoplasm if known)
795.06	Papanicolaou smear of cervix with cytologic evidence of malignancy
795.16	Papanicolaou smear of vagina with cytologic evidence of malignancy
795.76	Papanicolaou smear of anus with cytologic evidence of malignancy
V10.0 – V10.9	Personal history of malignancy (screen for recurrences, subsequent primaries, and/or subsequent treatment)

Certain *International Classification of Diseases, 9th Revision, Clinical Modification* (ICD-9-CM) codes used by medical records departments for discharge diagnoses identify cases of neoplasms that are reportable to the Surveillance, Epidemiology, and End Results (SEER) Program. Casefinding procedures should include the review of medical records coded with the values in the most current list available from SEER.

cases. Sometimes, a hospital programmer can modify the disease index report (electronic or hard copy) to identify the nonhospital cases if the hospital database has a designator in its database. Other times, the only practical means to identify the case as a nonhospital case is the lack of an actual medical record for the patient at the hospital.

Advances in hospital information systems are such that many hospitals use an enterprise-wide system that captures and stores records for inpatient and outpatient encounters, as well as radiation and medical oncology appointments. Some hospitals, however, maintain separate databases for inpatient, outpatient, radiation, and medical oncology records. The central registry and the hospital registrar should confirm with the programmer that all appropriate records are being reported to the central and hospital registries, whether from one extract program or multiple programs.

Hospital registrars should request that the programmer assigned to updating the extract program for the electronic disease index provide the registrar and the central registry with a copy of the programmed extract criteria for inclusion in their policy and procedures. The extract criteria should be reviewed carefully against the list of reportable ICD-9-CM codes to ensure that all required codes are being reported to the registry. Sometimes it is necessary to meet with the programmer to perform this comparison. In addition, the registrar and central registry staff should check the monthly disease index to ensure that patients with the newly identified codes are being included in the extract files. If no qualifying records are included in the monthly disease index file for any of the new codes, the registrar should ask the programmer to query the hospital information system to confirm that the extract program is working correctly.

For example, effective October 1, 2009, the code V10.9 was replaced by V10.90 and V10.91. If the extract program has not been modified appropriately, the patients coded to V10.90 and V10.91 are not being reported to the registry. Although the code V10.9 is no longer used as of October 1, 2009, the programmer should be instructed to keep that code in the extract criteria in case the central registry or the hospital registry requires that extract files for earlier months or years be resubmitted.

Because the central registry must identify patients with a past or present indication of a reportable disease, the central registry and the hospital registry may need different disease index reporting programs, with the central registry output file including both analytic and nonanalytic cases for the hospital registry. Examples of nonanalytic patients that the central registry needs to review includes the following patients: (1) those who may be presenting at the hospital for further management of the disease, (2) those who have a mention of a history of disease, or (3) those who are being seen at service/clinic that the hospital registry may not include in its definition of analytic cases. Therefore, the central registry disease index file may be much larger than the hospital registry's version.

Hospital registrars customizing their disease index for the hospital registry effort must take into account several factors. Most disease indices include other hospital services, such as emergency department visits, radiology encounters, cardiology testing encounters, and other services for that facility such as an endoscopy suite. The range of services can vary widely, and may include many specialty areas and clinic type services. It is essential to filter the medical indices by these options, or at least include them in the report. The common designations are by patient type major (acute/inpatient, outpatient), patient type minor (acute, day or outpatient surgery, outpatient services, psychiatric unit, home health), and service codes (outpatient surgery,

endoscopy procedures, emergency department, laboratory, radiology). Such ordering will assist the hospital registry in only reviewing the appropriate cases, minimizing time spent reviewing cases that are not meant to be included in the hospital casefinding process.

For example, if the facility does not perform casefinding from outpatient radiology tests, as that is not required by the CoC, then this service should be excluded from the report for hospital registry casefinding. (It still needs to be included in the report provided for central registry casefinding quality control.) Including the discharge code (home, transfer to another hospital, skilled nursing facility, expired) when running this report may assist both the hospital and the central registry in determining whether the patient was sent to another facility. Including procedure codes on the hospital registry casefinding report may help the hospital registry distinguish an analytic case from a nonanalytic case, such as a patient with a history of a cancer who is currently not under treatment, as seen by the procedure codes. Any help in distinguishing between cases that need to be reviewed and those that can be eliminated without a review can save the hospital registrar an enormous amount of valuable time. An in-depth review of the medical record indices criteria also can save valuable time for the hospital registrar.

On October 1, 2013, the *International Classification of Diseases, 10th Revision, Clinical Modification* (ICD-10-CM) codes will replace the ICD-9-CM code set. Reportability lists, extract programs for the hospital registries, and casefinding systems must be modified accordingly.

Availability of Electronic Sources and the Casefinding Process

For many central registries and hospital registries, electronic reporting and/or processing of casefinding source records are not yet possible. Processing hard-copy sources is more labor intensive because of the need to perform manual searches in the central registry database of each source record; however, the actual process of casefinding remains the same. Registries should check at least annually, if not more frequently, about whether sources have become available in an electronic format.

Regardless of whether a casefinding source is hard copy or electronic, each source record must be compared against the central registry database to answer the following three questions:

- Is the patient already in the central registry?
- Is the tumor reported for this patient?
- Does the tumor need to be reported from this facility in the form of an electronic NAACCR abstract?

The end result of the casefinding process is to create suspense lists for each facility of the cases for which the central registry expects an abstract. Cases remain on the suspense list for the facility until an abstract is received or until documentation is provided on the case informing the central registry that the case, on medical record review, is not reportable.

With electronic sources and the capability to process electronic sources, the central registry can expand its casefinding activities without adding more casefinding staff. The expansion of activities may include more frequent audits or audits with larger sample sizes of CoC hospital casefinding, and the addition of more nonhospital casefinding sources being processed.

A similar process takes places in the hospital registry but includes another process, which is follow-up. The questions for the hospital registry would include the following questions:

- Is the patient already in the hospital registry?
- Is the tumor reported for this patient?
- If the tumor is already in the hospital registry, does this provide new treatment information that must be added? Does this provide follow-up information that must be added?

Implementing Electronic Reporting of Casefinding Records

All registries, central and hospital, should pursue the submission of electronic casefinding records. More cancer registry database management systems are adding functionality for processing electronic casefinding records, and more health care facilities are implementing information systems capable of providing electronic files. For a central registry, it can take several years to achieve 100% electronic reporting from all facilities. The SEER Puget Sound registry in Seattle developed a regional electronic pathology reporting system in 1993 when several high-volume pathology laboratories in the Pacific Northwest implemented paperless systems and the last major laboratory in the region began submitting electronically in 2009.

One of the more difficult aspects of developing an electronic casefinding reporting system is negotiating the release of electronic data from each reporting facility. State reporting laws, reporting agreements between the central registry and the healthcare facilities, confidentiality agreements, transmittal and destruction procedures, security policies, and institutional review board approval are elements critical to negotiating release of electronic data. Often the negotiation activity takes more time and effort than the actual technical activities to implement electronic reporting by a facility.

The following items should be accomplished by the central registry before beginning negotiations:

1. Update state reporting rules, if necessary.
2. Update reporting agreements with the facilities to include provisions for electronic reporting. The agreement could include requirements for electronic reporting based on the facility's volume of reports.
3. Establish and maintain secure mechanisms for data transfer. Portable media, such as CD-ROMs and flash drives, should be avoided, as should unsecured e-mail systems. The central registry should investigate current standards for confidential file transfers and set up a system meeting those standards. For central registries that are departments within a larger organization (e.g., department of health, university system, cancer center), there may be information technology (IT) staff available from another department to help set up a system.
4. Define the frequency of reporting. This can be a function of a facility's volume of reports, with the frequency options being daily, weekly, or monthly. Monthly submissions may be the easiest to set up initially and monitor. After electronic reporting has been in place for a year, the central registry could request more frequent submissions based on the previous year's volume.
5. Define the data items for reporting and acceptable formats. Most state reporting rules do not yet include a mandated standard format for reporting; however, the central registry should have recommended formats to provide to the reporting facilities. If the reporting facilities cannot produce a file in one of the recommended formats, the central registry should consider whether to proceed with whatever format the facility can provide or continue with hard-copy reporting.

Review the NAACCR *Standards for Cancer Registries, Volume V: Pathology Laboratory Electronic Reporting*[5] for a detailed list of pathology reporting data items. The following list serves as a starting point for defining needed data items from disease index files.

a. Facility identifiers, such as National Provider Identifier (NPI), particularly if a facility provides records for more than one hospital
b. Patient identifiers: last name, first name, middle name, suffix, sex, date of birth, Social Security number
c. Patient address: street, city, state, zip, telephone number
d. Patient fields (additional): birthplace, race, occupation, insurance
e. Physician identifiers: last name, first name, NPI
f. Physician address: street, city, state, zip, telephone number
g. Date of service: visit date for outpatient disease index records, admission date for inpatient disease index records
h. Disease codes (allow for 20 occurrences in discrete fields)

After the data items are defined, establish a fixed column position format and a spreadsheet format that will work for the central registry software. The registry may need programming support to transform files submitted by reporting facilities into a format that the central registry software can process.

The programming support needed at the central registry for the ongoing processing of electronic casefinding records represents a smaller overall cost to the central registry than performing casefinding manually from hardcopy source documents.

Minimizing Disruptions in Reporting Source Documents

The central registry needs to survey data providers annually about upcoming changes to systems. When hospitals and pathology laboratories change vendor products or move from an in-house developed system to a vendor product, the facility staff may not remember to include the cancer reporting extract programs in the minimum specifications for the internal migration. Annually, the central registry should ask data providers if there will be any major system changes in the upcoming year.

Hospital registrars need to have representation at health information system stakeholder meetings either by being a member or ensuring that the HIM director has a list of items that the registry receives electronically or in hard-copy format, or both. Changes in systems can cause a serious disruption for casefinding, subsequently impacting the timeliness of abstracting.

Casefinding Timeliness

The planned use of the data and the reporting agencies to which the central registry reports determine the time frame for when casefinding, abstracting, and reporting must be done. Historically, the primary use of central registry data has been to support surveillance reporting on incidence, treatment, and survival. Under this model, time frames were determined based on when a complete year of incident cases would be available. The following current standards, from the *Standards for Cancer Registries, Volume III: Standards for Completeness, Quality Analysis, Management, Security and Confidentiality of Data*[7] reflect time frames supporting surveillance reporting.

- The NAACCR standard for reporting is that at least 95% of the expected cases of reportable cancer occurring in residents during that year should be reported within 23 months of the close of a diagnosis year.
- SEER central registries are required to provide complete counts of new cases for a calendar year within 22 months of the end of that calendar year.
- CDC's goal in its NPCR is that 90% of expected cases be available within 12 months of the close of the diagnosis year, and that 95% be available within 24 months.
- The CoC requires that 90% of cases be *abstracted* within 6 months of the date of first contact.

Currently, the timing of casefinding varies by central registry. Some central registries perform casefinding on

pathology reports on a monthly basis for every reporting facility, and process other casefinding sources, such as disease index files, in quarterly, semiannual, or annual batches. In this manner, the disease index file processing serves as a quality-control cross-check on histologically confirmed casefinding from pathology reports and as the primary means of initially identifying nonhistologically confirmed cases.

There is no mandated timeliness requirement for casefinding in a hospital. The convention is that casefinding precede abstracting. Most hospital registry staff try to case find pathology reports concurrently. The timeliness of performing this process depends on the hospital's abstracting time frame. If the hospital registrar abstracts near the 6-month deadline, there can be 5 to 6 months of cases identified from pathology included on the suspense file, and 3 to 5 months of cases identified from the disease index on the suspense file. Casefinding from the disease index typically lags behinds casefinding from pathology reports. However, abstracting at a 6-month timeframe is not ideal. Many hospital registries have opted to abstract concurrently. Under this process flow, pathology reports are reviewed concurrently, and the disease index must be reviewed monthly, as soon as the HIM department director indicates coding for the month has been completed.

Rapid case ascertainment is a consideration when specific case types are needed for epidemiologic protocols and for cancer conference presentations and clinical trials at hospitals. This rapid case ascertainment is also used for concurrent abstracting. Using this method, cases are usually identified for the central registry within 15 to 30 days after diagnosis or hospital admission. For example, the Rapid Case Ascertainment (RCA) Shared Resource at the Yale Cancer Center identifies new cancer cases in Connecticut within weeks of diagnosis. Similarly, the North Carolina Central Cancer Registry has an RCA system identifying cases within 1 month of diagnosis. Hospital registrars who perform concurrent abstracting, identify cases daily on receipt of the pathology report, and initiate the abstract within a day or two of the hospital or outpatient surgery discharge. This is especially true if the case is to be presented at cancer conference.

Typically, rapid case ascertainment is available only for a limited number of cases. For the majority of cases, central registries wait for hospital registries to submit abstracts and then the central registries pursues the nonhospital cases. This delay in reporting limits the use of the data.

As central registries and pathology laboratories partner to implement timely electronic reporting of pathology, more central registries will be able to perform rapid case ascertainment on greater volumes of cases. If the pathology laboratory has patient address as part of its database and its transmission to the central registry, incident cases from the pathology submission can be identified during the casefinding process. The core elements of an incident case are available from pathology reports describing biopsies and resections. An expanded casefinding model that identifies new incident cases from electronic pathology reports and also initially registers the cases from the minimal information available from pathology report is a model that would enable central registries to provide incident data sooner to meet the clinical and scientific needs of the future.

The SEER Puget Sound registry in Seattle has implemented such a system, referring to it as two-tier reporting. The first-tier report is the identification and registering of a new incident case from the process of casefinding the electronic pathology reports. The following minimum data items are coded from the pathology report(s): patient identifiers, address at diagnosis, diagnosis date, site, histology, laterality, available collaborative stage data items, available treatment data items, and healthcare provider (hospital, physician, or both). This first-tier report functions as a placeholder for the second-tier report: either an abstract from a hospital or information from a physician on a nonhospital case, sufficient to complete the case. The central registry generates suspense listings for the reporting hospitals and physicians, and the first-tier reported cases remain on the suspense listings until the hospitals and physicians officially report the cases.

The central registry of the future must broaden its base by identifying and obtaining cases at an earlier date to make the central registry data useful to clinicians. Two-tier reporting is one example of a paradigm shift in registry operations with the goal of the central registry being able to respond more quickly to the changing needs of the users of registry data.

This is similar to the shift in hospitals, where more timely data are needed by both the physicians and the administration.

Monitoring Casefinding Sources

Ensuring the timely submission and processing of casefinding sources is fundamental to ensuring timely abstracting. Whether the central registry performs 100% of the casefinding for a facility or audits the casefinding performed by the facility's staff, there should be a system in place for monitoring the receipt of casefinding sources and providing feedback to facilities of delinquent or incomplete sources. Similarly, hospital registries should monitor the receipt of their casefinding sources, particularly if they are dependent on other departments for those sources. At a minimum, the type of source, the date of receipt, the date range of included data, and the volume of received records should be maintained in a table, spreadsheet, or database. This will also help identify sources that do not provide useful information, or routinely identifies cases already found through other means. It will help the hospital registry choose the best casefinding sources and not waste time on others. In-

stances of decreased volume, either for a month or from year to year, should be investigated and reasons for those decreases documented. If the decrease was due to an error or problem, the casefinding data should be resubmitted as soon as possible. Examples of common problems include the following:

- Missed submission for a month
- Files from a previous submission re-sent for the current submission
- A data provider, such as a pathology laboratory, submits early one month and then in the following month fails to include the missed days from the previous submission: For example, a data provider submits data on June 25 because of an upcoming several week vacation and then on August 5 submits the file for July pathology reports, but neglects to submit the pathology reports for June 25 to 30.
- Failure to include the new ICD-9 codes that are implemented annually every October in the disease index extract programs: This is especially problematic if the extract programs specify individual disease codes instead of ranges of codes, such as 140.00 to 209.39. With a range, any new code created within that range will automatically be included in the extract program. For example, in October 2005, the code V58.1 (encounter for antineoplastic chemotherapy and immunotherapy) was replaced by V58.11 and V58.12. Extract programs that limited the selection criteria to V58.1 needed to be modified; however, extract programs using the range V58.00 to V58.99 automatically included the new disease codes.
- Failure by the data provider to run all expected extract programs for a given month: A secondary contact person running the extracts may inadvertently omit running one program, for example, if a pathology laboratory has separate extract programs for surgical and cytology reports.

These problems are most easily rectified when the central registry identifies the problem early and may be impossible to rectify if the problem remains undetected for a long period. If the problem is not identified within a year and the facility has changed information systems, the data may not be retrievable at all.

Tables 11-2 and 11-3 show simple grids used for recording the date of receipt for pathology submissions and disease index submissions from reporting facilities.

Monitoring the receipt of a casefinding file is the first step toward ensuring timeliness of reporting. The central registry should also monitor the volume of the monthly submissions. Abnormal increases or decreases should be investigated as soon as possible. An abnormal increase could indicate that cases had been missing in previous submissions. In Table 11-4, the volume of records substantially increased in December 2009. In discussions with the hospital registrar, the central registry learned that a new medi-

Table 11-2	Pathology Casefinding Source Reporting by Facility and the Month Required to Be Reported for 2009					
Institution	**Jan**	**Feb**	**Mar**	**Apr**	**May**	**Jun**
County general hospital	2/12/09	3/20/09	4/29/09	5/26/09	6/11/09	7/21/09
Community hospital	2/2/09	3/2/09	4/6/09	5/4/09	6/1/09	7/6/09
University hospital	2/2/09	3/2/09	4/7/09	5/7/09	6/9/09	7/20/09
Pathology laboratory Inc.	2/11/09	3/10/09	4/15/09	5/13/09	6/12/09	7/15/09
Health maintenance organization	2/17/09	4/10/09	4/10/09	5/11/09	7/8/09	7/8/09
Physicians' clinic	2/12/09	3/3/09	4/8/09	5/6/09	6/2/09	7/6/09

Table 11-3	Disease Index Casefinding Source Reporting by Facility and the Month Required to Be Reported for 2009					
Institution	**Jan**	**Feb**	**Mar**	**Apr**	**May**	**Jun**
County general hospital	3/16/09	3/16/09	4/9/09	6/12/09	6/16/09	7/30/09
Community hospital	3/24/09	4/15/09	5/15/09	6/19/09	7/15/09	8/17/09
University hospital	4/20/09	4/20/09	4/20/09	7/21/09	7/21/09	7/21/09
Health maintenance organization	3/17/09	4/14/09	4/14/09	5/27/09	6/16/09	7/21/09
Physicians' clinic	3/20/09	4/17/09	6/1/09	6/18/09	7/16/09	8/18/09

Table 11-4	Disease Index Casefinding Source Reporting by Month for 2007 to 2009 for Community Hospital														
Inst	**Year**	**Sum**	**Average**	**01**	**02**	**03**	**04**	**05**	**06**	**07**	**08**	**09**	**10**	**11**	**12**
060	2007	1,585	132	123	152	142	111	120	138	128	123	126	134	143	145
060	2008	1,592	132	137	119	140	128	132	118	108	151	139	128	145	147
060	2009	2,042	170	131	107	113	142	127	124	156	178	167	198	145	**454***

*Significant increase in volume of records compared to previous months. Must be investigated and verified, with documentation of reason for increase.

cal oncology center affiliated with the hospital opened in December, resulting in the increased volume.

In addition to checking the total volume of records submitted by month for disease index files, the central registry should develop reports to assess the completeness of reporting by disease code within the month. Table 11-5 is an example of a Source Record Report, which tallies source records by facility, date, and codes so that potential problems in the submission of casefinding sources from a facility can be identified. In this example, the hospital had lower than expected counts for the ICD-9-CM prostate code of 185, considering that the hospital is located in a county with one of the greatest rates of prostate cancer. The hospital registrar and hospital programmer compared the list of reportable ICD-9 codes with the codes being extracted by their disease index reporting program. They discovered that the central registry was receiving 185 codes only when the patient had another reportable code in the disease index record. In other words, the central registry was not receiving records when the only reportable code was 185. Because the majority of prostate cancer patients at this facility did not have a secondary cancer code, the result was that most of the prostate cases were not being submitted. The hospital programmer rewrote the extract program and resubmitted the data for 2007 to 2009. Table 11-6 shows the results of the resubmission for code 185.

Effective monitoring of casefinding sources may identify problems with casefinding earlier than retrospective casefinding audits.

Table 11-5		Disease Index Casefinding Source Reporting by Disease Code and Month for Community Hospital before Resubmission											
Code	Year	Year Sum	01	02	03	04	05	06	07	08	09	10	11	12
185*	2007	235*	12	23	22	14	18	24	20	15	17	18	22	30
	2008	56*	6	6	7	3	7	3	6	6	6	2	2	4
	2009	24*	7	4	2	2	0	3	1	2	2	0	2	0

*Counts for site code 185 by year show a decrease in 2008 and 2009 indicating potentially missed cases.

Table 11-6		Disease Index Casefinding Source Reporting by Disease Code and Month for Community Hospital after Resubmission											
Code	Year	Year Sum	01	02	03	04	05	06	07	08	09	10	11	12
185*	2007	249*	15	25	25	15	18	25	22	16	17	18	22	31
	2008	242*	21	22	20	23	21	15	22	19	20	20	20	19
	2009	220*	24	18	17	14	14	19	13	22	16	16	25	22

*New counts for site code 185 by year have now been corrected for 2008 and 2009 after investigation of the issue shown in Table 11-5.

Casefinding Audits and Death Clearance

As stated earlier, the central registry should pursue casefinding from pathology reports because most cancers are histologically confirmed; however, if the central registry has a means to processes disease indices electronically, such processing provides a cross-check on the pathology-based casefinding and provides a means for the central registry to identify the nonhistologically confirmed cases.

As stated previously, the expansion of casefinding into all types of nonhospital facilities would ensure more complete reporting; however, the central registry's ability to do so is limited by the financial resources available. Therefore, the registry should consider the following items when developing the casefinding methods for nonhospital facilities:

- The cost of accessing each type of nonhospital facility
- The quality of the data and the number of new incidence cases that would be obtained from each type of nonhospital facility
- The impact on the future use of the data if a decision is made not to collect data from a specific type of nonhospital facility

Central registries can use audits to obtain information on the above considerations for the nonhospital sources to determine the best use of central registry staff in performing nonhospital casefinding activities.

Auditing of hospital casefinding is a required activity. Central registries in the NPCR program must conduct casefinding and/or reabstracting audits from a sample of casefinding sources for each hospital-based reporting facility at least once every 5 years.[8] As stated earlier, some central registries perform 100% casefinding of hospital sources, independent of the casefinding performed by the hospital registries, effectively auditing every hospital every year.

All central registries are required to perform death clearance, which is the process of using the death certificates as a casefinding source. Death clearance serves as a regional casefinding audit in that one would expect the majority of cases to be identified from routine casefinding sources and processing. Death certificate files are similar to disease index files except that the causes of death are coded using the *International Classification of Diseases, 10th Revision* (ICD-10) coding scheme. The standard setters (SEER, NPCR, and NAACCR) have set benchmarks related to the volume of cases identified by death certificates only. The contractual standard for SEER registries is that no more than 1.5% of cases can be identified by death certificate only. NAACCR has standards of 3% for gold certification and 5% for silver certification.

A high death certificate only rate is typically a reflection of problems in routine casefinding procedures or casefinding source files, and the central registry needs to identify whether the problems are related to one of the following:

- The central registry's reportable list, used by all reporting facilities, is incomplete.
- One or more newly identified facilities have not begun reporting.
- A known facility has failed to report all required cases.

Death clearance provides the central registry with an annual opportunity to assess the effectiveness of its casefinding procedures. The central registry can also provide the hospital registrar with the identity of the specific cases missed during the hospital's routine casefinding procedures. This provides the hospital registrar an opportunity to determine why cases were originally missed and to improve their future casefinding processes.

Identifying New Sources

Because of the increasing capability of physicians to diagnose and/or treat patients in nonhospital settings for cancer, there is a growing need for the central registry to develop procedures for identifying new sources of cases. The procedures should include the following:

- Contacting state government agencies that license healthcare facilities and practitioners
- Contacting professional societies and associations
- Obtaining the NPI downloadable file[9] and searching by taxonomy code for individuals and organizations of interest within a geographic region; common examples include:

282N0000X	General Acute Care Hospital
291U0000X	Clinical Medical Laboratory
261QX0200X	Oncology Clinic/Center
261QX0203X	Oncology, Radiation Clinic/Center
207ND0900X	Dermatopathologist

- Reviewing pathology reports from tertiary care hospitals that require the original slides be reviewed by their own pathologists before the patient appointments for consultation; these pathology reports may have a "referred by" or "received from" statement identifying new reporting facilities or dermatopathologists within the region that might be potential new sources for cases
- Reviewing results of death clearance

Melanoma cases are difficult for registries to capture because dermatopathologists read their own slides. Because of the difficulty of capturing melanoma cases, for example, central registries should obtain listings of dermatologists in the region and survey them either by mail or telephone as to the pathology laboratory they use to process the biopsy or resection specimens. A similar survey could be made of urologists for capturing bladder and prostate cases. Such surveys can result in the identification of out-of-state pathology laboratories being used by in-area medical practitioners. These out-of-state facilities should be contacted to initiate reporting procedures.

Hospital registrars need to be proactive about anticipating the need to identify potential new casefinding sources. With new services opening, such as outpatient medical oncology and radiation oncology services, registrars need to confirm that they are receiving appropriate casefinding sources from the new units or affiliated practices.

Summary

Cancer registration is a dynamic field. Since 2001, there have been several changes to reporting requirements impacting casefinding:

2001	Expansion of the collection of hematopoietic diseases
2004	Inclusion of benign and borderline brain and central nervous system tumors
2007	Implementation of new multiple primary/histology (MP/H) rules
2010	Implementation of *2010 Hematopoietic and Lymphoid Neoplasm Case Reportability and Coding Manual,* which includes three histologies with proposed changes in behavior from /1 (borderline malignancy) to /3 (malignant)[10]

With each new reporting requirement, reporting rules, casefinding sources, and casefinding procedures must be reviewed to ensure that they adequately address the new requirements. This applies to the central registry, as well as the hospital registry.

In addition to the changes in reporting requirements, there are continual advances in information technology. Casefinding is one area in which further automation is needed at both the central registry and hospital level to enable registries to process multiple casefinding sources in a cost-effective manner in the pursuit of attaining timely and complete incidence reporting.

References

1. Seiffert, J., et al. *Standards for Cancer Registries, Volume III: Standards for Completeness, Quality Analysis and Management of Data.* Springfield, IL: North American Association of Central Cancer Registries, 2002.
2. Fritz, A., Percy, C., Jack, A., et al., editors. *International Disease Classification of Diseases for Oncology,* 3rd ed., U.S. final version, 2000 (ICD-O-3). Geneva, Switzerland: World Health Organization, 2000.
3. Johnson, C. H., Adamo, M., editors. *SEER Program Coding and Staging Manual 2007* (NIH Publication No. 07-5581). Bethesda, MD: National Cancer Institute, 2008.
4. Commission on Cancer. *Cancer Program Standards 2009,* revised edition. Chicago: American College of Surgeons, 2009.
5. Havener L, editor. *Standards for Cancer Registries, Volume V: Pathology Laboratory Electronic Reporting, Version 3.0.* Springfield, IL: North American Association of Central Cancer Registries, July 2009.
6. *International Classification of Diseases, 9th Revision, Clinical Modifications (ICD-9-CM),* 6th ed. Atlanta: Health and Human Services Department, Centers for Disease Control and Prevention, Centers for Medicare and Medicaid Services, 2009.

7. Hofferkamp, J., editor. *Standards for Cancer Registries, Volume III: Standards for Completeness, Quality Analysis, Management, Security and Confidentiality of Data.* Springfield, IL: North American Association of Central Cancer Registries, August 2008.

8. National Program of Cancer Registries, *Program Manual, Version 1.0.* Atlanta: Centers for Disease Control and Prevention, 2009.

9. Centers for Medicare & Medicaid Services. "National Provider Identifier Standard (NPI) Data Dissemination. Dissemination of Data from the National Plan and provider Enumeration System (NPPES)." Available at: http://www.cms.hhs.gov/NationalProvIdentStand/. Last accessed July 2010.

10. Johnson, C. H., Adamo, M., Peace, S., editors. *2010 Hematopoietic and Lymphoid Neoplasm Case Reportability and Coding Manual.* Bethesda, MD: National Cancer Institute, 2010.

chapter 12

General Principles of Abstracting

Melissa Pearson, CTR
Lois Dickie, CTR

One of the most important functions of a cancer registry is to provide an accurate account of the cancer experience by identifying and collecting information on all eligible cancer patients. The cancer registry abstract provides the means for the systematic and standardized collection of information for individuals diagnosed with cancer. An abstract is an abbreviated record that identifies the patient, the disease, the cancer directed treatment, and the disease process from the time of diagnosis until the patient's death.

The abstract also serves as the basic format to promote standardized data. The abstract is designed to allow the cancer registrar to meet the requirements for data collection by providing the structure for the data items that are to be collected, the length of the data field, and the valid codes that can be assigned to a particular data item. In cancer registries today, the abstract is in electronic database form with the ability to generate a paper version of the abstract. The data items collected in the abstract are categorized into six different sections, which are listed in Table 12-1. An example of an abstract with the common data items distributed among these different sections can be found in the accompanying review guide.

The abstract is the basis for the rest of the registry's functions. Without the summary data of a patient's cancer experience, no other registry function can take place. Data collection and abstract development should be based on the three major objectives of any cancer registry, which are listed in Table 12-2. One of the major responsibilities of the cancer registrar is the preparation of these abstracts.

Abstracting Process

The process of abstracting involves more than completing the abstract. The complete abstracting cycle requires the appropriate and thorough identification of all eligible patients and the gathering of pertinent information about the case.

The information must then be coded into a standardized data set, and steps must be taken to ensure the data are accurate and complete. Finally, the data must be submitted to the governing agencies to which the cancer registry is required to report. The cancer registry may report to one or more governing agencies, such as the Commission on Cancer (CoC) of the American College of Surgeons (ACoS), the Surveillance, Epidemiology, and End Results (SEER) Program, or a regional or state central cancer registry. How each step in the abstracting process is accomplished depends on the reporting requirements in effect for each agency and the procedures in place at each individual institution.

The cancer registrar is primarily responsible for performing the abstracting. Abstracting requires particular skills on the part of the cancer registrar. The cancer registrar must not only have a background in cancer registry operations, but must have medical knowledge of cancer, how it is diagnosed, and how it is treated. To do this competently, the cancer registrar must have knowledge of anatomy and the terminology used by clinicians, and an understanding of the cancer disease process. The cancer registrar works in a tremendously dynamic field. Cancer management is continually changing as advances in technology and more sophisticated tests provide more detailed information about the cancer. The cancer registrar must remain informed about the latest diagnostic and treatment methods through continuing education programs and self-directed learning.

The accuracy and completeness with which abstracting is performed is directly related to the value of the registry. Users of cancer registry data must be confident that the abstracted information is a true representation of the patient's demographics, diagnosis, and treatment. Reliable data are fundamental to a variety of research efforts, including those aimed at evaluating the effectiveness of cancer prevention, control, or treatment. It is the cancer registrar's responsibility to ensure the availability of com-

Table 12-1	Common Sections in a Cancer Registry Abstract
Patient identification	
Cancer identification	
Stage of disease at diagnosis	
First course of treatment	
Outcomes	
Case Administration	

Table 12-2	Three Major Objectives of a Cancer Registry
1. Identify and accession all cases meeting the criteria for inclusion in the registry in a manner that allows useful retrieval of the data.	
2. Develop and implement a quality-control program that will ensure data of unimpeachable quality.	
3. Disseminate the data while maintaining the patients' confidentiality.	

plete, timely, and high-quality cancer data that accurately represents the cancer burden.

Many of the components of the abstracting process such as casefinding, the suspense system, coding, staging, and quality control are discussed in more detail in other chapters of this textbook. This chapter provides a brief discussion related to abstracting.

Standards for Data Collection

Using standard data collecting rules and data definitions promotes uniform data. The primary value of data lies in the ability to compare the institution's data with data from other databases. Collection of the items to be compared must be made in the same manner using the same rules. For example, the CoC has published the *Facility Oncology Registry Data Standards (FORDS),* a data collection manual for CoC-accredited cancer programs.[1] This manual must be the basis of the data collection efforts of all CoC-accredited cancer programs. Use of the manual ensures that data collection is the same in all institutions and makes comparison of data more relevant. Each governing agency produces a data collection manual containing the rules and instructions for data that is submitted to their database. The cancer registry must ensure that all data collection efforts meet the reporting requirements of each governing agency to which it reports data.

It should be recognized from the beginning that accuracy and consistency are of utmost importance. Methods of ensuring the accuracy of data should be established early. Quality control begins at the time of abstracting by following the data standards. The cancer registry's procedure manual also serves as an important resource for ensuring consistent data collection. The procedures should provide direction for handling special or difficult issues that are specific to the institution. When data have been collected in a consistent manner, errors can be identified and corrected more easily. The procedures should also have a place to document changes in reporting and data collection requirements over time. Reports and studies containing cancer registry data will often span many years. Knowing when requirements changed during that time frame can assist in interpreting the results of the reports.

Abstracting requires the use of a variety of reference manuals. Some are necessary for proper abstracting, whereas others serve to aid in the process. The reference manuals a cancer registrar uses may vary depending on the requirements of the governing agency to which the registry reports. At a minimum, the registry should have pertinent medical reference books such as anatomy and medical terminology textbooks. The registry should also secure the latest information regarding regional or state registry requirements. Table 12-3 lists the widely used coding and staging manuals.

The cancer registrar must take an active approach in monitoring updates from the publishers of data collection manuals and incorporating changes in data collection standards. Because cancer registry data are so specialized and coded in such detail, manuals and coding instructions are continually being evaluated. Periodically, revisions to manuals are released. It is important that these revisions are incorporated so that the most current information is being used to collect the data.

Abstracting Time Frame

The abstracting time frame defines the interval of time between a patient's initial contact with the institution with a reportable diagnosis and the completion of the abstract. Abstracting timeliness encompasses a delicate balance between making information available as soon after contact as possible and providing complete diagnosis and treatment information that may not be completed until several months later. Availability of information and intended use

---

Table 12-3	Widely Used Coding and Staging Manuals

Cancer registrars may be required to use more than one staging and data collection manual depending on the governing agencies to which the registry reports. As of 2010, the standard coding and staging manuals used in hospital and central cancer registries are as follows:

- *2007 Multiple Primary and Histology Coding Rules Manual*
- *AJCC Cancer Staging Manual,* 7th edition
- *Collaborative Stage Data Collection System,* version 2
- *Facility Oncology Registry Data Standards,* Revised for 2010
- *International Classification of Disease for Oncology,* 3rd edition
- *SEER Coding and Staging Manual*
- *SEER *Rx – Interactive Antineoplastic Drugs Database*
- *SEER Hematopoietic Database and Manual*
- *SEER Summary Staging Manual 2000*

of the data are key factors in determining the abstracting time frame. The users of the data must be considered when making this decision. It is important for the cancer committee, administration, or other healthcare professionals to have access to current statistics collected in the cancer registry. As healthcare environments change, analysis of cases diagnosed or treated in the institution has become increasingly important to administrators.

Each governing agency specifies the maximum time frame for completing the abstract for each case of cancer. For institutions accredited by the CoC, the abstract must be completed within 6 months of the date of first contact with the institution.[2] A patient can enter into the care of the institution at any point in time during the disease course, which may be months or even years after the initial diagnosis. Therefore, abstracting timeliness is based on the date of first contact with the institution as opposed to the date of diagnosis. For completion of the abstract, typically, the complete workup, cancer staging, and planned first course of treatment have been determined within this 6-month period. For treatment that has not been completed, special codes and data items are available in the abstract to indicate that the treatment was recommended. This allows the abstract to be marked complete within the required time frame while waiting for treatment to be completed. In addition to the CoC requirements, each state central cancer registry also has established time frames for when abstracts must be completed that may differ from the CoC requirements.

Many cancer registries strive to abstract cases as soon as possible, abstracting cases within 2 to 4 months, as opposed to the maximum time frame of 6 months of the date of first contact. This not only allows for the availability of more timely information, but allows for flexibility in the event of unforeseen issues or problems that could cause the cancer registry to become delinquent in abstracting. Software conversions, computer problems, staffing vacancies, preparation of submission files, and the addition of special projects are situations the cancer registry must anticipate and plan for in determining the schedule for completing abstracts.

Some cancer registries find it more desirable to concurrently abstract cases. Concurrent abstracting is a process of completing the abstract as information becomes available. Information can be abstracted when a patient is discharged from the hospital and then information from later visits or from outside sources can be added as it becomes available. Concurrent abstracting can have many benefits. Key information about cancer cases can be more readily accessible for reports. The abstract will also have the benefit of being reviewed several times before being marked complete, which can increase data quality. However, the cancer registrar must make sure that the most definitive information has been recorded. For example, the stage that was based on the information available at the time of discharge may change if additional studies are performed after discharge. With any abstracting process, it is critical to establish a procedure for tracking abstracts that are waiting for more complete information and ensuring that additional information is added to the abstract. Some treatment may be done in freestanding facilities, or the cancer registrar may need to contact the physician to obtain additional information for case completeness.

Methods for obtaining information within a shorter period are continually being explored. Current data collection and submission mechanisms result in data being collected and reported retrospectively. Aggregated state- and national-level data may not be available for use until 2 years after the year of diagnosis, by which any analysis would be based on past performances. The need for more readily available, real-time information is continually increasing. In certain studies using cancer data, the need for this information demands that selected information be reported soon after diagnosis, usually before the entire abstract can be completed.

The rapid case ascertainment (RCA) study protocols and the CoC's Rapid Quality Reporting System (RQRS) are two examples where selected information is reported shortly after initial contact, which is usually before the standard abstracting time frame. RCA is an acceleration of the central cancer registry's reporting process for selected cancers, reducing the reporting time for selected information such as demographics, physicians, and pathology report findings. RCA supports population-based epidemiology research, and facilitates cancer prevention and control research that requires early contact with patients. The CoC's RQRS enables accredited cancer programs to report data on patients with breast and colon cancer concurrently to facilitate quality improvement measures that will encourage good-quality, evidence-based care in a timely manner at the local level. The RQRS allows for the collection of minimum data elements necessary for breast and colon cancers to support ongoing quality-assurance programs and to evaluate and compare variations in care that are delivered to these patients. These breast and colon cancer cases are extracted in a separate file from the registry's database and transmitted to the RQRS on a locally determined schedule, which can be as soon as the day after diagnosis, allowing for real-time quality-of-care assessments.

Regardless of the method used for completing the abstract, a procedure must be in place to ensure the cancer registry abstract is complete within the required time frame specified by each governing agency. The procedure must also take into consideration other activities that may affect the abstracting time frame, such as participation in the RCA or RQRS programs, or other special studies. It is important that all these requirements be taken into consideration when determining the most feasible process for completing the abstract. The procedure should also include the process for identifying cases with incomplete information and ensuring that information is added to abstract once it is available. It is important to ensure data (especially patient treatment) are complete and accurate, and an established procedure will document the process. Analysis of first course of therapy cannot be made until all data are collected and recorded.

Suspense System

Before an abstract can be prepared, cases that are eligible for the database must be identified. This process, called *casefinding* (or *case ascertainment*), identifies all potential cases for inclusion in the cancer registry database through a systematic review of pathology reports, disease indices, and treatment summaries. Potential cases that are identified are maintained in the suspense system until the final determination is made that the case is reportable and the case is ready to be completely abstracted.

In most cancer registry software systems, the suspense system consists of partial abstracts that contain minimum information about potential cases. This typically includes patient name, patient identifier, date of diagnosis or date of first contact, and primary site.[2] The cancer registrar enters this information into the cancer registry database and saves the case as a suspense case, which is a potentially reportable case awaiting completion. Cases are often identified from multiple casefinding sources. For example, the cancer registry may receive a pathology report for a patient and the same patient will be listed on the disease index. The automated suspense system in the cancer registry software allows for the information identified from multiple casefinding sources on the same patient to be consolidated into one partial abstract.

Each case in the suspense system must then be reviewed in more detail to determine whether it is reportable. Before the final determination is made, a review of the complete medical record or other source documents may be required. If reportable, the case is abstracted. If not, the case is removed from the suspense system. For a person with more than one primary cancer, a separate abstract is prepared for each independent cancer diagnosis. The Multiple Primary and Histology Coding Manual should be used to make a determination as to how many abstracts should be prepared. The cancer registry software should be able to generate a listing of all suspense cases. This allows the cancer registry to monitor the number of cases waiting to be abstracted and ensure that identified cases are completed within the required time frame.

Abstract Sections and the Data Set

The information that follows is an overview of certain items included in cancer registry abstracts and where the information can be found in the health record. The data items the cancer registry is required to collect are deter-mined by the governing agencies to which the cancer registry reports. A complete list and definition of each data item can be found in the *FORDS* or other appropriate data manuals.

Patient Identification

The patient identification section consists of the following data items that identify the patient or descriptors: accession number, sequence number, medical record number, Social Security number, patient's name, patient's address at diagnosis, place of birth, date of birth, race, Spanish origin, sex, primary payer at diagnosis, comorbidities and complications, and the physicians who were involved in the diagnosis and treatment of this cancer.

Most of the information to complete the patient identification data items is usually found on the admission registration form or the institution's cover sheet (face sheet) for a patient's health record. The date of birth and Social Security number are important for matching cases or avoiding duplicates, updating follow-up information, and matching deaths from state death listings.

Demographics

The demographic data collected by cancer registrars refer to selected population characteristics that are used in cancer research and also by healthcare providers for marketing purposes. Commonly used demographics used in cancer research include race, age, sex, and geographic location. By collecting consistent demographic data over time, researchers will be able to follow trends. The collection of accurate demographic information is an important function of the cancer registrar, and every effort should be taken to collect these data items.

Most of the information needed to code demographics will be found in the admission form or the cover sheet. Other locations where this information may be found are the history and physical or in the physician consultation notes.

Accession Number

The accession number is a unique nine-digit number assigned to the patient. It is usually generated by the computer software. The first four digits of the number indicate the year in which the patient was first seen for cancer in the reporting institution. The rest of the number is the sequential order in which the patient was identified by the registry or abstracted into the database. For example, if a patient had a positive biopsy in January 2010 and was the first case identified in 2010, the accession number would be 20100001. It is important to assign accession numbers that include the year in which the patient was first seen in the institution. If, somehow, the patient was not identified for inclusion into the registry until a later year, the accession number should still begin with 2010. Because the accession number identifies the patient, the same number is used for all additional primaries that the patient may develop, regardless of the year in which subsequent reportable tumors occur.

Sequence Number

The sequence number identifies separate primaries for each patient. The sequence number allows the registry to identify patients who have multiple primaries. Sequence numbers range from 00 to 88, as well as code 99, and are divided into two groups. Sequence numbers in the range of 00 to 59, as well as code 99, are to be used for histologies with a behavior code of 2 (in situ) or 3 (malignant). If the patient has only one malignant primary cancer, the sequence number is 00. If the patient has more than one malignant primary cancer, 00 is changed to 01 to indicate that this is the first of several or more malignant primaries. Each subsequent primary is labeled according to the sequence in which it occurred.

Sequence numbers in the range of 60 to 88 are assigned to histologies with a behavior code of /0 (benign) or /1 (borderline). This range includes the nonmalignant central nervous system tumors. The rules for this range of codes are the same in that a code of 60 is assigned if the patient has one and only one nonmalignant primary tumor and should be changed to 61 if the patient is diagnosed with a subsequent nonmalignant primary tumor. When determining the sequence number, these two groups of codes are assigned independent of each other.

Notably, the sequence number indicates the number of primary cancers the patient has had in his or her lifetime, not just the number of primary cancers diagnosed or treated at the reporting institution. For example, if a patient is diagnosed or treated at the reporting institution for lung cancer and has a history of breast cancer diagnosed and treated elsewhere, the institution would assign the lung cancer a sequence number of 02 to reflect the fact that it is the second primary for the patient.

Physicians and Institutions Involved with the Case

The names of all physicians involved with the case (such as surgeons and referring, consulting, and following physicians) should be recorded. This information is useful in obtaining additional information regarding complete first course of treatment and follow-up or patient status for outcome reporting. This information can also be used in administrative reports about physician activity or referrals.

Cancer Identification

The cancer identification section contains data items that describe the disease and contains additional administrative information: class of case, facility referred from, facility referred to, date of first contact, date of initial diagnosis, primary site, laterality, histology, behavior code, grade/differentiation, diagnostic confirmation, tumor size, regional lymph nodes examined, and regional lymph nodes positive. The data elements "facility referred from" and "facility referred to" establish patterns of referral, which can be used by administration to identify patient migration patterns. Categories of patients referred from certain areas can be further defined and analyzed by creating subgroups using age, ethnicity, primary payer at diagnosis, and so on. This information can be used in developing marketing strategies and in program planning.

The admission history, physical examinations, radiology studies, and laboratory studies performed during the current admission and any earlier admissions are the sources of information used to determine the site, histology, and stage. The admission history and physical may provide clues to where the workup was done before admission. The admitting diagnosis is used to determine whether the diagnosis of cancer has already been made and the patient is being admitted for confirmation or whether the diagnosis is currently unknown. For some sites, the physical examination may provide information about laterality. It is important to look for copies of, or reference to, outside studies in the patient's record.

Class of Case

The class of case data item categorizes cases for analysis purposes and is used to indicate the type of interaction the patient had with the reporting institution. Class of case identifies the case as either analytic (codes 00–22) or nonanalytic (codes 30–49 and 99). The codes can be used to identify which patients were seen for initial diagnosis, for first course of treatment, or were seen after their initial diagnosis and treatment. Analytic means that the reporting institution participated in initially diagnosing and/or delivering all or part of the first course of treatment. Assigning class of case correctly has a significant effect on the administrative reports that identify the use of the institution's service areas.

Class of case is one of the criteria for determining whether a case should be included in the database. The CoC requires class of case 00 to 22 to be abstracted. Depending on the governing agencies the cancer registry reports to, the cancer registry may be required to collect some of the nonanalytic class of case categories. For example, for complete case ascertainment, central cancer registries may require that cases in the 30 to 38 range be abstracted and reported to the central database. Cancer registries must be sure that all of the requirements of the governing agencies being reported to are met.

Date of Initial Diagnosis

The date of initial diagnosis is an extremely important data item in the abstract. The data of initial diagnosis serves as a reference date for the cancer as it is the first time a medical practitioner confirms the presence of cancer. Quite often, it is the date of a pathology report, but it may also be based on a laboratory value, radiology report, or physical examination of the patient before biopsy. The cancer registrar should look for ambiguous terms that indicate a diagnosis—for example, terms such as *suspicious* and probable in reports and studies. A complete list of ambiguous terminology is defined in the *FORDS* to ensure consistency in establishing the date of diagnosis.

Primary Site and Histology

The primary site and histology data items identify, confirm, and support the body organ or tissue where the tumor originated and the cell type of the primary tumor. The pathology report contains the most definitive information about the histology and is helpful in assigning the correct ICD-O-3 codes for the primary site, histology, behavior, and grade. In addition, physical examinations, radiologic studies and endoscopic evaluations (such as a colonoscopy) may also lend information for determining the primary site.

Coding the primary site and histology as specifically as possible is essential. For most cancers, the staging scheme and surgery codes that are to be used are based on the primary site. For certain types of cancers, the staging scheme is determined by the histology. For example, lymphoma and Kaposi sarcoma of any primary site are schemes that are histology dependent.

Stage of Disease at Diagnosis

The section for stage of disease at diagnosis contains the data items that identify, confirm, and support the assigned stage of disease: surgical diagnostic and staging procedure, American Joint Committee on Cancer (AJCC) clinical and pathologic TNM elements, SEER Summary Stage 2000, and Collaborative Stage data elements. The staging information must include the assessment of three components: tumor (T), node (N), and metastasis (M), which have numerical subsets. In effect, the system is a shorthand notation for describing the clinical and/or pathologic anatomic extent of a particular malignant tumor at diagnosis. A clinical or pathologic stage group is determined from these three components.[3] Cancer registrars use the data elements in the Collaborative Stage Data Collection System (CS) to record specific information about the cancer. This information can then be derived into the AJCC TNM and SEER Summary Staging systems that would meet the needs of all of the various agencies that use staging information.

The most common and accurate method to stage most cancers is the pathologic examination of the resected tumor. The physical examination provides information about physical findings, symptoms, and palpable areas of involvement by tumor. Radiologic studies often provide the clinical information to stage a patient. Depending on the location of the primary site, endoscopic evaluations

are another clinical tool to document information for stage of disease. If the patient is deemed unresectable, this may be the only information to base the stage of disease. The discharge summary should summarize all clinical and pathologic findings together with the stage of the cancer. However, the cancer registrar should make certain that all of the necessary information has been included. Often, all of the workup may not be completed or the final pathology report may be awaiting the results of a consultation. This could result in a different diagnosis and stage assignment.

First Course of Treatment

This section contains data items that describe the surgical procedures, radiation therapy, chemotherapy, hormonal therapy, immunotherapy, hematologic transplant and endocrine procedures, as well as palliative procedures. All treatment information should be recorded according to the definitions in the data collection manual.

Determining first course of treatment can be difficult. First course of therapy is the treatment that is either given or planned at the time of initial diagnosis. Setting a limit of time for initiation of treatment is no longer appropriate. Some treatment regimens may take a year or more to complete. An example of an extended first course of treatment plan would be a patient diagnosed with inflammatory carcinoma of the breast. The patient is diagnosed by biopsy and treated with several cycles of chemotherapy (which may take 5 months or longer). At that time, a mastectomy may be done. After the patient has recovered from the mastectomy, radiotherapy may be given. If all of this treatment was planned when the patient was initially diagnosed, it should be included in the first course of therapy.

The opposite situation can also happen. A patient may come in with a primary tumor of the colon. Diagnostic workup may include liver function studies and other tests that indicate no metastatic disease. Surgery would be complete removal of the primary tumor. If, at the 6-week postoperative checkup, liver function studies are abnormal and a scan shows hepatic metastases, the patient would be placed on chemotherapy. The chemotherapy was not planned at the time of initial diagnosis. The chemotherapy was given because of disease progression or recurrence. The second course of therapy is treatment initiated either because the disease did not respond to the first treatment, or because the disease progressed or recurred.

Outcomes

The outcomes section consists of the follow-up data items: date of first recurrence, type of first recurrence, date of last contact or death, vital status, cancer status, following registry, follow-up source, and next follow-up source.

The date of first recurrence has increased in importance as quality of survival is being studied more intensely. In some cases, the goal may be to delay recurrence rather than to prevent it. The date of first recurrence is determined by a physician and always follows a disease-free interval (the patient must be completely free of disease before a recurrence can be recorded).

If a date of first recurrence is reported, the type of first recurrence must also be recorded. This may be local recurrence, which is recurrence of the primary tumor itself, regional recurrence, which is recurrence beyond the limits of the organ of origin, or distant recurrence, which is disseminated recurrence or recurrence that is remote from the original primary tumor.

Follow-up data include the name, address, telephone number, and relationship of a relative, friend, or neighbor who is most likely to know how to locate the patient. Multiple listings for contacts are common. The name of the spouse should be recorded for married adults and the next of kin for children. These data items can usually be found on the institution's registration form or cover sheet (also called the *face sheet*). These items are used to obtain follow-up information.

Follow-up information on the initial abstract includes the last date the patient was known to be alive or the date of death at the time of abstracting. The status of the cancer must be recorded. This information is updated at least annually according to CoC accreditation requirements.[2] The institution's cancer committee may choose to require more frequent follow-up for some sites.

Case Administration

The case administration section contains override flags and identifies coding systems used to abstract the case, the version of coding manual that was used to abstract the case, the reporting institution, and the abstractor who coded and abstracted the data.

Text Documentation

A complete abstract includes coded data items and typed text. Text serves to summarize the cancer patient's medical experience, and numerical codes collapse the information into assigned data fields. Data comparisons rely on coded information for analysis and statistics. When comparing a large number of cases, tabulating numeric codes is more feasible than attempting to use the text. To validate that the coded data items are correct, text must be included to support this information.

Text should be an accurate, concise summary of the patient's cancer. There are certain qualities that text should have to ensure that it is useful and attains its purpose. Text should validate, at a minimum, the following critical data items: age, sex, race, sequence number, stage, date of diagnosis, primary site, laterality, histology, behavior, grade, and dates and types of all treatment modalities. Text should also clarify difficult coding decisions and validate unusual situations such as a rare site and histology combination.

The central cancer registry also relies on complete and thorough text to reconcile duplicate cases and confirm the accuracy of the coded data items. Patients that are seen at more than one facility are reported by each of those facilities, resulting in more than one record for that primary cancer. The central cancer registry must compare each record and merge the records into one case with the best information available for that cancer. It is likely that there will be a discrepancy in the coded data items because the information available to each reporting facility may vary. The central cancer registry uses the text to decide which code is the most accurate or which reporting source most likely had the most complete and final information. The CoC does not require that text be recorded or reported. Therefore, guidelines for reporting text documentation will be provided by the central cancer registry.

Standards for a Complete Abstract

The abstract is not limited to the information available in the patient's medical record. A complete abstract contains both text and coded information, and provides a complete picture of the patient's cancer. Before marking the abstract as complete, a visual review should be done to ensure that all required data fields have been completed according to the data standards. In addition, the data fields should represent the most specific information, such as the most specific cell type or stage. Data fields that are coded to unknown, have a default code, or are auto-filled should be closely inspected. A review at the time of abstracting, and when the information from the medical record can be recalled, promotes the completeness and accuracy of the data. The abstract should also reflect a logical sequence of events. For example, first course of treatment cannot be before the date of diagnosis, and the treatment recorded should be in alignment with the treatment guidelines for the stage and diagnosis. If not, then the text should verify that the treatment recorded is correct and complete.

All pertinent information related to the diagnosis and treatment of the cancer that can be obtained should be included in the abstract. This includes care delivered outside of the institution. In many instances, the physician or institution that delivered this care must be contacted directly to request additional information. The registrar must be proactive in recognizing when additional information may be available and taking the necessary action to obtain and report this information.

The follow-up process, as well as studies and reports using the data, can result in the identification of missing or more detailed information, but often this is after the abstract has been reported to other agencies. Also, patients may enter the institution at any time during their disease course, which may not be until there is a recurrence or progression of disease. New information should be reviewed carefully to determine what applies to the original diagnosis, stage, and treatment, and that which may be a result of disease progression. The abstract should reflect the most complete information about the original diagnosis and treatment. Most cancer registry software systems provide separate data fields to record subsequent treatment should the registry elect to do so. There is no time limit for making revisions that yield more complete and accurate information, as long as the information meets the reporting and timing requirements.[1]

Quality Control of Cancer Data

Quality control must be an integral part of every activity performed in the cancer registry. With the cancer registry data being the basis of many other activities, there must be assurance that the data are reliable and accurate. Cancer registry data should not be released for use unless it has undergone extensive quality review. Releasing information that contains errors could have detrimental results for the user of the data by providing potentially misleading information. Strategies for ensuring accurate data are numerous. The most common methods are visual review, computerized data edit checks, physician review of abstracted data, reabstracting audits, and targeting specific areas of review through the generation of reports from the cancer registry database.[4]

Quality control begins at the time of abstracting by having trained and knowledgeable staff performing the abstracting and by following the established data reporting standards. Visual review at the time of abstracting was discussed earlier in this chapter but can be done anytime there is interaction with the abstract, such as when updates from subsequent visits or from follow-up information are available. Anytime there is interaction with the abstract, the potential to identify missing or erroneous information is increased, especially if the review is performed by someone other than the original abstractor.

Edit checks is a process in which a computer program compares the coded data with the rules for abstracting. Any conflicts are displayed as a potential error that needs to be verified or corrected. Most cancer registry database systems have the capability to run the edits program against the data at the time of abstracting. Edit checks can also be run on a set of cases, such as all cases abstracted within a particular time frame. The ability to utilize the edit checks program to identify errors and correct the data should not be ignored. Most edits identify errors in which a correction is required, for example, a conflict between the stage and behavior code. Any edit errors identified should be thoroughly investigated before bypassing the edit, signifying that the coded information is correct.

There are many types of errors that edits are not able to identify. For example, the edits program cannot compare with the original source document and determine that a different subsite of the primary organ should be the primary site. The cancer registry should be utilizing multiple methods of quality control to evaluate the accuracy of the data. Physician review and reabstracting audits are common methods for comparing the abstracted data to the original source document and the abstracted text. These reviews usually include only a selected number or percentage of cases based on the focus of the review.

Quality-control activities have many benefits beyond identifying errors and correcting the data. Often, consistent errors and areas in need of further staff training can be identified. This can lead to better quality at the time of abstracting and the need for fewer corrections during later review. Quality-control activities also demonstrate the high level of quality, reliable information to the users of the data and further increase the value of the cancer registry data.

Data Submission and Dissemination

The primary purpose for expending the amount of effort required for data collection is to use the data to evaluate and monitor the burden of cancer. Cancer registries should be continually providing data to support the need for reliable cancer information of the medical community, government agencies, legislators, and the general public. For that to be accomplished, data collected at the patient care level must be reported to the agencies that are in need of this information. Agencies that receive data from outside sources in North America are listed in Table 12-4.

Table 12-4   Agencies That Receive Data from Facilities in North America
Canadian Cancer Registry (CCR)
Commission on Cancer's National Cancer Data Base (CoC/NCDB)
Centers for Disease Control and Prevention's National Program of Cancer Registries (CDC NPCR)
North American Association of Central Cancer Registries (NAACCR)
Surveillance, Epidemiology, and End Results Program (SEER)
State or territory central cancer registries

The agency the cancer registry reports to depends on several factors, including the geographic location of the institution and CoC accreditation status. It is possible that a cancer registry will be required to report data to more than one agency. An institution that is accredited by the CoC will report data to the National Cancer Data Base (NCDB), as well as the central cancer registry. The central cancer registry may report data to North American Association of Central Cancer Registries (NAACCR), NPCR, or SEER, or possibly all three agencies. Each agency has a specific purpose for requiring that data. Therefore, the data collection and reporting requirements for each agency will differ. For example, a population-based cancer registry, such as the state's central cancer registry, is interested in identifying all cases of cancer within the defined population. Therefore, reporting nonanalytic cases in addition to analytic cases will be required.

Reporting schedules will also differ. The NCDB conducts an annual call for data whereby the most recent year's data, together with other cases specified in the call for data, are submitted. Many central cancer registries require that data be submitted on a shorter, more frequent basis, such as monthly or quarterly. For example, cases abstracted in the first quarter of the year will be required to be submitted in October of that same year. The cancer registry has the responsibility of meeting the requirements for each agency the data are reported to and for submitting the data according to the defined reporting schedule.

Summary

The most valuable database is one that is complete with flawless information. The labor that goes into abstracting the data from the health record is offset by the usefulness of the data. It is important to remember that the data input must be accurate for the data output to be reliable. Registry data and the outcomes can be used as internal or external benchmarks. The ability to produce reports beneficial to physicians, researchers, administrators, and other healthcare professionals is of paramount importance to the future of the registry.

References

1. American College of Surgeons (ACoS) Commission on Cancer (CoC). *Facility Oncology Registry Data Standards (FORDS), Vol. II: Standards of the Commission on Cancer.* Chicago: American College of Surgeons Commission on Cancer, 2002 (Revised for 2010).
2. American College of Surgeons (ACoS) Commission on Cancer (CoC). *Cancer Program Standards Manual, Vol. I: Standards of the Commission on Cancer.* Chicago: American College of Surgeons Commission on Cancer, 2002 (Revised for 2009).
3. Edge, S., Byrd, D., Compton, C., et al., editors. *AJCC Cancer Staging Manual,* 7th ed. New York: Springer, 2009.
4. Hofferkamp, J., editor. *Standards for Cancer Registries, Vol. III: Standards for Completeness, Quality, Analysis, Management, Security and Confidentiality of Data.* Springfield, Ill: North American Association of Central Cancer Registries, August 2008.

ICD-O and MP/H Rules

April Fritz, RHIT, CTR

According to the dictionary, a *code* is a set of symbols arranged systematically for easy reference. The purpose of coding is to express a concept symbolically, allowing similar concepts to be grouped for the purposes of information retrieval. For example, take the concept of the color red. Red has many different names: rose, carmine, ruby, sanguine, cardinal, cherry, salmon, and vermillion, just to name a few. A data analyst who wanted to review cases that involved the concept of red would have to remember all the different synonyms to gather every case of "red." However, if the original data collector had a system in which all of the different synonyms of red had the same code and such a code was assigned at the time of data collection, it would be straightforward for the data analyst to retrieve all cases that represented "red" by looking for a single code.

The act of coding is the process used to transpose text to codes. Most coding begins with a nomenclature, or a system of names. In the previous example, that nomenclature would have classified the major color groups for red, blue, yellow, and so forth, under which would be the lists of synonyms that represented the various color concepts. For cancer registries, the codes and disease nomenclature identify where the cancer started (the topography) and what the tumor is (morphology).

International Classification of Diseases for Oncology—Coding of Neoplasms

History of Coding Neoplasms

As early as 400 B.C., the Egyptians used codes. The Greeks, following Hippocrates' teachings, were the first to attempt to classify diseases into groups (the four humors).[1] In the seventeenth century, John Graunt in London recognized the need for classifying diseases,[2] and William Farr (1807–1883) of the Registrar General's Office in England, the first medical statistician, labored for better, more uniform classification of diseases.[3]

In 1891, the International Statistical Institute formed a committee, headed by Dr. Jacques Bertillon, to prepare a classification for causes of death, and the first edition of the International List of Causes of Death was published in 1900.[4] Details of this early history and the beginning of the publication of the list are well documented in the introduction of the *International Classification of Diseases* (ICD), 1955 revision, published by the World Health Organization (WHO) in 1957.[5]

In the United States, a committee of the American Medical Association was convened to develop a nomenclature of diseases. This nomenclature was based on the one published by the Royal College of Physicians in 1869. In 1903, *The Bellevue Hospital Nomenclature of Diseases* was published. Between 1903 and 1933, eight other nomenclatures and coding books were developed in the United States. In 1933, the first edition of the *Standard Nomenclature of Diseases* was published, and in 1942, the first edition of the *Standard Nomenclature of Operations* was included. These two nomenclatures became the *Standard Nomenclature of Diseases and Operations* (SNODO), 4th edition, published by the American Medical Association in 1952.[6]

SNODO

SNODO's code structure consisted of a code for the topography (site), a hyphen, and a code for the etiology (cause). Although no one knew the etiology of cancer, the series of codes beginning with 8 was used for new growths, and various histologic types were filled in. The origin of the morphology section code numbers beginning with 8 developed from this.

By itself, coding did not provide access to data; it was coupled with indexing—a manual system of recording cases with similar codes in the same section of the index. For example, an index card was prepared for every code of major body sites. Medical records having the same site codes were indexed on the same card. The disease or procedure code was written in the column labeled with the first digit of the code. When beginning a study for a physician, one had to identify the appropriate code and go through all of the site cards for that code looking for entries for the specific disease or procedure. This was time-consuming, but it was the only system available at the time. The same coding and indexing system was used for cancer registries. The fifth edition of SNODO was the last edition ever published or used.[7]

After World War II, when the WHO was formed to deal with the health problems of the United Nations, it was given the responsibility for revising the ICD. Chapter 2 of ICD has always been assigned to neoplasms, including malignant neoplasms (cancers), benign neoplasms, in situ lesions, uncertain as to whether benign or malignant, and so forth.

Neoplasms are usually described first by their topographic site, the place in the body where the cancer originated (lung, breast, bone marrow, colon, etc.); next by their behavior, that is, whether they are malignant, benign, in situ, or otherwise classifiable; and then by the cell type, also called the morphologic or histologic type, as determined by a pathologist using a microscope. The neoplasm chapter of the ICD is principally a topographic code that takes the behavior into account. Few specific morphologic types are included: melanomas, lymphomas, leukemias, and multiple myeloma. Pathologists objected to this because they wanted to be able to identify, for example, whether a lung tumor was an adenocarcinoma, squamous cell carcinoma, small cell carcinoma, or some other histologic type. These tumors acted just as differently within the lung as various types of cancers acted in different parts of the body.

MOTNAC

In 1951, the American Cancer Society assigned a committee, principally composed of pathologists and statisticians, to develop the *Manual of Tumor Nomenclature and Coding* (MOTNAC).[8] This code book contained only a three-digit code, two digits for morphology and the last digit, preceded by a period, for the behavior. Tumor registries assigned as a topography code whatever was used in their hospital, either SNODO or ICD.

In the early 1960s, hospitals in the United States began using the ICD for coding morbidity and mortality because it was easier to use and had more current terms, but it was still not ideal. When the *International Classification of Diseases, 1965 revision* (ICD-8), was published,[9] users in the United States found that it did not meet the coding needs of hospital health records departments. Two adaptations of ICD-8 were published in the United States. One was *International Classification of Diseases, Adapted for Use in the United States* (1967; ICDA-8).[10] The other adaptation was developed and published by the Commission on Professional and Hospital Activities (CPHA) in Ann Arbor, Michigan. This book, *Hospital International Classification of Diseases Adapted* (H-ICDA)[11] was used for coding by those hospitals that were members of CPHA, as well as others who preferred H-ICDA over ICD-8.

SNOP

The College of American Pathologists decided in the early 1960s to develop a code for all pathologic terms, not just neoplasms. The culmination of their efforts was the *Systematized Nomenclature of Pathology* (SNOP), published in 1965.[12] It had been agreed ahead of time that when the book was finished, the people interested in cancer could use the neoplasm sections (sections 8 and 9) from this book and publish their own code book just for neoplasms. So in 1968, the American Cancer Society published the *Manual of Tumor Nomenclature and Coding, 1968 edition* (MOTNAC).[13] It consisted of a topography section based on the neoplasms chapter of ICDA-8 and a morphology section adapted from sections 8 and 9 of SNOP.

ICD-O

In the early 1970s, the WHO started preparing for the ninth revision of ICD. While they were doing this, physicians expressed a desire to have a cancer supplement that included morphology. They looked around for a suitable morphology code structure and finally selected MOTNAC. After extensive field testing in the leading countries of the world, a practice WHO had never tried before, the *International Classification of Diseases for Oncology* (ICD-O) was published in late 1976.[14] Naturally, the topography of ICD-O was based on the neoplasms chapter of ICD-9.

The ICD-O is a 10-digit code consisting of four digits for topography and four for morphology, followed by a slash (/) and a single-digit behavior code indicating whether the tumor is malignant, benign, in situ, or otherwise classified. Most cancer registries around the world collect only those tumors that are malignant (/3) or in situ (/2).* Pathologists may use /6 (malignant, metastatic) or /9 (malignant, uncertain whether primary or metastatic). The registry, however, reports these neoplasms as C80.9, "unknown primary site," unless a primary has been determined through other diagnostic means. The sixth or last digit of the morphology code is for grading or differentiation and describes how much or how little a tumor resembles the normal tissue from which it arose. Acceptable sixth digits for solid tumors are 1, 2, 3, 4 and 9.

ICD-9 and ICD-9-CM

The ninth revision of the *International Classification of Diseases* (ICD-9) was published in 1977, with the morphology code numbers (M-codes) included in the alphabetic index and listed numerically in the back of Volume 1 (pages 667–690).[15]

ICD-9 encompasses two volumes: the tabular list (codes in sequential order) and the alphabetic index (alphabetic listing of terms and corresponding codes). ICD-9 was used by vital statistics offices for coding death certificates through 1998. However, it was not adequate for the multiplicity of other uses for coded data, such as health care review, reimbursement, and scientific studies. A clinical modification for the United States was published, the *International Classification of Diseases, 9th Revision, Clinical Modification* (ICD-9-CM), which added a third volume containing both a tabular list and an alphabetic index for operations and procedures.[16]

The ICD-9-CM is a numeric classification system. The tabular list is divided into 17 chapters; some are classified by condition and others by site. There are also two supplementary chapters with special classifications: V-codes (factors influencing health status and contact with health services) and E-codes (external causes of injury and poisoning).

Each chapter of the tabular list is further subdivided into sections, categories, subcategories, and subclassifications. Sections are groups of three-digit code numbers such as "Diseases of other endocrine glands" (250-259). A category within the section is one three-digit code number, for example, diabetes mellitus (250). At the four-digit level are subcategories of code numbers that further delineate the category, such as diabetes mellitus with ketoacidosis (250.1). A fifth digit is required in some categories within the tabular list. The five-digit code numbers are called *subclassifications*. Using the example of diabetes, the subclassification 250.10 is diabetes mellitus with ketoacidosis, adult onset,[17] as shown in Table 13-1.

The ICD-9-CM index is an alphabetic listing of diagnoses. These diagnoses are listed by main terms followed by modifiers and subterms, for example:

Diabetes, diabetic (mellitus) with ketosis, ketoacidosis 250.1[17]

---

*In the United States, cancer registries have been federally mandated since 2004 to collect benign and borderline tumors of the central nervous system in addition to the invasive (/3) and in situ (/2) cancers.

Table 13-1	Stylized Representation of Section of *International Classification of Diseases, 9th Revision, Clinical Modification* (ICD-9-CM) Tabular List	
Division	**Code**	**Meaning**
Section	250-59	Diseases of other endocrine glands
Category	250	Diabetes mellitus
Subcategory	250.0	Diabetes mellitus without mention of complication
	250.1	Diabetes with ketoacidosis
Subclassification	250.10	Adult onset

The main word or term of the disease or procedure must be located in the alphabetic index to select the proper code in ICD-9-CM. Usually only nouns are indexed. Modifiers and subterms must be reviewed carefully because they may affect the choice of the most appropriate code associated with the diagnosis. The most specific code must be selected, for example, 250.1 for diabetes with ketoacidosis, not simply 250. The code must be verified in the tabular list. Before the final code selection is made, all instructional notations, punctuation, symbols, and other coding conventions must be reviewed to determine the accuracy of the code selected.

Coding conventions used in ICD-9-CM include punctuation, symbols, typefaces, abbreviations, and other notations such as "includes" and "excludes" notes. Each of these tells the coder something about the code. These conventions must be followed to correctly code a diagnosis. Only one of the abbreviations in ICD-9-CM—NOS (not otherwise specified)—is used to code neoplasms in ICD-O. The tabular list of ICD-O contains no inclusions or exclusions to be reviewed that are not also printed in the index.

In ICD-9's alphabetic index under the term *neoplasm,* anatomic sites are listed alphabetically. For each site there are five columns indicating the behavior: malignant, benign, and so on. The coder selects the appropriate column based on the description in the medical record. In ICD-O, all primary cancers use the same anatomic site codes, and the behavior is indicated by adding a fifth digit to the morphology code after the slash.

ICD-O was successfully introduced in 1976 and has been used not only in cancer registries throughout the United States but in the rest of the world as well. It has been translated into all the major languages of the world. The Surveillance, Epidemiology, and End Results (SEER) Program of the National Cancer Institute adopted ICD-O as its official code book for coding the site and histologic type of neoplasms,[18] and other standard setters in the United States, Canada, and the rest of the world have designated ICD-O as the official reference for coding neoplasms.

SNOMED

In 1977, the College of American Pathologists published an extensive revision of SNOP, entitled the *Systematized Nomenclature of Medicine* (SNOMED).[19] It incorporated the neoplasm section as presented in the first edition of ICD-O. SNOMED has been used for coding in many pathology laboratories all over the world.

Although there had usually been a 10-year interval between revisions of the ICD, the WHO wanted the 10th revision to be a major one, so they extended the interval between revisions to 15 years. However, oncologists were anxious to add new terminology and classifications to ICD-O, especially for lymphomas. A working party was formed by WHO to revise ICD-O. It was again decided to base the topography on the forthcoming 10th revision of ICD (ICD-10). There was a major change in the codes, because WHO had decided it was necessary to go to an alphanumeric code to have sufficient room for expansion. Therefore, the topography section of ICD-O-2 contains C-codes. Many people thought this meant cancer, but it was purely coincidental. The first chapter of the *International Statistical Classification of Diseases and Related Health Problems, 10th revision,*[20] used the letters A and B for infectious and parasitic diseases, and because neoplasms were always coded in the second chapter, the next available letter of the alphabet was C.

ICD-O-2

The second edition of ICD-O was published in 1990.[21] Some people started using it immediately, mostly foreign countries that had not used the first edition of ICD-O and were anxious to begin coding their data. The SEER Program implemented ICD-O-2 for their 1992 data, after holding extensive training programs. Widespread use of ICD-O-2 by U.S. cancer registries began in 1993. The introduction and instructions in the beginning of ICD-O-2 were very detailed and clear, so it is not necessary to repeat them here.

The primary difference between ICD-O and ICD-O-2 is that the topography of ICD-O-2, which is based on ICD-10, has an alpha character C in front of the three digits, and the numeric digits range from 00.0 to 80.9. New morphologic terms were added, and the lymphoma section was expanded to include terms used in the Working Formulation and some foreign classifications, such as the Kiel classification for lymphomas. The introduction and instructions at the beginning were expanded. The last few pages of the book list the new morphology code numbers, terms, and synonyms. The final page is important because it lists the terms in the second edition that had been changed to malignant. Added to the grading or differentiation column in ICD-O-2 were codes for T and B cells when diagnosed for lymphomas and leukemias.

A new edition of SNOMED, now called the *Systematized Nomenclature of Human and Veterinary Medicine* (SNOMED International) was published in 1993.[22] This edition was published in four volumes by the College of American Pathologists. Volume 1 includes the morphology sections 8 and 9 of ICD-O-2. SNOMED International was the final printed version of this code scheme. Subsequent versions of the codes—*SNOMED Reference Technology* (RT)[23] and *SNOMED Clinical Terms* (CT)[24]—have been published in electronic format for use in computerized coding systems. Each new version of SNOMED has retained compatibility of the morphology sections 8 and 9 of ICD-O.

ICD-10

The United States implemented ICD-10 for coding death certificates in 1999. However, with the availability of computers and other electronic mechanisms to assist with coding, it has become more complicated to change existing programs and hardware and to retrain coders. Studies have demonstrated that ICD-10 is not adequate to code morbidity in medical facilities, so a clinical modification of ICD-10 was necessary. The National Center for Health Statistics, which now operates under the Centers for Disease Control and Prevention (CDC), is involved in the development, as well as the Centers for Medicare and Medicaid Services (formerly the Social Security Administration), because of their oversight of payments for hospitalization. Following comments on the initial draft, an updated draft of the clinical modification of ICD-10[25] was released in June 2003 for public viewing. As of early 2010, the ICD-10-CM implementation date has been established for the United States as October 1, 2013.

Concurrent with the implementation of ICD-O-2 in North America, there were significant advances in the diagnosis of neoplasms, particularly the hematopoietic diseases (diseases arising in the lymphatic system and bone marrow). In particular, new cytogenetic techniques contributed considerably to the body of knowledge about lymphomas, leukemias, and other bone marrow conditions. As a result, the nomenclature for these diseases expanded and data collectors were unable to easily assign codes to the new terminology. Once again, the WHO assembled a task force in 1998 to assess whether new codes for the lymphomas and leukemias should simply be added to ICD-O-2 or whether a new edition was warranted. After receiving comments from many national registries, the decision was made to develop a new edition.

ICD-O-3

In addition to incorporating the WHO classification of hematopoietic and lymphoid neoplasms,[26] the editors of the new edition included the terminology of other WHO publications such as the *Histological Typing of Tumors*[27] series, known to pathologists as the "blue books" because of the cover color for the series' first edition. After a limited international field trial in 1999 and further refinements of the morphology codes, introduction, and index, the third edition of the *International Classification of Disease for Oncology*[28] was published in late 2000 with implementation set by the North American Association of Central Cancer Registries (NAACCR) as beginning with cases diagnosed on or after January 1, 2001.

There were no changes to the topography code structure between ICD-O-2 and ICD-O-3; ICD-O-3 continues to be based on ICD-10. However, some terms changed behavior code, affecting their reportability. Eleven terms changed from borderline (/1) to malignant (/3), and therefore reportable to all cancer registries. These include all of the refractory anemias, polycythemia vera, and several other hematopoietic diseases. Six neoplasms previously coded as malignant, the various cystadenomas of the ovary and pilocytic astrocytoma, were changed from malignant (/3) to borderline (/1), making them not reportable as of 2001 diagnoses. However, by agreement among North American standard setters, pilocytic astrocytoma will continue to be reported as a malignancy because of its significance as a childhood tumor and the effect that excluding those cases would have on incidence rates over time. The principal impact of the third edition was the inclusion of about 780 morphology terms and synonyms, roughly two-thirds in the first part of the list (M-8000-M-9580) and one-third in the lymphomas and leukemias section.

To reflect contemporary pathology practice and terminology, a number of acronyms were added to ICD-O-3 as synonyms of the terms they represent. For example, one of the primary morphology terms for breast cancer is "ductal carcinoma in situ," but it is commonly reported as "DCIS." Both terms are coded to M-8500/2 in ICD-O-3. On the other hand, ICD-O serves as a reference manual for legacy data as well, so virtually all terms from older classifications have been retained. Terms that are truly archaic, such as lymphosarcoma, are marked with [obs] as an indication that use of the term is discouraged because better, more definitive and descriptive terms are available. Another example in ICD-O-3 is the term "hepatoma," which is marked with [obs] because the preferred terminology is now hepatocellular carcinoma, of which there are four distinct and separately coded subtypes.[29]

Another issue that arose from the inclusion of certain new codes was the correct coding of tumors that contain multiple histologic types, in particular, the new combination codes 8523/3, infiltrating duct mixed with other types of carcinoma, and 8524/3, infiltrating lobular mixed with other types of carcinoma. These two codes are intended to describe a single lesion containing multiple histologic types. They should not be used to code multiple independent tumors of differing histologic types in the same primary site. This same principle applies to other combination codes in

ICD-O-2 and ICD-O-3. The evolution of coding over three editions of ICD-O requires a solid understanding of the implications of adding new codes or combining old codes and how those changes and data conversions affect incidence reporting in population-based registries.

A number of side issues related to the implementation of ICD-O-3 were identified during the development process, all of which are related to the increasing reliance of cancer registries on electronic databases. These included timely revision of cancer registry software to accommodate ICD-O-3 codes, development of reference tables incorporating the new codes, storage of ICD-O-3 codes in cancer registry databases, and converting ICD-O-2 codes to ICD-O-3. Because of NAACCR's efforts to standardize data collection and data transfer, a task force was formed for the first time to prepare guidelines for implementing ICD-O-3. Conversion tables for ICD-O-2 to ICD-O-3 and vice versa, as well as conversion between ICD-O-3 and ICD-9 were developed, together with a new primary site/histology table listing the histology codes most commonly associated with each primary site. The guidelines published by the task force[30] included recommendations for implementation and storage of the codes, and recommendations for collecting or no longer collecting cases with codes that changed behavior, as well as alternatives for coding and storing cases when a registry's software installation might be delayed. The work of this task force set the standard for coordinated implementation of later changes in the cancer registry data set, such as Collaborative Staging, the 2003 treatment codes, and the 2007 Multiple Primary and Histology (MP/H) coding rules.

Figure 13-1, adapted from the introduction of the *International Classification of Diseases for Oncology,* Third Edition

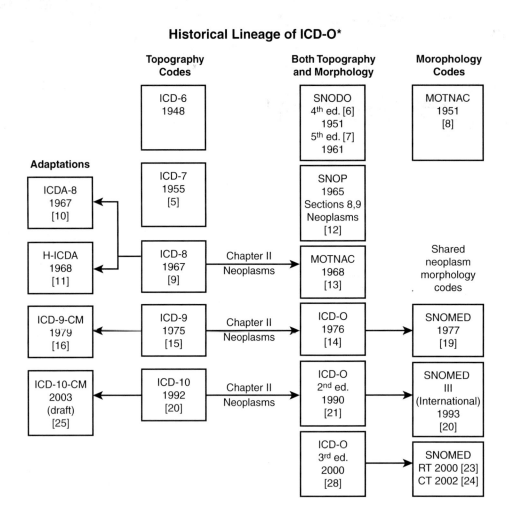

Historical Lineage of ICD-O*

Note: Dates shown are publication dates, not implementation dates.

*Adapted from Table 1. Coding of Neoplasms 1946–2000: Historical Lineage of ICD-O.
International Classification of Diseases for Oncology, third edition, 2000[28]*. Page 2.*
Numbers in [brackets] refer to the publications cited at the end of this chapter.

Figure 13-1. Illustrates the Coding Texts That Directly Led to the Development of ICD-O

(ICD-O-3), shows all the code books used for neoplasms for the past seven decades.

Table 13-2 shows how the code structure for neoplasms has evolved from MOTNAC (1951) to ICD-O-3.

Since the publication of ICD-O-3, work has continued on the WHO blue book series, and the fourth edition of the *WHO Classification of Tumours of Haematopoietic and Lym-*

phoid Tissues was published in 2008.[31] This edition added another 33 terms to ICD-O-3 and changed three codes from /1 borderline behavior to /3 malignant, and therefore reportable. The new hematopoietic and lymphoid terms are listed in Appendix D of the *Hematopoietic and Lymphoid Neoplasm Case Reportability and Coding Manual*[32] published by the SEER Program and effective for use with 2010 diag-

Table 13-2	Evolution of Code Structure from *Manual of Tumor Nomenclature and Coding* (MOTNAC) and *Standard Nomenclature of Diseases and Operations* (SNODO) to *International Classification of Diseases for Oncology, Third Edition* (ICD-O-3)		
Publication Year	**Reference**	**Code**	**Meaning**
1951	MOTNAC[8]	00.6	Infiltrating duct carcinoma
1961	SNODO, 5th ed.[7]	190-8191F	Carcinoma of breast, infiltrating, differentiated
1965	SNOP[12]	0402 8503	Breast, right, infiltrating duct carcinoma
1967	ICD, 1965 ed.[9]	174	Malignant neoplasm of breast
1967	ICD-A[10]	174	Malignant neoplasm of breast
1968	H-ICDA[11]	174.0	Primary malignant neoplasm of breast
1968	MOTNAC 1968[12]	174.9 8503	Breast [NOS], duct carcinoma
1976	ICD-O[14]	174.4 M-8500/33	Breast, upper outer quadrant, infiltrating duct carcinoma, poorly differentiated
1978	ICD-9-CM[16]	174.4 M8500/3*	Malignant neoplasm of breast, upper outer quadrant; *optional morphology code: infiltrating duct carcinoma
1976	SNOMED[19]	T-04004 M-8500/33	Breast, upper outer quadrant, NOS, infiltrating duct carcinoma, poorly differentiated
1992	ICD-10[20]	C50.4 M-8500/3*	Malignant neoplasm of breast, upper outer quadrant; *optional morphology code: infiltrating duct carcinoma
1990	ICD-O-2[21]	C50.4 8500/33	Breast, upper outer quadrant, infiltrating duct carcinoma, poorly differentiated
1993	SNOMED Int.[22]	T-04004 M8500/3 G-F503*	Upper outer quadrant of breast [NOS], infiltrating duct carcinoma, *optional grade code: poorly differentiated
1996	SNOMED RT[23]	T-04024 M85003 G-F503*	Upper outer quadrant of right breast (body structure), infiltrating duct carcinoma (morphologic abnormality); *optional grade code: poorly differentiated (grade)
2001	ICD-O-3[28]	C50.4 8500/33	Breast, upper outer quadrant, infiltrating duct carcinoma, poorly differentiated
2002	SNOMED CT[24]	T-04024 M85003 F-02901*	Upper outer quadrant of right breast (body structure), infiltrating duct carcinoma (morphologic abnormality); *optional grade code: poorly differentiated histologic grade finding (finding)
2003	ICD-10-CM[25]	C50.41 M-8500/3*	Malignant neoplasm of right (female) breast, upper outer quadrant; *optional morphology code: infiltrating duct carcinoma

Diagnosis: poorly differentiated infiltrating duct carcinoma of upper outer quadrant of right breast.
SNOP, *Systematized Nomenclature of Pathology;* ICD-A, *International Classification of Diseases, Adapted for Use in the United States;* H-ICDA, *Hospital International Classification of Diseases Adapted;* NOS, not otherwise specified; ICD-9-CM, *International Classification of Diseases, 9th revision: Clinical Modification;* SNOMED, *Systematized Nomenclature of Medicine.*

noses and later. The diagnoses that changed from borderline to malignant are:

> Myeloproliferative neoplasm, unclassifiable/myelodysplastic/myeloproliferative neoplasm unclassifiable (9975/3)
>
> T-cell large granular lymphocytic leukemia/chronic lymphoproliferative disorder of NK cells (9831/3)
>
> Langerhans cell histiocytosis, NOS (9751/3) (It should be noted that several previously nonreportable Langerhans cell codes [9751/1, 9752/1, 9753/1], and code 9754/3 were collapsed into code 9751/3.)

As more volumes of the WHO blue books are published, it is likely that new disease entities will be described and new ICD-O morphology codes will be assigned. In early 2010, the International Agency for Research on Cancer, the cancer division of the WHO, convened a committee to review proposed code additions and changes based on the new editions of the WHO blue book series and gather them into an update to ICD-O-3. There are no plans at present to publish a fourth edition of ICD-O until the neoplasms chapter of ICD-11 is completed. That work is expected to take 3 to 4 years.

Basics of Coding Neoplasms

Just as the first edition of ICD-O had established, ICD-O-3 has a 10-digit code comprising a code number for topography (site), a code number for morphology (tumor type), a code for behavior, and a code for grade or differentiation. In ICD-O-3, the alphabetic index is used for coding both topography and morphology (the same as in ICD-O). The topographic terms begin with "C" and the morphologic terms with "M-," although recording these two characters and the punctuation (decimal point or slash separators) in a database is optional. Whereas in ICD-9 it is necessary to verify in the tabular list all code numbers found in the index to review any exclusions or other coding instructions, it is not necessary to do so in ICD-O because there are no special instructions in the numeric section that would alter the code number selected in the alphabetic section.

The coding guidelines for topography and morphology, and the instructions for use at the beginning of ICD-O-3 are very detailed and should be reviewed carefully before coding is attempted. Refer to ICD-O-3 for the specific rules of topography and morphology coding. These parts of the book are often overlooked by users, especially those with computerized registries, because software vendors include both code numbers and terms in their systems. Most software programs allow an operator to key a number, after which the term appears on the screen, or to enter the term, after which the corresponding number appears. The simplicity of the computerized look-up system can result in coding errors. The coding rules at the beginning of ICD-O must be studied before beginning to code. A related issue that bears comment is the importance of the "matrix principle." ICD-O is very flexible for coding the topography, morphology, and behavior of a particular neoplasm. When a data collector is dependent on a computerized system for assigning the code, some of that flexibility is lost. Therefore, it is important to remember that the purpose of the code is to describe what the pathologist says about the tumor, including a different behavior if so stated by the pathologist. The "matrix principle" allows the data collector to change the behavior code from what is printed in the book or included in a reference table in a computerized cancer registry system to truly represent in coded form what the pathologist described.

Summary

The quality of registry data depends on the care registrars take in reviewing available information and selecting the most accurate codes to represent the data they collect. To accurately code the primary site, histologic type, behavior, and grade or differentiation, a registrar must know every section in the coding book. This is especially important for coding rules and conventions as detailed in the instructions for use at the beginning of ICD-O-3. Most studies conducted by researchers, physicians, and others require, at a minimum, one of these elements as a parameter for case selection. If the codes are incorrect, the results of the studies will be flawed and the credibility of the registry damaged. Accuracy must be the operational word for coding site and histology.

Multiple Primary and Histology Coding Rules

The MP/H coding rules were implemented in the United States and parts of Canada after a 4-year effort by the cancer registry standards setters. The rules were effective for cancer diagnoses on and after January 1, 2007, and replaced all previous rules for determining how many primaries a case represented (and how many abstracts to prepare) and how to code the histology field on an individual abstract.

The MP/H Task Force was sponsored and chaired by staff of the National Cancer Institute's SEER Program. The task force consisted of representatives from the CDC National Program of Cancer Registries (NPCR), NAACCR, the National Cancer Registrars Association (NCRA), the American College of Surgeons (ACoS) Commission on Cancer (CoC), the American Joint Committee on Cancer (AJCC), 15 U.S. central registries, and several Canadian cancer registries. Specialty pathologists and clinicians provided physician guidance to the task force during the initial discussions, as well as the review and revision of the proposed rules. As part of the process, the task force consulted with the editors of ICD-O-3 to clarify the definitions of various ICD-O-3 codes and ensure that the new rules would properly overlay the morphology coding rules in ICD-O-3.

The material in this chapter is an overview of the MP/H rules; it is not intended to replace them. The rules themselves are provided in the document "The 2007 Multiple Primary and Histology Coding Rules"[33] (available from www.seer.cancer.gov/tools/mphrules). The rules can be downloaded as a single PDF document or in nine sections. Once downloaded, they can be printed or accessed electronically on the computer screen without having to log on to the Internet.

Why Were MP/H Rules Needed?

Rules for determining the number of abstracts to prepare—in other words, multiple primary rules—were first established more than 30 years ago when the SEER Program was established. A number of changes in medicine have occurred in three decades, and it became apparent that updated multiple primary rules were necessary. Among the changes are:

- The development and widespread use of computed tomography and magnetic resonance imaging scans: These noninvasive imaging techniques can provide almost as much information as exploratory surgeries that were previously needed to make a diagnosis.
- The development of advanced laboratory procedures, such as cytogenetic testing, tumor markers, and molecular markers, which provide the pathologist with more information about the tumor than ever before
- An explosion of clinical and pathologic information stored in the medical record: For a registrar, it is sometimes difficult to sort out what is descriptive detail and what is prognostically important and should be captured in the cancer abstract.

In addition, the publication of the ICD-O-3 in 2000 presented some challenges and some benefits to the registry world. The primary benefit was that registrars could code many new diseases and conditions that had been identified as a result of medical advances in the decade since the second edition was published. However, many of the new terms included in ICD-O-3 were limited in their use or the circumstances of their use were not well explained. Because code rubrics were limited, particularly in the lymphomas and leukemias section of ICD-O-3, some codes had to be placed where space was available, and this caused problems because the codes were no longer hierarchical.

As a result of all these changes, the cancer registry standards setters were finding it challenging to continue revising or patching the existing rules as medical practice and diagnosis evolved. It was difficult to train new registrars on the existing rules because there was no priority to the rules and there were so many exceptions to remember. For the same reasons, it was not possible to write a computer program to automate application of the rules in central registries.

Two separate issues emerged: where the information in the medical record was incomplete, there were problems deciding how many primary cancers there were for the case; and there were, in some cases, too many potentially codable descriptive histology terms in the pathology report. These issues presented data quality, consistency, and reproducibility problems both for counting of incidence in central registries and for identification of individual cancers in facility-based registries. The rules needed to be the same for both types of registries.

The MP/H coding rules implemented in 2007 were a collaborative effort to update the way primary cancers are counted and to code their histologic cell types in the United States and Canada. Furthermore, the task force realized that the overall data quality in cancer registries could be improved by developing standardized, consistent sets of rules for both "high-volume" (common) cancers such as breast, colon, and lung, and "high-risk" (problematic) cancers such as melanoma, urinary tract, and kidney.

As mentioned earlier, there are nine sections to the rules. The following paragraphs describe the sections and provide some background, but the rules themselves are not repeated in this chapter. It is important that the reader/coder review and understand the MP/H coding rules as given in the official documentation.

- *Cover, Table of Contents, Preface:* The one-page preface describes the basics of the MP/H rules and lists the participants in the project, the site-specific sets of rules, and information about further training on the rules.
- *MP/H Coding Rules General Instructions:* The general instructions include equivalent terms, definitions, and ambiguous terminology that apply to all of the rules sets, as well as the priorities for determining multiple primaries and how to use the rules for determining the histologic type for each abstract. *This is the most important section for a new registrar to read and understand.*
- *Terms & Definitions MP/H Coding Rules:* This section is the supporting information for the site-specific rules themselves. It includes an introduction, equivalent terms, definitions, histology tables, priority guidelines, and anatomic illustrations for each of the nine sets of rules for specific organs or body systems, plus the "other sites" set of rules that covers all other organs except the hematopoietic diseases and Kaposi sarcoma. See Table 13-3 for a list of the rules sets. *This section must be used in conjunction with the MP/H coding rules in the selected format.*
- *Multiple Primary Rules and Histology Coding Rules formatted:* The 10 sets of rules have been developed in three formats—text, matrix, and flowchart—for users with different learning styles. The concepts expressed in the rules are the same, only the format is different, so registrars can select the format that makes the rules most understandable and workable for the individual. See Figure 13-2 for a comparison of the three formats for the same rule.
  - **Text**—full sentences similar to other coding manuals

Table 13-3	2007 Multiple Primary and Histology (MP/H) Site-Specific Rules Sets

- Head and neck
- Colon
- Lung
- Malignant melanoma of skin
- Breast
- Kidney
- Urinary tract (renal pelvis, ureter, bladder and other urinary)
- Brain and central nervous system, malignant
- Brain and central nervous system, benign/borderline
- Other sites (organs and body systems not included in one of the rules sets above)

TEXT FORMAT

M2. A single tumor is always a *single* primary. *
Note: The tumor may overlap onto or extend into adjacent/contiguous site or subsite.

MATRIX FORMAT

Rule	Site	Histology	Timing	Behavior	Notes/Examples	Primary
SINGLE TUMOR					1. Tumor not described as metastasis 2. Includes combinations of in situ and invasive	
M2	Single				Tumor may overlap onto or extend into adjacent/contiguous site or subsite	Single*

FLOWCHART FORMAT

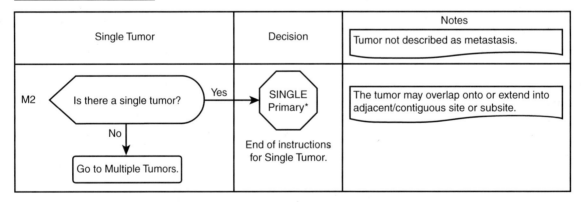

Figure 13-2. Comparison of Formats for Example Rule M2. Note: This example is from the multiple primary rules. The histology coding rules use the same formats.

- **Matrix**—tables with labeled columns defining the elements of the rule's concept and the result (one primary, more than one primary, or the correct code)
- **Flowchart**—similar to a computer program, stating the rule as a question and then indicating what to do, based on whether the answer to the question is yes or no
- **Appendices**—This section contains the names of MP/H Task Force members, CoC Clinical Advisory Panels, and board of directors of the Central Brain Tumor Registry of the United States

Important MP/H Concepts

Important MP/H concepts include:

- *The MP/H rules apply to 2007 diagnoses and forward.* The rules should not be applied to pre-2007 diagnoses. However, a pre-2007 diagnosis must be considered when the patient has a new tumor diagnosed in 2007 or after. For example, a patient had a head and neck cancer in 2005 and now enters hospital in 2010 with "recurrence." The registrar must apply the head and neck rules to determine whether the 2010 diagnosis is a new primary.

- *The MP/H rules apply to solid tumors only.* The rules do not apply to Kaposi sarcoma or to lymphomas, leukemias or other hematopoietic diseases. A separate set of rules for lymphomas and hematopoietic diseases, discussed later, was implemented in 2010.
- *The MP/H rules do not apply to casefinding, staging, or other registry purposes.* They are strictly for determining how many abstracts to prepare and how to code the histology for each abstract. Conversely, rules from other registry activities should not be used to determine multiple primaries or histology codes.
- *Site-specific sets of rules are complete in themselves.* Each set of rules is self-contained, meaning that the rules are accompanied by a set of definitions, equivalent terms, and other guidelines. Do not mix rules from one site-specific set with another.
- *Rules are in hierarchical order.* The individual rules within each set are in priority or hierarchical order. The rules say, "Take the first rule that applies and then STOP." Do not continue to search for a rule that might be better for the case.

Using the MP/H Coding Rules

The main principles to follow in using the coding rules include:

1. *Read the General Instructions.* The general instructions apply to all sets of MP/H coding rules unless exceptions are made in the site-specific rules.
2. *Review the case to determine the primary site(s).* Review the medical record to identify the location of the tumor(s). In most cases, this is apparent from the pathology report and imaging, but it may be necessary to read the entire record for references to more than one tumor.
3. *Go to the appropriate set of site-specific rules and read the Site-specific Equivalent Terms, Definitions, Tables and Illustrations.* Based on the primary site(s) indicated in the medical record, review the guidelines, definitions, and rules for the appropriate site-specific set of rules. If necessary, assign the primary site code(s) to the case and then look at the headers for the rules sets to find the site codes included.
4. *Apply the Multiple Primary Rules first.* If there is any question whether the case is more than one primary site, use the multiple primary rules. Within each set of site-specific rules are three modules based on how many tumors are indicated in the medical record: Unknown if Single or Multiple Tumors, Single Tumor, and Multiple Tumors.
   A. Count the number of primary cancers described in the medical record. Do not count metastatic sites or microscopic spots (foci) of tumor. Use only the module pertaining to the number of primary tumors identified.
      - If there is only one tumor, use the "Single Tumor" module and complete a single abstract.
      - If there is more than one tumor, use the "Multiple Tumors" module and follow the instructions that will indicate whether to complete a single abstract or more than one abstract.
      - If the number of tumors cannot be determined, use the "Unknown if Single or Multiple Tumors" module, which defaults to completing a single abstract.
   B. Read through the module starting with the first rule. If that rule does not apply, keep reading until the *first* rule applicable to the case is found, which will say how many abstracts to prepare. Don't waste time reading any further.
   C. Open the abstract (if a single abstract is indicated) or the first abstract (if multiple abstracts are indicated by the rules) and move on to the histology coding rules. Focus on one abstract at a time.
5. *Use the Histology Coding Rules for the first abstract.*
   A. In priority order, review the pathology report(s) for the case, if available, then cytology reports, then the rest of the medical record for any statement of a cell type.
   B. If there is more than one pathology report, code the histology from the final diagnosis of the most representative tumor specimen. The "most representative tumor specimen" is the specimen that contains the greatest amount of tumor, which may not be the most extensive resection of the primary site. The "Final Diagnosis" is the pathologist's summary of findings for the case and may include comments, a cancer protocol or pathology checklist, or in some cases, an amended diagnosis after consultation. Do not use information from the gross or microscopic description of the specimen unless indicated in the histology coding rules.
   C. Note the keywords in the diagnosis and go to the appropriate module in the histology coding rules. If there is only one tumor, use the "Single Tumor" module. If the multiple tumors module of the multiple primaries rules said to complete a single abstract for a case having multiple tumors, use the "Multiple Tumors Abstracted as a Single Primary module." Remember to focus on determining the histology code for one abstract at a time if the case has multiple primaries.
   D. Read through the module starting with the first rule. If that rule does not apply, keep reading until the first rule that applies to the case is found, which will say what histology code to use. Don't waste time reading any further. Finish the abstract and move on to the next abstract.

Both the multiple primaries and the histology coding rules have now been applied to the case. Most cancers are single primaries. The multiple primary rules will apply to about 10% of solid tumor cases in the average cancer registry, and the histology coding rules will apply to between 15% and 25% of individual abstracts.

Hematopoietic and Lymphoid Neoplasm Case Reportability and Coding Rules

This long title for the supplement to the MP/H coding rules is usually shortened to "Heme MP/H Rules." Implemented for cases diagnosed in 2010 and forward, the heme MP/H rules are a continuation of the concepts that were first presented for solid tumors in 2007. This new set of rules covers the malignant lymphomas, leukemias, myeloproliferative and myelodysplastic neoplasms in the ICD-O-3 morphology code range 9590 to 9992. The coding rules are presented in the same three formats—text, matrix, and flowchart—as the solid tumor rules, although there are a few substantial differences between the heme and solid tumor rules.

- The heme rules cover not only counting of multiple primaries and histology coding for individual cases, but also case reportability, primary site coding, and grade coding. The reason for the extra rules is to resolve longstanding issues with these diseases, such as which of the hematopoietic neoplasms are reportable to cancer registries, to answer questions about the appropriate primary site code to use for certain types of neoplasms, and to indicate the correct code to use in the sixth digit (grade/differentiation) position of the ICD-O-3 morphology code. With the exception of the case reportability instructions, the new sets of rules are also provided in the same three formats.
- Just as with the solid tumor MP/H rules, the heme rules replace all previous rules, coding guides, and reportable lists for lymphomas and hematopoietic diseases.
- The heme rules include new disease entities and codes from the 2008 *World Health Organization Classification of Tumours of the Haematopoietic and Lymphoid Tissues,* which added about 32 new primary terms to ICD-O-3. This is the first formal update to ICD-O-3 since the initial errata were published in 2001 and 2002. The WHO Classification made a few additional terms reportable, including myeloproliferative and myelodysplastic/myeloproliferative neoplasm, unclassifiable; T-cell large granular lymphocytic leukemia and chronic lymphoproliferative disorder of natural killer (NK) cells; and all the variants of Langerhans cell histiocytosis.
- Determination of multiple primaries has always been challenging. Previous documentation consisted of lists or charts of histologies that were considered distinct entities, and therefore subsequent or multiple primaries. However, previous lists did not address transformations, which are a process where a disease changes from one cell type to another as a result of continued mutation or the effects of therapy. Transformations from one disease to another, such as a refractory anemia with excess blasts (RAEB) transforming into acute myeloid leukemia (AML), are reportable as two primaries effective with 2010 diagnoses. (Formerly, the transformation to AML would be recorded on the RAEB abstract as follow-up, but the AML would not be counted as a new entity in the year it was diagnosed.)
- In addition to the coding manual documentation of the rules, there is a separate hematopoietic database that serves as a companion reference of abstractor information. It is important to understand that the heme database supplements the rules but does not replace them. Neither the coding manual nor the heme database is intended to be used as a stand-alone product. Table 13-4 lists the contents of each product.

The official documentation and program files can be downloaded from the SEER Program Web site (http://seer.cancer.gov/tools/heme/index.html). They will not be repeated in this chapter. The coding manual itself (the four sets of instructions and rules) is imbedded in the hematopoietic database and can be accessed electronically once it has been downloaded. A wealth of training materials is available from SEER, the NAACCR, and the NCRA.

There are four steps to using the heme MP/H rules.

1. *Determine whether the case is reportable.* Refer to the 10 case reportability instructions. The instructions are in text format only and are not hierarchical. Pay attention to the notes in this set of instructions. If rules 1 to 9 do not apply to the case, use the heme database to determine reportability.

2. *Determine how many primaries to abstract.* The 13 Multiple Primary (M_) rules are hierarchical. Start with M1 and keep reading until a rule applies to the case. If a transformation is mentioned, refer to the heme database to verify. If rules M1 to M12 do not apply, use the multiple primary calculator feature in the heme database to determine how many abstracts to prepare.

3. *Code the primary site and histology.* The Primary Site and Histology (PH) Coding Rules are the largest section and address problematic coding rules and terminology. There are 41 rules in 9 modules, but only a maximum of three or four modules will be necessary to code a case. Module 1 contains three general rules that apply to all cases. Modules 2 to 6 are histology specific; applicable codes are listed in the header for each module. Module 7 is the primary site rules for lymphomas. Module 8 is general histology rules for all neoplasms. Modules 1 to 8 are not hierarchical: use Module 1 first, then go to the appropriate histology-

Table 13-4	Contents of Hematopoietic and Lymphoid Neoplasm Case Reportability Documents

Heme MP/H Coding Manual
- Case Reportability Instructions
- Multiple Primary Rules (M_)
- Primary Site and Histology Coding Rules (PH_)
- Grade Coding Rules (G_)
- Appendices
  - Glossary
  - A. History and list of obsolete terms
  - B. Histology Lineages
  - C. Lymph Node/Lymph Node Chain Reference Table
  - D. New Histology Terms and Codes and Newly Reportable Hematopoietic Diseases
  - E. Histology "NOS" Table
  - F. Master Code Lists

Hematopoietic Data Base—Specific Diseases
- Definition of disease entity
- Synonyms
- Definitive diagnostic methods
- Transformations
- Abstractor notes
- Treatment types
- Genetic testing and immunophenotyping
- Multiple primaries calculator
- Casefinding lists—ICD-9-CM and ICD-10

MP/H, Multiple Primary and Histology; NOS, not otherwise specified; ICD-9-CM, *International Classification of Diseases, 9th revision: Clinical Modification;* ICD-10, *International Classification of Diseases, 10th revision: Clinical Modification.*

specific module (2–6). Rules within the modules are hierarchical. Module 9 consists of two rules to be used only if previous modules do not apply. Refer to the heme database when instructed in the rules.

4. *Code the grade of the neoplasm.* There are 11 hierarchical rules for coding the sixth digit of the ICD-O-3 morphology code. These rules say when to code the grade/differentiation as 9 (for all myelodysplastic neoplasms and some others), 5 (T cell), 6 (B cell), 7 (non-T non-B), and 8 (NK cell).

These four steps complete the reportability, primary site, histology, and grade for the case. Additional information about diagnostic and therapeutic procedures and other aspects of the abstract is available in the hematopoietic database.

Summary

The MP/H coding rules were developed by the North American standards setters to provide guidelines for determining the number of primary malignancies (multiple primaries) and the histology code for each primary. The MP/H rules handle situations that are not covered in the ICD-O-3 coding rules and are intended to improve the overall quality of cancer registry databases by providing a standardized set of rules to be used by both facility- and population-based registries. The first set, implemented in 2007, covered all solid tumors, excluding Kaposi sarcoma. The rules for benign and borderline central nervous system tumors developed when those tumors were made reportable in 2004 and were merged into the solid tumor rules. In 2010, rules for reportability, multiple primaries, primary site and histology coding and grade coding for the lymphoid and hematopoietic diseases were implemented to supplement the solid tumor rules. The MP/H coding rules will continue to evolve as more sites are extracted from the "other sites" rules and additional sets of site-specific rules are developed.

Additional Information

- SEER MP/H continuing education module (www.training.seer.cancer.gov)
- Beginning and advanced training for MP/H rules (webcasts and PowerPoint presentations: http://seer.cancer.gov/tools/mphrules/training.html)
- Online training for Hematopoietic and Lymphoid Neoplasms coding rules (http://seer.cancer.gov/tools/heme/training/index.html)

References

1. Huffman, E. K. "The Standard Nomenclature of Diseases and Operation." In *Manual for Medical Record Librarians* (pp. 207–244). Berwyn, IL: Physician's Record Company, 1960.

2. Greenwood, M. *Medical Statistics from Graunt to Farr* (p. 28.). New York: Cambridge University Press, 1948.

3. Registrar General of England and Wales. *Sixteenth Annual Report, 1856* (p. 75). London: Wellcome Library, 1856.

4. Bertillon, J. "Classification of the Causes of Death" [abstract]. *Transactions of the 15th International Congress of Hygiene and Demography* (pp. 52–55). Washington, DC, Department of State, 1912.

5. *Manual of the International Statistical Classification of Diseases, Injuries and Causes of Death, 1955 revision*, Vols. 1 and 2. Geneva, Switzerland: World Health Organization, 1957.

6. Plunkett, R. J., Hayden, A. D., editors. *Standard Nomenclature of Diseases and Operations*, 4th ed. Philadelphia: The Blackiston Company; American Medical Association, 1952.

7. *Standard Nomenclature of Diseases and Operations*, 5th ed. New York: McGraw-Hill; American Medical Association, 1961.

8. *Manual of Tumor Nomenclature and Coding*. Atlanta: American Cancer Society, 1951.

9. *International Classification of Diseases, 1965 Revision*, Vols. 1 and 2. Geneva, Switzerland: World Health Organization, 1967.

10. *International Classification of Diseases, Adapted for Use in the United States*, Vols. 1 and 2 [PHS Publication No. 1693]. Washington, DC: U.S. Department of Health, Education and Welfare; Public Health Service; National Center for Health Statistics, 1967.

11. *International Classification of Diseases, Adapted*, Vols. 1 and 2. Ann Arbor, MI: Commission on Professional and Hospital Activities, 1968.

12. *Systematized Nomenclature of Pathology*. Skokie, IL: College of American Pathologists, 1965.

13. *Manual of Tumor Nomenclature and Coding*. Atlanta: American Cancer Society, 1968.

14. *International Classification of Diseases for Oncology*. Geneva, Switzerland: World Health Organization, 1976.

15. *International Classification of Diseases, 1975 revision*, Vols. 1 and 2. Geneva, Switzerland: World Health Organization, 1977.

16. *International Classification of Diseases, 9th revision: Clinical Modification*, Vols. 1–3. Ann Arbor, MI: Commission on Professional and Hospital Activities, 1978.

17. *International Classification of Diseases, 9th revision: Clinical Modification*, Vols. 1–3 (p. 159). Ann Arbor, MI: Commission on Professional and Hospital Activities, 1978.

18. Young, J., Percy, C. L., Asire, A. J., editors. *Surveillance, Epidemiology and End Results: Incidence and Mortality Data, 1973-1977* [National Cancer Institute monograph 57]. Washington, DC: U.S. Department of Health and Human Services, National Institutes of Health, 1981.

19. *Systematized Nomenclature of Medicine*, Vols. 1 and 2. Skokie, IL: College of American Pathologists, 1976–1977.

20. *International Statistical Classification of Diseases and Related Health Problems, 10th Revision*, Vols. 1–3. Geneva, Switzerland: World Health Organization, 1992.

21. Percy, C., Van Holten, V., Muir, C., editors. *International Classification of Diseases for Oncology*, 2nd ed. Geneva, Switzerland: World Health Organization, 1990.

22. *The Systematized Nomenclature of Human and Veterinary Medicine*, Vols. 1–4. Skokie, IL: College of American Pathologists, 1993.

23. Spackman, K. A., Campbell, K. E., Cote, R. A. *SNOMED RT: A Reference Terminology for Health Care.* Northfield, IL: College of American Pathologists, 2000.

24. SNOMED Clinical Terms (SNOMED CT). Northfield, IL: College of American Pathologists, 2002.

25. *International Classification of Diseases, Tenth Revision, Clinical Modification* (ICD-10-CM), U.S. National Center for Health Statistics, June 2003. Available at: http://www.cdc.gov/nchs/about/otheract/icd9/icd10cm.htm. Accessed January 29, 2004.

26. Jaffee, E. S., Harris, N. L., Stein, H., Vardiman, J. W., editors. *World Health Organization Classification of Tumors. Pathology and Genetics of Tumors of Hematopoietic and Lymphoid Tissues.* Lyon: IARC Press, 2001.

27. *International Histological Typing of Tumours*, 2nd ed. Geneva, Switzerland: World Health Organization, 1981–2000.

28. Fritz, A. G., Percy, C., et al., editors: *International Classification of Diseases for Oncology*, 3rd ed. Geneva, Switzerland: World Health Organization, 2000.

29. Fritz, A., Percy, C. "Introducing ICD-O-3: Impact of the New Edition," *Journal of Registry Management*, 2000;27(4):125–132.

30. *ICD-O-3 Implementation Guidelines.* Springfield, IL: North American Association of Central Cancer Registries, November 27, 2000. Available at: http://www.naaccr.org/StandardsandRegistryOperations/ImplementationGuidelines.aspx, last accessed August 2010.

31. Swerdlow, S. H., Campo, E., Harris, N. L., et al., editors. *WHO Classification of Tumours of Haematopoietic and Lymphoid Tissues*, 4th ed. Lyon: International Agency for Research on Cancer, 2008.

32. Johnson, C. H., Adamo, M., Peace, S., Percy-Laurry, A., editors. *2010 Hematopoietic and Lymphoid Neoplasm Case Reportability and Coding Manual.* Bethesda, MD: National Cancer Institute, 2010. Available at: www.seer.cancer.gov/tools/heme/index.html, last accessed August 2010.

33. Johnson, C. H., Peace, S., Adamo, P., Fritz, A., Percy-Laurry, A., Edwards, B. K. *The 2007 Multiple Primary and Histology Coding Rules.* Bethesda, MD: National Cancer Institute, Surveillance, Epidemiology, and End Results Program, 2007.

Cancer Staging

Donna M. Gress, RHIT, CTR

In 1929, the League of Nations' World Health Organization introduced the concept of describing disease by stage or the extent of the disease. The first primary site so described was cancer of the cervix. Staging is a common language developed by medical professionals to communicate information about a disease to others. The disease can be any acute or chronic disease such as cancer, diabetes, acquired immunodeficiency syndrome (AIDS), cardiovascular disease, or rheumatoid arthritis. This is mainly for the purposes of treatment, disease management, and prognosis.

Staging for cancer has evolved over many years. Many groups have developed different staging systems. Some cover all cancer sites. Others are limited to particular ages, histologies, sites, study groups, or medical specialties. This chapter discusses common staging systems and the various classifications within these systems, based on staging at different points in time of a patient's care. The most common staging systems used in hospital and central registries are reviewed.

Cancer staging is historically based solely on the anatomic extent of cancer, and it remains primarily anatomic. However, an increasing number of nonanatomic factors about a cancer and its host provide critical prognostic information and may predict the value of specific therapies.[1]

Staging is a shorthand method for describing disease. A coded format, such as a numerical system with increasing values meaning more involvement or severity, ensures understanding of the system. A general definition for staging is the grouping of cases into broad categories based on extent of disease and other nonanatomic factors that play a role in treatment and prognosis. These broad stage categories consist of more detailed information. There are detailed elements describing how far the tumor has spread from the organ or site of origin (the primary site), the involvement of regional lymph nodes, and distant metastatic spread. Nonanatomic characteristics about a case also play a role in describing the disease and can be part of how they are grouped into categories. These additional factors personalize the information for that patient and provide further information for individualized or personalized prognosis. Thus, staging transforms specific information from each patient's cancer into groups that can be studied or evaluated for prognostic significance.

Different staging systems exist to serve different purposes. Some staging systems, such as Summary Stage, have broad categories that rarely change over time, providing a simple grouping that has longitudinal stability. These are mainly used by population registries. They are less complex than other systems and were developed for epidemiologists who want some information on stage but do not need the more detailed information. They can also be useful when a series of cases is so small that only general categories can produce enough data for a meaningful analysis. Some staging systems, such as the historic Surveillance, Epidemiology, and End Results (SEER) Extent of Disease (EOD), are more detailed, but capture data only once. They put together the best information from the diagnostic workup and the pathologic examination of the resected specimens. Another type of staging system, the American Joint Committee on Cancer (AJCC) stage, provides the more detailed information but also adds in assigning the stage at different points in time. This allows analysis of cases at the same point in time, such as the stage determined by the diagnostic workup and then the stage after surgical resection. This can meet the decision-making needs of clinicians choosing the appropriate treatment methods and the evaluation of those results. This type of staging needs to be flexible enough to change when data analysis proves it is necessary. This provides forward flexibility and clinical utility for choosing treatment and estimating prognosis for individual cancer cases. This type of system is used by clinicians to guide patient care.[2]

Purposes of Staging

There are several reasons for staging cancer cases. It is important for the medical practitioner to adequately assess the extent of cancer to treat the disease in the most appropriate manner. Understanding the extent of disease assists the physician in determining the most appropriate treatment to cure the disease, decrease the tumor burden, or relieve symptoms.

Staging is also used to indicate prognosis. Data from historical sources can provide an estimate of the expected survival rate for a particular cancer with a corresponding extent of disease. Histology, grade of the tumor, age, sex, race, and the efficacy of therapy play a part in determining the patient's prognosis and quality of survival.

Staging provides a means of comparing local institutional experience with national data. It can be used to compare treatment results based on common criteria for extent of disease. Staging expedites the exchange of data and assists in the continuing research on cancer. The health information record is the primary source of documentation for staging information.

General Guidelines for Staging Systems

The following list includes general guidelines for staging for all systems:

- Rules for assigning the stage, including timing rules, ensure consistency in the data.
- Stage grouping can be applied only to cancers that are alike in site, histology, or both.
- Accurate and complete assessment of the cancer is necessary before staging.
- A few cases are unstageable. The unknown stage category should be assigned only after all efforts to

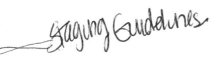
identify the extent of disease have been exhausted, or the site or histology does not meet criteria for staging.

- It is mandatory to stage uniformly using the same staging system to compare data or results.
- It is important to seek further information if staging information is unclear to ensure the quality of data.

The following list includes general guidelines for AJCC staging:

- Stage may be defined at a number of points in the care of the patient. These stage classifications further refine the information comparing patients at the same point in time. These classifications include clinical, pathologic, post-treatment (post-rx), retreatment, and autopsy.
- When there is doubt about assigning the correct stage, select the lower (lesser) category.
- Staging is revised as medical science progresses. It is important to use the most current edition of a staging system. Changes to a new edition are effective with diagnoses at the beginning of a year.
- It is important to verify physician staging. Request substantiation if a physician's staging does not correlate with the information in the health information record.
- Stage documentation in the cancer registry started with breast in 1982, and lung and colon were added in 1986, according to the Cancer Program Standards of the Commission on Cancer (CoC). It became mandatory to start staging all sites in January 1991.
- Stage documentation in the health information record by the managing physician started with cases diagnosed after January 1, 1995, by the CoC Cancer Program Standards. Although staging forms are not required, they are helpful in determining and documenting the stage. Please refer to the CoC Standards for the current requirements.

Sources of Information for Staging

Many sources in the health information record must be examined to determine the stage. These sources are part of the diagnostic workup for the disease and also the assessment after surgical treatment. Many of the tests in the diagnostic workup may be done on an outpatient basis or in a physician's office.

Physical Examination

For most cancers, the report of the physical examination should include the location of a tumor, including site and subsite, direct extension of the tumor to other organs or structures, and palpability and mobility of accessible lymph nodes. The probability of distant site involvement, such as organomegaly, pleural effusion, ascites, or neurologic findings should be stated. Many signs and symptoms may indicate distant site or metastatic involvement. In a breast cancer case, for example, the physical examination should describe the exact location of the tumor mass, clinical size of the tumor, and the condition of the skin surrounding the tumor, including changes in skin color and texture, and attachment or fixation of the mass. The examination should include the entire axilla and other regional nodal areas including the supraclavicular nodes.

Tumors of the head and neck area are evaluated with a general examination of the face and neck. The eyes, skin, ears, and nasal cavity should be examined in addition to mucosal surfaces of the nasopharynx, oral cavity, oropharynx, hypopharynx, and larynx. Digital and bimanual palpation of the oral cavity, oropharynx, and neck should be included in the physical examination.

Some organ sites are not easily examined clinically. A patient suspected of having a gastrointestinal tumor should have external palpation of the liver and abdomen. Female patients should have both a digital rectal examination and a pelvic examination. Male patients should have a digital rectal examination. Patients with suspected lung cancer should have an assessment of cervical and supraclavicular nodal areas.

In all cases, other than lymphomas, nodes must be described by a clinician as "involved" to be considered to contain cancer. For example, if it is stated that nodes are enlarged, they are not considered to contain cancer until there is a physician's clinical determination based on size, matting, or fixation, or until there is cytologic or pathologic confirmation.

Radiologic Procedures

Radiographs and scans are useful for staging purposes. Radiologic reports should define the location of the cancer, the size of the tumor, involvement of adjacent structures, or existence of distant disease. They can help determine the resectability of the tumor. All radiologic reports should be reviewed to determine the extent of disease. The CoC of the American College of Surgeons (ACoS) lists some common terms that are to be interpreted as evidence of tumor involvement and another list of terms that are to be interpreted as no tumor involvement. It is important to refer to the current publication for the list.[3]

Radiographs

The most common radiograph is the chest film, which is used for a variety of purposes. The posteroanterior and lateral chest x-ray procedures are simple methods of detecting lung cancers or lesions metastatic to the lung from other primary cancer sites. The radiograph can show the tumor size, location, obstruction, pleural effusion, or invasion of adjacent structures such as the chest wall or mediastinum.

Mammography is an x-ray technique used to diagnose abnormalities in the breast. Usually, two views are taken of each breast, and the radiographs are examined for lesions or microcalcifications. The mammogram is useful in localizing suspicious nonpalpable lesions. The area of concern is visualized while the breast is in the mammography unit. The radiologist injects dye or inserts a special hookwire needle into the suspicious area. The surgeon is then able to excise the abnormal area.

The most common x-ray procedure used for the diagnosis of colon cancer is the barium enema. The large colon is filled with a barium solution and multiple x-ray films are taken. Polyps, as well as constricted and obstructed areas, can be seen. The upper GI (gastrointestinal) series is useful in diagnosing lesions of the pharynx, esophagus, stomach, and small intestine.

One common radiologic examination used in the study of the urinary tract is the KUB, a frontal film of the abdomen used to examine the kidneys, ureters, and bladder. Several other urinary tract x-ray examinations use a contrast medium (a radiopaque substance to delineate and define the contour of the structures). The intravenous pyelogram follows the injection of the contrast media into a vein and displays the path of the media through the kidneys, ureters, and bladder. A retrograde urogram is performed by inserting a cystoscope into the ureteral meatus, inserting a catheter through the cystoscope, and adding a contrast solution to study the renal pelvis and ureters. The location and size of tumors of the urinary tract can often be defined through these x-ray studies.

An angiogram is an x-ray study of the vascular system that is used to diagnose some cancers. A cerebral angiogram helps define the blood supply to brain lesions. Lymphangiograms are useful in the study of the vessels of the lymphatic system. They were used as a staging workup for lymphomas before the widespread availability of Computerized axial tomographic (CT) scanning and magnetic resonance imaging (MRI).

Scans or Imaging

CT scanning is used for the examination of many parts of the body. The scan's images show cross-sectional "slices" of the body that are each a millimeter thick. A composite image is created by the computer. The CT scan gives an accurate picture of the extent of disease and helps identify tumors at an early stage. CT scans are performed both with and without contrast media. CT scans can be taken of the head, chest, abdomen, pelvis, or the whole body. When a case is staged, the entire report should be reviewed for correct interpretation of the areas that are involved or not involved with tumor. Enlarged lymph nodes may also be seen on the CT scans.

Diagnostic nuclear medicine examinations or scans are used to identify abnormalities in the brain, salivary glands, thyroid, heart, lung, kidney, liver, spleen, and bone.

The patient is given a radioisotope that emits gamma rays and permits the radiologist to see abnormal structures or functions. Bone scans can show metastatic lytic (destructive) lesions or blastic (overgrowth of bone) lesions of bone. For example, breast and prostate cancers are known to metastasize to the bone. Therefore, a bone scan may confirm or rule out the distant spread of disease. Liver and spleen scans can show the presence and size of a tumor. Brain scans can indicate the location of a tumor, size, and associated vascular structures.

MRI uses magnetic fields to provide images of body tissues. MRI can be used to look at all parts of the body, including the brain, the heart, blood vessels, the spinal cord, and the extremities. An MRI system can create axial images, as well as images in the sagittal plane and coronally or any degree in between. Combining radiofrequency (pulsing) energy and different levels of magnetic fields processed with highly sophisticated computers, MRI scans produce detailed and clear pictures of body parts. Intravenous contrast liquid can be used to improve the appearance of some body tissues within an image.

Ultrasound

Ultrasound produces sound waves that are beamed into the body causing return echoes that are recorded to "visualize" structures beneath the skin. The ability to measure different echoes reflected from a variety of tissues allows a shadow picture to be constructed. The technology is especially accurate at seeing the interface between solid and fluid-filled spaces.

Endoscopy

An endoscopic examination involves using an instrument to examine internal passages or the inside of hollow organs or viscera. This can be effective in the nasopharynx, pharynx, larynx, esophagus, stomach, large bowel, bladder, and parts of the lungs. The common endoscopic procedures used in cancer diagnosis are discussed in this section.

A bronchoscopy is the examination of bronchi in the lungs. The scope can be inserted through the oral or nasal cavity. The pharynx, larynx, and trachea can be seen as the bronchoscope goes through to the bronchi. Using the flexible bronchoscope, the interior segmental and subsegmental bronchi can be visualized. The endoscopist looks for irregular bronchial folds, mucosal thickening, stenosis, friable tissue, and many other abnormalities such as a tumor mass. Normally, biopsies or bronchial washings are obtained during a bronchoscopic examination.

A proctoscopy is often done using a rigid scope. A sigmoidoscope is more flexible and can be used to observe the colon into the descending colon at greater than 30 cm. In the past, rigid sigmoidoscopes were often used, but they have been replaced with flexible sigmoidoscopes. Flexible scopes allow greater visualization of the sigmoid colon. A

neuro neuroendocrine tumors

fiberoptic colonoscope is a flexible instrument that examines the colon to the cecum. Often, the physician will photograph and biopsy any abnormalities or suspicious areas seen during colonoscopy.

A cystoscope is used to examine the interior of the bladder. It is inserted through the urethra, so the urethra can also be examined. Abnormalities can be surgically removed or electrocauterized during the cystoscopic procedure.

The entire endoscopic procedure report must be read to obtain pertinent information. Endoscopic reports define certain observations, tumor location, pertinent findings, diagnosis, or the impressions of cancer. For example, colonoscopy reports should state the distance of the abnormality from the anal verge. Esophagoscopy reports should state the distance of the abnormality from the incisors to help determine the exact location of the tumor. Any biopsies or washings sent for microscopic examination should be noted. It is important to review the pathology and cytology reports to confirm the diagnosis of cancer.

Some endoscopic procedures can be accomplished through natural openings in the body. Others must be performed through incisions into the body. For example, thoracoscopy is used to examine the pleural cavity. The instrument is inserted through an intercostal space. Mediastinoscopy is performed through an incision and allows visualization of the area between the lungs. The mediastinal lymph nodes that are examined for potential involvement by metastatic cancer can determine the unresectability of a lung cancer.

Laparoscopy, performed through an incision in the abdominal wall, allows the visualization of intra-abdominal structures. Laparoscopy is useful in gastrointestinal and gynecologic malignancies to diagnose both the primary organ and metastatic involvement. Some surgeries can be completed as laparoscopic or laparoscope-aided procedures. A culdoscopy incision is made through the posterior vaginal wall and allows visualization of the cul-de-sac.

The endoscopic retrograde cholangiopancreatogram (ERCP) allows direct visualization and contrast x-ray films of the ampulla of Vater and the duodenal mucosa. ERCP is helpful in diagnosing both pancreatic and bile duct cancers.

Prognostic Factors (Site-Specific Factors) or Prognostic Features

Specific biological properties of the cancer may be an important key in prognostic systems for patient management. It is important to record this information. Some of these factors have been validated, and guide patient care and prognosis, whereas other factors are still under investigation. As more of these nonanatomic prognostic factors are fully validated, they will be incorporated into staging systems.

The main categories of prognostic factors include descriptions or diseases, pathology report information, laboratory tests, and genetics. The descriptions or diseases can be tumor location, human papillomavirus, or Crohn's disease. The pathology report information can include tumor-infiltrating lymphocytes, mitotic rate, or nodal extracapsular spread. Some of the common laboratory tests include carcinoembryonic antigen (CEA), cancer antigen 19-9 (CA 19-9), serum chromogranin A (CgA), lactate dehydrogenase (LDH), Ki-67 growth fraction, and prostate-specific antigen (PSA). The more common genetic tests are microsatellite instability, kit gene mutation, human epidermal growth factor receptor 2 (HER2), KRAS gene mutation, and 18q loss of heterozygosity (LOH). It is important to read each chapter in the *AJCC Cancer Staging Manual* to determine the important factors, and to review the information in the Collaborative Stage (CS) Data Collection System Coding Instructions for the data collected in the Site-Specific Factors of each schema.

These prognostic factors are also referred to as tumor markers. Cytologic tumor markers are tumor-specific substances in the blood serum or other tissues that can assist in determining the presence or absence of cancer. They can help determine the initial tumor burden in both the primary site and distant sites. Tumor markers can be helpful in monitoring for recurrence. Care should be taken to seek this information to assist in determining stage.

The most common factors used for prognosis in breast cancer are the estrogen receptor (ER) assay and the progesterone receptor (PR) assay. Both are steroid hormone receptors. ER and PR assays are used to estimate the potential response to endocrine, or hormone therapy. They help in the determination of prognosis and the management of patients with breast cancer. Pieces of breast cancer tissue are analyzed in the laboratory to determine the ER and PR assays. The presence of ERs or PRs, or both, denotes whether the cancer is growing in the presence of either or both naturally occurring hormones.

CA-15-3, a tumor-associated glycoprotein, is found in the serum. It can be useful in monitoring the presence of metastatic breast cancer and the patient's response to chemotherapy.

PSA, a proteolytic enzyme, is used as a screening mechanism for prostate cancer. It can monitor the presence of metastatic disease in patients who have undergone a radical prostatectomy. Increased PSAs can also be found in aging patients and in association with benign prostatic hypertrophy and prostatitis.

One oncofetal antigen, CEA, has been used for many years to monitor colon, lung, breast, and pancreatic cancers. Increasing serum levels of CEA may indicate disease recurrence many months before clinical manifestations.

Cancer antigen 125 (CA-125) is a glycoprotein associated with ovarian carcinoma cells. Increased levels appear in about 75% of patients with ovarian cancer and may be associated with tumor burden and recurrence. CA-125 is used to monitor patients for residual or recurrent disease.

immunoglobulins - multiple myeloma, Waldenstrom

alpha-Fetoprotein (AFP) is an oncofetal antigen that is useful in monitoring patients with nonseminomatous testicular cancer and certain types of ovarian cancer. Human chorionic gonadotropin (hCG) is a hormone that can be detected to assess the prognosis and to monitor treatment response in patients with germ cell tumors, breast cancer, choriocarcinoma, and testicular carcinoma.

Flow cytometry has become an important clinical test to determine cellular DNA ploidy (the number of sets of chromosomes in a cell) and S-phase (the percentage of cells in active DNA synthesis). In flow cytometry, cells are stained with a special dye and then analyzed in a flow cytometer by using a laser beam to measure the fluorescence of cells. The results are charted in a histogram showing the distribution of DNA in the cells.[4] Results of flow cytometry are helpful to determine prognosis, monitor treatment response, and document tumor recurrence. Tumors demonstrating an abnormal number of chromosomes, such as tetraploidy, polyploidy, or aneuploidy, are more likely to be aggressive than tumors that are diploid (i.e., have the normal two sets of chromosomes).[5] Tumors with a low S-phase have a better prognosis.

Surgical Reports

All surgical procedures should be noted in a written operative report. Pertinent observations from operative procedures should be noted, including the location of the tumor and any direct extension, nodal involvement, or metastatic spread. Information from the operative or procedure report supplements the information noted in the pathology report. The operative report should state whether the procedure was considered curative or palliative. If a palliative procedure is done, a biopsy may be performed on any residual tumor.

Noncancer-directed surgeries such as cystotomy, gastrotomy, laparotomy, and thoracotomy may contribute information on involvement of organs, tissues, or lymph nodes that were not resected. Bypass surgery may be performed to create a passage around a tumor, often for palliation of symptoms. Bypass surgeries such as esophagogastrostomy, gastrostomy, and urethrostomy may provide information on the extent of tumor involvement.

In summary, cancer-directed surgery reports should describe the removal, location, size, and extent of the tumor. Observations of regional lymph nodes, adjacent structures, and organs should be included. The pathology report will confirm the presence or absence of tumor in resected specimens.

Pathologic Examinations

The most common and accurate methods of diagnosing cancer include microscopic examination of either tissues or cells. Cells examined are usually obtained from fluid around the suspected site of cancer. Tissues examined are usually removed from the primary or metastatic site of a cancer.

Many kinds of biopsies are available to remove tissue for a cancer diagnosis. An aspiration biopsy is obtained by using a needle to suction fluid, cells, or tissue into a syringe. A bone marrow biopsy is the removal of bone marrow from one of the body's larger hollow bones.

Excisional biopsies attempt to remove the entire tumor. Incisional biopsies remove only a portion of the tissue. Often, the biopsy specimens are quickly frozen, thinly sliced, and examined to determine the presence or absence of cancer cells (frozen sections). Permanent sections are then made, and the diagnosis from the permanent sections should take precedence over frozen section reports.

Surgical resections involve removing more tissue from the body, including margins of normal tissue or regional lymph nodes, or both. The pathologist can often determine some of the staging information by examining the primary tumor, surrounding tissue, and regional nodes when there is a "total" resection of the tumor. The information from a total resection takes precedence over biopsy reports and operative notes.

Quite often, there are several tissue samples, biopsies, or surgical resections for one cancer. When staging a cancer, it is important to review all pathology reports for the clinical diagnosis, gross description of the specimen, and postoperative diagnosis.

The gross description of the specimen should include the total size of the tumor. Both the gross and microscopic descriptions should state whether the surgical margins are involved by tumor. The pathology report should contain information about the primary site and the spread of disease in surrounding tissues. It is important to note all areas, organs, or structures involved with tumor.

The pathology report contains the histologic type of cancer and the grade of the tumor (how closely the cancer cells resemble normal tissue). Grade is normally expressed as grade I through IV or as well differentiated, moderately differentiated, poorly differentiated, and undifferentiated, respectively.

The final diagnosis of the histologic type takes precedence over preliminary reports and frozen sections. The microscopic description takes precedence over the gross description. Occasionally, pathologic specimens are sent to other centers for consultation, and the final pathology report may not be signed until all consultations have been returned.

The most important information in a pathology report includes source of the specimen, primary site, tumor size, histologic type of cancer, grade of tumor, and the extent of disease within the organ of origin and beyond. The type, size, location, number of lymph nodes removed, and number of nodes containing tumor should be noted. This information is often required for accurate staging.

Pieces or chips of tumor should not be added together to determine tumor size. Multifocal and multicentric are synonymous terms. The size of the largest of the multifocal tumors should be used for staging, and the multiple tumors should be noted. In AJCC, this is done with the descriptor "m," as in T1 (m).

Autopsy reports are a type of pathology report that contains detailed information about organs and structures of the body. They are considered the most complete pathology reports. In summary, pathology reports, or reports of tissue, contain information about biopsies, frozen sections, tissue aspiration or biopsy of bone marrow, surgical specimens, and autopsies.

Cytology reports describe the microscopic examination of cells in body fluids such as sputum, bronchial washings and brushings, pleural fluid, peritoneal fluid, spinal fluid, aspirations from bone marrow, and cervical smears. The Papanicolaou (Pap) smear, used for detection of abnormal cervical cells, is probably the most widely known cytology specimen. Cells can also be obtained by fine-needle aspiration to diagnose cancers of the liver, pancreas, breast, and lung. The most common ways of obtaining cells include brushing the lining of an organ, puncturing a cavity and removing fluid, scraping the lining, or using a swab to obtain secretions.

Thoracentesis is a puncturing of the thoracic, or chest, cavity for the removal of fluid. Paracentesis is the puncture of the abdominal cavity for removal of fluid.

There may be multiple cytology reports. It is important to note the source of the specimen, the histologic description, and pertinent findings, together with interpretations.

Progress Notes and Discharge Summaries

Progress notes summarize diagnostic findings and patient status on a daily basis. The progress notes should be read to supplement and clarify information from laboratory tests, radiology tests, endoscopies, procedures, and histologic reports. The final progress note or the discharge summary should summarize all diagnostic, surgical, and pathologic findings. The stage of cancer should be stated.

Disease Process of Cancer

According to the theory of cancer growth or the natural history of cancer, cancer originates in a single cell. The cell continues to divide and grow in the organ of origin, spreads to adjacent tissue or regional lymph node drainage areas, and then spreads to distant organs or structures. Cancer can spread directly from the organ of origin through the bloodstream into distant organs without involving adjacent organs and regional lymph nodes.

Many cancers go through a matured course, advancing in tumor size or involvement to regional nodal involvement and eventually to distant metastasis. Small tumors can metastasize, with the first sign of the cancer being the metastatic disease.

Staging Systems

The commonly used staging systems by the national groups are explored in this section. They include CS Data Collection System, AJCC Stage, and Summary Stage. Other common staging systems and the historical staging system of SEER EOD are also discussed.

Requirements for Staging

Different staging systems are used for different purposes. Each large database determines the best staging system for its purpose as discussed in the introduction.

The National Program of Cancer Registries (NPCR) of the Centers for Disease Control and Prevention (CDC) collects cancer data nationally through state cancer registries. It was established in 1992 by Congress. NPCR uses Summary Stage, as derived by the CS Data Collection System.

The CoC of the ACoS requires the AJCC staging system be documented on all applicable sites and histologies. The CoC requires the use of the CS Data Collection System and its derived stages for all cases. These data are collected in the National Cancer Data Base (NCDB).

The SEER Program of the National Cancer Institute (NCI) collects cancer data from designated population-based cancer registries in various areas of the country. SEER uses the codes from the CS Data Collection System and the derived stages for their database.

Collaborative Stage Data Collection System

The AJCC, in collaboration with the ACoS/CoC, the NCI/SEER program, the CDC/NPCR program, North American Association of Central Cancer Registries, NCRA, Canadian Council of Cancer Registries, and Canadian Partnership Against Cancer, has developed a CS Data Collection System for use beginning with cases diagnosed on or after January 1, 2004. CS version 2 (CSv2) started with January 1, 2010, cases. The CS system was developed to assure the collection of a unified dataset in all registries and to permit a translation or other method of conversion between the TNM (primary tumor, regional lymph nodes, and distant metastasis) staging system of the AJCC and the SEER Summary Stage System.[6] CS resolves rule issues for timing, and combines clinical and pathologic data for a best stage. CS is based on a modified EOD system, utilizes rules based on AJCC TNM, and includes all elements necessary for derivation of AJCC TNM and Summary Stage.

Nine data items are used to accommodate the main part of CS; six of the data items include information on tumor size, primary tumor extension, regional lymph node involvement, and distant metastasis, and the other three fields determining the staging basis for the size and extension of the primary tumor, regional lymph node, and metastatic involvement. Six site-specific factors (formerly known as tumor markers) were also part of the CS dataset in version 1, and have now expanded to 25 site-specific factors in CSv2, as the importance of these items became apparent. The CS system includes a computer algorithm to derive the AJCC T, AJCC N, AJCC M, AJCC Stage Group and AJCC T, AJCC N, AJCC M descriptor fields (clinical, pathologic, or y pathologic), as well as Summary Stage 1977 and Summary Stage 2000. For cases diagnosed on or after January 1, 2012, CSv2 has a set of data fields that collect the pretreatment (pre-rx) stage information, which is the same as the AJCC clinical stage, and derive the AJCC pre-rx stage. These will be a set of the nine main data fields described earlier. This can be captured on all patients. For cases diagnosed on or after January 1, 2012, CSv2 also has data fields to collect the post-rx stage information, which is the same as the AJCC y pathologic stage. This will include only six of those nine main data fields, eliminating the three descriptor fields for the stage basis. Post-rx stage information is collected only after neoadjuvant therapy, which is systemic or radiation therapy followed by surgical resection. It is not appropriate after other forms of treatment. The requirements for completing the pre-rx and post-rx data fields will be determined by each of the standard setters. Registrars will follow the requirements of the standard setters to whom they report.

CS does not have multiple versions that begin and end within certain time frames, as is common with other staging systems. When a new version is released, the previous version and all existing data are brought up to the newest version. There is an automatic conversion of data where necessary to bring all data up to the current coding structure. Sometimes a few cases must be manually reviewed to update to the newest version, and those conversion specifications are clearly outlined in the release documentation.

Purpose of Collaborative Stage

The purpose of CS was to eliminate the discrepancies in staging guidelines among the major staging systems and, therefore, develop one common staging system. This common system, CS, could be utilized by everyone to meet their individual needs. CS is a data collection system or tool and is itself not a staging system. Before CS, many registrars would stage the same case with as many as three different sets of staging systems all with their different codes and rules. CS would allow the cancer registrar to record one set of facts, by one set of staging rules, instead of recording the same information in multiple staging systems with conflicting and confusing rules. This would reduce confusion and errors, and increase the accuracy of the information. It also saved time, as it takes longer to use three sets of coding

manuals, referencing their individual rules before assigning any of those staging system codes. This was a major step forward for recording cancer stage information.

The CS algorithm translation (or deriving of AJCC and Summary Stage) eliminates duplicate data collection by registrars reporting to clinical (facility-based) and epidemiologic (population-based central) registries, addresses the concerns of clinicians for more clinically relevant data, as well as the public health sector's concerns about data reproducibility over time, and provides a higher degree of compatibility between the systems that would expand data-sharing opportunities.[2]

Best Stage

Best stage is a mixture of information sources, using the best or most definitive information. This can be information from the resected specimen or information from imaging tests. This is not an AJCC definition, but the system used in CS. It is also the system used in Summary Stage. Priority is given to pathologic information over clinical information, especially when the pathologic information disproves the clinical information. If further extent of disease is found clinically that was not examined pathologically, it can be used over pathologic information. The information coded is always the best evidence of the most extensive disease.

Pretreatment Stage

Pretreatment (pre-rx) stage is the same as the AJCC clinical classification. This is applicable for all cases, though requirements for collection will vary by agency. Some may collect it only on cases treated with neoadjuvant therapy, whereas others will collect it for all cases.

The timing rule for pre-rx staging will match the pure definition of clinical staging, using the first treatment as the cutoff. Anything before treatment (surgery/systemic/radiation treatment) is pre-rx, and anything after treatment does not belong to pre-rx.

There can be an exception for inclusion of studies in pre-rx staging. Workup that is planned to take place before treatment and is delayed until after treatment because of unusual circumstances, but within the hospitalization or within 2 weeks, may be included in the clinical staging. This must be the unusual case, the exception, and must be used with caution. This can be applied to any of the T, N, or M elements.

The need for pre-rx stage has been clearly identified. It can be used for monitoring of appropriateness of treatment, because treatment is based on clinical stage, and national treatment guidelines can be used to assess the appropriateness. It is the only point in time when all cases can be compared, because pre-rx (clinical) stage takes place before treatment and all cases can be compared regardless of treatment. It also allows for the monitoring of the stage at the time of diagnosis (pre-rx stage), which can be assessed if screening programs are identifying cases at an earlier stage, and can help assess whether diagnosis at a late stage indicates lack of access to screening programs.

Post-treatment Classification

Post-treatment (post-rx) classification is the same as the AJCC y pathologic (yp) classification. Post-rx classification is obtained on patients who have received systemic or radiation therapy followed by surgery, and includes information obtained during surgical resection and the pathologic review of tissue.

This is applicable only for cases receiving neoadjuvant therapy (systemic/radiation followed by surgery), though requirements for collection will vary by agency. Some may require it on all cases treated with neoadjuvant therapy, whereas others may limit it to certain sites.

The M component should be classified by the M status defined clinically or pathologically before therapy, according to the rules of *AJCC Cancer Staging Manual,* 7th edition. The M category for patients treated with neoadjuvant therapy is the category assigned in the clinical stage, before initiation of neoadjuvant therapy. Identification of distant metastases after the start of therapy in cases where pretherapy evaluation showed no metastases is considered progression of disease. If a patient was designated to have detectable distant metastases (M1) before chemotherapy, the patient will be designated as M1 throughout. If a patient presents with M1 before neoadjuvant systemic therapy, the stage is considered Stage IV and remains Stage IV regardless of response to neoadjuvant therapy.

CSv2 will not derive a yp stage group. Just the T, N, and M elements will be derived. This will be called the post-rx classification. It will not be called a stage since a stage group will not be assigned, just the T, N, and M elements.

The need for post-rx classification has been clearly identified. It can be used for evaluation of the response to neoadjuvant therapy, which requires the starting point (pre-rx stage) and the ending point (post-rx classification). These data are currently available only if the cancer registry documents both the AJCC clinical and y pathologic stages. This will provide nationwide data on a large number of cases, providing valuable information to clinicians and researchers.

American Joint Committee on Cancer Staging System

The concept of a classification system that would encompass all aspects of cancer distribution in terms of primary tumor (T), regional lymph nodes (N), and distant metastasis (M) was first introduced in 1958 by the International Union Against Cancer, or Union Internationale Contre le Cancer (UICC), for worldwide use. The American Joint Committee for Cancer Staging and End Results Reporting (AJC) was established in 1959. The AJC changed its name to the American Joint Committee on Cancer (AJCC) in 1980. Staging systems were developed to be consistent with the practice of medicine in the United States and used the basic premise of the TNM system: Cancers of similar histology or site of origin share similar patterns of growth and extension. This group published a series of site-specific staging systems from 1962 until 1974. The AJCC published the first edition of the *Manual for Staging of Cancer* in 1977. Every 6 to 8 years, a new edition is published with updates and new chapters for additional cancer sites. Table 14-1 provides information regarding the publication usage of all the staging manuals. This manual is sold throughout the world and published in many languages. It is not confined to use in the United States.

The AJCC staging system is based on the evaluation of the T, N, and M components and the assignment of a stage grouping. The T element designates the size and invasiveness of the primary tumor. The numerical value increases with tumor size and extent of invasiveness. For example, a small lesion confined to the organ of origin would be coded as T1; larger tumor size or deeper extension into adjacent structures, tissues, capsules, or ligaments as T2; larger tumor size or extension beyond the organ of origin but confined to the region as T3; and a massive lesion or one that directly invades another organ or viscera, major nerves, arteries, or bone as T4.

The N component designates the presence or absence of tumor in the regional nodes. In some sites, there is an increasing numerical value based on size, fixation, or capsular invasion. In other sites, numerical value is based on multiple node involvement, or number or location of the regional lymph nodes. The sixth edition of the *AJCC Cancer Staging Manual* added identifiers to the breast cancer chapter to indicate the absence or presence of isolated tumor cells (ITCs) or small-cell clusters in regional lymph nodes usually detected by immunohistochemical or molecular methods.[7]

The M component identifies the presence or absence of distant metastases, including lymph nodes that are not regional. The seventh edition of the *AJCC Cancer Staging Manual* added the concept of ITCs in metastatic sites. Circulating tumor cells are those found in blood, whereas dis-

Table 14-1	AJCC Cancer Staging Manual Publication Usage History
First edition	1978–1983
Second edition	1984–1988
Third edition	1989–1992
Fourth edition	1993–1997
Fifth edition	1998–2002
Sixth edition	2003–2009
Seventh edition	2010–

seminated tumor cells are those found in bone marrow or other structures.[8]

The stage group is assigned using the table listed in each chapter. Stage 0 reflects minimal involvement, usually carcinoma in situ, whereas Stage IV indicates either greatest tumor involvement or distant metastasis. Some of the stage groups have subdivisions, based on survival rates, and are listed as IIA, IIB, and so on.

The stage group may also include other factors besides T, N, and M that are used to assign the appropriate group. These factors play a role in the patient's treatment and prognosis. The most common additional factor in the past has been grade. For the seventh edition of *AJCC Manual for Staging of Cancer,* this was expanded and now includes tumor location, mitotic rate, and many other factors.

The general rules for the AJCC staging system are defined in the *AJCC Manual for Staging of Cancer.* Before staging a cancer, the appropriate site-specific staging system must be determined. Certain sites include only specific tumor histologic types. Some sites require microscopic confirmation to verify the histology.

The point of evaluation determines the staging basis or classification. The clinical and pathologic staging classifications are defined for each site in the *AJCC Manual for Staging of Cancer.* Rules applicable to one site do not necessarily apply to another. For some chapters, the other classifications are also defined. The general rules for all of the classifications are detailed in Chapter 1 of the seventh edition.

Clinical Classification

The clinical classification is based on evidence acquired before the initiation of primary treatment. The clinical stage is used to select the primary treatment, usually based on national treatment guidelines. It is the only point in time when all patients can be compared, as all patients do not receive surgical treatment and, therefore, will not have a pathologic classification.

Clinical assessment uses information from the history, physical examination, imaging, endoscopy, biopsy of the primary site, and biopsy of a single node or sentinel nodes as part of the diagnostic workup, surgical exploration, and other relevant examinations.

The timing rule states that clinical staging includes any information obtained about the extent of cancer before initiation of definitive treatment (surgery, systemic or radiation therapy, active surveillance, or palliative care) or within 4 months after the date of diagnosis, whichever is shorter, as long as the cancer has not clearly progressed during that time frame.[9]

Pathologic Classification

The pathologic classification is based on information acquired before treatment, supplemented and modified by the additional evidence acquired during and from surgery,

particularly from pathologic examination of resected tissues. The pathologic stage is used mainly for survival or prognostic data.

The timing rule states that pathologic staging includes any information obtained about the extent of cancer through completion of definitive surgery as part of first-course treatment or identified within 4 months after the date of diagnosis, whichever is longer, as long as there is no systemic or radiation therapy initiated or the cancer has not clearly progressed during that time frame.[9]

Post-therapy or Postneoadjuvant Therapy Classification

Cases for whom systemic or radiation therapy, or both, is given before surgery (neoadjuvant) or for whom no surgery is performed may have the extent of disease assessed at the conclusion of the therapy by clinical or pathologic means (if resection is performed).

The yc prefix is used for cases with a clinical stage assigned after the systemic or radiation therapy, or both. The yp prefix is used for cases with a pathologic stage assigned after a surgical resection following the neoadjuvant (systemic, radiation, or both) therapy. The yp stage can be utilized in conjunction with the clinical stage to assess the response to neoadjuvant therapy.

Retreatment Classification

The retreatment classification is based on recurrence information after a disease-free interval and is used to select appropriate further treatment. Biopsy confirmation is important, if clinically feasible.

Autopsy Classification

The autopsy classification is based on the postmortem examination for a patient for whom cancer was not evident before death. It includes all clinical and pathologic information obtained at the time of death and autopsy.

Stage Groupings

Cases of cancer with similar prognoses are grouped based on their classification, such as clinical or pathologic. The stage group includes the T, N, M, and sometimes additional nonanatomic factors. In the seventh edition of the *AJCC Cancer Staging Manual,* the Stage Grouping was renamed Anatomic Stage/Prognostic Groups to signify this inclusion of additional information in some sites to assign the group.

There are specific rules to assigning the stage group, the most important of which is that the pathologic stage may utilize a clinical M to assign the group. Pathologic M0 is an impossibility because it implies that it was pathologically proved that the patient had no metastatic disease in all tissues of the body.

Summary Stage

Summary Stage is based on the theory of cancer growth described earlier in this chapter (see Disease Process of Cancer). The SEER Summary Stage Manual 1977 was the first publication. The SEER Summary Stage Manual 2000 was the second publication and was effective with cases diagnosed on or after January 1, 2001. It includes Summary Stage for all sites and histologies including the reportable hematopoietic diseases.

Intraepithelial, noninvasive, or noninfiltrating cancer is described as in situ. In situ tumors fulfill all microscopic criteria for malignancy except invasion of the basement membrane of the organ.

A localized tumor is confined to the organ of origin without extension beyond the primary organ. There can be no evidence of metastasis elsewhere in the body. Descriptive terms such as *perineural invasion, lymphatic invasion,* and *blood vessel invasion,* when applied to tissue from the organ of origin, imply local involvement.

Regional disease can be regional extension, regional nodes, or regional NOS (not otherwise specified). *Regional extension* of tumor is direct extension to adjacent organs or structures. *Regional nodes* is spread to regional lymph nodes. When assigning this stage, it is important to establish that the cancer has spread beyond the organ of origin. *Distant spread* must be ruled out based on all scans, physical examinations, and clinical impressions available in the health information record.

Areas of tumor in lymph node drainage areas are considered regional nodes involved with cancer. Nodes in a specimen of unknown original location are considered regional nodes. Most often, discontinuous or noncontiguous growth is recorded on the abstract as being positive for evidence of distant disease. Discontinuous growth that is thought to be regional disease must be handled on a site-specific basis.

If the cancer has spread to parts of the body remote from the primary tumor, it is considered distant disease. Common metastatic sites include bone, brain, liver, lungs, and distant lymph nodes. More difficult or controversial areas include some of the following examples: malignant cells in cytologic examinations of fluid from a thoracentesis or paracentesis are indicative of regional or distant disease; liver involvement may be mentioned as both "regional" and "distant" for some sites such as the pancreas, transverse colon, or hepatic flexure. If there is direct or contiguous spread of tumor into the liver, the appropriate regional stage is used. When involvement of the liver is discontinuous or there are multiple diffuse lesions, the distant stage is appropriate. The method of spread to these structures indicates whether it is regional or distant.

There are several common routes of tumor spread (Figure 14-1). Direct extension occurs when the cancer first invades the organ of origin, extends through the organ wall, invades adjacent connective tissue, and eventually extends to neighboring organs and structures. Tumor can also spread through the vascular and lymphatic systems because they transport fluids throughout the body. Malignant cells invade the lymph or blood vessels in the primary site and pass through the lymphatic or vascular system to other sites in the body. They can become entrapped in lymph nodes or enter blood vessels and implant in adjoining organs or sites supplied by those blood vessels. Lung and liver are common sites of metastasis because blood flows directly through them.

Cancer cells can also spread by implantation that occurs when tumors perforate serosal surfaces and disseminate into body cavities. The cancer cells may implant on the lining of the thoracic or abdominal cavities. Sometimes there is insufficient information to assign a stage, such as in cases without diagnostic workups or cases for whom there is ambiguous or contradictory information.

Other Common Staging Systems

Gynecologic Staging

The International Federation of Gynecology and Obstetrics (FIGO) adopted the first classification of clinical extent of disease for cervical cancer in 1937. The AJCC and UICC have approved the use of FIGO classifications, adapting the FIGO stage to the TNM system and stage groups.[10] These groups work closely with FIGO in adopting their recommendations for the current staging manual.

Pediatric Staging

The AJCC staging manual is intended for adult malignancies. The pediatric community has developed its own staging based on cooperative groups and clinical trials. They include the Children's Oncology Group, the Pediatric Oncology Group, and many others.

Colon and Rectum Staging

In 1929, Dukes described a staging classification for cancer of the rectum. Simpson and Mayo modified Dukes' scheme for colon cancer in 1939. Astler, Coller, and others made further modifications. The Dukes staging system and its modifications are rarely used today, and are listed in the *AJCC Cancer Staging Manual* for historic comparison. The seventh edition of the manual is probably the last time this comparison will be offered.

Lymphoma Staging

The Ann Arbor staging classification for lymphoma was originally developed in 1971 for Hodgkin's lymphoma. It was subsequently updated and applied to non-Hodgkin's lymphoma as well. AJCC and UICC have adopted the Ann Arbor classification as the official system for classifying Hodgkin's and non-Hodgkin's lymphoma, with the exception of cutaneous lymphomas.

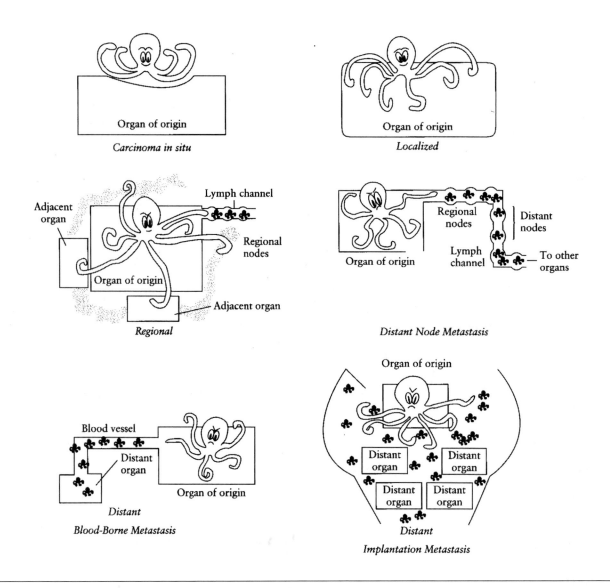

Figure 14-1. Interpretation of Spread of Disease. Reprinted with permission of the Surveillance, Epidemiology, and End Results Program, National Cancer Institute.

Other Site-Specific Staging

Other site-specific staging systems were originally developed but then abandoned as AJCC gained acceptance. For example, the American Urological Association (AUA) had its own staging system for prostate cancers, but with the publication of the *AJCC Manual for Staging of Cancer*, 4th edition, urologists mainly abandoned the AUA staging and adopted the AJCC staging system for worldwide uniformity.

Historical Surveillance, Epidemiology, and End Results Extent of Disease Coding

SEER EOD coding had gone through several revisions and included schemes for all sites of cancer, until it ended December 31, 2003, and SEER switched to CS. For his-

torical purposes, it is important to understand its structure. It became the basis of the coding structure for CS, though CS is based on AJCC staging rules. The EOD coding scheme consisted of a 10-digit code. It incorporated three digits for the size of the primary tumor, two for the extension of the tumor, and one more as a general code for lymph node involvement. Four more digits were used after these six: two for the number of pathologically positive regional lymph nodes and two more for the number of regional lymph nodes pathologically examined. The code was based on clinical, operative, and pathologic information, providing a best stage similar to the concept in Summary Stage and in CS.

As the depth of invasion increased in a site, the extension code increased. The extension code also included distant extension. If there were distant metastases, all information about local or regional extension was lost.

As the involvement of lymph nodes increased in a site, the lymph node code increased. Regional node involvement was classified by size, location, laterality, or number of nodes involved depending on the schema. The lymph node code also included distant nodes. If there were distant nodes involved, all information about regional nodes was lost.

The extent of disease coding schema recorded the number of regional nodes found positive for cancer at pathologic examination. The number of regional lymph nodes pathologically examined was also recorded. Regional lymph nodes were listed for each applicable site so that the regional nodes determined to be positive and the total number examined could be accurately coded and not include lymph nodes not in the immediate area of the primary site. Regional lymph nodes do not apply to sites such as the brain, lymphoma, and the hematopoietic system.

Time Frames for Staging

CS developed a common time frame for staging so that it could derive Summary Stage and AJCC Stage information. CS is based on combined clinical and operative/pathologic assessment, and includes all information available through the completion of surgery(ies) in the first course of treatment or within 4 months of diagnosis in the absence of disease progression, whichever is longer.[11] Summary Stage uses the same time frame as CS. The AJCC clinical staging includes any information obtained about the extent of cancer before initiation of definitive treatment or within 4 months after the date of diagnosis, whichever is shorter, as long as the cancer has not clearly progressed during that time frame. AJCC pathologic staging includes any information obtained about the extent of cancer through completion of definitive surgery as part of first-course treatment or identified within 4 months after the date of diagnosis, whichever is longer, as long as there is no systemic or radiation therapy initiated or the cancer has not clearly progressed during that time frame.

These time frames work together, because the CS evaluation data element specifies whether the tumor size/extension, regional nodes, or metastasis at diagnosis were evaluated on a clinical basis, pathologic basis, or as the y pathologic staging basis.

This agreement by the different staging systems on time frames for staging has enabled the registrar to code one set of facts and have those facts (through the CS algorithm) derive both the AJCC stage elements, each with their staging basis (time frame), and an AJCC best stage group, which uses these mixed staging basis elements and also the Summary Stage information.

Common Issues with Staging

Common issues with staging include:

- The rules for each CS staging schema must be reviewed, as there are site-specific differences from the general rules.
- CS applies to all sites and histologies. The AJCC staging system applies only to specific sites and histologies. The CS system will derive the AJCC information as appropriate.
- The rules for each AJCC chapter must be reviewed, as there are site-specific differences from the general rules.

Some cases of cancer are difficult to stage appropriately. Problem situations include the following:

- Diagnostic tests done on an outpatient basis with results not documented in the hospital health information record
- Tests and biopsies done in a physician's office and sent to freestanding laboratories for assessment
- Conflicting information about the exact location, size, and involvement of the tumor

It is important to discuss these cases with the managing physician to obtain an accurate assessment of the information, assign the correct CS codes, and derive an accurate stage.

Summary

Many resources are available for staging cancers. The registry should have adequate access to appropriate references. The CS Coding Instructions and the current edition of the *AJCC Cancer Staging Manual* provide comprehensive guidelines, and it is impossible to accurately record the stage information without these resources. They should be routinely reviewed at the time of abstracting to verify the staging information.

The current CoC Cancer Program Standards regarding staging should be reviewed carefully. It is important for the registrar to understand the AJCC stage to ensure accuracy and completeness of the CS data and the AJCC stage information. It is imperative that staging be correct when registry data are reported and analyzed.

The patient's treatment is based on the stage, and many national treatment guidelines are available. The prognosis of the disease can be estimated by the stage and other prognostic factors. In certain stages of disease, quality-of-life issues may influence treatment decisions. The stage of disease is used in research studies and in the analysis of cancers. The survival by stage data over the years influences subsequent editions of the *AJCC Cancer Staging Manual*.

References

1. Edge, S. B., et al. *American Joint Committee on Cancer Staging Manual,* 7th ed. (p. 3). New York: Springer, 2009.
2. American Joint Committee on Cancer. *Collaborative Stage Data Collection System Coding Instructions, Version 2. Collaborative Stage Workgroup* (p. I-1). Chicago: American Joint Committee on Cancer, 2010.
3. Commission on Cancer. *Facility Oncology Registry Data Standards (FORDS) Revised for 2010* (p. 17). Chicago: American College of Surgeons, 2010.
4. Sklar, J. "Principles of Molecular Cell Biology of Cancer; Molecular Approaches to Cancer Diagnosis" (p. 96). In V. T. DeVita, S. Hellman, S. N. Rosenberg, editors. *Cancer Principles and Practice of Oncology,* 4th ed. Philadelphia: J. B. Lippincott, 1989.
5. Zackon, I., Goosby, C. "A Clinician's Guide to Flow Cytometry" (pp. 14–36). In *Contemporary Oncology.* Montvale, NJ: Medical Economics Publishing, 1994.
6. American Joint Committee on Cancer. *Collaborative Stage Data Collection System Coding Instructions, Version 2. Collaborative Stage Workgroup.* Chicago: American joint Committee on Cancer, 2010.
7. Greene, F. L., et al. *American Joint Committee on Cancer Staging Manual,* 6th ed. (p. 227). New York: Springer, 2002.
8. Edge, S. B., et al. *American Joint Committee on Cancer Staging Manual,* 7th ed. (p. 11). New York: Springer, 2009.
9. Edge, S. B., et al. *American Joint Committee on Cancer Staging Manual,* 7th ed. (p. 4). New York: Springer, 2009.
10. Edge, S. B., et al. *American Joint Committee on Cancer Staging Manual,* 7th ed. (p. 377). New York: Springer, 2009.
11. American Joint Committee on Cancer. *Collaborative Stage Data Collection System Coding Instructions, Version 2. Collaborative Stage Workgroup* (p. I-4). Chicago: American Joint Committee on Cancer, 2010.

Treatment

Louise Schuman, MA, CTR

"The goal of cancer treatment is to completely destroy or control the growth of neoplastic cells without significantly affecting the viability and function of host cells," claims the *Elsevier Guide to Oncology Drugs and Regimens.*[1] There are three major forms of cancer treatment: surgery, chemotherapy, and radiation therapy. Hormonal therapy is used in the treatment of many cancers. Immunotherapy is being used increasingly often. Chemotherapy, hormone therapy, and immunotherapy are known collectively as *systemic therapy* as opposed to surgery and radiation, which can be termed *local treatment.* Each of these forms of treatment are discussed in this chapter.

Cancer treatment can be curative or palliative. Curative treatment is defined as the probability of long-term survival after adequate therapy. Palliative treatment is defined as being used for patients with no hope of long-term survival. Treatment is given to alleviate pain or other conditions that are causing discomfort. Types of palliative treatment and some of the conditions for which it is given are discussed later in this chapter.

Local Treatment

Surgery

Surgery has been the mainstay of cancer treatment for centuries. As medical science progresses, surgery has become less and less invasive. In the past, almost all surgery involved making a large incision into the body to provide direct access to otherwise inaccessible organs. This exploratory surgery, called a *laparotomy* when it involves abdominal organs, is used to explore the abdomen to determine the extent of disease and the possibility of resectability of the primary cancer. Surgery to the chest is called a *thoracotomy.* If it is determined that the primary tumor is resectable, it is removed with as wide a margin of normal tissue as possible. The primary tumor is often removed with its attendant lymph nodes, as well as adjacent organs, which may be believed to be involved with the cancer. In some cases, if the tumor cannot be completely resected, it can be debulked. In debulking, the surgeon removes as much of the tumor as possible to decrease the tumor burden for later chemotherapy or radiation therapy.

Surgical Techniques

Laparoscopy

Today, minimally invasive surgery has become more prevalent. The most common minimally invasive surgery is laparoscopy in which the surgeon places a minimal amount of small openings in the abdomen. The surgeon then places a camera and other instruments to explore the abdomen, and, if believed to be resectable, to remove the cancerous organ and possibly its lymph nodes. This type of surgery decreases patient morbidity, and reduces recovery time and hospital

days. It is less debilitating and may decrease costs by necessitating a shorter hospital stay. It can be used for many sites including colon and kidney. Sometimes a diagnostic laparoscopy is performed to determine the possibility of resection. If the tumor is believed to be resectable, an open laparotomy may still be performed, particularly for tumors that cannot be adequately viewed by the laparoscope.

Natural Orifice Transluminal Endoscopic Surgery

The most recent form of minimally invasive surgery is NOTES (natural orifice transluminal endoscopic surgery). NOTES involves accessing the abdominal cavity through one of the body's natural orifices such as the mouth, the anus, vagina or urethra. A flexible endoscope is advanced into the peritoneal cavity, and the surgery is performed using conventional endoscopic instruments.

Robotics

Another recent advance in the way surgery is performed is the use of robotics. This consists of three components: a surgeon's console and a patient-side robotic cart with four arms manipulated by the surgeon, and a high-definition 3D vision system. One of the arms is to control the camera, and the other three are to manipulate the instruments. The camera has high-definition three-dimensional vision system. The surgical instruments mounted on the robotic arms are inserted into the body through cannulas—slender tubes that are designed to be inserted into a body cavity. Robotic surgery cuts down on the number of medical personnel required for a procedure. Generally, one surgeon, one anesthesiologist, and one or two nurses are needed. As with other laparoscopic surgery, robotic surgery allows for smaller incisions, less pain, shorter hospital stays, and faster recovery time. However, robotic surgery is believed to offer more precise movements than the traditional laparoscope because the instruments are more like the human hand, and thus are more flexible. It has been speculated that, in the future, robotic surgery will permit a surgeon to operate on a patient who is many miles away.

Radiofrequency Ablation

Surgeons can remove cancerous growths in other ways. One of these is radiofrequency ablation (RFA). Tumors are destroyed using heat energy. A needle is inserted through the skin into the tumor using imaging techniques such as ultrasound or computed tomography (CT), and radiofrequency waves are sent down through the needle to the tumor to heat the tumor for 10 to 15 minutes to slightly more than 100°F. It is hoped that the heat will destroy the cancer cells, as well as tissue immediately surrounding the tumor. This procedure is usually done as an outpatient procedure and requires no hospital stay. Although this procedure is usually used to eradicate liver cancer, primary or metastatic, it has been used successfully to treat lung cancer in patients with early-stage disease who are unable to withstand surgery. A current clinical trial has used this technique on 126 patients with inoperable lung cancer, more than 50 percent of whom are still alive at 5 years.

Laser Ablation

Another form of ablation is laser ablation. The term *laser* is an acronym for *l*ight *a*mplification by *s*timulated *e*mission of *r*adiation. Laser therapy uses high-intensity light to treat superficial cancers such as basal cell carcinoma of the skin or early stage of cancers such as cervical, penile, vaginal and nonsmall-cell lung cancer. Most often laser therapy is combined with other forms of treatment such as chemotherapy or radiation therapy. A form of laser therapy is photodynamic therapy. A photosensitizing agent is injected into a patient and is absorbed by all the cells in the body. After 2 days, the agent is found mostly in the cancer cells. Laser light is then used to activate the agent and destroy the cancer cells. In clinical trials, laser light is being used to treat cancers of the brain and prostate, as well as other cancers.

Endocrine Surgery

Surgical ablative therapy is used primarily for patients with prostate cancer who have become hormone refractory. Bilateral orchiectomy is coded as endocrine surgery, not as surgery to the primary site. Bilateral oophorectomy was considered an important tool in treating premenopausal women with advanced breast cancer, especially if their tumors were estrogen positive. However, this has fallen out of favor and is rarely, if ever, seen now.

[handwritten: hormone positive]

Cryosurgery

Cryosurgery was an almost outmoded form of treatment. It involves the freezing of targeted cancer tissues by applying extremely cold temperatures using liquid nitrogen or argon gas to the tumor to destroy it. The freezing process causes changes on the cellular level. Postfreezing tissue includes ischemia and necrosis. Cryosurgery was used originally for melanoma but then started to be used by some practitioners for prostate cancer. It lost favor, but some major cancer centers are again using it for treating different types of cancer. Some of the cancers being treated by cryosurgery are retinoblastoma and small AIDS-related Kaposi's sarcoma lesions. Researchers are evaluating its use to treat breast, colon, and kidney cancer, and are exploring its use as part of multimodality treatment.

Radiation Therapy

Radiation therapy damages the genetic material in cancer cells, and thus limits their ability to reproduce. Normal cells are also affected, but they retain the ability to successfully replicate themselves. Whereas chemotherapy is systemic, radiation therapy is targeted to specific areas. Chemother-

apy has the possibility of preventing distant metastases. Radiation therapy is useful for preventing local recurrence.

Radiation therapy can be delivered in many ways. The most widely used is external beam radiation, which is delivered by a linear accelerator that produces high-energy electrons. External beam radiation is also known as *teletherapy*.

External beam radiation can be delivered in various ways. Three-dimensional conformal radiation therapy uses computers and special imaging techniques to show the exact shape of the tumor so that the radiation oncologist can precisely focus the electron beam to the size and shape of the tumor.

Intensity Modulated *[handwritten: iMRT]*

Intensity-modulated radiation therapy is becoming much more common. This is a specialized form of three-dimensional conformal therapy that breaks up the beam into many "beamlets," which can then be adjusted to further limit the amount of radiation being given to surrounding normal tissue. For this reason, sometimes higher doses of radiation can be given, potentially increasing the chance for cure.

Image Guided

Image-guided radiation therapy uses imaging taken just before the patient is treated every day. These images are compared with previous images to determine whether the treatment needs to be adjusted to accommodate for tumor movement.

Stereotactic

Stereotactic radiosurgery is a form of external beam therapy used for treatment of brain lesions. A stereotactic frame is attached to the patient's skull to provide highly accurate landmarks that allow for the localization of intracranial targets. The lesions must be less than 4 cm and have the potential to respond to a single large dose of radiation as the treatment is usually given for a period of one day.

GammaKnife

GammaKnife therapy is a form of stereotactic radiosurgery that uses cobalt energy. It is expensive to purchase and maintain because it requires a highly shielded space, and the cobalt must be replaced after 7 years.

CyberKnife

With CyberKnife radiation therapy, a miniaturized photon linear accelerator, usually 6 megavolts (6 MV), is mounted on a highly mobile arm, and a set of ceiling-mounted X-ray cameras provide real-time data on patient position and target exposure during treatment.

Proton Beam

Proton beam therapy uses linear accelerators that deliver energy beams of up to 250 MV and are used to reach deep-seated tumors.

Orthovoltage

Orthovoltage was the forerunner of linear accelerators. This type of external beam radiation uses lower energy photons for tumors that are either on or very close to the skin. The energy of the beam is low, which is the reason it cannot be used for deeper tumors. Because electron beams can now do the work of orthovoltage, the use of this type of treatment is becoming increasingly rare.

Total Body

Although most radiation therapy is directed to a single targeted area of tumor, total body irradiation (TBI) has been used as a form of systemic treatment for more than 100 years, although it is not used often now. TBI uses low- or high-dose external beam radiation to treat the entire body usually for a few fractions over a few days. When it is used, it is generally part of the prestem cell transplant procedure for leukemia and lymphoma.

Brachytherapy

Radiation can be instilled into the body using brachytherapy, derived from the Greek word for "short distance." Sealed radioactive sources are placed in or near the tumor and are left in for a short time or permanently depending on the type of tumor. Brachytherapy is often used in conjunction with external beam radiation. Low-dose-rate brachytherapy involves the longer placement of radiation into the tumor area. High-dose-rate brachytherapy uses more powerful radiation sources given through a catheter, usually in multiple doses once or twice a day or once or twice a week.

Brachytherapy is given intracavitarily by placing applicators filled with a radioactive substance into a body cavity in close proximity to the target tissue and is a temporary application. It is widely used in the treatment of cervical cancer and occasionally for endometrial cancer.

With interstitial brachytherapy, radioactive seeds are placed directly into tumor tissue either temporarily or permanently. This is most commonly used for the treatment of prostate cancer.

Since 2002, a select group of patients with breast cancer have been able to receive radiation directed to the tumors with a process called *MammoSite radiation*. After lumpectomy, a catheter is placed inside the lumpectomy cavity. A balloon is inserted through the catheter and inflated with saline. High-dose radiation is then given through the catheter for a period of 10 to 15 minutes, often twice a day. Treatment is completed in 5 days. The treatment is limited to patients at least 45 years old (in some facilities, the minimum age is 50) with a node-negative tumor 3 cm or less with negative surgical margins.

Two other forms of brachytherapy that are used much less often are transluminal and mold therapies. With transluminal therapy, a radioactive source is placed directly into a body lumen such as the esophagus to treat the surface area and the adjacent tissue. With mold therapy, an applicator that contains an array of radioactive sources is used to deliver a uniform dose to the skin or mucosal surface.

Radioisotopes

Radiation can be given internally with radioisotopes. The most commonly used is I-131, which is given to patients with thyroid cancer after surgery to ablate any remaining thyroid tissue. It is given in therapeutic doses ranging from 100 to 200 millicuries (mCi).

Phosphorus (^{32}P) is used for polycythemia vera, malignant ascites, or malignant pleural effusion. Strontium 89 (^{89}SR) is an analog of calcium and concentrates in osteoblastic cancer lesions. For that reason, it is used primarily for patients with bone metastases.

Strontium 90 is coded as brachytherapy, and because it is used to treat bone pain, it should also be coded as palliative care.

Hyperthermia

Hyperthermia involves heating the tumor to 41°C to 43°C or the whole body to 40°C to 42°C to exploit the weakness of the tumor compared with normal tissue. Hyperthermia is used primarily in conjunction with radiation therapy so that the radiation becomes more cytotoxic than it would be by itself. There are various ways to heat the tumor or the body, but hyperthermia is not frequently used.

Systemic Therapy

Chemotherapy

Paul Ehrlich, a German scientist, is credited with launching chemotherapy in 1910 when he created a drug to cure syphilis. The first cancer chemotherapy was developed in the 1940s with the use of nitrogen mustard to treat lymphoma.

Each type of drug may act on the cancer cell in a different phase of its DNA function. Some drugs are phase specific; that is, they affect cells primarily during a specific phase of the cell cycle. Other drugs can kill cells during any phase of the cell cycle. The mechanics of action of some drugs is unknown.

Types of Chemotherapy

There are different types of chemotherapy agents.

1. Antimetabolites of which there are three kinds:
   a. Folic acid antagonists such as methotrexate
   b. Purine analogues, such as fludarabine, pentostatin, and thioguanine
   c. Pyrimidine analogs, such as capecitabine, cytarabine, and gemcitabine
2. Vinca alkaloids, such as vinblastine and vincristine
3. Taxanes, such as Taxol and Taxotere
4. Type 1 topoisomerase inhibitors, such as irinotecan and topotecan
5. Alkylating agents, the oldest of chemotherapy drugs, such as chlorambucil, busulfan, and dacarbazine
6. Platinum agents, such as cisplatin, carboplatin, and oxaliplatin
7. Antitumor antibiotics, such as daunorubicin and dactinomycin

Routes of Administration

Intravenous

Chemotherapy can be administered in many ways. Probably the most common is continuous intravenous infusion, which requires chronic venous access, a continuous infusion pump, and an appropriate drug reservoir and drug vehicle. Because only a fraction of tumor cells are cycling at one time, continuous infusion exposes the cancer cells to the drug over a longer period and over more of the cell cycle. The use of continuous infusion has been shown to decrease or alter the toxicity of a number of chemotherapeutic agents.

Intraperitoneal

Chemotherapy can be given intraperitoneally. This exposes the tumor in the cavity to higher doses for longer periods that can safely be given with systemic treatment such as continuous infusion. This method is used now primarily for ovarian carcinoma, but the parameters for treatment are under consideration; it is generally thought to be best used for small-volume residual disease either as first-line or salvage treatment. This route of administration was used years ago for ovarian carcinoma. It seemed to fall out of favor, but it is again being used.

Intra-arterial

Intra-arterial therapy is also known as *chemoembolization* when it is given with therapeutic microspheres such as Gelfoam. The Gelfoam is infused with the chemotherapeutic agent and then inserted through a catheter into the selected artery. It is most widely used in the treatment of primary liver cancer and liver metastasis. The blood supply must be accessible and the drug(s) must be infused into the appropriate artery feeding the tumor to be effective. Sometimes chemoembolization is done without the use of chemo-

therapeutic agents. In that case, it is not considered cancer-directed treatment and is not abstracted as such. There are specific coding guidelines in *Facility Oncology Registry Data Standards (FORDS)*.

Intraventricular and Intrathecal

Intraventricular and intrathecal therapy is a way of injecting drugs into the central nervous system to circumvent the blood–brain barrier. This is given by way of lumbar puncture or intraventricular reservoir such as the Omaya reservoir, an implantable, closed delivery system.

Oral, Intramuscular, and Topical

Some drugs are taken orally, such as capecitabine (Xeloda) and temozolomide (Temodar); other drugs are injected directly into the muscle. A few agents are given topically for diseases such as mycosis fungoides.

It should be noted that chemotherapy drugs are usually given in combination called *regimens or protocols*. Each drug in the regimen should be effective alone against the specific cancer being treated but should increase the effectiveness of the other drugs.

Biologic Therapy

Biologic therapy, also known as *immunotherapy* and *biologic response modifiers* (BRMs), uses the body's immune system to fight cancer. The immune system consists of cells and organs that defend the body against infection or disease. BRMs can perform many functions to treat cancer or promote the body's ability to recover from other cancer treatments such as chemotherapy or radiation therapy. BRMs are being used alone or in combination with other forms of treatment.

As with chemotherapy, there are different types of BRMs:

1. Interferons (IFNs) of which there are three types:
   a. IFN-α, the most widely used in cancer treatment
   b. IFN-β
   c. IFN-γ

The IFNs can improve the way a patient's immune system fights cancer cells. They may also act directly on cancer cells by slowing their growth or turning them into more normal cells. IFN-α has been approved for use with hairy cell leukemia, melanoma, chronic myeloid leukemia, and AIDS-related Kaposi's sarcoma. It may also be effective in treating kidney cancer and non-Hodgkin's lymphoma.

2. ILs, like IFN, are a naturally occurring cytokine. There are many ILs, but the most commonly used is IL-2, which stimulates the growth and activity of many immune cells that can destroy cancer cells. IL-2 is approved for the treatment of metastatic kidney cancer and metastatic melanoma.
3. Colony-stimulating factors (CSFs) are also known as *growth factors.* These CSFs do not fight cancer but rather

encourage the growth of bone marrow stem cells that can be destroyed by cancer treatment, particularly high-dose chemotherapy. By using CSFs to stimulate bone marrow stem cell production, the doses of chemotherapy can be increased. There are different types of CSFs:

a. Granulocyte colony-stimulating factor (G-CSF) and granulocyte-macrophage colony-stimulating factor (GM-CSF) can increase the number of white blood cells, reducing the risk for infection. They can also be used in preparation for bone marrow or stem cell transplants.

b. Erythropoietin is used to increase the number of red blood cells, thereby reducing the need for red blood cell transfusion.

c. IL-11 stimulates the growth of platelets, reducing the need for platelet transfusions during cancer treatment.

4. Tumor necrosis factor is a cytokine protein molecule whose mechanism of action is not known. It is not widely used.

5. Cancer vaccines are used to boost the immune system and can be used as preventative medicine or as treatment. Probably the most well-known preventative vaccine is the recently developed Gardasil, which protects against two types of human papillomavirus (HPV) that cause the majority of cervical cancers. Its use has recently been expanded to prevent HPV-associated vulvar and vaginal cancers. The Food and Drug Administration (FDA) has not yet approved any treatment vaccines, although clinical trials are under way to study the effect of treatment vaccines on multiple kinds of cancer including bladder cancer, melanoma, multiple myeloma, kidney cancer, and many others.

Other Systemic Therapy

Targeted therapy is being used more frequently. This includes monoclonal antibodies that identify and bind to specific antigens on cancer cells inducing an immunologic response. Such drugs include rituximab (Rituxan), which is now a mainstay in the treatment of non-Hodgkin's lymphoma, and trastuzumab (Herceptin), which is used to treat patients with breast cancer whose Her-2/Neu gene is positive. Both of these are coded as chemotherapy.

Small molecule inhibitors such as imatinib (Gleevec) have proved effective in the treatment of chronic myelogenous leukemia and malignant gastrointestinal stromal tumors (GIST). Gleevec is coded as chemotherapy.

Apoptosis-inducing drugs such as bortezomib (Velcade) are used in the treatment of myeloproliferative disorders. Apoptosis is cell death. Velcade is also coded as chemotherapy.

Hormones

Hormones are used to treat hormonally sensitive tumors such as breast cancer, prostate cancer, and endometrial cancer.

Antiestrogens. Estrogens have been shown to stimulate the production of a substance that acts on the surface of the cancer cell that produced it. Antiestrogens, such as tamoxifen, can inhibit cell proliferation, and thus inhibit growth factor stimulation of breast carcinoma.

Aromatase inhibitors, such as aminoglutethimide (AG), inhibit the formation of estrogens and androgens, and thus have been found to be of use in metastatic breast and prostate cancer. Arimidex is often used as first-line treatment for postmenopausal women with estrogen receptor–positive breast carcinoma.

Antiandrogens. Antiandrogens are used primarily for the treatment of metastatic prostate cancer because they inhibit the nuclear binding of androgens. Flutamide and bicalutamide (Casodex) are the most commonly used.

Luteinizing hormone–releasing hormone (LHRH) analogs produce a medical form of castration. If used for long periods, they will cause irreversible testosterone suppression. Common LHRH agonists are leuprolide (Lupron) and goserelin (Zoladex).

Androgen blockade combined with the drug ketoconazole is known to interfere with androgen synthesized in the adrenals and the testes. This has shown an increase in survival time in patients with metastatic prostatic carcinoma.

Antiandrogens and LHRH analogs may be used as initial treatment for prostate cancers. These agents will not cure cancer but have been known to keep patients alive and with a good quality of life for very long periods. Sometimes they are given after the initial diagnosis of prostate cancer to shrink the tumor in preparation for radiation therapy.

Adrenocorticoids. Adrenocorticoids most commonly used are prednisone and Decadron (dexamethasone). Others are cortisone acetate, hydrocortisone, prednisolone, and methylprednisone. These are noted to have an antitumor effect as single agents, as well as reduce adverse effects, such as hemolytic anemia or immune thrombocytopenia. For this reason, they may be given in low doses for a long period. When adrenocorticoids such as prednisone and Decadron are given with chemotherapy for non-Hodgkin's lymphoma, Hodgkin's lymphoma, leukemia, multiple myeloma, and other hematopoietic and lymphoproliferative disorders, they are coded as hormonal treatment. In the case of myeloma and other hematopoietic disease, they may be given as single agents and are coded as hormonal treatment.

Thyroid Replacement. When levothyroxine (Synthroid) or liothyronine (Cytomel) is given to patients with thyroid cancer after a total thyroidectomy for papillary carcinoma, those should also be coded as hormonal treatment.

Megace. Megestrol (Megace) is a hormonal agent that was used in the past as treatment for certain cancers, particularly breast cancer. However, now it is most often used as an appetite stimulant for all patients, including cancer patients. The registrar should determine the reason Megace is prescribed before coding it as cancer treatment.

Bone Marrow Transplantation

Most chemotherapy is destructive to normal bone marrow, which limits the dosage that can safely be given. In certain cases, extremely high doses of chemotherapy must be given to totally eradicate disease or to prevent recurrence. Such high doses completely kill the normal bone marrow cells. This is used primarily for hematopoietic disease. Before receiving the high dose of chemotherapy, stem cells are harvested to be transplanted to the patient after the completion of chemotherapy.

There are three types of transplant. In autologous transplant, the patient's own bone marrow cells, or most commonly stem cells, are used. Allogeneic transplant uses donor cells from another person. Allogeneic transplants use stem cells from a matched relative. A form of allogeneic transplant called *syngeneic* uses the stem cells of an identical twin. If no relative is a donor match, the patient receives cells from a matched unrelated donor from the National Marrow Donor Program.

Palliative Therapy

As noted earlier, palliative therapy is used for patients with no hope of long-term survival. Radiation therapy is often used to alleviate the pain of metastases or to emergently relieve an obstruction caused by a cancer encroaching on a vital organ. The aim of palliative radiotherapy is to relieve symptoms quickly to ease suffering or to prevent morbidity such as paralysis if the tumor is pressing against the spinal cord.

There are many forms of palliative treatment to relieve the symptoms caused by the cancer or by the treatment of the cancer. As stated, radiation can be one form of palliation, as can chemotherapy and surgery. Antibiotics may be used to treat infection brought on by a weakened immune system. Prednisone may be used to treat radiation-induced pneumonitis. There are treatments for dyspnea, ascites, candida and herpes infections, anorexia, and mucositis. Much palliative treatment is for pain. When abstracting, palliative treatment should be coded. If surgery, radiation, chemotherapy, or any form of conventional treatment is given palliatively as part of the first course of treatment for cancer, that treatment should be recorded and coded as first-course treatment and also coded as palliation.

Ancillary drugs are also used to treat manifestations of cancer. One such drug is zoledronic acid (Zometa), which is a biphosphonate. This drug is used to treat hypercalcemia or to lessen the complications of bone metastasis such as fractures or pain. It works by slowing down the effects of osteoclasts, which can be secreted by cancer cells to dissolve portions of the bone. This and other ancillary drugs are not to be coded as cancer treatment.

Complementary and Alternative Medicine

Complementary and alternative medicine (CAM) is an emerging field in the treatment of cancer and its symptoms. CAM is defined by the National Center for Complementary and Alternative Medicine (NCCAM) as "a group of diverse medical and health systems, practices, and products that are not presently considered to be part of *conventional medicine. Complementary medicine* is used together with conventional medicine. *Alternative medicine* is used in place of conventional medicine."[2] Some of the CAMs currently being studied by the NCCAM and the National Cancer Institute are as follows:

1. Acupuncture to reduce the symptoms of advanced colorectal cancer
2. Combination chemotherapy and radiation therapy with or without shark cartilage for patients with unresectable lung cancer
3. Hyperbaric oxygen therapy with laryngectomy patients
4. Massage therapy for cancer-related fatigue
5. Chemotherapy compared with pancreatic enzyme therapy plus specialized diet for the treatment of pancreatic cancer
6. Mistletoe extract and chemotherapy for the treatment of solid tumors

Note that all of the complementary therapy is used with conventional therapy. As NCCAM's definition explains, alternative medicine is used in place of conventional medicine.

Unproven Treatment

Alternative medicine used to be called "cancer quackery." It was not uncommon in the past for nonphysicians and even some licensed medical doctors to make claims for miracle cures. There are many interesting reports of how these practitioners preyed on cancer patients desperate to find a cure for their disease. Two of the most widely known hoaxes were Krebiozen and Laetrile.

Krebiozen was said to have been manufactured from the serum of horses inoculated with a mold that causes an equine disease called *lumpy jaw.* Laetrile, which came later, was derived from apricot pits.

The danger of unproven cancer treatment is that patients may spend a great deal of money and time on worthless treatments while refusing conventional treatment that could cure them or at least prolong their lives.

There are still alternative treatments being used by patients, occasionally with the use of conventional treatment as well. When a patient chooses this type of treatment, it should be coded as unproven treatment.

Support Services

Cancer patients need not only effective treatment but support services as well. Often they need physical or occupational therapy. Laryngectomy patients, for example, require speech therapy. Patients with colon cancer with an ostomy need support from the enterostomal therapist.

Cancer patients can get pastoral care. Many facilities offer support groups, which provide group sessions for patients with a specific type of cancer, or even for the children or caregivers of cancer patients. The American Cancer Society offers patient information, as well as support groups such as Reach for Recovery for breast cancer patients and the Lost Chord for laryngectomy patients. The Social Services department of a hospital may provide help to find skilled nursing facility placement or hospice care. This department may be useful in directing the patient to find financial assistance and home health care. The cancer patient must be treated as a whole person, not just a disease to be treated.

Multimodality Treatment

Although all these treatments—surgery, chemotherapy, radiation, and immunotherapy—have been discussed separately, it is often the case that these different forms of treatment are given in combination called *multimodality treatment*. Just as chemotherapy often works best with a combination of drugs, most treatment is more effective with the use of more than one form of treatment. Often surgery is followed by radiation or chemotherapy, or both. Radiation and chemotherapy may be given together. Multimodality treatment is, in fact, the mainstay of cancer treatment.

Neoadjuvant Therapy

Systemic treatment (chemotherapy, immunotherapy, hormone therapy) or radiation therapy can be given before planned surgery, in which case it is called *neoadjuvant*. The purpose of neoadjuvant therapy is to shrink the tumor to increase the possibility of resectability, decrease the morbidity of surgery, and protect bodily functions that otherwise might be impaired.

Adjuvant Therapy

Systemic therapy or radiation therapy given after surgery is called *adjuvant therapy*. The purpose of adjuvant therapy is to control macroscopic residual tumor or possible microscopic residual tumor and to prevent recurrence.

It is important for the cancer registrar to learn the natural history of the cancer being abstracted and to understand the usual treatment for that cancer. A good source of information is the National Comprehensive Cancer Network (NCCN), which provides guidelines for the treatment of most cancer sites. There are many excellent resources for cancer registrars on the Internet. Many of them are listed at the end this chapter. The registrar should use caution when researching information on the Internet that the information comes from reliable Web sites.

The treatment of cancer is an important and large topic that fills volumes and volumes. This chapter has given an overview of the main types of therapy used to treat cancer patients curatively, palliatively, and supportively. The information provided by cancer registrars to the medical community is vital, and has been and will continue to be used in fighting cancer.

Thanks to David Okun, MD, for the use of reference material from his personal library. Thanks to Earl S. Schuman, MD, FACS for information regarding minimally invasive surgery.

References

1. The Elsevier Guide to Oncology Drugs and Regimens. Elsevier, Inc. Huntington NY 2008. www.oncologydrugguide.com
2. National Cancer Institute—http://www.cancer.gov/cancertopics/pdq/cam/cam-cancer-treatment

Resources

National Guideline Clearinghouse—http://www.guideline.gov/browse/summaryarchive.aspx

http://www.rtanswers.org/dictionary/index.aspx

Chemo Care—http://www.chemocare.com/search.asp (search for Zometa)

OncoLink—http://www.oncolink.org

MammoSite—http://www.mammosite.com

Chemo Care: What Is Complementary Medicine?—http://www.chemocare.com/complementary_medicine.asp

American Society for Radiation Oncology—http://www.astro.org

Mayo Clinic—http://www.mayoclinic.com/health/search/search (search for stem cell transplant)

National Cancer Institute: Cancer Vaccines—http://www.cancer.gov/cancertopics/factsheet/Therapy/cancer-vaccines

WebMD: Orchiectomy—http://www.webmd.com/prostate-cancer/orchiectomy

National Cancer Institute: Biological Therapies for Cancer: Questions and Answers—http://www.cancer.gov/cancertopics/factsheet/Therapy/biological

National Cancer Institute: Hyperthermia in Cancer Treatment: Questions and Answers—http://www.cancer.gov/cancertopics/factsheet/Therapy/hyperthermia

Surveillance, Epidemiology, and End Results—http://www.SEER.cancer.gov

Cancer Lynx: The Relationship Between Mind, Body and Soul—http://www.cancerlynx.com

Michigan State University, Department of Chemistry—http://www.cem.msu.edu/,cem181fp/cryosurgery/index2/html

Wikipedia: Laparoscopic Surgery http://en.wikipedia/org/wiki/Laparoscopic_surgery

National Cancer Institute: Radiofrequency Ablation Making Inroads as Cancer Treatment—http://www.cancer.gov/nci-cancerbulletin/NCI_Cancer_Bulletin_071905/page3

Cancer Treatment Watch—http://www.cancertreatmentwatch.org

National Cancer Institute: Cryosurgery in Cancer Treatment: Questions and Answers—http://www.cancer.gov/cancer-topics/factsheet/Therapy/cryosurgery

American College of Surgeons Commission on Cancer—http://www.FACS.org/cancer

http://cancernet.nci.nih/gov/

PubMed—http://www.ncbi.nih.gov/sites/entrez?tool5infotrieve

PubMed—www.pubmed.gov

National Comprehensive Cancer Network—http://www.nccn.org

American Cancer Society—http://www.cancer.org

Suggested Readings

Brock, P. *Charlatan: America's Most Dangerous Huckster, The Man Who Pursued Him, and the Age of Flimflam.* New York: Crown, 2008.

Firlik, K. *Another Day in the Frontal Lobe: A Brain Surgeon Exposes Life on the Inside.* New York: Random House, 2007.

Gawande, A. *Complications: A Surgeon's Notes on an Imperfect Science.* New York: Picador, 2003.

Groopman, J. *How Doctors Think.* Boston: Houghton Mifflin Company, 2007.

Chu, E., DaVita, Jr., V. T. *Physicians' Cancer Chemotherapy Drug Manual.* Sudbury, Mass: Hones & Bartlett Publishers, 2007.

Perry, C., editor. *The Chemotherapy Source Book,* 2nd ed. Baltimore: Williams & Wilkins, 1997.

Clifford Chao, K. S., Perez, C. A., Brady, L. W. *Radiation Oncology. Management Decisions.* Philadelphia: Lippincott Williams and Wilkins, 2002.

Price, P., Sikora, K. *Treatment of Cancer.* New York: Oxford University Press, 2002.

Ponsky, J. L. "Natural orifice transluminal endoscopic surgery: Past, present and future." *Journal of Minimal Access Surgery,* 2007;3(2):43–46.

chapter 16

Monitoring Patient Outcome: Follow-up

Kathleen M. Rogers, CTR

The primary purposes of effective, complete, and lifetime follow-up of each cancer patient is to ensure continued medical surveillance, evaluate the success of therapy, identify new primary malignancies, and monitor the health status of the population under investigation. Follow-up information also provides the documentation of residual disease or its spread, recurrences, subsequent therapy, and vital status.

Outcome and end-results data enable researchers, physicians, and others to assess clinical standards and quality of care. Follow-up information must be comprehensive. Successful follow-up must be maintained to produce survival data. Accurate follow-up data enables hospitals and central registries to compare outcomes with national, regional, or state statistics. The follow-up system can promote optimal patient care and provide a valuable record of patient outcomes.

Health professionals may initiate follow-up, but often it is the responsibility of hospital cancer registrars to carry out. In the United States, follow-up is required for hospitals to receive accreditation for cancer programs by the American College of Surgeons (ACoS) Commission on Cancer (CoC).

All reportable cases require follow-up, with the following exceptions:

- Residents of foreign countries
- Cases that are reportable by agreement
- Patients whose age exceeds 100 and their last contact exceeds 12 months
- Patients diagnosed on or after January 1, 2006, and classified as Class of Case 0

Most cancer registry software will calculate follow-up rates to the latest standard for all cases, as well those diagnosed within the last 5 years, to determine accurate follow-up rates for the ACoS CoC accredited cancer programs.[1]

Types of Follow-up

Active Follow-up

There are two main types of follow-up: active and passive. Active follow-up is a term referring to the cancer registry sending follow-up letters to the physician to obtain information on an individual patient. This is the most common method of obtaining patient follow-up. For those cases in which follow-up is not successful in obtaining information from the patient's physician, or in those cases when there is no physician information available, follow-up letters are sent directly to the patient or the patient's next of kin. Contacting the patient directly allows the registry to obtain follow-up information, as well as to encourage the patient to maintain regular contact with his or her physician.

Some registries prefer to contact the patients directly by telephone. This method allows them direct contact with patients and may enhance the quality of information

obtained by asking questions relating to any recurrences, subsequent therapy received, as well as update contact information. Registrars must be cautious when making telephone calls to be compliant with Health Insurance Portability and Accountability Act (HIPAA) regulations. They may not leave any confidential information on an answering machine, and should speak directly to the patient so as not to breach patient confidentiality. This policy should be cleared with the cancer committee, hospital administration, and/or governing agencies.

Methods to Perform Active Follow-up

First, physicians may be sent a list of patients due for follow-up. Because follow-up is required on an annual basis, this list would contain names of those patients who have not been seen or contacted for more than a year. The physician may use this list to initiate a patient contact if necessary. Some patients are seen by their physician on an annual basis. Many registries wait at least a month past the due date to allow time for the patient to be seen and the information to be available in the patient's medical record. This will make it easy for the physician to complete the information in the requested letter.

Second, central registries may send of list of patients who are due follow-up to those hospitals or reporting agencies that were involved with the initial diagnosis or treatment of these patients. The hospital cancer registrar should review the patient's medical records to determine whether the patient has been seen or had direct contact with their facility. If the hospital does not have or is unable to obtain current follow-up information, they may contact the patient, patient's physician, or next of kin for additional information.

Third, registry staff may directly contact patients to obtain follow-up information. The most common method of contact is by letter or by telephone. These contacts should be made in accordance with the registry guidelines.

Finally, registries may conduct or support active research programs that involve patients, such as in a case–control study. The results of these contacts regarding patient status can be reported to the registry.

It is hoped that these active methods will prompt provider/patient interaction. The follow-up information collected is needed for cancer surveillance and to calculate survival statistics.

Passive Follow-up

Passive follow-up methods are primarily used to determine the patient's vital status, a current date last known to be alive, and the date and cause of the patient's death. Passive methods usually involve computerized searches of nonregistry files. Cancer registrars use various methods, linkages, and Web sites to conduct passive follow-up.

Some registries perform passive follow-up on a routine basis. This allows them to have follow-up information concurrently without waiting for the patient to come due for follow-up. They include:

- Checking the obituaries in the local newspaper
- Checking with the hospital's home care and hospice department for a listing of those patients who have died
- Receiving reports from freestanding Radiation Oncology or Medical Oncology Centers
- Checking the hospital database for readmissions unrelated to the cancer, such as emergency department visits, laboratory or radiology tests

Passive Follow-up Sources (include but not limited to)

Armed Forces locating services
Bureaus of Vital Statistics
County assessor offices
County welfare departments
Death indexes or searches
Department of Motor Vehicles
Embassies or consulates
Employers or unions
Halls of records (recorded marriages and births)
Health Care Finance Administrations
Hospices
Insurance companies
Local, county, or state records
Other registries (e.g., hospital, central, or state)
Professional organization directories
Public housing and public utilities
Religious organizations
Schools and alumni groups
Social Security Administration
State boards of certification and licensure
Visiting nurse and home care agencies
Voter registration

Generally, most linkages are performed in the central registry. Central registries are required to do a death clearance at the end of each calendar year on all residents of their state or territory who died during that year. The central registry will link their entire database of "live" patients with mortality files in state departments of vital statistics. These linkages may be done monthly, quarterly, or yearly to identify cases in which registry patients have died and provide the date, location, and cause of death. Other information may also be available on the death certificate such as birth date, birthplace, occupation, race, religion, and next of kin.

Another passive method is linkage with state Department of Motor Vehicles (DMV) records. Depending on the agency, a variety of data may be available for all licensed drivers. The date of last renewal should be available, and in some cases, dates of any traffic violations. These dates can be used to verify patient status "alive" on these particular dates. In 1997, a new federal law went into effect to restrict the use of driver license information. The interpretation of who has access to these records is left up to the discretion of the individual state.

Medicare linkage is extremely valuable primarily for people older than 65. These files contain the most recent date of visit to any physician or hospital for any cause for which Medicare is billed.

Voter Registration records contain names of all registered voters. Because elections generally occur at least every 2 years, these may be valuable records to update the dates a patient was last known to be alive, as well as update address information.

National Death Index (NDI) began in 1979, and records the date and location for all deaths in the United States. The use of the National Death Index can be expensive if many patients and many years of death are to be searched. Beginning in 2009, state central registries are exempt from these fees.

A successful linkage is with the Social Security Epidemiological Vital Status Data (SSEVSD), which contains an individual's Social Security earning data. If the patient is deceased, the date of death is given. This linkage provides excellent results for patients with accurate Social Security numbers.

Social Security Death Index Web site is a good source for central registries and hospitals to perform passive follow-up for individual cases.

Data Items Needed

Patient identifying information is needed to facilitate follow-up efforts. The more complete and accurate patient information available, the easier the follow-up process. The needed items will vary depending on the method of follow-up (active, passive, or both) and depending on the source of the information. For example, when seeking active follow-up from a physician, the data items will have to include the physician name, address and telephone number, as well as the patient's name and date of birth.

Core Data Items Needed for Successful Follow-up

Patient's full name
Date of birth
Social Security number
Date of diagnosis
Primary site(s)
Cancer status
Date of last contact or death
Place of death
Cause of death
Autopsy
Recurrence type (if applicable)
Subsequent therapy (if applicable)

Methodologic Issues

Many methodologic issues are associated with performing follow-up. Name changes or incorrect spelling of names may complicate patient identification or successful linkage. Typographical errors in the patient's Social Security number and/or date of birth also add to the number of missed or unlinked patients. Linking names between the registry and other sources may be problematic. The more accurate and complete the identifying information is in each database or list, the more successful the linkages will be. Computer linkage programs also vary by registry; some require exact linkages, whereas others are more sophisticated, incorporating probabilistic matches. A policy is needed in each registry regarding how closely one matches names in two files to be considered a match. These decisions will influence the amount of manual work necessary to complete the task and the amount of error that is acceptable. If matching criteria are too exact, many matches may be missed because of inexact spellings, and so on. "Possible" matches will require the registry to do manual review. If the matching criteria are too loose, many "false" matches may result in the wrong patients being linked together.

Time Frame Requirements

Each registry must decide how often to follow patients. The ACoS CoC requires follow-up information be obtained at least annually for all living analytic patients included in the cancer registry database. Those patients for whom no follow-up information is obtained within 15 months are considered lost to follow-up. The National Cancer Institute's Surveillance, Epidemiology and End Results Program uses 19 months as the "lost to follow-up" date. Thus, there is fairly good agreement that follow-up should be performed on an annual basis, with several months to complete follow-up before the case is considered lost.

The CoC of the ACoS requires accredited cancer programs to meet two follow-up standards[1]:

- Maintain an 80% follow-up rate for all eligible analytic patients from the cancer registry reference date.
- A 90% follow-up rate must be maintained for all eligible analytic patients diagnosed within the last 5 years, or from the cancer registry reference date, whichever is shorter.

The follow-up rate is calculated on all eligible patients, both living and dead.[1]

Confidentiality

The issues of confidentiality must be emphasized when obtaining patient data, especially follow-up information. Cancer registries must have policies and procedures in place regarding patient and physician contact stipulations. Some facilities require physician approval before any patient contact can be done.

Costs

The costs of maintaining follow-up is dependent on the follow-up methods the registry utilizes, as well as the size of the follow-up file. Performing "active" follow-up is more expensive than performing passive follow-up because of the fact that it is labor intensive.

In an active follow-up system, most of the work can be performed by the physician's office, as well as the registry staff. Most registries are electronic, and their software is capable of generating physician and patient follow-up letters. Staff will be needed to process these letters, as well as update the database when letters are returned to the registry with updated follow-up information. When mailing follow-up letters to patient, families, or friends, stamping "Address Correction Requested" on the envelope is useful. The U.S. Postal Service will usually return the letter with a forwarding address within a certain period. For those letters that are returned unopened, or for those cases in which no good address information is available, staff will need to perform telephone calls or online searches of various Web sites. This will require numerous staff hours.

Passive follow-up relies primarily on linkages to other computerized files or Web sites to obtain current follow-up information. Some agencies charge fees to link with their database. Reconciling possible matches will require substantial staff hours.

In both active and passive follow-up systems, there will be costs for computer time, supplies, telephone calls, and postage, among other tasks.

Follow-up Letters

Follow-up letters should be developed for each type of contact. These letters represent the facility and must be approved by the appropriate hospital committees, the hospital administration, and/or the cancer committee. All letters should identify the hospital and registry, either by using hospital stationery or printing the information in the letter. The registry telephone number should be included.

Letter content depends on the type of contact. Letters to nonmedical contacts should be written in a language that is easily understood. Registrars should always exercise caution in mentioning the word *cancer* in the letter. Some patients have in situ or benign tumors, or in some cases, the physician or next of kin has determined not to tell the patient he or she has cancer for various reasons. It is recommended to use a separate follow-up letter for these cases, or include a statement such as "our facility is performing follow-up on patients with cancer or other benign or cancer-related conditions." Facilities should modify follow-up letters to meet their needs. All letters need to be cleared by

the cancer committee, hospital administration, and or governing agencies. Samples of successful follow-up letters are provided in Figures 16-1 through 16-5.

Follow-up Letter Samples

Physician Letters (Figure 16-1)

- These letters are sent to the patient's physician (primary care, surgeon, radiation oncologist, medical oncologist, urologist, gynecologist, dermatologist, etc.)
- Include patient's name, date of birth, diagnosis, primary site, etc.
- Ask the physician to provide date of last contact, cancer status, recurrence status, as well as any subsequent therapies.

Community Hospital
2222 Hope Lane
Anywhere, ZZ 00000

Date of letter: 11/17/04

James Smith, M.D.
123 Any Street
Anytown, XX 99999

Dr. Smith,
Community Hospital is required to perform annual follow-up of all patients diagnosed or treated with cancer at our facility. Our records indicate that this patient is, or was previously under your care. We would appreciate receiving the latest information you have on this patient. All the information you provide is kept strictly confidential.

Thank you for your prompt attention to this matter. Please do not hesitate to call the Cancer Registry if you have any questions or concerns.

Sincerely,
Betty Smyth
Manager, Cancer Registry
(222)999-0000

Patient; John Smith
SSN; 222-22-2222
Date of Birth; 1/1/1920

Primary Site; Colon
Date of Diagnosis; 9/9/2009
Accession Number: 200900555

Date of Last Contact:		Patient Status: ( ) Alive ( ) Dead	
Date of Death:	Cause of Death:		Place of Death
Disease Status			
( ) Evidence ( ) No Evidence ( ) Recurrence/Mets ( ) Unknown			
Recurrence Date:		Site(s);	
Subsequent Treatment			
Surgery (Date and Type)			
Radiation (Date, Site and dosage)			
Chemotherapy (Date and agents)			
Hormone Therapy (Date and agents)			
Other (specify)			

Figure 16-1. Physician Follow-up Sample Letter

Community Hospital
2222 Hope Lane
Anywhere, ZZ 00000

Mm/dd/yyyy

Care Convalescent Home
1234 Any Street
Anytown, XX 99999

Community Hospital is required to perform annual follow-up of all patients diagnosed or treated with cancer or certain cancer related diseases. Our records show that the patient listed below was a resident at your facility. To complete our records, we would appreciate you providing us with the following information. If you have any questions, please contact the patient follow-up registry at (111)222-3333.

Sincerely,

May Day
Manager, Cancer Registry

RE: Doe, John
Date of Birth: 1/2/1920
Diagnosis: Colon Cancer

1. Is this patient still residing at your facility: _____ Yes _____ No
    If no
            Date transferred _____ Where transferred _____
            Date of death _____ Cause of death _____
                                        Place of death _____

2. Status of disease:
    _____ Evidence of disease _____ No evidence _____ Unknown

Comments: _____
_____

Patient's Attending Physician
    Name _____Phone ( ) _____
    Address _____

Figure 16-2. Nursing Home Follow-up Sample Letter

Nursing Home Letters (Figure 16-2)

- These letters are sent to the nursing home that the patient is currently residing in or was last known to reside.
- Oftentimes these letters arc completed by nonphysicians, so the language should be written in a language that is easily understood.
- Include patient's name and date of birth.
- Request information regarding whether patient is still a resident, date and place of transfer if applicable, or date of death.

Patient Letters (Figure 16-3)

- Address these letters directly to the patient. It is not necessary to provide any additional demographic information because this is going to the patient.
- Ask the patient to update his or her contact information, as well as provide next of kin contact information.
- Ask the patient the status of his or her cancer or benign condition (evidence or no evidence).
- Ask the patient to provide any additional or current treatment he or she is receiving.

Community Hospital
2222 Hope Lane
Anywhere, ZZ 00000

Mm/dd/yyyy

John Doe 4545
Mockingbird Lane
Fort Knox, YY 99999

Dear Mr. Doe:
Community Hospital is interested in the health and well-being of its patients long after their encounter with the hospital/clinic. We would appreciate it if you would take a moment to complete the brief questionnaire below. Your response will contribute to the improvement of patient care and will be kept strictly confidential.

Thank you for your time.

Sincerely,
Follow-Up Coordinator

1. What is the status of your cancer or benign disease?
   _____ Free of disease   _____ Not free of disease

2. Have you had any further treatment for the condition for which you were treated?

   _____Yes   _____No
   If yes, please give date(s) and describe _____
   _____

3. Are you under the care of a personal physician or have you had a physical examination within the last year? If so, may we have your physician's name and address?

   Name:_____   Phone ( )_____
   Address:_____City_____State_____Zip:_____

If the patient is deceased, please give the date and place of death:
_____

Signature _____   Date _____

Figure 16-3. Patient Follow-up Sample Letter

- Include name and contact information of his or her physician(s).
- At the bottom of the letter, provide a line for the patient's signature and date.
  *Note: The date is the date the cancer registry will use to update their follow-up with the patient as the last known alive, not the date the letter was sent and not the date the letter was received back by the cancer registry.

Patient's Next of Kin (spouse, relative, friend, etc.) Letters (Figure 16-4)

- Provide only the patient's name
- Ask recipient to provide their last date of contact with this patient
- Provide updated patient contact information
- Provide name and contact information of patient's physician(s)

Community Hospital
2222 Hope Lane
Anywhere, ZZ 00000

Mm/dd/yyyy

Jane Friendly
2222 Main St
Anytown, ZZ 11111

Dear Jane Friendly,

The staff of Community Hospital are interested in the health and well-being of all our patients. Unfortunately, we have not been able to contact:

John Smith III

For the purposes of follow-up, we are anxious to communicate with a number of our former patients. If you have any knowledge of the whereabouts of this patient, we would appreciate it if you would complete the information at the bottom of this page and return it to us in th eneclosed return-addressed envelope. Please be assured that all the inforation you provide will be kept strictly confidential. If you have any questions, please feel free to contact us at (222)111-5555.

Thank you for your assistance.

Betty Smyth
Patient Follow-up Coordinator

Please provide information on: JOHN SMITH III

Current Address: _____

Telephone Number: _____

Patient's current condition: Doing well _____   Not doing well _____

Comments:_____ _____

_____

Figure 16-4. Relative or Friend Sample Follow-up Letter

Cancer Registry Letters (Figure 16-5)

- These letters are sent to any facility that was involved with the diagnosis or treatment of this patient to determine whether they have current follow information.
- Include patient's full name, date of birth, Social Security number, date of diagnosis, and primary site.

It is important to use direct phrasing in an understandable language to obtain a response. Contacts must understand what information is being requested, as well as be assured that all information provided will be kept strictly confidential.

Follow-up Responses

When follow-up letters are returned, the return address on the envelope or the updated address in the follow-up letter should be verified against the current address shown in the registry. Update files to reflect the patient's current contact information.

All follow-up letters should provide a space for the date and signature of the person completing the follow-up request. If the date is blank, the date stamped on the return envelope or the date the letter was sent can be recorded as date of last contact. Do not record the date of last contact as the date the letter was received in the registry because it may have been in the mail system for a few days.

If a patient has multiple primary cancers, all records should be updated with the date of last contact. Letters should provide a space to enter the cancer status of each primary separately.

One of the most important duties when performing follow-up duties is to record the type of follow-up requested (physician, patient, nursing home, etc.) and the source of the follow-up information. This will assist in expediting follow-up on this patient for the next time by identifying a reliable follow-up source.

Community Hospital
2222 Hope Lane
Anywhere, ZZ 00000

Mm/dd/yyyy

Little Town Hospital – Cancer Registry
2222 Main St
Anytown, ZZ 11111

An integral part of our hospital cancer program at Community Hospital involves performing annual follow-up of our patients. We believe following patient is being seen at your institution. Would you be so kind as to provide me with the following information for our registry.

Patient; John Smith   **Primary Site;** Colon
SSN; 222-22-2222   **Date of Diagnosis;** 9/9/2009
Date of Birth; 1/1/1920   **Accession Number:** 200900555

Status of Patient
( ) Alive   Date of your last contact __/__/____ (MM/DD/YYYY)
                       ( ) Normal Activity w/o symptoms   ( ) Bedridden
                       ( ) Symptomatic but ambulatory   ( ) Unknown

( ) Dead   Date of Death __/__/____ (MM/DD/YYYY)
                       Cause of Death _____Place of Death _____
                       Autopsy   ( ) Yes ( ) No

Cancer Status   ( ) Evidence   ( ) No Evidence   ( ) Unknown

Recurrence   Date of Recurrence __/__/___Type of Recurrence _____

Subsequent Treatment(s)
       ( ) Surgery Date /__/____   ( ) Chemotherapy Date __/__/____
       ( ) Radiation Date __/__/____   ( ) Hormones Date __/__/____
       ( ) Immunotherapy Date __/__/____ ( ) Other Date __/__/____

If treatment is checked please provide additional information here (regimen, rads,surg etc.): _____
_____

Thank you for your assistance,

Betty Smith
Manager, Cancer Registry

Figure 16-5. Cancer Registry Sample Follow-up Letter 80/90

Summary

Follow-up ensures continued medical surveillance and monitors the health status of patients. Follow-up is essential to evaluate outcomes of cancer care. The course of disease or new malignancies can be tracked, and clinical standards and outcomes can be assessed by researchers and others, with accurate and timely data.

Confidentiality is extremely important, especially when working with follow-up. Follow-up policies and procedures must be developed and approved by the cancer committee or governing agencies.

Follow-up information should be obtained at least annually for all living patients included in the cancer registry database. The CoC requires accredited cancer programs to meet two standards in regard to follow-up: Maintain an 80% follow-up rate for all eligible analytic patients from the cancer registry reference date, and 90% follow-up rate must be maintained for all eligible analytic patients diagnosed within the last 5 years or from the cancer registry reference date, whichever is shorter. Adequate staffing, equipment, and work areas must be provided for the registry to manage follow-up operations.

A follow-up system contributes to a worthwhile record of patient outcome. Accurate survival data are possible only if successful follow-up is maintained.

Reference

1. Commission on Cancer of the American College of Surgeons. *Cancer Program Standards 2009 Revised Edition.* Chicago: American College of Surgeons, 2009.

chapter 17

Data Linkage and Record Consolidation

Judy Jacobs Williams, RHIT, CTR
Ruth Maranda, LPN, CTR

Data Linkage

What Does It Mean to "Link" Data?

Data linkage is the process of matching data from different sources and is based on identical or similar data items from each source. It is not enough to be able to electronically import data into a database from different sources. There must be a process for matching (linking) and then consolidating incoming data for linking to be successful.

Cancer registry software applications may include an automated matching process, defined for both demographic and tumor matching. Demographic matching is accomplished by using either "deterministic" or "probabilistic" methods. These two methods are discussed later in this chapter.

The standard in North America for tumor matching is the Surveillance, Epidemiology, and End Results (SEER) Multiple Primary Rules. New rules for determining multiple primaries were introduced in 2007. Primary site and histology matching can be complex, often requiring the use of multiple sets of rules to conclusively determine a match or nonmatch. For this reason, registrars should be familiar with the multiple primary/histology rules and have access to either the online manual or a hard copy of the manual.

The process of combining the matched data is called *record consolidation;* this is also discussed later in the chapter. The purpose of record consolidation is to ensure that all tumor record data for a patient is counted only once, meaning that the record will not contain duplicated data.

Electronic Patient Matching

Electronic patient (demographic) matching is the key to successfully linking data files. The two methods of electronic patient matching are deterministic and probabilistic.

Deterministic

Deterministic matching is simple. Records in two data files must have an exact match on key fields to be considered the same patient. The data in each file must contain unique identifying information for each patient record. The data files must not contain large amounts of missing or erroneous key data fields, such as social security number, sex, or name. A match cannot be made if one data file is missing a critical data field. Therefore, this method is successful only when both data files have accurately recorded key data fields used to assign the match.

Probabilistic

Probabilistic demographic matching relies on a match score or "weight" created by comparing key fields in the patient records. A computerized matching algorithm is run on the incoming data file and creates a match score for each record that is based on the mathematical likelihood that identical *or* similar field values indicate a match.

Examples of fields used in a probabilistic matching algorithm are name, date of birth, social security number, and/or medical record number. The basic premise of the probabilistic system is that the higher the score, the closer the match probability. Probabilistic is the preferred method of demographic matching because it allows a match even if all fields are not exactly the same. For example, if a birth date is different by one day in a patient record in an incoming data file, the match to the patient record in the database can still be made by the probabilistic matching algorithm, which then assigns a score in the appropriate matching range. Scores are usually divided into ranges indicating a match, a nonmatch or an undetermined match. Reasons for an undetermined match include one key data field different or missing critical data fields. An example of an undetermined match is when all information on the patient matches exactly, except for the last name. Undetermined matches require manual review to resolve. A match indicates that the incoming record is the same patient as contained in the database. A nonmatch indicates that the incoming record is a new patient for that particular database.

Sources of Electronic Data Used for Linkage

Facility Electronic Health Record

In today's world, many facilities either currently use electronic health (or medical) records or have plans for a paperless record. These electronic records are commonly referred to in today's world as EHR (electronic health record) or EMR (electronic medical record). Those facilities that are not electronic may be in the process of converting their paper records to electronic records. The EHR software should provide data export based on diagnosis codes, date of admission or discharge, or both. This data file may need to be converted into a file format compatible to import into the registry database.

Pathology Laboratory

A vital part of any cancer registry abstract is pathology information, including College of American Pathologists (CAP) protocols. Many choices are available to import pathology data into the registry database. This may take the form of a direct import or an interface program. An import from pathology should include, at minimum, primary site information, text, and staging elements.

Physician Office/Clinic Including Outpatient Oncology

Perhaps the most difficult data to collect are physician office data. An electronic data linkage such as a direct import into the registry database is often possible; however, the problem with physician office data is often the completeness and accuracy of the data. An alternative option that has worked well is the use of Web-based programs that contain a minimal dataset. In this type of program, physician office staff use the Internet to access the program, enter the data, and upload it to a file, which is then imported into the registry database.

Central Registry

Central registries accept data files from many different reporting sources, such as facility registries, freestanding or nonhospital facilities, physician offices, pathology laboratories, and death certificate files. Before the acceptance of new data files, central registries first perform patient linkage. This process is crucial to identifying potential patient duplicates. Most central registries today have an automated program to link patient data.

Central registries occasionally return patient follow-up or death information to the hospital registries in an electronic file format. The hospital registry should be able to import the data to incorporate into the registry database for updates, changes, or both. Ideally, hospital registry software should include a method for linking and consolidating the data.

Record Consolidation

Record consolidation is the process of combining data from two or more records for the same patient and tumor to produce a single "best" value for each patient and tumor variable. Record consolidation involves a series of processes that include editing, determining the best information for demographic and tumor consolidation, and final acceptance of the consolidated record.

Consolidation is performed to ensure that each cancer is counted only once, and that the combined record includes the best information available from all sources. Consolidating multiple records received on a cancer patient is a challenging function of central cancer registries that is essential for ensuring data quality. Consolidation is a necessary process for central registries because they receive multiple record sources, multiple submissions for each cancer, and variations in quality and completeness of records received. Hospital registries that import data also must rely on record consolidation to successfully combine imported data into the patient abstract in the database.

Failure to consolidate records correctly leads to undercounts or overcounts in the data, which may affect the cancer incidence rate. Improper consolidation would also hamper the ability to compare different regions with each other or with national or international data.

The logic of record consolidation is closely related to both code assignment and data editing. When data from multiple sources pertaining to the same person or case are combined, inevitable discrepancies appear between infor-

mation in the database and the new data. Some discrepancies represent new information (e.g., a more detailed morphology), and some are erroneous (a misspelled name). Consolidation rules determine which data inconsistencies can be resolved automatically and when to assign precedence of one code over another.

The following terms are used in record consolidation:

1. *Source Record:* This is the record that is received by a central registry from a reporting hospital, physician's office, pathology laboratory, or clinic, or a death certificate. A hospital registry may receive electronic data files containing (source) records from an EMR, a pathology laboratory, or a physician's office. The terminology used in a hospital cancer registry for source record is "abstract."
2. *Patient or Case:* This refers to an individual person with one or more primary cancers or reportable neoplasms. "Patient" describes the consolidated demographic record for a central registry and a hospital registry abstract.
3. *Tumor:* This is the complete set of information on a single primary cancer or a reportable neoplasm, compiled from one or more source records and for a central registry, from one or more facilities. Tumors are counted in incidence surveillance. This is the central registry consolidated tumor record or section of the hospital registry abstract that describes each single primary cancer for a person.
4. *Consolidation:* Record consolidation is the process of combining data from two or more records for the same patient and tumor to produce a single "best" value for each patient or tumor data fields.

Why Is Record Consolidation Necessary?

A central cancer registry may receive reports of cancers from many different sources. Hospital/clinic cancer registries, private pathology laboratories, radiation therapy centers, and other sources all provide cancer information to a central registry. These records are called *source records.* A single patient may have only one source record or any number of combinations of types of source records. In addition, multiple source records may be submitted for the same cancer. Checking for logical consistency among reports when multiple sources submit information on the same cancer is an important quality-control function.

In addition, multiple source records for a patient need to be consolidated into one distinct record so that cancers are counted only once to accurately describe the incidence of cancer. A hospital registry may receive electronic data files from different departments in the facility. It is necessary to combine the incoming data into the patient's abstract in the registry database.

Consolidation of Records

Record consolidation is not demographic or tumor linkage, as discussed earlier in this chapter. The functions of record consolidation are frequently misassigned to the term *record linkage,* which refers to data linkage. Although their methods are similar, using pieces of information to identify distinct groups, their function is different. Data linkage is the process of identifying and matching patient and tumor data. *Record consolidation* then combines data field values and decides the best value for each data field.

Record consolidation follows data linkage in the processing cycle. It is imperative that all of the records on a patient, and only the records for that patient, are used to determine the number of tumors a patient has and which information should be used.

Central cancer registries have the common objective of building a centralized database of the most accurate patient and cancer information available to measure cancer incidence in a defined population. Even though all registries have this primary objective in common, each is unique in terms of its population base, reporting sources, legislation, and resources available to accomplish its goals.

Hospital cancer registries have the same goal; however, the hospital registry's population is its patients.

The following questions should be considered when designing or updating a registry's record consolidation system:

> How many cancers are reported to the registry annually?
>
> What are the reporting sources, and how reliable are they?
>
> How can the most accurate data be obtained?
>
> What kinds of hardware and software are available to the registry and at what cost?
>
> What are the available resources for money, staff, or time schedules?
>
> How will record editing (data quality assurance) be performed?
>
> What are the greatest strengths of the registry, and how can they best be used to offset the weakest elements?

Given the consideration mentioned earlier, there are still universal elements to the process of record consolidation: standard rules, preprocess editing, tumor linkage, consolidation, and final editing of consolidated data. The process of editing records is critical to ensuring that the correct data are stored in the registry database. Data editing is discussed in Chapter 8.

Types of Record Consolidation

Automated

The benefits of an automated record consolidation system are significant. First is the ability to consistently apply consolidation rules uniformly to all cases. Most registry software programs today provide an automated record consolidation process. If the registry software does not provide a record consolidation function, external applications can be developed and used to build the logic, assuring that cases will be processed consistently. The second benefit to an automated record consolidation system is the financial and time savings for staff. While implementation and maintenance costs are involved in automating the consolidation process, it is much less than the ongoing cost and time involved in manually consolidating cases. The third benefit to an automated record consolidation system is the ability to systematically monitor the effects of changes in consolidation rules.

Manual

When consolidating cases manually, the results of consolidation can be different based on the reviewer's experience in consolidating source records, the caseload, and the special case-finding (ascertainment) or coding rules within the registry. Unusual situations are especially prone to different outcomes when consolidating records manually.

During record consolidation, all records for a patient must be adequately reviewed to accurately implement the rules for determining number of primary tumors. Six critical data items have been identified as necessary for determining the number of primary tumors: topography (primary site), laterality, histology, behavior code, diagnosis date, and sequence number. In some situations, more information is needed, such as history of prior cancers, physician comment, and other textual explanations that are not coded fields.

All cancer registries use a variety of manual and automated approaches to accomplish tumor linkage and consolidation. This process can be referred to as a *suspense system.*

Choosing the Best Value

As best practices for choosing data values are not yet defined, cancer registries use a variety of methods to determine which data value to use in the consolidated record. The decision as to what method best suits the registry is based on the time and resources available, the accuracy of the incoming data, the priority of the data item, and the specificity needed for use of the consolidated data value.

Data fields that are critical for patient and tumor linkage must be consolidated accurately for continued database maintenance and for valid cancer surveillance and research.

The critical patient data fields are name, address (both current and at the time of diagnosis), date of birth, sex, social security number, vital status, and date of death. The important fields for tumor identification include primary site, laterality, histology, behavior, diagnosis date, diagnostic confirmation code, stage of disease, and treatment. Accuracy in tumor data consolidation is essential for reporting cancer incidence rates by type of cancer, diagnosis year, and stage of disease. These fields also are used for identifying appropriate records for research studies and for describing the cancer burden in a population.

Record Consolidation Rules

The following is a list of rules used to make record consolidation consistant:

- **Most frequent.** This rule applies when there are multiple incoming records for the same patient. The most frequent value for a data field will be chosen. An example is date of birth: record 1 = 01/01/1940; record 2 = 01/01/1941; record 3 = 01/01/1940. In this case, the consolidated date of birth is 01/01/1940.
- **Hierarchy.** This rule uses a hierarchy to decide the consolidated code value. Hierarchy rules mean that certain codes are to be used before others. Example: record 1 class of case field value = "2"; record 2 class of case field value = "1." In this case, the consolidated code value would be "1" because code "1" has the highest priority in the hierarchy rules for this field.
- **Highest value.** This rule will assign the highest value to a consolidated data field. An example is highest surgery code: record 1 surgery code = 20; record 2 surgery code = 22. In this case, the consolidated value would be 22.
- **Time submitted.** There are rules to use the data from the first submitted record or the last submitted record. Some registries use the data value from the first record received, assuming that information gathered closest to the date of diagnosis of the cancer is most likely to be correct. Others choose the most recently reported value, surmising that a later reporting source has had the opportunity to gather all available information.
- **Known over Unknown.** This rule will use a known value over an unknown value for consolidation. Example: sex = 9 (unknown) for record 1; sex = 1 (male) for record 2. The consolidated value will be 1 (male).

Another way that registries can decide which consolidated value to use is to identify which incoming record appears to be most accurate and use that entire record. Specific algorithms can also be constructed to select data item values based on the characteristics of the reporting source (class of case, hospital vs. nonhospital report, reputation or accreditation of the reporting facility, etc.). Whenever registries base their decisions on assumptions about the relative quality of data sources, periodic evaluations should be conducted to determine whether the logic used for the algorithms is correct.

Consolidation Accuracy versus Specificity

To determine the final data values for the consolidated record, the registry must determine the level of specificity that is required to provide useful data. All registries consider accuracy to be the fundamental goal because all other functions are meaningless without accurate data.

Two balance points that are moderated by cost and timeliness must be considered:

- Accuracy versus Specificity
- Automatic versus Manual Review

There is a difference between being *accurate* and being *specific.* For example, recording "lung" as the primary site of a cancer is accurate; recording "upper lobe of the lung" is accurate and also more specific. The following are methods that may be used by the Central Cancer Registry:

- A registry may choose to be accurate but not specific. Based on a variety of factors, including use of the data and registry resources for staff review, being specific may be cost prohibitive for all data items. A registry will need to decide whether the cost and time to obtain specific information for a particular data item is worthwhile.
- As discussed earlier in this chapter, an automated record consolidation system will be able to choose one value over another when there is a discrepancy between specific values. In this situation, the data value may be more specific, but may not be accurate and may still require manual review.

The decision to choose accuracy or specificity, or a combination, is based on registry requirements and resources available. Automatic consolidation is using the software to automatically add single admission events. The software looks at the name, social security number, date of birth, sex, site, and histology, as well as doing edit checks as determined by the central registry to determine whether this case has passed the edits and does not require a person to review it. If errors occur, the case is reviewed by a staff member to determine what corrections are needed or whether an override edit should be used. This method is using your computer as a full-time employee to do case editing.

Manual review of 100% of cases submitted to the central cancer registry is time consuming and costly because of the added staff needed to complete the task in a timely manner. A combination of these two methods decreases staffing needs and still maintains the integrity of data.

Using Text Produces Quality Data

High-quality text information is critical for accurate record consolidation. Text may be the only place where vital information about the patient and the primary tumor are documented. This type of information is usually not found in coded data items, such as a physician's comments on the history of other cancers or comments from the pathology report that will indicate the number of lesions, the exact site, or whether the tumor represents a metastasis or recurrence. All of these factors are very important in correct coding and staging.

Rules for Determining the Number of Primary Tumors

Determination of the number of primary tumors must adhere to national or international standards if registry data are to be comparable. North American registries follow the SEER Multiple Primary and Histology Coding Rules implemented January 1, 2007. Multiple primary rules should be made a part of the record consolidation system to provide comparability in incidence rates.

International registries follow rules for determining multiple primaries established by the International Agency for Research on Cancer (IARC). It should be noted that there are significant differences between the SEER Multiple Primary and Histology Coding Rules and the IARC rules.

Importance of Consistency in Consolidation

Variations in record consolidation among registries have a detrimental effect on the ability to fully use registry data. When a central cancer registry fails to correctly and consistently link and consolidate records, cancers will be overcounted or undercounted in that geographic area. Hospital cancer registries might overcount their facilities' cancer

treatment if patient duplicates are abstracted. Overcounts occur when the same patient is counted more than once, or the same tumor is recorded multiple times for the same patient. Conversely, undercounts result from false-positive patient linkages or from misapplication of the multiple primary rules resulting in multiple primary cancers combined into a single primary. Improper consolidation also occurs when linked records contain conflicting information for a particular data item and the incorrect value is chosen. When this type of error occurs in demographic data items, it can result in misleading age trends used to make recommendations for screening programs or incorrect identification of disease excesses in small populations. Errors in tumor information, such as primary site or histology, can affect a patient's treatment or eligibility for a research study, as well as the results of that study.

The proper use of data linkage and record consolidation greatly enhances data collection and usage for all cancer registries.

Resources for Linkage and Consolidation

More information on linkage and consolidation is available from the following resources:

NCRA *Guidebook on Informatics,* May 2009

Additional online resources include:

North American Association of Central Cancer Registries (NAACCR) Web site: http://www.naaccr.org
SEER Web site: http://www.seer.cancer.gov
IARC Web site: http://www.iarc.fr

chapter 18

Quality Control

Mildred N. Jones, BA, CTR
Judy H. Andrews, CTR

The need for quality in consumer goods and products is constant. Consumers demand that quality products be made available. Governments legislate those products be made and sold in a particular manner. Restaurants are graded by health inspectors, building construction must pass inspection several times before occupancy is permitted, and even doughnuts on the production line are inspected for consistency in shape. Quality measures are everywhere.

Yet how do registries, which create data, evaluate quality? Activities must be in place to ensure a good job is being performed, but with hundreds of data fields, how can data be evaluated and ultimately improved on? This chapter deals with the components of an effective data quality management program within a cancer registry. The objectives of this chapter are as follows:

- Introduce general concepts of quality and quality control.
- Review the standard quality-control methods currently utilized by cancer registries.
- Highlight tools that can be used in providing feedback to the data collection community.

Modern statistical quality-control (SQC) practices can be applied to the cancer registry system; therefore, three broad categories of quality-control methods are presented: acceptance sampling, process control, and designed studies. In addition, five characteristics of specific quality-control methods are described. Lastly, a brief summary is made of some of the current industrial methodologies, including Six Sigma. Quality plus efficiency should be the goal of all registries.

What Is Quality?

Quality is typically defined as fitness for use.[1] If the overall features and characteristics of a product fulfill the needs of its users, it is of high quality. In this instance, the product is data, and it fulfills the needs of the users, whether they are physicians, administrators, researchers, or data users from organizations such as National Cancer Institute (NCI) Surveillance, Epidemiology, and End Results (SEER), North American Association of Central Cancer Registries (NAACCR), National Cancer Data Base (NCDB), among others. Quality characteristics must be operationally defined and quantifiable. An operational definition includes both the type of measurement and the limits of acceptability. An example is that "90 percent of all cases must be abstracted within 4-6 months from the date of first contact." The measurement is that cases are abstracted within 4 to 6 months from date of first contact. The limit of acceptability is that this occurs at least 90% of the time. This is an example of a quality measure evaluated by the Commission on Cancer (CoC).

Quality control is a carefully planned set of activities. Registry coordinators and database managers, from facility and population-based registries, perform quality control by monitoring the prescribed activities and taking appropriate remedial action as necessary to positively affect future quality. An annual control plan required by the CoC for hospital cancer registries is an example of quality control. The plan is established by the hospital's Cancer Committee to monitor compliance on a variety of registry activities. As required by the CoC, the plan is as follows[2]:

- Set the review criteria.
- Set the quality-control timetable.
- Specify the quality-control methods, sources, and individuals involved.
- Identify the activities to be evaluated.
- Define the scope of the evaluation.
- Establish the minimum quality benchmarks.
- Maintain documentation of the quality-control activity.

The plan can guide the steps of the registrar's quality improvement process and provide oversight on various registry activities. On the other hand, quality assurance monitors the processes and methods used to ensure quality. The facility, central registry, or other government agency develops a philosophical approach to ensure quality.

Categories of Quality

In general, three major categories of quality exist: quality of design, quality of conformance, and quality of performance. The three categories are connected through a feedback loop; design affects process capability and conformance, which, in turn, affects performance. Review of performance can result in redesign; then the cycle resumes.

Quality of design relates to the restrictions and functions mandated by the design of the system. One example of design decision that can influence quality is data item selection. Data items with vague definitions tend to be less reliable than those with clear definitions. Quality of conformance is the degree to which the product adheres to the design specifications and tolerances. Clearly defined data items can still be collected poorly. Quality of conformance is influenced by both the characteristics of the raw data (e.g., medical records) and the abstractor's skills. Quality of performance is the degree to which the final form of the product or service meets the needs of the consumers. This may include the registry's available data, as well as its reliability and how it is presented in published reports. The most reliable data cannot compensate for failing to publish the data in a usable format.[3] In summary, quality of design ensures that the fundamental intent is correct; quality of conformance is that the product itself is reproduced accurately; and quality of performance is that the end product is useful.

Quality-Control Program for a Cancer Registry

As briefly discussed earlier, each registry should have an overall quality program that includes specific quality-control activities. Comprehensiveness, establishment of standards, feedback, data on data quality, and cost versus benefit should be considered when developing the program.

The quality-control program of a registry should be comprehensive. Monitoring activities should take place in all areas of the registry, not simply data collection. However, a distinction should be made between quality control of registry operations and quality control of data. Registry operations have a much broader scope, and include complete casefinding, timely reporting, policies and procedure manuals, and staff training. Quality control of data is limited to the specific characteristics of the information reported (i.e., accuracy).

Comprehensiveness also means involvement of all staff in the registry. Although specifically designated staff may be responsible for the performance of standard quality-control procedures, the entire registry should be involved in the identification and solution of problems. Data processing and computer programmers also play important roles.

Physicians, too, contribute to the quality improvement processes in hospital registries. Despite the variance of CoC requirements across facility types, physician review of registry data is integral to the quality-control program. A multidisciplinary team of physicians is tasked with review of registry data and functions in accordance with the quality-control plan. This added dimension allows for growth in the relationship between clinician and registrar, and can provide greater understanding about capabilities and constraints in documentation and coding. The CoC also maintains an online best practices repository for registrars, which includes quality improvement resources and tools.

Establishing uniform standards of quality is an essential part of the process. Governing agencies, some mentioned previously, will determine standards of quality; however, individual facilities can also identify standards of quality. Registries are held accountable to meet these uniform standards once they have been discussed, approved, and distributed. The registry should be able to explain why the minimum level of accepted quality is set at a particular level, describe the consequences of what occurs when the level is not met, and create a plan to address the problem. For instance, in one central registry, the minimum acceptable threshold of completeness for a reporting facility is 97%.[4]

Another important component in any quality-control program is communication and feedback. Feedback to the data collectors to effect a change is essential. This marks the difference between quality control (i.e., the mechanics of improving quality) and quality assurance (i.e., an organization's broader philosophical approach to quality).[3]

Figure 18-1 above illustrates the communication system. Guidelines or standards are established; performance is measured according to those standards; outcomes are analyzed; and research and training is utilized to ensure the desired outcomes. Modifications of the guidelines can be made by the accrediting bodies should the need arise.

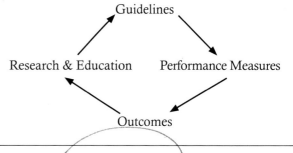

Figure 18-1. Determinates of Quality

Some time ago, researchers studying melanoma patients found that patients with very thin melanomas were expiring because of their disease. The question was raised as to why early-stage patients were expiring at a rate greater than later stage patients. On further analysis of the registry data, it was determined that the depth of the tumor had been miscoded by abstractors. Hospital registries were notified of the issue and instructed to review their data. Abstractors received re-education, and appropriate changes were made. The data were resubmitted to the central registry, and accurate research could continue. In this instance, the end user, researchers, identified the problem. Although the quality-control plan is important, identifying a problem as it arises and utilizing the Determinates of Quality to solve it is essential for proper use of the data.

Another important element of a quality-control program is the collection and maintenance of data on data quality. It is helpful for the registry to maintain data on a variety of quality characteristics over time. For example, a hospital registry may record the completion of clinical staging on a quarterly basis, or a central registry may maintain the timely submittal rate for counties by month. Only by consistently measuring such indicators and maintaining them can trends be identified and communicated. If the staging completion rate has been consistently 90%, but dips the following quarter to 80%, the problem can be quickly addressed.

In addition, the design of any quality-control program must be based on a balance of the costs and anticipated benefits. The registry's budget needs to include adequate funding for designated staff, as well as quality-control activities. Consideration should be given to the possible outcomes that result from a particular quality-control activity, and the associated decisions and actions. If no action will result, regardless of the outcome, then the value of the quality-control activity should be reconsidered. For example, if the primary payer data field is to be evaluated for accuracy and completeness, but no change will result regardless of the findings, then the quality measure should be reconsidered. Written procedures, including a schedule for routine edits and reports with feedback to the data collectors, should be documented. Quality-control activities should be part of a planned, coordinated effort and not unrelated, sporadic activities.

Statistical Quality Control

Several principles of modern SQC can also be applied to the cancer registry field. These are acceptance sampling, process control, and designed studies. Newer registries tend to utilize acceptance sampling and, over time, shift to process controls and designed studies as they gain more experience and system stability. A brief description of each principle is listed in the following sections.

Acceptance Sampling and the kp Rule

Acceptance sampling refers to the inspection and acceptance of the data. In traditional industrial acceptance sampling, a sample of a batch of incoming material is inspected, and batches of raw material are accepted or rejected based on the results of the sample. William Deming is widely credited for improving production in the United States. He believed that inspection should be all or none and refers to this as the kp rule.* Deming's basic premise is that the inspection of 100% of cases should be done only if the cost of inspection is less than the cost of internal and external failures that could be avoided by doing the inspection. In other words, if the avoidable failure costs are less than the inspection costs, then inspection should not be done.

In the case of cancer registries, very inexpensive forms of inspection should be done on all cases (computerized edit checks), and more expensive forms of inspection (visual edits) should be targeted for specific groups of cases. Hospital registries may focus on a new abstractor or cases affected by data collection standard changes. Central registries may choose to review cases with rare primary site/histology combinations or cases from a hospital whose reporting is inconsistent. Chronic lymphocytic leukemia (CLL)/small lymphocytic lymphoma (SLL) are good examples. There may be instances where the cases are coded as CLL, but the rules mandate they be coded to SLL. Periodic review of such abstracts would likely improve the correct classification of the site/histology.

Process Control

In contrast with acceptance sampling, process control methods are used to monitor the state of a process and determine statistically whether it is in control or out of control, and may thus require action. Edit checks can be used to illustrate the difference between acceptance sampling and process control. In acceptance sampling, cases that fail the central registry edits are sent back to the facility to be corrected, and if the rate of rejection increases, the cases will be sent back indefinitely at this greater rate. Process control edits, in contrast, would identify the increase in rejections and notify the

central registry that intervention needs to take place. As a result of this intervention, training could be focused on a particular area and the rejection rate should decrease back to its normal level, together with the cost of correcting the cases.

In addition to edit rejection rates, other examples of process control methods are monitoring the percentage of death certificate–only (DCO) cases, reviewing historical data to evaluate the case incidence completeness of the registry, reviewing the use of "unknown" codes to monitor data completeness, and reviewing the lag time in reporting to evaluate timeliness.

Designed Studies

Designed studies are used to estimate aspects of the current level of quality and do not directly change the level of quality. A designed study can effect a change in the level of quality if the results of the study are communicated to registrars and registry staff with ensuing actions identified and carried out. Reabstracting studies are an example of a designed study and are discussed in detail in an upcoming section. Other examples of designed studies are comparative coding and independent case ascertainment (ICA) studies.

During the planning phase, thought should be given to developing studies that can meet dual objectives. With the expense of the resources involved in conducting studies, evaluating more than one attribute is a cost-saving advantage.

Five Characteristics of Data Quality

The categories of quality provide the framework for a comprehensive review of registry activities, but to ensure sound data, five aspects of data quality must be addressed. Accuracy, case completeness, data completeness, timeliness, and consistency are the major characteristics of data quality, and they are discussed in detail.

Accuracy

The accuracy of the data is perhaps the most commonly thought of characteristic of data quality. Accuracy can be described in such terms as consistency, reliability, validity, reproducibility, and concordance. Methods to assess accuracy include edit checks, visual editing, and recoding audits. A description of each of these processes follows.

Computerized Edit Checks

Computerized edit checks is an extremely cost-effective way of assessing the quality of the registry data. Routine and automated edit checks should be applied to 100% of the registry's cases. There are four types of edit checks: range and allowable code checks, interitem checks, interrecord checks, and interdatabase checks.

---

*kp rule refers to "k" as the average cost to find a conforming item from the additional supply to replace a detected nonconforming item and "p" as the average proportion of nonconforming items in the lots.

The codes for sex show the range and allowable edit checks that exist for this data field.

Code	Sex
1	Male
2	Female
3	Hermaphrodite
4	Transsexual
9	Unknown

A code outside of those listed above would be considered unallowable and would, therefore, fail the edit check.

Interitem edit checks examine data items within a particular patient's abstract. For example, a male patient should not be reported with a gynecologic cancer, and a patient should not be receiving treatment before the date of diagnosis.

Inter-record edit checks examine data items between related records. A patient may have more than one primary or have been reported by more than one facility. Demographic identifiers (name, birth date, sex) should be the same for all abstracts.

The last type of edit check, interdatabase, compares data from the abstract with other sources in the central registry database, such as death certificates or data from special studies. Caution must be observed when accepting data from another source as the definitive answer. Some registries keep both items clearly marked and delineate source origin. For instance, birthplace from the reporting facility and birthplace from the death certificate are maintained in the database in two separate fields.

Feedback to the reporting source on the results of edit checks is invaluable in identifying problem areas that could be addressed. Review of the results could also lead to possible revision of the edit at the central registry level.

Visual Editing

Visual review of the abstracts is another method to detect possible inaccuracies. This should be performed by a qualified staff member, who manually compares the text with the coded data items to identify coding errors or other inconsistencies. Such editing will detect errors that may not be identified by computer edits. Incongruity between text and coding could be identified in this manner. Accurate, complete, and succinct text documentation by the abstractor is critical. If the text does not support a code, it is impossible to determine veracity and may require time-consuming follow-up with the source document or reporting facility. For instance, the surgical code may not match the descriptive surgical text. The surgery would need to be researched. At the facility, abstractors should visually review their cases once they are complete. Some central registries conduct 100% review of every abstract, whereas others do sampling of their incoming abstracts or review only a set of data items.

Although visual editing is an excellent method for detecting errors, it can be relatively expensive on the central registry level to conduct, because it is staff dependent and time consuming. In addition, because it is dependent on humans, it can be subjective, and not all editors will identify the same errors. To be the most effective, visual editing procedures should be standardized, and documentation of the errors detected should occur.

Registries can identify global errors through data query processes. Miscoding of information on an individual or registry level can be identified visually via the data query or report. Rather than visually editing hundreds of abstracts, a data query can be generated showing the desired comparative data. Differences can then be easily identified. For example, a query is generated for all breast surgery cases. The surgery codes are compared with the operative text for congruity. Should the code and the text be mismatched, then further investigation takes place. Likewise, a query of prostate cases with histologic grade coded as 2 or less and Gleasons score coded as 007 or greater would identify a miscoding for one of these data fields.

Recoding Audits

Recoding audits provide verification that coding guidelines and rules are correctly applied by the data collectors. Samples of submitted abstracts are collected and reviewed by an experienced quality-control staff member who recodes an abstract based on the text provided. Results are tabulated and feedback is given to the data collectors. This is an excellent way to identify areas for training. For example, if a number of registrars have incorrectly coded the core biopsy for patients with breast cancer, training should be given to clarify any misinterpretations. Having abstractors code from the text of submitted abstracts reinforces the importance of complete, clear text documentation, as well as accurate coding. For a central registry, this is a fairly cost-effective method of determining whether there is consistent application of coding rules.

A Pareto diagram can be a good way to present findings from a recoding audit. The diagram helps identify areas that need attention by ranking them in decreasing order of occurrence. Thus, the data items with the most errors will be listed first, the second will be next, and so on. Focusing on reducing the areas with the most errors will do more for overall improvement than reducing the smaller ones. If a registry determines that the majority of errors fall in class of case, then class of case will be the focus.

Reabstracting Studies

Reabstracting studies assess the quality of the collected data by having a qualified staff member reabstract a sample of cases from the medical record documents. Reabstracting is performed to:

- Estimate rates of agreement between the registry data and the information in source documents.
- Identify problems in the interpretation and coding of specific data.
- Develop standard guidelines and rules for abstracting ambiguous situations.

A comparison is then made between the data that were originally abstracted and that of the reabstracted case. Data items that do not agree can then be further classified as to minor or major discrepancies. An example of a minor discrepancy would be a correction to the subsite of a primary, such as sigmoid colon (C18.7) to descending colon (C18.6). A major discrepancy would be a correction to an entirely different site code, such as sigmoid colon (C18.7) to liver (C22.0).

This is a resource-dependent activity, and facilities and central registries must purposefully establish their plan for reabstracting cases. Some hospital registries may randomly choose cases from their top five sites. Some central registries may conduct a prescribed number of audits or studies per year, selecting hospitals by perceived need (i.e., the hospitals with large caseloads or those hospitals with questionable data quality). Cases are randomly identified for study inclusion. After the cases have been reabstracted and the data items compared, it is imperative that the results be communicated to the abstractors. This can be done in a simple table summarizing the findings. Again, the feedback loop is critical for improvement in data quality at both the hospital and the central registry levels.

Case Incidence Completeness

Case incidence completeness is a second characteristic of data that must be monitored. Inclusion of all reportable cases by hospital and central registries is essential. Also, a process to detect duplicate cases must be established. In hospitals, patients routinely return for care but at times utilize different first or last names. Patients can also have been treated at multiple facilities. For central registries, a mechanism must be in place to detect possible duplicates, and to link them appropriately or eliminate them as the situation requires. Case incidence completeness can be evaluated through casefinding audits, DCO, historical data review, and ICA.

Casefinding Audits

Casefinding is a critical function of the cancer registry. Identification of reportable disease is key to complete data reporting of volume. Casefinding audits can be performed by both hospitals and central registries. A hospital may perform a casefinding audit on disease indices, pathology reports, autopsies, radiation oncology logs, and so on. The hospital will define the scope and particular time frame for the review. Although all of the radiation oncology logs are reviewed, perhaps a quarter of the disease indices is sampled. A central registry will also perform audits to ascertain whether a facility is complete. For a central registry, the number of months reviewed for each source depends on the size of the hospital. For a hospital with a small caseload, it is possible to conduct a review of all months of all available sources, but a larger hospital may require a sampling. One way to avoid duplication in the sample would

be to review pathology reports for the months of March, June, September, and December, and the medical record disease indices for the months of January, April, July, and October. Review of radiation oncology records would be performed for the months of February, May, August, and November. All autopsies would be reviewed. This would yield a good indication if there were cases missed.

Results can be calculated based on the number of missed cases divided by the total number of cases identified, then multiplied by 100 to get a percentage. See the following formulas followed by examples:

Completeness rate (%) = 100 − [(missed cases/total number identified) * 100]

Example: 100 − [(1 missed case/300 cases identified)*100] = 99.67%

Missed rate = (# missed total/ # identified)*100

Example: (1 missed case/300 identified by pathology + disease index = 0.00334) * 100 = 0.3%

Independent Case Ascertainment

The ICA method assesses completeness using estimations from an independent survey of cases or from independent sources. This most costly method is not commonly utilized but provides the most direct estimate of completeness. As with the death certificate method, some types of cases may be over- or under-represented. For example, if the external source of case ascertainment was a radiation oncology clinic, then cancers that are treated by radiation would likely predominate.

ICA studies can be complex to design and analyze because there are several levels of sampling. Hospitals may form one level. Within selected hospitals, case reporting sources such as pathology, disease indices, and radiation oncology may form other levels. If the sampling schemes include stratification, the intensity may differ among strata, and all of these design features need to be considered when calculating correct estimates of completeness.

Death Certificate Only

Another method to assess case completeness is the monitoring of the DCO rate. This is a reportable case for which the only information the central registry has is a death certificate. The NAACCR has issued standardized guidelines for the interpretation of a DCO. To calculate the DCO rate, use the following equation:

$$DCO\ rate = \frac{Total\ \#\ of\ DCO\ cases\ for\ a\ given\ year}{Total\ \#\ of\ incident\ cases\ for\ the\ year}$$

The denominator is determined by the standard setter for that particular registry.

Theoretically, a central registry with a high percentage of DCO cases is less complete than a registry with a lower percentage of DCO cases.

Historical Data Review

A third method to evaluate case completeness is the historic data method. This involves comparison of the number of cases expected based on previous years or on standard incidence rates with those observed. As with the DCO method, the historical data review does not provide a definitive measure of completeness, but both methods are relatively inexpensive and could indicate changes in case completeness over time. Table 18-1 demonstrates an example of a historic data review for two sister hospitals from 2004 through 2009. The completion percentage shows a decrease in 2009 for Hospital A based on the pattern from previous years. The database manager would need to identify reasons for the decrease in case frequency, or perhaps conduct a casefinding audit. For example, if physician practice has changed over the calendar year, volume could have been impacted; however, that would need to be substantiated.

Historical review by primary site can pinpoint which kinds of cases are not being identified. Table 18-2 shows a central registry report with a decrease in calendar years 2008 and 2009. Case collection appears to be incomplete and requires further investigation.

Historical data review can be a useful tool for case incidence completeness for both hospital and central registries.

Data Completeness

Just as accuracy and case incidence completeness is important, so is data completeness. Data completeness is the comprehensiveness of the data set collected, the specifica-

tion of code values (as opposed to blanks and "unknown" codes), and the avoidance of omissions (overlooking additional therapy or follow-up information). Utilization of computerized edit checks and process controls can monitor the frequency of unknown or ill-defined codes.

Text Documentation

Text documentation is a vital aspect of data completeness. Text must be dated, complete, and succinct. The source of the data should be identified, especially because patients are treated in multiple settings. One patient may very well be seen initially for a biopsy at an independent outpatient facility, followed by surgery at the hospital, chemotherapy at the physician's office, and radiation therapy at a standalone facility. Text must tell "the story" in readable language that supports the coding. It must be easy to follow not only for the abstractor, but for the central registry staff and any physician reviewing the abstracts. Abstracts reviewed during CoC survey are subject to evaluation for compliance with treatment management guidelines and completeness of data. With regards to the central registry, text impacts the efficiency and accuracy of data processing, particularly for defining critical data elements in the diagnosis, workup, and staging of patients. Unknown values, incorrect coding, or incongruity between codes cannot be resolved quickly through visual editing if the central registry must contact the facility for corrections. Facilities must then retrieve source documents to either validate a code or resolve an unknown code.

Unknown Values

Unknown values, especially in key data items, pose a problem to data analysis. Monitoring the use of unknown or ill-defined codes through process controls such as a report

Table 18-1	Historical Data Review Case Frequency					
	2004	2005	2006	2007	2008	2009
Hospital A	3,432	3,511	3,624	4,025	4,139	3,289
Hospital B	1,801	1,901	1,981	2,124	2,216	2,307

Table 18-2	Historical Review by Primary Site						
				Year			
Primary Site	2004	2005	2006	2007	2008	2009	Total
Colorectal	417	398	412	423	378	264	2,292
Lung	548	562	580	607	555	387	3,239
Melanoma	251	270	271	278	275	86	5,531
Breast	665	650	682	755	740	519	4,011
Ovary	53	58	57	63	58	43	332
Prostate	534	548	631	673	615	345	3,346
Total	2,468	2,486	2,633	2,799	2,621	1,644	14,651

of unknown site, race, sex, or stage by abstractor and facility can help identify areas in need of training or a potential reabstracting audit. Many data items will have a code for a situation that is truly unknown, and registries will have legitimate uses for such codes. The use of unknown or ill-defined codes can be tracked weekly, monthly, or annually depending on the circumstances (e.g., a new abstractor at a facility). Reports should be able to list cases with specific unknown codes for review. Edit checks can be used to require that certain fields are not left blank. If an abstractor uses unknown codes appropriately and judiciously, the rates should be relatively stable over time. If an unusually high rate of unknown codes is discovered, the rate may indicate that sources of information may have been overlooked. Conversely, if rates of unknown value codes suddenly decrease dramatically, this, too, should be investigated, as it may indicate an abstractor is making unsupported assumptions about the data. Table 18-3 shows a brief snapshot of variables, or data fields, and the instances of unknown or missing values. The data field with the greatest number of missing values is grade. Having 42% of the grade for tumors coded as unknown should trigger review for coding errors. This may be an error at the abstract level, or it may have been missed in the medical record. Text documentation of grade in the abstract could allow for quick and efficient review. Lack of documentation would require a medical record review.

Timeliness

Timeliness is the degree to which various stages of the registration process occur on schedule. It is an important quality-control characteristic, particularly for registries actively participating in research studies and those that publish annual statistics. For hospitals that publish annual reports on their cancer programs, without timely data, the annual report or the timeline for the report could be severely impacted. Another example of a timeliness process control would be a report that tracks cases by date of diagnosis against the date received in the central registry (lag-time report). Data that are accurate and complete may not be as useful to the central registry if there is a significant lag time between date of diagnosis and date reported. Consistent monitoring of monthly timeliness reports can detect delays in reporting before a large backlog occurs. By generating a monthly report, both the hospital and the central registry can quickly see how well each meets their timeliness standard. If corrective action is needed, such as having central registry staff abstract cases at cost to the facility, this can be done before the burden becomes too great. In Table 18-4, Facility A reports little more than half of their required cases within 6 months. By 18 months, they report 89%, and although this is significantly better, the facility has not yet reported approximately 45 cases. Some hospitals report out more cases than the previous year, as their volume increases, and their average can be greater than 100%. Through scheduled monitoring, early intervention can occur to maintain timeliness.

Consistency

Coding consistency is a difficult characteristic to assess and monitor. It is reliant on individuals within the registry and, thus, is subject to human bias. For this reason, registries may never attain 100% consistency in their coding, but designed studies can be helpful in achieving high levels of consistency.

Table 18-3	Variables with Missing, Unknown, and Unspecific Data Values		
Submission: MM/DD/YR		**Total Abstracts Accepted: 55**	
Variable		**Count**	**Percent**
Histology (8000, 9590, 9800)		0	0%
Primary Site (C809, missing)		1	2%
Primary Site (fourth digit 9, selected sites)		10	18%
Laterality (9, missing)		2	4%
Grade (9, missing)		22	40%

Table 18-4	Timeliness/Lag-Time Report of Cases Submitted						
Timeliness				**2008 Diagnosis Year**			
Name	**Total Abstracts**	**Within 6 Months**	**% Average**	**Within 12 Months**	**% Average**	**Within 18 Months**	**% Average**
Facility A	555	330	60%	472	85%	494	89%
Facility B	461	423	91%	458	99%	482	104%

Comparative coding is one way to monitor consistency. A reliability study uses a set of standardized medical charts or other source documents that are abstracted by a sample of data collectors. The results are then analyzed. Because the data collectors code from the same set of documents, differences in coding can be readily detected. At that point, education and training can be targeted for those areas in disagreement. This method can be utilized by central registry quality-control staff, as well as by abstractors in hospital facilities, to determine consistency in coding.

Reliability studies are particularly useful when new data fields or changes in coding are introduced. These situations are highly likely to increase the variability of coding among staff members. Such a study will help identify where the documentation is unclear and lead to clarifications to increase the consistency in coding.

Quality-Control Methods

The five quality characteristics have been discussed, as well as examples for acceptance, process control, and designed studies. The matrix in Table 18-5 illustrates how these three methods of SQC methods can be used to evaluate data quality in the cancer registry. As mentioned earlier, some studies can address multiple quality characteristics, if designed properly.

Industrial Quality Control

Three methodologies utilized in the industry are benchmarking, total quality management (TQM), and Six Sigma. This section will endeavor to briefly describe these methodologies and their uses.

Benchmarking

Benchmarking is the process of improving performance by continually identifying, understanding, and adapting outstanding practices and processes found inside and outside an organization. Benchmarking focuses on how to improve any process by using best practices rather than simply measuring the best performance. The key to benchmarking is not to apply resources to just beat the new benchmark, but instead to learn about how best performance is accomplished. Obtaining adequate measurements before implementation is critical. Equally important is measuring the project's operational effects and financial cost/benefit after the project has been completed.[5]

The CoC Cancer Program Practice Profile Reports (CP[3]R) offers such benchmarking. The CoC requires hospitals to examine their data based on predetermined National Quality Forum measures. Benchmarking is available by facility type or geographical location—on a state, regional, or national level. This comparison data can be communicated to the facility's Cancer Committee for discussion and possible improvement recommendations based on best practices.

One central registry benchmark focuses on the allowable rate for the number of unknown or ill-defined sites. An established goal is to have less than 2.5% of the cases coded to C76 or C80, excluding DCO cases. For example, a registry reporting 1.65% of their cases as C76 or C80 would meet the goal or benchmark. Failing to achieve the benchmark requires a thorough evaluation and a plan for improvement.

Total Quality Management

Industrial quality control has supplied many concepts to the healthcare environment including TQM in hospital settings. One example that has received considerable attention is the Joint Commission on Accreditation of Healthcare Organizations' (JCAHO's) 10-step Quality Improvement Program Components. Although they may have been originally designed to apply to any hospital, they can also be a good basis for the development of a cancer registry quality improvement program. The 10 steps are listed in Table 18-6 tracking a registry example in the follow-up arena.[6]

Table 18-5	Quality Control Matrix[3]		
Quality Characteristic	**Acceptance Sampling**	**Process Control**	**Designed Study**
Accuracy	Visual review Computer edit checks	Edit rejection rates	Recoding audit
Case incidence completeness	Casefinding audit	DCO percentage Historical data review	ICA study
Data completeness	Computer edit checks Data Query CoC survey review	Use of "unknown" Monthly central registry reporting	Reabstracting studies
Timeliness	CoC survey review	Lag time in reporting	—
Data consistency	—	—	Reliability study

CoC, Commission on Cancer; DCO, death certificate only; ICA, independent case ascertainment.

Table 18-6	Joint Commission on Accreditation of Healthcare Organizations (JCAHO) 10 Steps[6] in a Cancer Registry Activity[3]

JCAHO 10 Steps	Example of a Cancer Registry Activity: Follow-up Services for Hospital Program Example
1. Assign responsibility	1. All follow-up activities assigned to a registrar
2. Delineate scope of care/service	2. Obtain last date of contact, recurrence and subsequent treatment on analytic cases, <100 years of age, residing in United States, since reference year
3. Identify important aspects of care/service	3. Aspects of follow-up service: (between two and four aspects) • Obtain follow-up within 12 months • Obtain recurrence information • Obtain subsequent treatment information • Maintain current patient contact information
4. Identify indicators	4. Patients falling within scope of care should have recorded follow-up dates within the last 12 months, at a rate of at least 80% (Only one indicator will be tracked for this example.)
5. Establish a means to trigger evaluation	5. Follow-up report is generated monthly
6. Collect and organize data	6. Data is maintained monthly; if follow-up rate decreases, gather data from the variety of methods used in follow-up to identify where the decrease occurred
7. Evaluate care	7. Analyze the data to establish why the decrease occurred
8. Take actions to improve	8. Create an action plan to address the follow-up method that has negatively impacted the rate; improve on that method of follow-up or engage additional resources in existing follow-up methods to improve rate
9. Assess the actions, document improvement	9. After the change is implemented, assess the rate and document results
10. Communicate results, relevant information	10. Communicate follow-up results to key stakeholders, that is, Cancer Committee

Six Sigma

The third data-driven methodology is Six Sigma. This highly efficient and highly sophisticated method is a measure of quality that strives for near perfection. It is a disciplined, data-driven approach for eliminating defects by always striving toward six standard deviations between the mean and the nearest specification limit in any process. It requires the project be put through the entire DMAIC process (Define, Measure, Analyze, Improve, and Control). Many of the tools used for Six Sigma have proved useful in conjunction with TQM. The basic premise of both methods is that data are needed to identify input, process, and output areas for improvement, and to ensure that quality improvements are not haphazardly implemented. Instead, resources are assigned to projects where it can be shown through data analysis that a difference can be made.[7] Suggested materials for additional reading on Six Sigma are listed at the end of the chapter.

Conclusion

This chapter has explained quality and categories of quality, the various types of quality control, including industrial and statistical, and has described the five characteristics of data quality used today. The registration process is rarely perfect, and a variety of errors can occur, but by developing and utilizing a quality-control plan, a registry can certainly limit the number of errors it generates. The registry requires a well-thought-out plan, resources to adequately carry out the plan, and understanding of the principles in practice behind quality control. Quality control allows the registry to produce accurate and useful information about cancer incidence and cancer care within its population.

References

1. Hilsenbeck, S. G., Glaefke, G. S., Feigl, P., et al. *Quality Control for Cancer Registries.* Bethesda, MD: U.S. Department of Health and Human Services, Public Health Service, National Institutes of Health, May 1985.
2. Commission on Cancer of the American College of Surgeons. *Cancer Program Standards, 2009 Revised Edition.* Chicago: American College of Surgeons, 2009.
3. Hilsenbeck, S. G. "Quality Control." In Menck H, Smart C, editors. *Central Cancer Registries: Design, Management, and Use.* Chur, Switzerland: Harwood Academic Publishers, 1994.
4. California Cancer Registry. *Cancer Reporting in California: Abstracting and Coding Procedures, Volume I.* Sacramento, CA: California Cancer Registry, March 2005.
5. "An APQC White Paper for Senior Management Based on Organizing and Managing Benchmarking," APQC, Houston, Texas 1995.
6. Joint Commission on Accreditation of Healthcare Organizations. *JCAHO: Accreditation Manual for Hospital, Volume 1—Standards.* Chicago: JCAHO, 1993.
7. Swinney, J. "Defining Six Sigma for Your Business or Organization." iSixSigma LLC; Bainbridge Island, WA, 2000–2005.

Additional Reading Materials

Six Sigma Method

Lean Six Sigma for Service
Michael L. George
McGraw-Hill
ISBN 0-07-141821-0
Copyright 2003

What Is Six Sigma Process Management?
Rowland Hayler, Michael Nichols
McGraw-Hill
ISBN 0-07-145341-5
Copyright 2005

Other References

The Six Sigma Way Powells
Peter S. Pande, Robert P. Neuman, Roland R. Cavanagh
McGraw-Hill, 2003
ISBN 0-07-135806-4

Six Sigma for Managers Powells
Greg Blue
McGraw-Hill, 2005
ISBN 0-07-138755-2

Six Sigma for Managers Powells (24 Lessons to Understand and Apply Six Sigma Principal in Any Organization)
Greg Blue
McGraw-Hill, 2002
ISBN 0-071455-48-5

Cancer Program Survey and Accreditation Process of the American College of Surgeons Commission on Cancer

M. Asa Carter, CTR

In an effort to standardize clinical cancer care, the American College of Surgeons' (ACoS) Committee on the Treatment of Malignant Diseases published minimum standards for cancer clinics and recommended the formation of cancer clinics in general hospitals. These minimum requirements for cancer program accreditation were first published in 1930. The early requirements are the model for the current multidisciplinary approach to cancer care that has become the standard in the United States for both Commission on Cancer (CoC)–accredited and nonaccredited facilities.[1]

Initial pilot test surveys of cancer clinics were performed in 1931 by one surgeon employed by the ACoS and one National Cancer Institute (NCI) employee who was made available as part of an NCI grant to the ACoS.

The first listing of the 140 approved cancer clinics was published in the ACoS Bulletin in 1933. At that time, accreditation was granted to 70% (140/200) of the surveyed cancer clinics. By 1955, 693 clinics had gained accreditation.

In 1965, the multidisciplinary CoC replaced the Committee on the Treatment of Malignant Diseases. The surveyor team has now grown to more than 40 volunteer physicians representing the full scope of the diagnostic and treatment specialties, as well as two Certified Tumor Registrars (CTRs).

The CoC surveys individual hospitals, integrated programs, freestanding facilities, and healthcare networks. The survey format and activity remains consistent, but the process may be tailored to accommodate complex healthcare settings. For example, the survey of a Network Cancer Program always involves more than one surveyor and a visit to more than one site in the network. The survey format has changed over time to keep pace with the advances in healthcare organization, operation, and technology, and to adapt to the CoC's increasing focus on the quality of care and outcomes rather than structure and process.[2]

The survey is designed to be both educational and evaluative. An interactive exchange with equal contributions from the surveyor(s) and program team is essential to a successful completion of the survey. This open format both assesses compliance with the standards and provides the program with an opportunity to benefit from the surveyor(s) experience so that future program activity can be enhanced. The survey process focuses on discussions with the multidisciplinary team to understand the following factors:

How clinical care is provided
How accuracy of data collection is assured
How quality of care and patient outcomes are evaluated and improved

The Program's Preparation for Survey

Cancer Committee Assesses Activity

Each cancer program is expected to comply with all of the standards throughout the 3-year accreditation cycle. The cancer committee assures the program's compliance with the standards and readiness for survey at any time. This is accomplished through the setting and monitoring of annual goals and the work of the program activity coordinators. Each activity coordinator ensures that the activity for a specified program area fulfills the requirements. These program areas include, but are not limited to, the following:

- Multidisciplinary discussion of treatment options for patients discussed at cancer conferences
- Evaluating and improving patient care through the completion of studies of quality and implementation of corrective actions or new programs[2]

The cancer committee performs an ongoing assessment of program performance throughout the 3-year accreditation period. Program activity can be recorded in the online Survey Application Record (SAR), as well as in facility documentation such as minutes of cancer committee meetings and facility developed tracking tools. The ongoing assessment enables the cancer committee to fulfill its leadership role for the program. The review ensures that activity of all areas is meeting the standards or provides an opportunity to identify and address problems as they arise.

The cancer committee identifies one team member to be the key contact for the survey. The key contact coordinates the arrangements and preparations for the on-site visit (Table 19-1). In smaller facilities, the cancer registrar

Table 19-1	Responsibilities of the Key Contact

Negotiates with the surveyor and committee members to identify a survey date and schedule
Provides information about the surveyor(s) to the cancer committee using the surveyor profiles
Coordinates development of the survey agenda
Coordinates meeting rooms and facility tours
Reviews the Survey Application Record; ensures accuracy of recorded information
Plans for and assembles documentation of program activity

is designated to be the key contact. Larger facilities or networks may assign this responsibility to the Cancer Program Administrator or a physician member of the cancer committee. In some programs, this may be an ongoing appointment, whereas in others the designation is made during the year prior to survey. Each cancer committee will choose the time frame that matches the program's organizational needs.

Using a Commission on Cancer–Trained Cancer Program Consultant to Improve Performance

In the early 2000s, the CoC added to the volunteer field staff by recruiting CTRs to become members of the CoC-trained Cancer Program Consultant Team. These registry professionals contract with programs to both help facilities establish and grow the cancer program in preparation for the initial survey, and to assist facilities that are currently accredited to improve their performance before the next survey.

Services provided by the consultants cover the full scope of cancer program activity including, but not limited to, the following:

- Guiding the cancer committee to understand their role
- Establishing the cancer registry
- Developing policies and procedures for the program and registry
- Designing and implementing the cancer program quality improvement program
- Evaluating cancer registry performance

When there have been changes to the program or program staff during the 3-year accreditation period, the cancer committee should consider contracting with a CoC-trained consultant to perform a program assessment and assist with implementing corrective action. This preemptive action may reduce or eliminate the identified deficiencies in the standards and improve the survey outcome.

Completing the Survey Application Record

The Web-based SAR is a primary source of program information and serves three purposes:

1. The program uses the SAR to track activities between surveys.
2. The surveyor uses the SAR to review program performance in advance of the on-site visit.
3. The CoC uses the SAR to report and analyze the activity and performance of all CoC-accredited programs.

The SAR provides a summary of demographic information, resources and services, and description of annual cancer program activity for the facility. Information recorded in the SAR is used by both the surveyor(s) and CoC staff to evaluate and rate the program's compliance with the standards at the time of survey; therefore, complete information is required to ensure an accurate assessment and accreditation award.

Except for the time immediately after the on-site survey, the SAR is available throughout the 3-year accreditation period. Information should routinely be added to the SAR to assist with the cancer committee's ongoing program assessment. The cancer committee should consider an annual SAR review as part of the cancer committee meeting agenda.

Annually, each CoC-accredited program is asked to update selected areas of the SAR. The areas to be updated are selected each year by the CoC Accreditation Committee. The information provided is designed to report the experience in CoC-accredited programs or evaluate performance with an eye toward future enhancements. [2]

Program staff review and update all information on the SAR before the survey. In preparation for survey, the program staff also record a numeric rating of the program's compliance with each standard. The rating is based on the time between surveys and is used by both the facility's cancer program team and the surveyor(s) to guide discussions during the on-site visit. [3]

The SAR update is completed at least 14 days before the scheduled survey date to allow the surveyor(s) adequate preparation time. If the SAR is not updated, the survey will be based on incomplete information that will affect the survey outcome and accreditation award. [3]

Preparing Survey Documentation

Documentation of program activity is to be available to the surveyor at least 14 days before the survey date. The documents are to be provided in electronic format and uploaded to the Survey Documentation area of the SAR. The system is designed to accept multiple formats that accommodate the most frequent document types. These are:

> Microsoft Corporation WORD documents. (.doc or .docx)
> Microsoft Corporation Excel (.xls)
> Microsoft Corporation Rich Text Format (.rtf)
> Adobe Systems Portable Document Format (.pdf)
> Joint Photographic Experts Group JPEG (.jpg)

Cancer Program Standards 2009 Revised Edition (pages 8 and 9) lists the materials that are to be provided in advance of the on-site visit. Table 19-2, a modified list of documents (page 9), is provided for the NCI-designated Comprehensive Cancer Center Programs. The documentation provided supports the information and rating of compliance reported through the SAR. [2]

Table 19-2	Documentation Provided to the Surveyor(s) from the Facility Undergoing Survey

Certificate or letter from accrediting body
Minutes of cancer committee or leadership body meetings and related attachments
Results of outcomes analysis(es) and methods of dissemination
Accession list for each of the 3 complete years in the 3-year accreditation period
Published annual report, if applicable

Presurvey Mechanics

Facility Communication

The CoC provides an initial survey notification to the cancer registrar at each program due for survey by July 1 of the year before the survey. The notification includes information about the target time frame for the survey, how to access the online SAR, the fee for survey, and how to request a survey extension and the extension deadline. [2] This notification is shared with the cancer committee so that survey preparation can begin.

Surveyor Communications

Confirming the Survey Date

Survey dates and schedules are planned well in advance to be sensitive to the needs of the surveyor(s), to allow all cancer program team members to participate in the visit, and to limit disruption to patient care. This may involve multiple concerns and requires the coordination of surveyor(s) and cancer program team member schedules, tumor board/cancer conference schedules, other survey activities, and travel plans. Every effort is made to accommodate the needs of both the surveyor(s) and facility. [5]

Most surveyors will make initial contact with the cancer registrar during November or December of the year before the survey. The cancer registrar provides the key contact's information to the surveyor so that the negotiation process can begin. As part of a network survey, one of the assigned surveyors is responsible for working with the key contact to negotiate the survey dates. The CoC provides the program with a survey confirmation notice once the date and time for survey are set.

Setting the Agenda

The on-site visit comprises a comprehensive review of all areas of the cancer program. This review requires at least 1 day (6 hours) to complete. Two or more days are required for surveys of Network Cancer Programs. [4]

The agenda is customized for each program, but each on-site visit includes:

A meeting with the facility's CEO or other key administrative staff

Discussion of program activity with the key members of the cancer program team, including the cancer program coordinators
Review of documentation
Facility tour (inpatient medical oncology unit or functional equivalent)
Participation in a cancer conference
Meeting with the cancer registrar
Quality-control review of cancer registry abstracts and pathology reports
Confirmation of data quality through medical record review
Summation conference

Other items may be added to the agenda by either the surveyor(s) or program in advance of the on-site visit. Additional items will depend on the program scope.

The agenda is provided to all members of the cancer program team in advance of the survey as a guide for survey preparation.

Surveyor Preparation

All documentation is thoroughly reviewed before the on-site visit. In addition, the surveyor(s) may review information posted on the facility Web site, which can provide a snapshot of the facility as a whole and the community it serves.

The surveyor(s) uses the facility ratings and supporting documentation to map areas to be discussed during the on-site visit. The surveyor may also begin to assign a rating of compliance to some standards, where appropriate.

The On-site Visit: Putting Your Best Face Forward

Discussing Program Activity

The survey is educational and evaluative. A discussion of program activity with all members of the cancer program team is essential to understanding the program organization, strengths, and opportunities for improvement. All team members are encouraged to describe their achievements and challenges, as well as plans and goals for their area of responsibility.

The coordinators present information about the key areas of program activity to which they are assigned. The cancer conference coordinator describes the committee's process to establish the annual cancer conference goals. A discussion of the monitoring activity, including the documentation of stage of the cases discussed, the results of the evaluation, and the methods to address areas that fall below the established goals enables the surveyor(s) to assess the cancer conference activity.

The coordinator for the quality of cancer registry data shares information about the development and implementation of the cancer registry quality-control plan. The discussion should include the areas of cancer registry operation targeted for evaluation, especially the evaluation of the quality of Collaborative Stage derived stage recorded in the cancer registry database. The quality-control findings and plans to address areas for improvement are also highlighted during the discussion.

The annual submission of data to the National Cancer Data Base (NCDB) and the methods to ensure the quality of the data submitted are also discussed. The quality of the data submitted at the most recent Call for Data, the NCDB edit report, and plans to review, correct, and resubmit the data to meet the requirements for Standard 3.7 are shared with the surveyor(s) by the coordinator.

The quality improvement coordinator describes the completed studies of quality and outcomes, and shares the plans for future studies. The process used to identify topics and study development is also discussed with the surveyor(s). The coordinator reviews past annual improvements to cancer care, as well as identifying the improvements planned for the current year.

The community outreach coordinator shares information about the screening and prevention activities completed since the last survey, plans for future programs, and the monitoring and assessment methods used to evaluate the current programs.

Learning from Cancer Conferences

Observing the multidisciplinary participation, discussing stage, and discussing treatment options during the conference assists the surveyor(s) to evaluate and rate the team approach to the provision of patient care.

Assessing the Quality of Care

The CoC provides each CoC-accredited program with information about their practice patterns for cases of breast, colon, and rectal cancer that meet the specific criteria for an established performance measure.

Each year the cancer committee reviews the performance measure data that are displayed in the Cancer Program Practice Profile Reports (CP³R) to monitor the quality of care and addresses instances of physician performance or inaccurate or incomplete data in the cancer

registry database. The committee records their review activities in the SAR.

Two weeks (14 days) before survey, the NCDB selects one of the performance measures for review and identifies for review a maximum of 25 cases from the most recent year of data submitted to the NCDB. The accession number, sequence number, diagnosis date, and diagnosis age for each case are added to the SAR. The registrar provides the medical record for each case for surveyor review during the on-site visit.

The surveyor(s) reviews the medical record to confirm specific information for each case as specified by the NCDB. This information is recorded in the SAR, and the surveyor discusses the findings with the cancer committee during the summation conference. This discussion provides the cancer committee an opportunity to acknowledge good performance or develop a plan to address identified issues.

Currently, this performance review has no impact on the program's survey outcome or accreditation award. However, facility performance against these measures will be part of the standards released in 2012.

Review of Additional Documentation

As part of the on-site visit, the surveyor(s) reviews additional documentation demonstrating the full scope of the cancer program activity. This may be accomplished during the meeting with the cancer program team members or as a separate activity. A listing of suggested additional documentation can be found in *Cancer Program Standards 2009 Revised Edition* (page 8). [2]

Touring the Service Areas

A tour of the facility enables the surveyor(s) to observe the care settings, multidisciplinary staff interaction, and communication with the patients. The surveyor(s) may review policies and procedures or interview area staff during the tour.

The inpatient medical oncology unit, or functional equivalent, must be part of the facility tour. The program may choose to include other areas such as the outpatient infusion center, oncology clinic, radiation oncology department, pathology department, pharmacy, or patient library. The scope of the tour is planned during the development of the survey agenda.

Evaluating Registry Operations

Time spent with the cancer registrar allows for an exchange of information and suggestions to improve registry operations. The meeting includes an evaluation of the cancer registry operations, such as the policy and procedure manual, suspense list, and data request log. The quality of the abstracted data recorded in the cancer registry data base is compared with the information found in the patient medical records.

At least 30 abstracts are reviewed to evaluate the timeliness of abstracting. Abstracts are selected from each year during the 3-year accreditation period. In addition, 30 pathology reports are selected for the review of the presence of the scientifically validated data elements for the sites that have been outlined in the College of American Pathologists (CAP) Cancer Protocols. As with the selection of abstracts, reports representing each year in the 3-year accreditation period are selected. As part of a network survey, 30 abstracts and pathology reports from each network location are evaluated. The review findings are shared with the cancer committee and the CoC to provide documentation of the surveyor(s) ratings for Standards 3.3 and 4.6. [1]*

Providing an Overview of the Findings

After the complete evaluation of the program, the surveyor(s) summarizes the findings of the evaluation for the cancer committee and other members of the cancer program team at a final conference.

The interactive format of this meeting allows the surveyor(s) to acknowledge the program strengths and identify the areas where program activity falls below the required levels. The cancer program team has an opportunity to respond to the identified deficiencies and provide additional documentation or information to resolve the ratings for the standard(s) before the conclusion of the on-site visit.

The surveyor(s) will offer suggestions for improving current program activity, describe ways to resolve the identified deficiencies, and share information on important CoC initiatives and upcoming activities. The surveyor(s) may also suggest that areas of the SAR be modified to offer more accurate or complete information about program activity.

Postsurvey Activity
Facility
Completing Final Changes to the Survey Application Record

The facility is allowed to make changes to the SAR during the 72 hours after the survey. Information that presents an accurate picture of the program and clarifies services offered by the facility is recorded by the cancer registrar or the key contact for survey preparation. Information needed to resolve issues with performance identified during the summation meeting should be added to the SAR at this time.

Evaluating Surveyor Performance

Within the 2 weeks after the survey, the cancer program team meets to discuss the survey experience and complete the online postsurvey evaluation form. The postsurvey evaluation collects information about the survey scheduling process, customer support provided by members of the Cancer Programs staff, as well as details on surveyor(s) performance. Completion of this evaluation is a required part of the survey and assists the development of educational programs for surveyors, together with the CoC-trained Cancer Program Consultants, and enhances the survey process and the overall improvement of the Accreditation Program of the CoC.

Surveyor(s)
Rating Program Activity

Once the SAR is closed to the facility for changes, the surveyor records comments about each standard and rates compliance based on the discussions and findings of the on-site visit. The surveyor completes the program assessment within the 2 weeks after the survey. The network cancer program surveyors discuss their findings and agree to one rating of compliance for each standard that is recorded in the SAR. The surveyor notifies the CoC by e-mail when the survey is complete. Miscellaneous paper documentation is shipped to the CoC for review and destruction.

Writing an Evaluation Summary

The surveyor(s) uses the surveyor comment page in the SAR to summarize the findings of the on-site visit. The surveyor(s) acknowledges the program strengths, describes areas that need improvement, and comments on exceptional program activities that may not tie directly to a standard.

Accreditation and Standards technical staff use the information provided in the summary to enhance the content of the Accredited Cancer Program Performance Report.

The Accreditation Process

Describing the Accreditation Awards

An Accreditation Award is granted to each program surveyed by the CoC. The awards range from Full Accreditation to Nonaccreditation. To be accredited by the CoC, a program must be in compliance with at least 29 (80%) of the standards set forth in *Cancer Program Standards 2009 Revised Edition.* [2]

---

*Standard 3.3: For each year between survey, 90% of cases are abstracted within 6 months of the date of first contact.

Standard 4.6: The guidelines for patient management and treatment currently required by the CoC are followed.

Programs with fewer than eight deficiencies receive a Three-Year with Contingency award and are expected to resolve the deficiency(ies) within 1 year. A program that is not currently accredited and identified to have a deficiency in one standard will receive the Accreditation Deferred status. This status allows the program to make corrections to the identified deficiency and receive accreditation without a resurvey. [2]

Programs with eight or more deficiencies receive Nonaccreditation. The programs are encouraged to make corrections to program activity and reapply for a survey at a future time. Historically, few programs receive Nonaccreditation. [2]

Completing the Technical Review Process

Each survey is evaluated by a technical staff member of the Accreditations and Standards Section. The SAR, the facility and surveyor ratings and comments, and all program documentation submitted by the surveyor(s) are included in this technical review of the survey. This independent review ensures that the CoC standards have been accurately and consistently applied to all cancer programs.

When a question about compliance surfaces, the technical staff member may follow-back with the program for clarification or confer with the surveyor(s) to confirm a compliance rating.

The technical staff member uses the special area of the facility's SAR to record comments and assigns a rating for each standard, and assigns an Accreditation Award to the program based on a consensus between the surveyor(s) and technical staff rating.

Confirming the Accreditation Award

The survey may also be referred to the Program Review Subcommittee of the Accreditation Committee for review and confirmation of the accreditation award. Annually, the Program Review Subcommittee chooses to monitor program performance with several standards, as well as other related issues. These standards are part of the SAR Annual Update process described earlier in this chapter.

The Program Review Subcommittee also confirms all Nonaccreditation awards by reviewing all survey information for each program. Occasionally, the program may want to appeal the Accreditation Award. This is appropriate when program activity was misinterpreted by the surveyor or technical staff reviewer, or when existing documentation of compliance was available, but not reviewed, at the time of the survey. The Program Review Subcommittee accepts documentation to appeal an Accreditation Award up to 45 days after distribution of the Accredited Cancer Program Performance Report. The Program Review Subcommittee reviews and confirms the Accreditation Award for each appeal that is submitted.

Understanding and Using the Accredited Cancer Program Performance Report

Within 45 days of the on-site visit, survey results and Accreditation Awards are available through the on-line Accredited Cancer Program Performance Report (Performance Report). The individualized Performance Report is prepared by the technical staff member after confirmation of the Accreditation Award. Each Performance Report has the following characteristics:

Provides facility and surveyor identification, and includes the date the survey was performed
Documents the Accreditation Award
Identifies the deficient standards
Provides a summary of the deficiency(ies) and the expected compliance
Identifies the contingency period and the date documentation of compliance is due
Acknowledges the commendation(s)
Provides comparison data by state, category, and overall for all programs surveyed in the period

Program Recognition

The CoC recognizes each accredited program by including the facility contact information, as well as resources and services, in the database of all accredited programs. The database is accessible from the Cancer Programs page of the ACoS Web site, http://www.facs.org/cancerprogram/index.html. The searchable database includes:

Facility name and address
Cancer center name, if applicable
Category of accreditation
Facility resource and service information
Special achievements, such as receiving the CoC Outstanding Achievement Award

Following survey, each CoC-accredited program is provided with a press kit and marketing materials that can be used to promote a new CoC Accreditation or continuing participation in the CoC Accreditations Program. Information describing the facility's Accreditation status can be shared with facility staff and the community by placing notices or advertisements in local newspapers and magazines, including the Accreditation status in reports or brochures, or posting information on the facility intranet or Web site.

What's on the Horizon for the Survey Process?

2012 will bring changes to the CoC standards for cancer programs, the SAR, and the on-site evaluation with the release of the newly revised manual. The standards are being restructured in the following ways:

> To identify numerous eligibility requirements that must be in place throughout the 3-year accreditation period to
> Address the continuum of care
> Focus on the quality of care provided
> Improve patient outcomes

Conclusion

The voluntary group of CoC-accredited cancer programs provides care to approximately 80% of newly diagnosed cancer patients each year while representing only 25% of the acute care hospitals in the United States and Puerto Rico.

The facility demonstrates a commitment to providing high-quality cancer care because it willingly participates in an objective external evaluation of its cancer program as measured against the standards of the CoC. The CoC acknowledges the facility's commitment through the assignment of the Accreditation Award.

References

1. American College of Surgeons Archives, Commission on Cancer, letter from Thomas S. Cullen to Franklin H. Martin, November 26, 1932, including copy of letter to Joseph C. Bloodgood (October 26, 1928).
2. Commission on Cancer of the American College of Surgeons. *Cancer Program Standards 2009 Revised Edition.* Chicago: American College of Surgeons, 2009.
3. *Commission on Cancer, Initial Survey Notification for 2010 Surveys.* Chicago: American College of Surgeons, 2010. Available at: http://www.facs.org/cancer/coc/initialsurvey.html. Last accessed August 2010.
4. *Commission on Cancer, Sample Survey Agenda and Required Documents.* Chicago: American College of Surgeons, 2010. Available at: http://www.facs.org/cancer/coc/surveyresources.html.
5. *Commission on Cancer, Surveyor Assignment for 2010 Surveys.* Chicago: American College of Surgeons, 2010. Available at: http://www.facs.org/cancer/coc/surveyorassignment.html. Last accessed August 2010.

chapter 20

Education

Donna M. Gress, RHIT, CTR

Lilly Grossman, BA

Louise Schuman, MA, CTR

Lillian Antonelli-Twal, MS, CTR

Education is essential for all careers. The cancer registry profession mandates a minimum of an Associate of Arts (AA) degree or its equivalent. This requirement began with those wanting to take the credentialing examination in 2010. As with many careers, the educational requirements have evolved through the years. In the early years of the profession, many registrars learned through training programs and workshops. Others came into the field through related allied health careers. Cancer registry classes have often been a component of the Health Information Management college curriculum. College classes for registrars have been offered in the past, with some oversight and input from National Cancer Registrars Association (NCRA). The formal college education for the registry professional became uniform with the publication of the first edition of this textbook, designed strictly for registrars, in 1997.

Formal Education

The Cancer Information Management program is designed for those interested in entering the cancer registry profession. Cancer registrars must possess the clinical and technical knowledge and skills necessary to maintain a registry. Cancer registrars manage the registry database consistent with medical, administrative, ethical, legal, and accreditation requirements of the healthcare delivery system.

The cancer registry database serves many purposes. The information collected and maintained by cancer registry professionals is used for research, quality management, and facility planning and marketing. The data collected are also used to evaluate the results of treatment and monitor patient outcomes and to report survival data. The information must meet national accreditation standards and be compliant with reporting timelines. Formal education programs teach the aspiring cancer registrar how to become proficient in these important tasks.

There are many types of formal education programs. There are prerequisite classes common to many allied health professions and core classes specific to the registry profession. These are examples of common classes for both the prerequisites and the core subjects. The exact class structures will vary with the college program.[1,2]

Prerequisites

There are college-level classes that must be taken for credit that registrars need as the building blocks to their more specialized cancer information education. The classes will vary according to the program, but all will encompass these general descriptions.

Human Anatomy and Physiology

It is essential for registrars to have a human anatomy and physiology foundation for their work, to ensure accuracy in data collection. This is the basic information necessary for a general understanding of the structure and function of the human body.

The topics covered include organization of the body, chemistry of life, body tissues, cells and membranes, blood, and human development and birth. The body systems include integumentary, musculoskeletal, nervous, lymphatic, sensory, endocrine, cardiovascular, respiratory, digestive, urinary, and reproductive organs.

Computer Basics in Health Care

Cancer registries utilize computerized databases and other software for analysis and reports. It is vital that registrars have an understanding of these systems. This course offers a general overview of computers and the Internet, and the role each plays in health care. It is important to learn the basics of hardware and software, and to have a general understanding of the most commonly used applications.

Medical Terminology

Registrars use the medical record and other medical documents to gather the information needed for the registry database. This class teaches how to break medical terms into prefixes, suffixes, and roots, and become familiar with the spelling and definition of common medical terms related to major disease processes, diagnostic procedures, laboratory tests, abbreviations, drugs, and treatment modalities.

Pathophysiology/Pharmacology

Understanding the various diseases in the body, not just cancer, assists a registrar in understanding all of the information in the medical record, not just related to the cancer diagnosis. It is important to have knowledge of these other processes because they can affect the cancer diagnosis and treatment. Emphasis is placed on the disease processes that affect the human body via an integrated approach to specific disease entities. The study of causes, diagnosis, and treatment of disease, as well as an understanding of the basic principles of pharmacology, is the basis of this class.

Biology/Introduction to Medicine

It is essential for registrars to have a basic understanding of biology to provide a good foundation for their work. This class explores the characteristics of the disease process, as well as the characteristics of cancer and other diseases.

Core Classes in Cancer Information Management

Core classes in cancer information management enable a registrar to learn the principles of cancer registry and all of the practical applications of those theories. The various functions of a registry are covered in detail to provide a strong foundation for the registrar's knowledge and future performance.

Cancer Registry Structure and Management

The basic concepts of the structure and management of cancer registries is the underlying foundation a registrar must learn and understand. It is important to have a basic knowledge of the types and purpose of cancer registries, confidentiality issues, and the role of standard-setting organizations in cancer data management.

Cancer Registry Operations

There are many processes to the functioning of a registry. This class provides an in-depth depiction of the systematic processes used in the daily operations of a cancer registry, including those to identify, code, maintain quality, and provide lifetime follow-up on cases. Detailed guidelines are provided on how to determine which cases meet eligibility requirements of state and national standards. Insight will be given as to the role the standards play in providing comparable data for analysis. There is a thorough explanation of the standards necessary for registry operations for approved cancer programs of the American College of Surgeons Commission on Cancer (CoC).

Cancer Disease Coding and Staging

One of the most important concepts for registrars to understand is the different types of cancer and how cancer grows and spreads. This class defines cancer, how it develops, and can invade other parts of the body and ultimately cause death. The hundreds of different types of cancer and benign tumors are discussed, together with how to classify these tumors utilizing globally recognized codes. Classification will help distinguish where the cancer initiated, what type of cancer, and how aggressive it may be. The class focuses on and provides instruction in data collection processes. The various components of a medical record, the principles of abstracting and coding, and cancer staging principles are explained. In this class, the student will learn about cancer histology and the components of the *International Classification of Diseases for Oncology,* Third Edition (ICD-O-3). Two major staging systems are reviewed extensively, the American Joint Committee on Cancer (AJCC) TNM and the Collaborative Stage Data Collection System. Historical staging systems are also explored, including the General Summary Staging and Extent of Disease (EOD) staging systems.

Abstracting Methods

The abstract forms the building block of the entire registry. The abstract is the place where the registrar enters all the information about the patient's diagnostic workup, treatment, and staging. It is the basic component on which everything is built. This class takes a systematic look at the source documents for data. The identification of cases that are eligible for inclusion in the cancer registry database and methods of documenting pertinent clinical information into each of the data fields according to established standards are discussed. This class usually includes the student independently abstracting complete cancer registry data elements. This is part of the professional practice experience required.

Oncology Treatment and Coding

Understanding the treatment for cancer and applying the correct codes to the various options is extremely important. This class provides an in-depth overview of available cancer treatment options, how treatment works to destroy or eliminate cancer, and how to code each. It includes a comprehensive review of surgery, chemotherapy, radiation therapy, immunotherapy, hormonal therapy, and other less frequently used treatment modalities. Treatment modalities are linked to the types of cancer for which they are used. The student must have a good knowledge of the natural history of the particular cancer being abstracted. To assist with this, there is a study of clinical pathways and nationally accepted treatment guidelines. These help the registrar to determine what types of treatment are found in medical records based on site, extent, and type of cancer. These guidelines also tell the registrar how to search for information that may not be found in the medical record. There are reviews of case summaries, where treatment identification and coding is performed. First line of treatment must be defined and identified. For each treatment modality, a detailed overview of coding references should be undertaken so that appropriate codes are assigned. After case summaries have been coded, it is important for registrars to determine whether the treatment for the case is complete or whether the case requires further research.

Follow-up, Data Quality, and Utilization

Follow-up information is vital to the cancer registry and provides the long-term outcome of the case. It is important to have accurate quality data so that it may be utilized to provide the information needed to assess the care and outcome of the cancer patient. Survival data for cancer patients is determined largely from the follow-up information provided by cancer registries. This course provides best practices for obtaining lifelong follow-up on appropriate cases. It also demonstrates the need for data quality and methods to ensure consistent, accurate data and outcomes. Statistics and epidemiology as it applies to the registry is explained. The student will learn how to use the data to provide information for clinical studies requested by staff physicians and administration. The structure and management of the database is also explored.

Professional Practice Experience

The curriculum for the cancer registry classes includes the important component of the professional practice experience. There is a requirement of 160 hours, which includes specific hours and tasks in different areas. (See the NCRA Web site for specifics on the requirements of this practicum.[1])

Accredited College Programs

The Accredited College Program identifies those education programs that meet and maintain standards for education for professional development in Cancer Registry Management. This may be either a certificate program or an associate's degree program. The accreditation status of education programs is contained in a roster maintained by the NCRA office. This contains the accreditation status of the program, the degree level, the current period of accreditation, and the year of its next scheduled reaccreditation review. NCRA publishes the names of accredited programs and those holding provisional status in the Online Guide to Formal Education in Cancer Registry Management on NCRA's Web site (www.ncra-usa.org).

As an Accredited College Program provider of cancer registry education, the program is given access to a variety of resources aimed at supporting and ensuring the growth of the program. There are different types of programs, either offering an associate's degree or a certificate. The programs also include online and traditional classroom. NCRA's Partners in Education (PIE) offers a Mentor Directory that allows students to search online for sites to complete their clinical work experience. Students who successfully complete an accredited Formal Education Program are eligible to sit for the Certified Tumor Registrar (CTR) Credentialing Examination. As of 2010, there are four eligibility routes to sit for the examination. This information is available at the NCRA Web site (www.ncra-usa.org).

Partners in Education

NCRA's PIE is a collaborative network between cancer registry professionals, cancer registry schools, and students. PIE offers valuable resources for current and promising cancer registry professionals, and can be used for students and experienced professional alike.

Students

Students enrolled in an Accredited Formal Education Program who want to complete the clinical can search a database to find a location that will conduct the clinical practicum. The clinical practicum must be done under the supervision of a CTR. It is important to understand the scope, time, and resources needed to complete a clinical practicum. Information about internship and the clinical requirement can be found by accessing the NCRA Web site (www.ncra-usa.org).

Mentors

Experienced CTRs are needed to assist with the clinical aspect of the Accredited Formal Education Programs. Experienced CTR's help students complete the requirements of the clinical practicum, which is a part of the eligibility to take the CTR examination. It is crucial to find experienced CTR's who can create a positive environment for new registrars and to expand the number of professionals entering the field. Information regarding how to become a clinical host can be found by going the National Cancer Registrars Association Web site (www.ncra-usa.org).

Continuing Education

Continuing education (CE) is vital for cancer registrars, as oncology medicine is an ever-changing specialty. There are new diagnostic tests and biologic markers, and changes to treatments are being developed constantly. To ensure that the most accurate and timely data are collected, registrars must keep their knowledge up to date. There are also changes to the data fields based on these medical changes, and registrars need to update their skills in understanding how to document this new information. The starting point to become an accomplished registrar is to be actively engaged in continuing professional education.

CE ensures that once certified in a profession, individuals will maintain high levels of performance in the practice of that profession. Each CTR is responsible for self-assessment of personal knowledge and understanding of the registry field, and further, a continued maintenance of those abilities through participation in appropriate educational programs. This is particularly important in the healthcare field, where advances in knowledge and technology occur at a rapid pace.

A registrar needs to incorporate many different subjects into their education. This can be site-specific information, new tests and treatments, computer skills, changes to the data items in the registry database, updates on coding and staging, management classes, and other subjects that will enhance the knowledge and skills needed by a registrar.

Maintaining Your Certified Tumor Registrar Credential

Although all registrars need to update their knowledge and skills through CE, there are specific requirements for CTRs. Registrars must complete 20 hours of CE credits every 2 years to maintain the CTR certificate. Many types of programs meet the criteria for CE credit. The credential can be revoked if the CE hours are not maintained and for other reasons.

Understanding Your Options

Many different activities can be used for CE. Some of them include attendance at cancer conferences, active participation in professional organizations, formal presentation of an original work relating to the cancer registry field to an audience, virtually attending or attending in person lectures, taking journal quizzes or completing case scenarios, publication of an article on the registry, and many other activities.

In addition, education programs come in a variety of formats and can be offered by different organizations such as national professional organizations, local organizations, and standard-setting organizations. These groups work to offer meaningful educational opportunities for cancer registrars. Often, these programs target specific communities within the cancer registry profession such as management courses, advanced abstracting courses, or even programs that help prospective employers find experienced registry staff. The cancer registry profession, like many, has a workforce with layered identities that need to be considered when offering and participating in educational programs.

Online Learning

With the increased use of technology in the learning environment, more and more organizations are offering opportunities for cancer registrars to obtain important education via the online platform. Technology is rapidly changing, which can make choosing an educational opportunity daunting. There are some key areas to consider when deciding on the type of online learning that works best for the participant.

There are basically two key types of online learning that define the type of interaction that will happen in a virtual learning environment. They are *synchronous* and *asynchronous* online learning.

Synchronous describes the type of online learning that happens in "real time" and involves coordinated live interaction with an instructor or facilitator. In a synchronous environment, the instructor and student are online at the same time exchanging information using a Web-based instructional platform.

Asynchronous learning describes an online learning environment that does not involve a coordinated live interaction between the instructor and participant. It can be described as a "self-directed" environment that depends on the participant to work through the training at his or her own pace.

Workshops and Conferences

Although online education has a great presence in today's education environment, there is much to be said for the benefits of in-person training. Many organizations offer a variety of educational opportunities like 1- or 2-day hands-on workshops, as well as industry conferences where credentialed cancer registrars can earn CE credits, network, and gain valuable professional development opportunities.

Professional Organizations

The NCRA is a membership-based, professional nonprofit organization that represents cancer registrars and is committed to being the premier education and advocacy resource for cancer registrars.

Involvement in a professional organization, such as NCRA, gives members access to the types of educational activities mentioned earlier in the chapter. Beyond access to education, involvement in the organization is also a valuable professional development resource. By being an active member in the organization, volunteer leaders build vital leadership experience that can greatly enhance career opportunities.

National Cancer Registrars Association Leadership Opportunities

NCRA is an organization that is led by a volunteer board of directors. The members of the board of directors actively seek committed, experienced, and credentialed cancer registrars to lead various types of education-driven committees.[1] The leaders of these committees are instrumental in the development and delivery of relevant education for cancer registrars.

Professional associations like the NCRA also depend on paid staff to support the volunteer leaders in their endeavors. The Education Manager is the staff person volunteer leaders look to for guidance on understanding the latest trends in adult education theory and instructional design. Combined, the volunteer leaders and staff form a team of dedicated professionals whose mission is to create meaningful educational opportunities.

Through the guidance of a strategic management plan, NCRA committee leaders and staff are tasked with developing educational opportunities that are relevant to specific groups of individuals in the profession. Understanding how these groups work and who they target is an important resource to gaining educational and professional opportunities. Table 20-1 describes the various committees and their roles in developing education.

Summary

Communicating the role and value of education to new and experienced cancer registrars is instrumental in developing a strong workforce. Many factors play a role in deciding what type of education to embark upon. From traditional educational opportunities to online learning and

Table 20-1	NCRA Board and Committee Structure for Education Projects

Board of Director Representative (voted in by membership)	Committee by Name (appointed by board representative)	Type of Education
Board Director of Education	CE Committee	The *Continuing Education Committee* reviews educational activities that the cancer registrars participate in to assure that the educational programs enhance the knowledge and expertise of the cancer registrar consistent with the advances in healthcare technology, the field of oncology, and changing registry standards.
	Program Recognition Committee	The *Program Recognition Committee* receives applications from organizations seeking CE hours for programs that they will be presenting. This committee reviews the program information to determine whether it meets the criteria for CE credits and awards the number of CE credits the program merits based on specific criteria.
	Alternative Methods Committee	The *Alternative Methods Committee* develops educational opportunities that can be accomplished as an individual. These are alternatives to attending workshops or meetings. The committee writes the quizzes for the *Journal of Registry Management*.
	Education Committee	The *Education Committee* is responsible for developing an education plan to meet the changing demands of the profession and the CTR credentialed individual, and is responsible for overseeing the development and delivery of *basic* and *advanced* education opportunities.
	CTR Exam Prep Committee	*CTR Exam Prep Committee* is comprised of workshops and Webinars. The mission is to provide a thorough and accurate review to assist candidates in preparing for the CTR Examination.
Professional Development Board Director	Formal Education Committee	The *Formal Education Committee* is responsible for the communication and outreach to Accredited Formal Education Programs.
	Formal Education Program Review Committee	The *Formal Education Program Review Committee* is charged with accrediting formal education programs for cancer registrars.

CE: continuing education.

involvement in professional organizations, each option is an investment in your future as a cancer registrar.

CE is a career-long investment and should be considered when entering the profession. Make an education plan and review it periodically. Develop personal goals and document milestones. Your investment in education will help bridge the gap between cancer research and a cure, and ensure a strong and competent workforce.

References

1. National Cancer Registrars Association Web site: http://www.ncra-usa.org/.
2. American Health Information Management Association: Distance Education Campus. Available at: http://www.ahima.org/ContinuingEd/Campus/default.aspx, last accessed July 2010.

chapter 21

Cancer Conference

Bonnie Quiñónez, BSB/M, RHIT, CTR

Accrediting bodies in the field of medicine began to emerge in the early twentieth century. The American College of Surgeons (ACoS), founded in 1913, created the Commission on Cancer (CoC) in 1922. The CoC modified the standards for approved cancer programs in 1954 and mandated that facilities establish *tumor boards,* currently referred to as *cancer conferences.* The 1966 *Manual for Cancer Programs* refers to a "consultative cancer conference" with a formal structure and preferred weekly sessions. Conferences were conducted for the purpose of discussion and treatment recommendations. The manual specified there should be a clear understanding that the ultimate responsibility remains with the patient's physician. Opportunities to participate in the clinical conference were expected to be extended to all members of the staff, as well as community providers, with an emphasis on presenting problem cases.[1]

The academic environment has historically used board-style meetings as part of the educational platform. Formal multidisciplinary discussions encourage the establishment of treatment plans based on current diagnosis and treatment standards in an effort to improve overall management of patient care. Cancer conferences, once referred to as "tumor site conferences" and often still referred to as "tumor boards," facilitate multidisciplinary discussions of the complex systemic disease, *cancer.* Consultative meetings similar to cancer conferences occur in facilities not approved by the CoC and further support the effectiveness of this type of discussion. In addition, many physicians view cancer conference as the equivalent to a second opinion and communicate the case presentation discussion to their patients.

Healthcare organizations and processes for consultative services have changed a great deal since the CoC implemented the requirement of cancer conferences. The CoC remains the regulating mechanism for cancer conferences in the United States. According to the American Society of Clinical Oncology (ASCO), "Tumor Board is used as the approach to treatment planning, consisting of different cancer specialists reviewing and discussing a patient's medical condition and possible treatment options."[2] This chapter serves to provide suggestions for developing and maintaining successful cancer conferences.

Definitions

Tumor Board versus Cancer Conference

Many physicians and cancer registrars use the terms *tumor board* and *cancer conference* interchangeably. The ACoS-CoC uses *cancer conference* as the preferred term to describe the multidisciplinary discussion meant to enhance patient care. A potential explanation for this name change is the evolution of multidisciplinary participation in case presentations and development of treatment plans based on multidisciplinary physician consensus rather than direction given by an established board of physicians.

Prospective and Retrospective

Prospective cases are presented for discussion at the time of initial diagnosis, with an emphasis on establishing accurate staging (clinical or pathologic), treatment options based on national treatment guidelines, and expected patient management plans. Prospective conferences may also include discussion of adjuvant therapy after the initial surgical treatment or treatment plans for a recurrence. The prospective approach is, in essence, a look forward, as opposed to the retrospective approach. Retrospective cases are discussed after the completion of all treatment, primarily for the purpose of education, and are not intended to influence the management of patient care. Careful scrutiny of the discussion content, questions, and suggestions occurring during the case presentation will provide the support for categorizing cases presented.

Institutions can benefit from both prospective and retrospective case discussions based on the established goals for each cancer conference (see Frequency and Format section later in this chapter).

Developing Cancer Conferences

Developing a cancer conference to fit the unique structure within each organizational environment requires flexibility, innovative thinking, and collaboration. Establishing a list of available resources and organizational needs will assist the Cancer Committee or other responsible parties in preparing effective cancer conference plans. In addition, administrative and physician support, as well as available monetary and physical resources, will further define the potential for cancer conference development.

CoC-approved programs are required to adhere to administrative and physician infrastructure requirements defined in the *Cancer Program Standards.* Registrars of CoC-approved programs should reference the current version of *Cancer Program Standards* when preparing recommendations. The major CoC Standards (revised, 2009) focusing on cancer conference requirements include:

- 2.3—Program activity coordinators
- 2.4—Meeting schedule
- 2.5—Duties and responsibilities
- 2.6—Cancer conference, frequency and format
- 2.7—Requirements for attendance
- 2.8—Prospective and retrospective case presentation
- 2.9—Cancer Committee reporting
- 4.6—Patient management guidelines

Potential Monetary and Physical Resources for Cancer Conference

- *Monetary support*
  - Catering costs for a cancer conference will depend on the scheduled meeting time, availability of on-site catering versus local catering deliveries, and access to educational grants through drug company representatives.
  - The Medical Education department may serve as a resource in providing sponsored physician CME events through current speaker lists and contacts.
- *Meeting site and room availability*
  - Consistency in meeting site and time limits confusion.
  - Room comfort and ease of accessibility encourage attendance.
  - Limited parking issues may detour physician attendance. Evaluate access to physician parking in relation to room location.
- *Equipment and technologies*
  - Virtual meetings have become cost-efficient alternatives of the face-to-face meetings. If this is the meeting of choice, coordinators need to be familiar with virtual meeting software and other related equipment.

American College of Surgeons Commission on Cancer Program Categories

The category of approval establishes the frequency and format requirements for cancer conference, currently detailed in Standard 2.6. Cancer registrars should reference the current edition of the CoC standards for program approvals for details.

Frequency and Format

Requirements for the frequency and format of cancer conference are detailed in CoC Standard 2.6 (revised, 2009). Determining factors used to establish the frequency and format include program category, number of annual analytic accessions, types of cases seen by the facility, need for consultative services, and need for educational activities.[3]

Types of Cancer Conference (Format)

Each institution will establish the cancer conference format based on the unique challenges within their facility. Successful cancer conferences require the application of a format structure that can be supported by the institution and facilitates discussions that provide the most benefit to the specific patient population. For instance, smaller community hospitals settings will have different oncologic consultative needs than do large metropolitan areas with multiple academic institutions and greater access to community oncology specialists.

Some examples of the most common cancer conference formats are as follows:

- *Departmental:* Cancer conference attendance and presentation is department specific.
- *Facility wide:* Cancer conference attendance and presentation opportunities are open to all members of the medical staff.
- *Network wide:* Cancer conference attendance and presentation opportunities are open to all members within a network. The attendees of a network cancer conference are based on the needs of the facility. Examples might include a cancer conference with participation from physician members of a Health Maintenance Organization (HMO), with multiple locations throughout a state or states.
- *Site focused:* Focus of cancer conference is on one specific primary site or discipline; examples include breast cancer conference or gynecologic oncology conference.
- *Academic/Teaching:* Examples include Ground Rounds, Daily Cancer Conferences,[4] or histology-specific conferences.
- *Community wide:* Cancer conference attendance and presentation are open to all healthcare professionals within the community.

Physician Presentation Format

Soliciting physician presenters for cancer conference should comprise all possible resources as applicable to the facility infrastructure and resources. The primary source for physician presenters begins with active medical staff rosters, physician members of Cancer Committee, and community oncologists. Administrative support will help increase participation of active medical staff; however, the best possible persuasion for physician participation is a quality and productive cancer conference. It is imperative that cancer registrars seek administrative guidance regarding attendance before establishing methods for recruitment of physician presenters, to avoid unintentional breaches in patient confidentiality.

The CoC requires facilities to present cases based on the five major sites seen at the facility. Reviewing site tables assist facilities to solicit physician presenters from the required specialties. For example, if one of the top five primary sites is cervical cancer, gynecologic oncologists need to be included as presenters and required attendance.

The CoC requires establishing the cancer conference format. Many facilities meet this by establishing a *template* for use when preparing case presentations to facilitate adherence to requirements for prospective case discussions. This case presentation material is prepared by the cancer registrar. In a few facilities, the physicians dictate this information.

The registrar can enter this presentation information into the registry database and print an abstract for use as the presentation material at cancer conference. This is the same information used in the registry abstract, and it is not efficient to enter the same information twice into two different formats, the meeting presentation materials and the registry database. It is more efficient to enter it once into the registry database. It also familiarizes the physicians with the information collected by the registry. Registrars should take notes during the cancer conference discussion of items to assist in abstracting such as verifying the primary site and histology, and documenting the American Joint Committee on Cancer (AJCC) stage and treatment plan. Documenting the treatment plan based on the discussion provides an excellent source of treatment data. The treatment plan will guide the registrar in knowing what information to seek. The plan can change, but it provides an excellent way to know the possible treatment options.

Example Items for Cancer Conference Presenter Format
(examples only, amount of information and number of items will vary by facility)

- Case identification (facility-preferred method of case identification, i.e., patient initials only or numeric values such as Case #1)
- History and physical examination (H&P) (facility-required information such as physical findings, chief complaint, and clinical AJCC/TNM elements)
- Laboratory results pertinent to the case
- Diagnostic radiology findings
  - Including discussion of clinical AJCC/TNM elements
- Pathology findings
  - Including discussion of applicable AJCC/TNM elements based on cancer staging rules of clinical versus pathologic
  - Biopsy only, no surgical resection, clinical AJCC/TNM
  - Surgically resected specimen, pathologic AJCC/TNM is discussed based on the resected specimens
  - Discuss College of American Pathologists (CAP) protocols where applicable
- Presenting physician discussion of AJCC Cancer Staging, including elements and category (i.e., clinical or pathologic)
- Discuss treatment options based on national treatment guidelines
- Optional point: confidentiality and protection of patient information (see Confidentiality section later in this chapter)

Cancer Conference Schedule (Frequency)

The frequency of cancer conference may be weekly or monthly, based on the category of CoC approval and the number of cases required for presentation. When weekly cancer conferences are required, greater physician resources are needed than that for monthly conferences. Teaching facilities or large cancer programs will have access to a greater number of physicians for rotating case presentation assignments. Additional examples of frequency might include bimonthly or quarterly meetings. The Cancer Committee must document the established frequency in committee minutes.

Information Technology

Advances in the field of information technology (IT) and use of IT in cancer conference have existed for many years. An article published in 1986 titled "A New Mechanism for Physician Participation in a Tumor Board" details the addition of teleconference in 1982 to meet multiple programmatic needs.[5] IT options are broad and include computers, telecommunications, Web-based technology, and other electronic modes of communication. Web-based meetings and telemedicine has become a common method of communication in many settings. Successful incorporation of advances in IT communication requires involvement from ancillary departments:

- Virtual meetings are a cost-efficient alternative to face-to-face meetings. If virtual meetings become the meeting of choice, coordinators need to be familiar with virtual meeting software.
  - The IT support staff must be included in developing an IT plan that can limit technical difficulties that hinder advancement and frustrate attendees and users.
  - The staff in charge of cancer conference must increase their familiarity with the IT advances to avoid interruptions and other problems during meetings.

Multidisciplinary Attendance

"Consultative services are optimal when physician representatives from diagnostic radiology, pathology, surgery, medical oncology, and radiation oncology participate in facility-wide or network-wide cancer conferences."[6]

Attendance requirements will encourage involvement of multiple disciplines improving the overall care for cancer patients. Considerations for required attendance should include an evaluation of the active staff physicians by specialty, available community physicians, primary sites seen within the facility, and access to outside affiliated physicians. Restrictions on attendance at cancer conference by nonstaff physicians are subject to the direction of the facility's administration. The cancer registrar should verify attendance guidelines with the Cancer Committee, facility's medical staff office, privacy officer, or other applicable source.

The CoC requires physician representation by surgery, medical oncology, radiation oncology, diagnostic radiology, and pathology. Physician participation is voluntary, and accommodating every physician schedule is not possible. The schedules for physicians active in the cancer program and dedicated to developing productive cancer conferences should be the registrar's first priority. The Cancer Committee is required to provide documentation of attendance requirements in committee minutes.

The specialties of primary care, internal medicine, family practice, and other physician specialties should be included as required attendance to encourage comprehensive discussions regarding early diagnosis and follow-up.

Nonphysician attendance by nursing, hospice care, social services, cancer registry, and other allied healthcare workers will enhance a total approach to caring for patients diagnosed with cancer.

Continuing Education

The Cancer Committee may decide to request continuing medical education credits (CME) for attendance at Cancer Conference in an attempt to provide an additional boost to overall physician attendance. A member of the Cancer Committee should be involved in the process of requesting CMEs, including providing input on the development of required goals and objectives for CME events. Continuing education credits should also be requested for other professionals to encourage their attendance. Examples of physician and other professional groups include:

- Accreditation Council for Continuing Medical Education (ACCME)
- Accreditation Council for Graduate Medical Education (ACGME)
- American Nurses Association (ANA) and the American Nurses Credentialing Center (ANCC)
- National Cancer Registrars Association (NCRA)
- American Association of Medical Dosimetrists (AAMD)
- American Society of Radiologic Technologists (ASRT)

Commercial Support

Additional consideration should be given when accepting commercial support for a Cancer Conference. Councils such as ACCME or ACGME have stringent guidelines to avoid any unethical influence by the sponsor. Medical Education staff can provide guidance regarding these endeavors. Disclosures and transparency by physicians participating in Cancer Conferences becomes crucial to the viability

of programs approved to grant CMEs, and diligence in this area is essential.

The decision by a Cancer Committee to make a Cancer Conference an "open" conference versus a "closed" conference can influence attendance and the acceptance of commercial support. (The issue of confidentiality is covered in a later section.)

Case Selection

Selecting cases for presentation requires evaluating and setting levels in three categories: required number of cases, discussion approach, and major sites within the facility:

1. Required number of cases: Establishing the expected number of cases to be presented each year requires an estimation of the total annual analytic caseload.
2. Required number of prospective cases discussed: This number would be 75% of at least 10% of the expected analytic caseload.
3. Major sites to be presented: Identify the five primary sites with the highest incidence count for the institution, and set requirements for case selection and presentation accordingly.

Multiple mechanisms are available to aid in selection of cases for presentation at cancer conference. Prospective case presentation requires the use of real-time identification resources to guarantee discussion of current patient management issues.

- Physician presenters will personally select the cases for discussion
- Evaluation of current in-house admissions with a diagnosis of cancer
- Evaluation of weekly pathology cases with a cancer-related diagnosis
- Cancer Registry involvement through disease index listings or other casefinding mechanisms

Other considerations for case selection include establishing the timeliness for notification of cases to be presented to the departments of pathology and diagnostic radiology. The registrar often serves as the intermediary for disseminating patient information on pending cases. When a case has been selected, all physicians who participated in the patient's care should be informed of the pending cancer conference and be encouraged to attend.

Confidentiality

Establishing cancer conference presentation formats should include defined rules for the use of protected health information (PHI) to avoid displaying PHI when possible. Safeguarding PHI includes diligent efforts in checking meeting rooms at the end of every cancer conference to ensure that all documents that contain PHI are removed. The electronic display of medical records might include the patient name or other information. In CoC-approved facilities, the Cancer Conference Coordinator can provide assistance in enforcing the Cancer Committee and facility rules for confidentiality. Registrars should consult their Cancer Committee and administrative personnel to evaluate the facility policy regarding confidentiality.

The rules regarding attendance at an *open* cancer conference should be established through Cancer Committee and administrative support such as the medical staff department or privacy officer. The requirement regarding signed confidentiality agreements by physician and nonphysician attendees should be established and documented for reference of registry staff. In addition, steps required in the event of a breach of confidentiality should be established.

Cancer Conference Documentation

For CoC-approved programs, documentation of cancer conference activity includes multiple items that can be prepared in a single report for review by cancer committee annually or more frequently. Items to include in annual Cancer Committee review are as follows:

- Meetings
  - Total number of meetings annually
  - Meeting format (multiple formats may occur)
- Primary sites discussed
  - List of primary sites discussed (compare sites presented with sites seen at the facility)
- Attendance
  - CoC and Cancer Committee required physician attendance by CoC and cancer committee direction
- Prospective or retrospective
  - List of the number of cases discussed prospectively
- Treatment planning
  - Documents the use of national guidelines in treatment planning
- AJCC/TNM
  - Documents the discussion of the AJCC/TNM elements, by clinical and pathologic categories

Software systems can easily provide a tool for tracking the documentation items. Examples of formats for use in cancer conference documentation are available in the CoC Standards, as well as through the CoC best practice repository via the CoC Web site.

Cancer Conference Discussions

The CoC *does not* require documentation of cancer conference discussions. If requests are made to the cancer registrars to document and retain cancer conference discussions, the request should be forwarded to the appropriate facility staff (i.e., Cancer Committee or Facility Privacy Officer). Extreme caution must be taken before agreeing to retain documentation of physician discussions during a cancer conference. Cancer registrars should familiarize themselves with the process of peer review within their respective state because the rules of discoverability vary. Cancer registrars should not assume that rules of discoverability cannot affect them, because the term "person most knowledgeable" describes the person having the most knowledge about a given subject, and this person can be called for deposition. The facility privacy officer should be involved in decisions regarding documentation of cancer conference discussions. In addition, physician participants in a cancer conference must be certain that all discussions will remain confidential. Any breach of this confidence poses the threat of limiting physician participation and serves as a possible liability.

Patient Management and National Guidelines

CoC Standard 4.6 (revised, 2009) requires the Cancer Committee to adopt national guidelines and monitor compliance to the guidelines within the facility. A large number of national guidelines are available for use; examples of national guidelines are provided on the CoC Web site. Inclusion of the adopted guidelines during presentation at a Cancer Conference is one way to document the use of national guidelines in treatment planning.

Summary

Cancer Conference provides an opportunity for physicians to hold multidisciplinary discussions to improve patient care. Advances in the treatment of cancer provide new and exciting topics for discussion during a cancer conference. Facilities that have conducted cancer conferences for many years should re-evaluate programs for adherence with CoC modifications and treatment advances, and may provide a new venue for discussions. The registrar continues to serve a pivotal role in the process of creating and carrying out effective cancer conference plans.

References

1. American College of Surgeons Commission on Cancer. *Manual for Cancer Programs* (p. 6). Cancer Clinical Program, I.C. Chicago: American College of Surgeons, 1966.

2. American Society of Clinical Oncology. "The Role of a Tumor Board in Cancer Treatment." ASCO Expert Corner. Available at: http://www.cancer.net. http://www.cancer.net/patient/All+About+Cancer/Cancer.Net+Features/Expert+Information+from+ASCO/ASCO+Expert+Corner%3A+The+Role+of+a+Tumor+Board+in+Cancer+Treatment. Accessed June 9, 2010.

3. American College of Suregons Commission on Cancer. *Cancer Program Standards* (Cancer Program Leadership, Standard 2.6, p. 27). Chicago: American College of Surgeons, 2009.

4. Bumm, R., Feith, M., Lordick, F., Herschbach, P., Siewert, J. "Impact of Multidisciplinary Tumor Boards on Diagnosis and Treatment of Esophageal Cancer." *European Surgery,* 2007;39(3):136–140.

5. Scholnik, A. P., Arnold, D. J., Gordon, D. C., Wiggins, J. D., Voorhees, E. G. "A New Mechanism for Physician Participation in a Tumor Board." *Progress in Clinical and Biological Research,* 1986;216:337–343.

6. American College of Surgeons Commission on Cancer. *Cancer Program Standards* (Cancer Program Leadership, Standard 2.7, p. 29). Chicago: American College of Surgeons, 2009.

Uses of Registry Data

Ann Griffin
Section Editor—Textbook

Jim Hofferkamp
Section Editor—Review Guide

chapter 22

Management Reports

Carol L. Kosary, MA
Linda Coyle, BS
Nicola Schussler, BS

The ultimate goal of every cancer registry is to enhance patient care and reduce the overall cancer burden by providing quality data to clinicians, researchers, legislators, administrators, and the public. The registry's overall success hinges on the success of two efforts: high-quality data management and effective reporting of cancer information to the broader healthcare community. The primary objective of this chapter is to provide cancer registrars with a framework for effective report writing. But first, it is necessary to define the types of information that a registrar may need to report.

- Physicians and hospital administrators compare cancer outcomes and survival rates against state, regional, and national data to evaluate treatment regimens and patterns of care provided to the hospital's patients.
- Hospital administrators use registry reports to justify or modify the allocation of resources for research, staffing, equipment, and physical facilities.
- Researchers and medical professionals request analyses to evaluate the efficacy of treatment modalities.
- The registry and organizations that fund the registry require management reports to evaluate the effectiveness of the registry in terms of completeness, accuracy, and timeliness.
- Central registries provide data and feedback to submitting facilities. This may include follow-up information on registered cases. It may also include feedback for the facility registrars showing results of computerized edits or changes made by registrars at the central registry.
- Registries publish periodic statistical reports to provide publicly accessible information for physicians, legislators, medical personnel, and the community. These are typically generated on an annual basis.

The registry must have clearly defined processes for responding to requests for data, statistics, and reports. A structured approach must be used to ensure that the response meets registry standards for quality and accuracy, and adheres to registry guidelines for the dissemination of data and statistics.

The obvious purpose of a report is to communicate information. This chapter describes steps to create reports that communicate an appropriate and effective message based on the registry's data. Figure 22-1 summarizes effective report-writing steps. This chapter includes discussions related to content, formatting, presentation, and distribution. Because these reports deal with cancer registry data, special consideration is given to quality control and confidentiality issues that must be considered in each step.

Identify the Audience

The question "Who is the intended audience?" must be investigated from several angles:

- **What is their level of knowledge?** This determines the level of detail, complexity, format, and use of medical terminology. Government officials and members of the public may not have the time to interpret or knowledge base to understand a highly detailed and technical report. For these groups, a direct format using plain language equivalents to medical terms may be appropriate. At times, it may be more important to be understood than to be precise. However, a report targeted to clinicians or cancer researchers may require detailed statistics and specific medical information to be persuasive.
- **Do they have the right to the requested data?** The release of the data may require written permission from registry management, an internal review board, hospital administration, or the registry's Health Insurance Portability and Accountability Act (HIPAA) privacy officer.
- **How will they use the data?** Will the data be included in a publication, presented at a conference, or included in an annual report? The person submitting the request may not be the true audience. Understanding the purpose of the request is necessary to ensure that the data are used appropriately and effectively.
- **What format would be most effective?** Would they be more likely to understand graphs, statistical tables, written text, or a combination of the three? Graphs may best show an administrator the current trends in patient care, whereas a researcher may prefer to review raw numbers in table form. If a researcher, do they require an extract of data to analyze in their own statistical software?
- **What method of distribution is appropriate?** By definition, reports designed for the general public

---

1. **Identify the audience.** What style of report will they understand? Do they understand medical terms and statistics?
2. **Define the purpose.** Write a clear and detailed objective statement.
3. **Identify the cases and data fields required.** Which patients, what years of diagnosis, which fields will answer the questions?
4. **Extract data and calculate statistics.**
5. **Choose the appropriate format for the audience and content.** Will you include tables, graphs, and/or narrative text?
6. **Edit and proof-read.** Verify statistics, data, and carefully proofread the text.
7. **Distribute, present, or publish the report.**

Figure 22-1. Overview of Report-Writing Steps

contain only nonconfidential analyses and, therefore, could be effectively distributed via the Internet. On the other hand, the electronic transmission of confidential reports requires that the data be encrypted and transmitted using secure methods. The transmission of confidential data must adhere to policies defined by the registry and all governing bodies. Local and federal governments have specific guidelines related to the encryption and transfer of confidential data.

Define the Purpose

The purpose of the report must be clearly understood and documented. Evaluate the request and determine the underlying need. What question or questions are you trying to answer? What information will be included? Complex questions may need to be addressed with multiple reports, rather than a single report that is too complicated to be understood.

To avoid misunderstandings and to ensure that the purpose is clearly understood, the registry should gather detailed information from the person submitting the request before developing the report. A standard request form should be used to help the requester organize their thoughts. Because the requester may not use terminology common to the registry, an iterative process should be used to ensure that an understanding has been achieved. This may involve rephrasing rather than repeating the request, avoiding industry buzzwords that the requester may only partially understand, and using visual aids such as a prototype of the report showing the layout and fields.

Identify the Data

Once the audience and purpose have been defined, the cohort of patients and data items to be used in the report must be determined by considering years of diagnosis, patient age, cancer site, record type, and other factors. If case selection is based on the value of certain data fields, such as cancer site or morphology, the codes for those fields should be clearly stated to remove ambiguity. Inclusion of the incorrect population may affect the results without being an obviously identifiable problem. People may believe that a mutual understanding of the terms has been achieved until they review detailed code lists.

The data items to be used include those used to limit the cohort, those that appear in the report, and those used to link various types of data together. It is important to understand which fields should be used to limit the data for the same reason that clear codes lists are important. Some limiters, like age at diagnosis, are fairly straightforward. However, there are many variants of stage, so limiting the cohort to stage II cancer can be defined many ways. The fields that are displayed on the report must help increase

the audience understanding, rather than being visual or mental clutter. Both the audience and the purpose affect this choice because some data that would be useless in a summary report would be of great interest in a detailed report designed to facilitate investigation. Both these data item decisions require knowledge of the data that have been collected, whether that is cancer data or management-related data about cancer collection in the registry.

The third set of data items needed, those that link the various types of data together, requires knowledge of the database. The requester and cancer experts frequently do not have this information. Also, depending on the setup in the registry and level of report desired, this issue may be more or less transparent to the person generating the report. If such linkages must be specified, it is important to understand how the data fits together so that all the data necessary can be correctly accessed.

Collection of Additional Data

As the earlier issues are being considered, it may become clear that the information desired is not typically collected by the registry. A request may have to be denied or rephrased if the data cannot be obtained for practical or legal reasons. However, it may also be possible to perform a study to collect the additional data. Studies are routinely done for both cancer research and registry operation purposes. Studies, like reports, need clearly defined goals and parameters. They have added complexity because one must decide what methods to use to collect the data and to ensure its reliability. Also, the data collected must be stored in such a way that enables access to the data, including the ability to link the study data to existing information in the registry when required.

Other considerations for special study include gathering the correct approvals and funding. Institutional review board (IRB) approval is necessary for studies involving cancer patients, whether or not direct contact is necessary. Obtaining this approval requires that the study be formally documented. Obviously the person or organization that made the initial request should be contacted first about any necessary funding. However, other sources of funding may also be available if the question is of interest to more than one group. This should be discussed with the requester because he or she may prefer to retain sole control of the requirements and data.

Data Extraction and Calculations

Some requests may be met with data listing or extracts. Other times, some type of statistics are required. Statistical methods should be carefully selected. Only statistics calculated using similar methods can be meaningfully compared. Chapter 24 describes statistical analysis in detail. Chapter 25 focuses on survival rates, which are frequently requested.

When constructing the logic for extracting the data, care should be taken that all the content specifications are being followed. For more complicated requests, it may be beneficial to start with a simpler version of the request that can be easily verified and then add complexity. This method can aid in the detection of flaws in the specifications or logic if an addition to the logic has an unexpected effect on the outcome. Unexpected results that cannot be explained by errors in logic should be investigated. These may be the result of a poorly designed question (the logic matches the request, but the request does not make sense), may indicate data quality issues in the database, or may accurately indicate an unexpected situation, such as a spike in cancer rates or decline in hospital reporting, that should be investigated in more detail.

Data Presentation

Accurate data that fulfill the request is useless if it is not presented appropriately. Reports also should be fully documented and capable of standing alone. Clear titles and explanatory footnotes should be included to ensure that the data in the report is not misunderstood. More complicated, related sets of reports may need an introduction or restatement of the request to provide context to the audience. Extracts should come with file descriptions including layout and field descriptions, as well as case counts or file size to help identify data corruption or the loss of data in transit.

Information one should incorporate includes, but is not limited to, a description of the included cohort, any specific exclusions, the period covered, the meaning of any codes displayed in the report, and a description of any simplifications made to improve the usefulness of the report, such as the collapse of data into a year range for earlier years. The source of the data and the number of events or cases being reported should be clearly evident. Text on the report should be easy to read, so avoid fancy fonts and stacked lettering. Contact information for the registry should also be included for all reports to be distributed to nonstaff members.

Complete, concise explanations of all terms used in the report should be included to ensure accurate interpretation of the data. It is better to underestimate the audience's understanding, as a misunderstanding could lead to an inappropriate response to the data presented.

The other part of data presentation is the actual structure chosen for the results of a report. Data may be presented as raw data in a file or a listing, tabulated, or represented graphically or in a figure. The structure selected should be one that increases the audience's ability to understand and use the information presented. Because tables and graphs are usually easier to understand and are more appealing, they should be used when possible, especially in reports to the public.

Tables

Tables present and summarize detail that would be cumbersome in narrative form. Exact values and comparisons among several variables are easier to interpret in tables.

Rows and columns in a table should be surrounded by as much white space as possible. Instead of using grid lines to divide cells, consider using white space. Shading or textured background can also be used for variety. If text is used within the table, keep it short. Numbers should be aligned on decimal points. Avoid leaving cells blank; instead enter a zero, a dash, or NA (not applicable). Subtotals are often useful to summarize categories of data within tables. They can be shown at the top or bottom of a column. Strive for an uncluttered look that leads the eye horizontally and vertically.

The simplest kind of table is a one-way classification showing only one variable. Tables can also have the form of two-, three- and four-way tables showing multiple variables. For example, a table might depict the distribution of breast cases by cell type, stage, menopausal status, and estrogen receptor status. Exceeding four variables usually results in tables that are difficult to interpret and should be avoided.

Graphs

Graphs or charts are a clear way to summarize detail, show relationships, illustrate trends, and make comparisons. Educators have long recognized that we learn about 10% from words we hear, 40% from the way they are said, and 50% from what we see. Because numbers are intangible, it can be hard to assimilate the meaning behind them. Graphs are attention grabbing and help to keep the audience interested in the data. They add meaning by condensing detailed information into easily absorbed pictures.

The kind of graph that should be used depends on the data being presented and the audience. For example, technical audiences are more experienced at interpreting complex charts. In addition to the documentation concerns mentioned, attention must be paid to the labeling of graphs. The x-axis (horizontal) of a graph should be placed horizontally and usually describes categories. y-Axis (vertical) labels should also be placed horizontally and usually show amount or frequency. Legends or keys should explain the symbols or colors used.

Line graphs are most effective for showing trends and change over time (see Figure 22-2). Most show an increment of time along the x-axis and the amount, frequency, or percentage on the y-axis. If more than one line is shown, use symbols to differentiate the lines. Generally, no more than four lines should be depicted on a graph.

Bar charts are most effective when comparing size or amount of a variable (see Figure 22-3). They can show

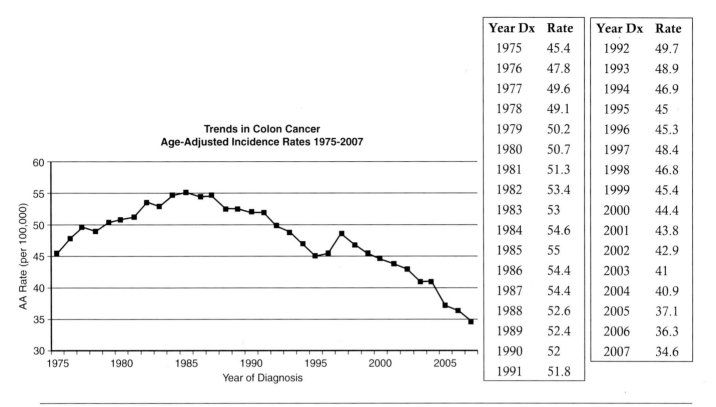

Year Dx	Rate	Year Dx	Rate
1975	45.4	1992	49.7
1976	47.8	1993	48.9
1977	49.6	1994	46.9
1978	49.1	1995	45
1979	50.2	1996	45.3
1980	50.7	1997	48.4
1981	51.3	1998	46.8
1982	53.4	1999	45.4
1983	53	2000	44.4
1984	54.6	2001	43.8
1985	55	2002	42.9
1986	54.4	2003	41
1987	54.4	2004	40.9
1988	52.6	2005	37.1
1989	52.4	2006	36.3
1990	52	2007	34.6
1991	51.8		

Figure 22-2. Sample Line Graph

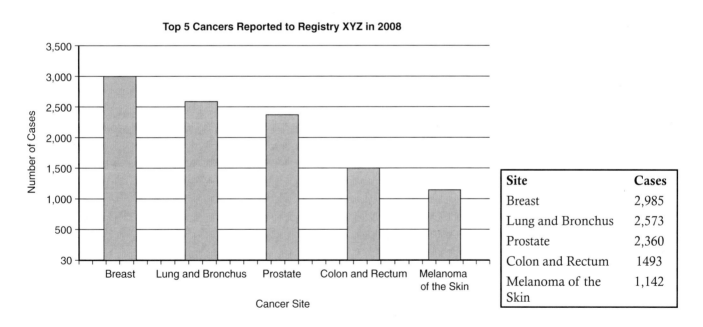

Site	Cases
Breast	2,985
Lung and Bronchus	2,573
Prostate	2,360
Colon and Rectum	1493
Melanoma of the Skin	1,142

Figure 22-3. Sample Bar Chart

differences in the magnitude of one item at various points in time. They are not as effective in showing trends over time. Bars can be filled or shaded with a pattern or color to show differences among the categories. The width of the bars should be uniform within the chart. Bars or groups of bars should be separated by space. Adjacent bars should depict related or comparable data groups. Avoid three-dimensional representations because they lead to misperceptions of the magnitude of the y-axis. Bars can be vertical or horizontal.

There are many kinds of bar charts. *Stacked columns* show parts of a whole where the length of the column is the sum of the totals in the segment. *100% columns* are all the same length, with the information in each column being

Facility	Count
Memorial Hospital	6712
General Hospital	3274
Community Hospital	2435
City Hospital	2323
Mercy Hospital	2846
Other	3124

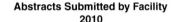

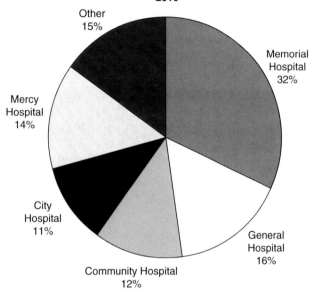

Figure 22-4. Sample Pie Chart

show as a percentage of the whole. *Paired bar charts* have two *y*-axes, with the 0 point in the center. These are often used to show simultaneous distributions, for example, cancer site for male and female patients. *Grouped columns* show related data sets that can be compared with the group. The number of columns in each group should be limited to four.

Histograms are used to show frequency distributions in bar form. They do not have space between the bars and are always vertically oriented. They are used for continuous variables, like age, and can show counts or percentages. Histograms are useful when it is more important to show the distribution of a variable rather than absolute numbers. *Frequency polygons* are used in similar situations but provide a different format. A line connects the midpoint of the top of each bar. This allows for several histograms to be shown on the same chart.

Pie charts provide a clear method of showing parts of a whole or percentages (see Figure 22-4). Try to limit the pie chart to no more than six slices with the smallest slice comprising no less than 2% of the whole. Slices can be "exploded" or pulled out to emphasize one component.

Pictorial charts make use of symbols that are strongly associated with the message of the chart. For example, us-

ing symbols of beds of various quantities effective shows the length of stay required by several types of surgery. Select symbols that are simple and easy to identify. Amount or volume is conveyed by the number of symbols.

Maps are often used in annual reports to visually represent patterns in the geographic area that is the focus of the report. Shaded maps are relatively easy to create. The differences in shading indicate varying concentrations of cases or events. The data displayed should be in terms of rates rather than counts, to show the relation between occurrences and population density. The map should be simple and easy to understand.

Color

Color can enhance data presentations and command the viewer's attention but should be used with care. Printed colors do not always appear the same way as colors on computer monitors. Sufficiently distinct colors should be selected and tested in both states to avoid this problem. No more than six or seven colors should be used in the same graph. The combination of colors, or palette, should be consistent over a series of related graphs. Remember the goal is to draw attention to the message, not to the colors, so some color combinations may not be suitable. Also, because many registries may be required to be compliant with Section 508, an alternate, complementary aid should be selected, such as symbols on the lines of a graph.

Data Comparison

It is important to understand that comparison data add credibility to a report. One of the long-standing requirements for cancer program approval by the Commission on Cancer is a review of registry data that includes the comparison of hospital data with regional, state, or national aggregate data. There are many potential sources of comparison data (pertinent links can be found on the NCRA Web site: www.ncra-usa.org). Each source contains a thorough description of the source of data, data collection guidelines, and statistical methods used. Footnotes and aids to interpreting the data enable registrars to group and analyze data in a way that allows valid comparisons. Possible sources include:

- State and regional registry publications of aggregate data
- *Cancer Facts and Figures,* published by the American Cancer Society
- The National Cancer Data Base, aggregated by the Commission on Cancer in conjunction with the American Cancer Society
- *Manual for Staging of Cancer,* published by the American Joint Committee on Cancer
- The MEDLINE database is available through the National Library of Medicine (www.nlm.nih.gov).

- Physician Data Query (PDQ), a database available through the National Cancer Institute (www.nci.nih.gov)
- *Cancer Incidence in North America* (CiNA+), published by the North American Association of Central Cancer Registries (www.naaccr.org)
- *Cancer Statistics Review,* published by the Surveillance, Epidemiology, and End Results (SEER) Program of the National Cancer Institute (more information about SEER can be obtained online at: http://seer.cancer.gov)

One should consider carefully whether comparative data are available for the information within the report. If not, can the report be modified so the data are more analogous to one of the available sources? Issues related to the validity of the comparison include:

- Similarity of population, including cohort definition and regional differences among populations
- Sufficient sample size to ensure accurate representation
- Completeness of and sources of casefinding
- Deduplication methods applied to the population data
- Reference date and data availability by year
- Currency of data with respect to incidence reporting, follow-up, and cause of death information
- Methods of data collection, coding, and statistical analysis used; changes to these over time
- Percentage of imprecise codes such as unknown, none, blank, not reported, and not otherwise specified

Many questions should be considered beyond these, of course. Variations of term definitions, how ambiguous data are handled, whether borderline cancers are excluded, rules for defining multiple primaries, and other policies related to determining a distinct incidence of cancer, counts for rare cancers, and site-specific questions related to grouping and inclusion are but a few.

Written Components

Some requests require more than just a table, graph, or set of numbers. For example, central registries generate documents such as state cancer profiles, which are a series of reports with narrative text describing the cohorts, statistic presented, and conclusions about those statistics. These may also be referred to as a report (as is the Cancer Report to the Nation). There are considerations for such a document, of any size, over and above those discussed in this chapter for individual reports.

An introduction to the data being presented is necessary to put the information that follows in context. This does not have to be lengthy but should be appropriate to the overall size of the document. The main part of the document may include a discussion of methods and results, comparisons with similar documents or past years, and conclusions supported by the data. There should be a summary to focus the audience on the main points of the document. One may also need a cover, title page, abstract, acknowledgements section, table of contents, list of figures and tables, appendices, reference section, and glossary, depending on the length, nature, and complexity of the document.

Similar to the steps for writing a report, one must determine the audience and purpose of the document. If a specific result is desired as an outcome of the document, it should be stated. One must also determine what data reports (statistics, graphs, tables, etc.) are needed to support the overall document.

Care must be taken if interpretations of the data are provided or conclusions about the data are presented. Registry procedures that could affect the data, such as reportability policies or data completeness, must be made clear as part of the discussion. Data analyses covering long periods must take into account changes in coding, staging rules, and treatment patterns. Demographic trends in the population that would affect the analyses must also be considered. For example, the proportion of elderly patients would affect the number of comorbid conditions. Other cultural or socioeconomic characteristics of the population that would impact the results should also be discussed.

Good writing practices should be applied. Larger documents should be outlined to ensure coverage of the desired topics and to aid in maintaining focus on those topics. Multiple drafts of most documents are necessary, and at least one draft should be reviewed by others to obtain comments about the clarity and content of the document. A clear message requires concise wording. Fancy words and overly verbose sentences can obscure the desired message or lose the interest of the audience.

Oral Presentations

Sometimes an oral presentation of the data is the more effective or desired vehicle. In these cases, intensive preparation is necessary to ensure a clear message and speaker confidence. Once again, the audience and purpose will drive the style of presentation. Certainly some audiences, such as administrators and physicians, have strict time constraints and appreciate clear and pointed presentations. Other situations, such as a presentation at a professional conference, may lend themselves to more detailed presentations.

As with writing, an outline helps to ensure the coverage of desired topics. This outline can be used as a basis for developing visual aids, such as slides or handouts. For these aids to be effective, they must be clear, concise, and easy to read. Slides especially should be brief, with more detailed information being spoken or provided in handouts.

Remembering that people only remember a fraction of what they hear, one should state the main points multiple times. The introduction to the presentation should clearly state the purpose and major points. The body of the address must be concise and relevant. A summation of the talk should reiterate the main points and desired results.

That is, tell them what you are going to say, say it clearly, and tell them what you have just said.

For presentations of any length, one must be aware of the audience's attention levels. Monotone speaking or simply reading from a script will quickly lose their interest. A variety of tone and rhythm will help keep them engaged. Intensive preparation will provide the speaker with a secure knowledge of the topic and will allow them to speak more naturally. Also, the speaker's interest in and enthusiasm for a subject communicates to the audience, so one should strive to keep the presentation fresh. In short, if the speaker is excited and can get the crowd united, then the goal can be obtained and the policy be changed. But if the speaker is a drone and speaks in monotone, the crowd will go to sleep and the old policy will keep.

Quality Control

All reports should undergo a quality-control review before being released. Quality control is a multifaceted process. A registry should develop guidelines or protocols for the review process. Different procedures should be defined for different styles of reports. A single-page frequency requires much less effort than a document detailing cancer rates in the state or rising treatment costs at a hospital.

The most basic quality control is, of course, maintaining the quality of the underlying data, which is discussed in Chapter 18. If the underlying data are of poor quality or are incomplete, no report generated from it can be satisfactory. The data within the report must also be reviewed to verify the accuracy of the results. Logic and statistical methods should be reviewed to ensure that appropriate selections were made and were correctly applied.

The report should also be reviewed for clarity. This includes the ease of reading tables and graphs, as well as any supporting or surrounding text. Terms should be clearly defined, and tables and graphs should be clearly labeled. The overall look of tables and graphs should be consistent with respect to fonts, symbols, and colors. Any codes used within the report or document should be defined. Most importantly, one should verify that the initial request has been satisfied and that the report will be comprehensible to the desired audience. Final results and any recommendations within document and reports should be stated clearly.

Another important consideration is to guarantee the protection of confidential data. If the report has confidential data, such as an extract or case listing, it must be treated with care. It may be wise to include a warning to the requester about their responsibility to protect the data. If the report is not supposed to have confidential data, then it should be reviewed to determine whether any counts are low enough to allow identification of an individual. Any such data point must be masked. For example, all cells with a count less than 5 may be marked with an asterisk, instead of the actual count. Be sure to clearly indicate what has been done if this is necessary. This is another area where the registry should develop specific policies.

Report Distribution

Once completed and having undergone a quality-control review, the report is ready for distribution. There are many methods of disseminating information, and multiple methods may be appropriate. Reports may be printed, such as a cancer facts sheet designed for distribution at conferences, or larger documents intended for publication. However, the ever-increasing belief that everything can be found on the Web dictates that most publications should be available in electronic form as well.

Reports may be distributed on the Internet via public or protected Web sites. Public Web sites allow access by anyone and should not be used for sensitive data. There are many levels of protected Web sites, and one should be familiar with the safeguards in place on a site before posting any data. Some Web sites merely restrict access by requiring a formal request for access or a set list of users. Other sites are fully encrypted and have security protocols in place. The safeguards on the chosen Web site must be appropriate to the sensitivity of the data within the report.

Reports may be distributed to the requester via e-mail or other electronic transfer methods if the report was designed as a response to a specific request. Remember to verify the e-mail address is correct before sending the report. One should also verify the report was received by the intended recipient.

If the report or extract includes sensitive data such as identifiers, scrupulous attention must be given to the protection of the data. This includes using high-level encryption protocols, ensuring secure transfers of data, sending passwords separately from the file itself, and similar security conscious steps. The registry, as the custodian of sensitive data, is responsible for its security. Policies should be clearly defined for data transfers of this kind. Also, if the recipient has responsibilities, these should be clearly detailed, and before the transfer of the report or extract, a signed statement of understanding and agreement should be obtained and should be kept on file.

Another method of report dissemination is to make an executable report available to the audience. If a registry manager needs to monitor the case completeness on a monthly basis, integrating an executable report into the registry data management system would allow the manager to generate the report as often and exactly when it is needed. This method can also be used to provide simple statistics on a Web site. One example of this is the Fast Stats Web tool maintained by the SEER Program (available online at: http://seer.cancer.gov/faststats). With this tool, the public can quickly generate simple statistics by site, race, sex, and age. This provides easy access to some commonly desired data without the delay of processing a formal request.

Types of Reports

Many different kinds of reports are routinely requested in a cancer registry. Registry managers have to monitor quality, completeness, and timeliness of the data, a task that is often supported by reports. Examples of these reports include:

- Frequencies of the cases received from the various data sources over times
- Frequencies of edit errors in the data
- Frequencies of missing or unknown values by field
- Timeliness of data sources (the amount of time it takes for the data to get to the registry).
- Timeliness of internal case management (the amount of time it takes to process the data once it arrives)
- Workload statistics related to outstanding tasks, including abstracts to be gathered, records to be consolidated, and edits to be resolved
- Workload statistics related to what tasks have been done in a given period by staff

Registries are frequently dependant on outside sources for data collection, quality, and completeness. Physicians answer questions about treatment provided to the patient, clarify the staging of a cancer, and provide other information. Registries exchange information about new primaries and patient survival for patients tracked in multiple registries, such as hospital, regional, and state registries. To maintain good relationships with those who provide such data, a registry must supply these sources with reports that provide a service. For example, a central registry may provide a hospital registry with better dates of last contact for all the patients they jointly track. A hospital registry may provide physicians with statistics to help justify a request for equipment or additional staff.

Registries receive requests for information from the public or government officials. These requests are frequently for statistics related to incidence, survival, or expenditure. Researchers request both statistics and raw data from the registries. These requests are the primary reason to collect cancer data. A registry must meet these requests in a timely manner with accurate data. The registry should also regularly produce reports or documents detailing cancer statistics and trends for public consumption. The only logical justification for the resources needed to support a cancer registry is that some benefit is received. The dissemination of information in these types of reports is the most important benefit the registries can provide.

Accessibility

Many registries may be required to comply with Section 508 of the Rehabilitation Act, which says that electronic information created with federal funding must be accessible to persons with disabilities. This applies to reports distributed in any electronic format, including Web pages, Adobe PDFs, spreadsheets, and other formats.

People with disabilities rely on assistive technology to access electronic information. Screen reading software and magnification software provide access to individuals with vision impairments. Individuals with mobility issues rely on assistive hardware such as touch screens, head pointers, and other devices.

To be compliant, reports must be in a format that can be interpreted by assistive software and accessible to individuals who are using assistive hardware. For example, every non-text element must also be conveyed in text so that a screen reader can convey the information. Row and column headers must be used in tables so that a screen reader can identify each cell to the user, and markup codes may be required if the table is complex.

In general, information that might be inaccessible to some users must be conveyed in an alternate manner. This rule applies to tables, graphs, and written material. It is important for report writers to become familiar with the best practices for developing accessible documents, and to get in the habit of using those practices when creating or revising a report. Nearly all modern graphing, report generating, and word processing software provide mechanisms for creating accessible documents. Resources for understanding and implementing Section 508 are available on the web at section508.gov.

Summary

The cancer registry is a rich resource of information with two primary responsibilities: to ensure the completeness and quality of data collection, and to guarantee that the data are used productively. To fulfill these responsibilities, the registry must develop effective methods to disseminate information based on the collected data. The registry must have clear procedures in place for report generation so they can produce timely, accurate, and clear reports. Converting data into useful information and disseminating it through effective reports is the principal reason for the existence of cancer registries.

chapter 23

Reporting to the Central Registry and the National Cancer Data Base

Sharon Labbate, CTR
Nancy Etzold, CTR

Reporting to the Central Registry

Central registries, also known as state cancer registries, are population-based cancer incidence reporting systems that collect, analyze, and disseminate information on all new cases of cancer. A statewide registry is the foundation for cancer prevention and control. This central repository of information is a valuable and essential tool for identifying populations at high risk for cancer, monitoring of cancer incidence trends and mortality, facilitating studies related to cancer prevention, evaluating cancer control initiatives, planning health care delivery systems, and developing educational awareness programs. It is dependent on complete, timely, and accurate reporting[1].

Confidentiality

Data obtained by central registries are for the confidential use of the individual state's Department of State Health Services, including persons, public or private entities that are necessary to carry out the public health interests of state legislature. The data are privileged and may not be divulged or made public in a manner that discloses individual identity of any patient. All reporting entities that comply with state legislature are immune from liability of furnishing the required information[1].

Disclosure

All data reported to central registries are available for use in aggregate form for analysis by the registry staff, cancer researchers, and the public. Reports of the incidence of cancer for the state can be generated. Public access to aggregate data is available through published reports or through the state registry, if in accordance with its data release policies and procedures[1].

The central registry may exchange patient specific data with the reporting facility, any other cancer-control agency, clinical facility, and pathology laboratories, and physician's offices for the purpose of obtaining information necessary to complete the abstract or follow-up information, provided that these agencies and facilities comply with the state registry's confidentiality policies. However, no facility-specific patient information can be released unless authorized under law[1].

Casefinding

Casefinding is a system for identifying all eligible cases. Facility sources used to identify cases include disease indices, pathology and laboratory reports, patient logs, and similar resources. Cooperation and a good working relationship between reporting personnel and other departments are essential for accurate case ascertainment. The reporter is responsible for identifying all casefinding sources under their

facility licensure and arranging access to these sources, for example, rural health clinics and surgery centers across town or off-campus[1].

Coding Instructions

Each state has created rules and guidelines to assure the consistent collection and coding of relevant cancer information. These guidelines and standards for cancer reporting have been established by the National Program of Cancer Registries (NPCR); Centers for Disease Control and Prevention (CDC); North American Association of Central Cancer Registries (NAACCR); Surveillance, Epidemiology, and End Results (SEER) Program of the National Cancer Institute (NCI); and the American College of Surgeons (ACoS[1]).

Editing Newly Abstracted Cases

The NAACCR standard edits are crucial to central registry reporting. Some central registries also require an additional state metafile to process cases. Hospital cancer registries that routinely perform standard NAACCR metafile edit checks spend less time reviewing cases before submission. It has become common practice for central registries to only accept cases that have passed edits[1].

Data Submission

As each central registry or state cancer registry determines the required process for submitting data, it is highly recommended to become familiarized with the central registry reporting policy and procedure manual before case submission. Typically, a designated person in the hospital cancer registry is assigned by the central registry to submit cases to the state. Contact the central registry pertinent to the state for any questions.

Preparation of the Central Registry File

The following steps provide a general overview to prepare a file to be submitted to the Central Cancer Registry. These steps may vary by facility and registry software processes.

1. Contact the cancer registry software provider for updates and assistance, if necessary, to enable submission of data to the central registry.
2. Good communication between the central registry and the hospital cancer registry is beneficial.
3. Verify that the most current edit metafile is activated in the cancer registry software.
4. Complete recording of all physician staging, treatment information, and other data pertinent to the cases being submitted.
5. Identify the population of cases in the hospital cancer registry database that are ready to be submitted to the central registry.

6. Once the population of cases is selected, ensure the standard NAACCR metafile, as well as any other additional state metafile that has been performed on the population.

7. Make adjustments to cases as needed, and rerun the selected population and metafiles until no edits remain.

8. Make sure cases are in the correct record layout accepted by the central registry (as specified by NAACCR or state central registry) before submission.

9. Depending on the type of cancer registry software, the date of submission and transmit code may be noted to the cases. Refer to the cancer registry software provider for details.

10. A file will be created and saved in the designated hard drive.

11. As most central registries provide online submission of data, the file created can be uploaded through the central registries Web portal. Please refer to central registry manual and/or contact central registry representative for details.

12. It is recommended to document the file submission to the central registry, including the number of new cases, corrections, follow-up, and deletion records, date, and file name.

Reporting to the National Cancer Data Base

The ACoS and the American Cancer Society established the National Cancer Data Base (NCDB) in 1989 to serve as a comprehensive clinical surveillance resource for cancer care in the United States. The two organizations jointly fund NCDB activities.

The NCDB helps to identify disparities in care at the local and national levels, further demonstrating that the NCDB influences patient care in 50 states including Guam and Puerto Rico, and impacts Americans of all regions and subpopulations.

The NCDB is a nationwide, facility-based oncology data set that currently captures approximately 70% of all newly diagnosed cancer cases in the United States annually and contains almost 26 million records from hospital cancer registries. Data on all types of cancer are tracked and analyzed. Data collected include patient demographics, tumor characteristics, extent of disease, and first course of treatment administered, disease recurrence, and survival outcomes[2].

Before initial survey, new programs are required to submit data to the NCDB for the most recent abstracting year completed. Data are submitted and errors/rejected records corrected prior to scheduling the initial survey. National standardized data item and coding definitions are specified in the CoC's *Facility Oncology Registry Data Standards (FORDS),* and national data transmission format specifications are specified by the NAACCR[3].

Data confidentiality is of prime importance. The NCDB has proactively worked to continually ensure and maintain compliance with the Health Insurance Portability and Accountability Act (HIPAA) of 1996 privacy regulations established by the federal government in 2003. Confidential patient and physician information are not collected[2].

Commission on Cancer Data Submission Requirements

Standard 3.6: Complete data for all analytic cases are submitted to the NCDB in accordance with the annual Call for Data[4].

All CoC-accredited cancer programs must fulfill this standard. Data submissions to the NCDB must be performed utilizing the CoC's secure online data submission application. Submission history is confirmed by the CoC and displayed in the Survey Application Record (SAR[4]).

Standard 3.7: Annually, cases submitted to the NCDB that were diagnosed in 2003 or more recently meet the established quality criteria and resubmission deadline specified by the annual Call for Data.

As part of its annual Call for Data, the NCDB will document the conditions that will cause the cases submitted to the NCDB to be rejected. Rejected cases do not meet specified data quality criteria.

Standardized, nationally accepted data edits are applied to all analytic cases submitted. The reporting registry is notified of the problematic cases through an edit report. The reporting registry must correct outstanding quality errors and resolve errors resulting in rejected records. Problematic cases diagnosed on 2003 or more recently are corrected and resubmitted by the deadline specified in the Call for Data. Resubmission history is confirmed by the CoC and displayed in the SAR[4] (see Figure 23-1).

The cancer committee monitors the resolution and resubmission of problematic cases (Standard 2.10).

Case Eligibility

Patients must have been initially diagnosed and/or received part of their first course of therapy at the reporting hospital *(analytic cases).* Cases to be submitted must meet the definition of Class of Case 00 through 22. All other Classes of Case will be rejected[5].

Editing Newly Abstracted Cases

The NAACCR standard edits form the backbone of the NCDB submission metafile and are recommended for use when new cases are abstracted (see Figure 23-2). Registrars should not have to spend large amounts of time cleaning data before submission. The prudent registrar will make a practice of reviewing data regularly (as individual cases are abstracted, daily, or weekly) using the standard NAACCR metafiles designed for hospital use[1].

Submisison Date	File Name	Submission Year	Records Submitted	Quality Accepted Records	Records with Data Quality Problems	Records Rejected
10/09/2008	SDMCACOS.DAT	2007	652	652	0	0
10/22/2007	06ACOS.DAT	2006	794	794	0	0
10/13/2008	SDMC2ACOS.DAT	2005	1	0	1	0
11/14/2006	2005ACOS.DAT	2005	1056	1056	0	0
11/11/2005	ACOS.DAT	2004	835	835	0	0
10/13/2008	SDMC2ACOS.DAT	2003	21	21	0	0
10/22/2007	2001ACOS.DAT	2003	1	1	0	0
12/02/2004	ACOS03.DAT	2003	639	639	0	0
10/13/2008	SDMC2ACOS.DAT	2002	654	654	0	0
10/22/2007	2001ACOS.DAT	2002	25	0	25	0
01/09/2004	02ACOS.DAT	2002	692	692	0	0
10/22/2007	2001ACOS.DAT	2001	589	0	586	3

Figure 23-1. Example of NCDB Data Submission History. From Commission on Cancer Web site. Copyright © 2010 by Commission on Cancer. Reprinted by permission.

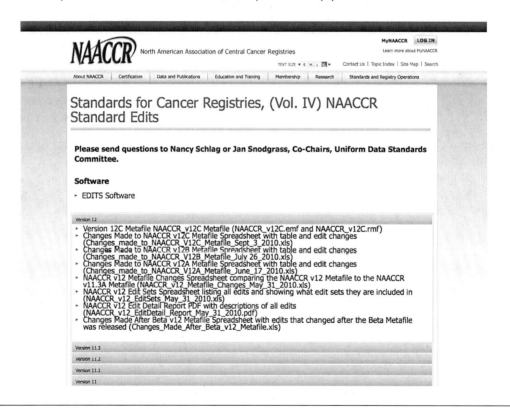

Figure 23-2. Standard Data Metafiles. From North American Association of Central Cancer Registries Web site. Copyright © 2010 by NAACCR. Reprinted by permission[3].

Instructions for downloading, installing, and running the GenEdits with the current NCDB Metafile can be found online at: http://www.facs.org/cancer/ncdb/datasubmission.html. Once downloaded and unzipped, the NAACCR's standard metafiles and configuration files will need to be updated only two to three times a year when revisions are posted[6]. This practice will assure the cleanest possible data for submission to the state and to the NCDB. Only a few newly written or modified edits may require attention at submission time, and only if the original data entry did not match the coding rules being checked by them[1].

Registry Plus Online Help: Integrated Edit Help and Easy-Click Cancer Manuals

The free Registry Plus Online Help application describes all standard edits with links to the item definitions they use and explanations for interpreting them. It has full copies of the *FORDS,* Collaborative Staging, Multiple Primary and Histology Coding manuals, as well as the NAACCR Data Dictionary, the SEER Coding Manual, and the introduction and histology sections of ICD-O-3. To install, Registry Plus Online Help is available at online at: http://www.cdc.gov/cancer/npcr[7].

Clinical Checks

Cancer registry data edits have traditionally focused on the assessment of valid codes and logical consistency of related items within reported case records. As part of its continuing effort to improve data quality, the CoC launched an initiative to extend the application of data edits to identify case records where reported treatment modalities are inconsistent with commonly recognized standards of care[8].

In this initial set of clinical checks, breast and colorectal cancer cases with specific tumor characteristics are identified, and the reported prognostic and treatment items for these cases evaluated. If the reported treatment does not appear to be consistent with widely recognized standards of care, the case record is flagged with a warning and included in the supplementary clinical report.

Breast or colorectal cancers reported to the NCDB that fail to contain known critical prognostic characteristics such as tumor size, hormone receptor (estrogen [ER] and progesterone receptors [PR]) status, and clinical and pathologic staging information are also flagged for review. These elements are critical to CoC-accredited hospitals in their assessment and evaluation of care provided to their patients.

The warnings reported as part of these clinical checks do not affect a cancer program's compliance with Standard 3.7. The clinical reports are provided as information by which CoC-Accredited cancer programs can assess the completeness of registry data for particular breast and colorectal cancer patients. Programs are encouraged to review these reports and resubmit case records that are updated or revised as a consequence of the assessment prompted by these reports.

What is evaluated by the clinical checks? Specifically, this set of clinical checks provides a case-by-case review of breast and colorectal cancer cases reported to the NCDB to identify cases that either fail to provide complete or sufficient information describing the tumor, or would appear to have incomplete or inaccurate treatment information reported in conjunction with a particular set of tumor characteristics. The three breast and three colorectal patient cohorts evaluated by this set of clinical checks are as follows:

- Patients undergoing breast-conserving surgery and who are younger than 70 should be considered for or receive radiation therapy.
- Patients with Stage I (tumor size > 1 cm and N0) and Stage II/III (any tumor size and N^+) with ER^- and PR^- breast tumors should be considered for or receive combination chemotherapy.
- Patients with Stage I (tumor size > 1 cm and N0) and Stage II/III (any tumor size and N^+), ER^+, or PR^+ breast tumors should be considered for or receive hormonal therapy (tamoxifen or a third-generation aromatase inhibitor).
- Patients who undergo surgical resection for primary tumors of the colon should have at least 12 regional lymph nodes pathologically examined.
- Patients who undergo surgical resection for Stage III (lymph node positive) colon cancer should be considered for or receive adjuvant chemotherapy.
- Patients with Stage II or III (T3/T4 and N0, or any T and N1) rectal cancer should be considered for or receive either preoperative or postoperative radiation therapy.

Notably, although the clinical checks on these six cohorts associate specific types of patient and tumor characteristics with particular treatment modalities, it is possible that some patients were provided appropriate and individualized care for their conditions that may not be consistent with these generalized standards of care. These clinical checks are designed with the intention of helping CoC-accredited cancer programs improve patient care by identifying cases that appear to have incomplete or inconsistent data.

Clinical Checks

- Prognostic and Staging Information Coding (Clin)
- Radiation with Breast-Conserving Surgery (Clin)
- Radiation with Rectal Cancer Surgery (Clin)
- Surgically Treated Nonmetastatic Colon Cancer (Clin)
- Systemic Treatment with Breast Surgery (Clin)[8]

Preparation of the National Cancer Data Base Submission File

1. Contact the cancer registry software provider for updates and assistance, if necessary, to enable submission of data to the NCDB.
2. Complete recording of all physician staging, delayed treatment, follow-up information, and other data pertinent to the cases being submitted.

3. Review the submission information online at: http://www.facs.org/cancer/ncdb/registrars.html. The document *Case Submission File Specifications and Format* describes the cases and items that must be submitted this year.

4. Run frequency counts of the facility's FIN, Archive FIN, NPI FIN, and NPI Archive FIN to make sure there are no invalid numbers. Edits cannot identify numbers that do not apply to accredited programs.

5. Run the data file(s) through the current NCDB Submission Metafile to be sure the cases are clean. Information for installing and running the GenEDITS Plus program can be found online at: http://www.facs.org/cancer/ncdb/edits.html

6. Check each file to make sure it contains the appropriate records to submit.

7. Make a note of the name of the submission file created. Make certain that it does not have an extension of .exe, .cmd, .dll, .sys, .bat, .src, .vbs, and .scr.

8. Submission files may be zipped (.zip) to reduce the time required to transmit the file to the NCDB. Compressed files will be recognized and managed appropriately on receipt.

Before National Cancer Data Base Submission

It is important to review the following information to ensure completeness of the National Cancer Data Base file submission.

- Have your CoC Datalinks User ID and Password available. If the username and password is not working, use the "hint" function on the Datalinks log-in page or e-mail: CoCDatalinks@facs.org.
- Note the location, drive, folder, and name of the submission file prepared for transmission to the NCDB.
- Instructions for registries making their own NCDB submissions or resubmissions, as well as instructions for registries allowing software providers to submit on their behalf are available online at: http://www.facs.org/cancer/ncdb/submit.pdf[9]

Summary

The cancer registry and the cancer registrar are the foundation of how data are provided to the central registry and to the NCDB. It is only through data submitted to the central registry and to NCDB that cancer data can be analyzed and outcomes established and assessed. A key element to the process of submitting data to the central registry and to the NCDB is to ensure data has been routinely verified through standard NAACCR metafiles, NCDB edits, and additional state metafiles on each abstract. This will provide greater efficiency and timely submission of abstracts to each entity. Another important element is to keep abreast of changes that occur with reporting functions, coding, and upgrades. Communication is an essential means to have the most current information available regarding changes.

References

1. Etzold, Nancy. May 2009. "Chapter 11: Reporting to the State Registry and the NCDB (National Cancer Data Base)." In *Guidebook on Informatics,* ed. Herman Menck, Wendy Scharber, Annette Hurlbut, and Robinson, Lisa, 85-94. Alexandria, VA: National Cancer Registrars Association.

2. Commission on Cancer, National Cancer Data Base. American College of Surgeons, Commission on Cancer. http://www.facs.org/cancer/ncdb/index.html (accessed December 22, 2010)

3. Standards and Registry Operations. North American Association of Central Cancer Registries. http://www.naaccr.org/StandardsandRegistryOperations/VolumeIV.aspx (accessed December 22, 2010)

4. Commission on Cancer, Cancer Program Standards Revised 2009. American College of Surgeons, Commission on Cancer. http://www.facs.org/cancer/coc/cocprogramstandards.pdf (accessed October 21, 2010).

5. Commission on Cancer, National Cancer Data Base Submission FAQ. American College of Surgeons, Commission on Cancer. http://www.facs.org/cancer/ncdb/callfordatafaq.pdf (accessed December 22, 2010)

6. Data Submission Instructions. Original and Resubmissions Beginning September 1, 2009. American College of Surgeons, Commission on Cancer. http://www.facs.org/cancer/ncdb/datasubmission.html (accessed October 21, 2010).

7. National Program of Cancer Registries. Centers for Disease Control and Prevention. http://www.cdc.gov/cancer/npcr (accessed October 21, 2010).

8. Commission on Cancer, National Cancer Data Base Quality Tools for Cancer Programs. American College of Surgeons, Commission on Cancer. http://www.facs.org/cancer/ncdb/qualitytools.html#cp3r (accessed October 21, 2010).

9. Data Submission Instructions. Original and Resubmissions Beginning January 1, 2011. American College of Surgeons, Commission on Cancer. http://www.facs.org/cancer/ncdb/submit.pdf (accessed December 22, 2010).

chapter 24

Statistics and Epidemiology

Wendy J. Langeberg, PhD, MPH

Statistics

Basic Concepts

Statistics are used to describe the characteristics of a *sample* of a population to infer the characteristics of the *population* from which the sample was drawn. For example, to describe the median age of diagnosis of breast cancer among women in the United States, one could gather information on *all* women diagnosed with breast cancer in the United States, but this would be costly, time consuming, and practically impossible. Instead, if a sample of women across the United States is chosen—a sample representative of the larger population—then the median age of diagnosis for this sample will reasonably represent the median age of diagnosis for the U.S. female population as a whole. Whereas statistics describe a population, statistical tests evaluate whether the characteristics of two populations differ. For example, statistical tests can help us determine whether the median age of diagnosis of breast cancer among U.S. women is different than among women in, for example, the United Kingdom.

Types of Data

Characteristics of a population can be described in two main ways: categorically or continuously. For example, to describe the age of a population, one might present the proportion of the population who is younger than 55 years old, 56 to 65 years old, and 66 years old or older. Here age is a categorical characteristic (or variable). Race, sex, and stage of disease are other examples of categorical variables. Age could also be described as a continuous variable, for example, by the average age or the range of ages in the population (e.g., the maximum and minimum values). Blood pressure, height, and tumor size are other examples of continuous variables.

Categorical variables can be further described as **nominal** ("named") or **ordinal** ("ordered"). Sex, smoking status, and race are examples of nominal data. We may assign the number 1 for women and the number 2 for men, but the number has no meaning; rather, these designations are just names for the categories. Stage of disease is an example of ordinal data. Here, the order of the numbers assigned to each category has a meaningful order: stage II is greater than stage I, yet it may not truly be twice the amount.

Continuous variables can be further described as **interval** and **ratio**. Interval data include numbers that begin from an arbitrary starting point, such as body temperature. Zero body temperature on the Fahrenheit scale is not the same as zero on the Celsius scale, and on neither scale is the zero value truly devoid of temperature; zero is just the starting point. In contrast, ratio data use a scale where zero means there is none, such as tumor size and height.

Frequency Distributions

Describing the frequency of characteristics such as age at diagnosis and race is the first step in understanding your sample or data set. To describe the frequency distribution for categorical data, one simply counts how many observations fit in each category; for example, how many men are in your sample and how many women. These counts can also be displayed as percentages; for example, maybe 55% of your sample is women and 45% are men. For continuous data, one would summarize the average values observed or describe the distribution in other ways that we discuss later in this chapter. One can also visually display the frequency distribution of data set. Here, we briefly touch on four simple diagrams for doing so: a pie chart, a stacked bar chart, a standard bar chart, and a histogram.

Charts such as those in Figure 24-1 can be used to show the percentage of the sample that falls into categories like sex or stage of disease. These charts show, among people diagnosed with cancer in North Carolina between 1990 and 1992, the proportion diagnosed at each stage of disease. The pie chart shows the proportion of the sample

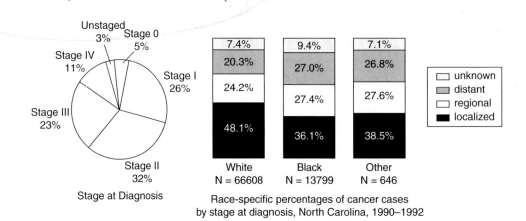

Stage at Diagnosis

Race-specific percentages of cancer cases by stage at diagnosis, North Carolina, 1990–1992

Figure 24-1. The Frequency Distribution of Categorical Data Using a Pie Chart and a Stacked Bar Chart

in each category as a slice of the pie. The bar charts show these proportions as a proportion of the bar, with a bar for each race. Pie charts and bar graphs are especially useful for nominal and ordinal data.

Categorical data can also be displayed in a **bar chart**, such as in Figure 24-2. Here, the number of patients in each category, rather than the percentage, is displayed. The bars of a bar chart do not touch, to signify that they have no quantitative relationship.

The frequency distribution of continuous data is often displayed using a histogram such as the one in Figure 24-3. Here, the x-axis is an actual number line and usually begins at zero. The bars of the histogram should touch, to signify they are continuous, quantitative categories. To create a histogram, one must first decide on how many "bins" to group the data into. For example, age at diagnosis might be grouped into the ranges 0 to 19, 20 to 39, 40 to 59, 60 to 79, and 80 or more years. The number of bins should be small enough to be informative but large enough to show the distribution or variation of the data. In addition, the bins should be mutually exclusive; that is, each person in a population should fit into only one bin. The y-axis is similar to that in a bar chart and displays the count (or frequency) or sometimes the proportion within each bin. In Figure 24-3,

tumor size is the x-axis, and the number of cases with tumor masses of that size is represented on the y-axis.

A histogram like the one shown in Figure 24-3 can take on several overall shapes, such as those shown in Figure 24-4. A "normal" distribution is bell-shaped and often occurs when looking at data in nature. For example, if we displayed the distribution of heights in a given population, most people's height would fall within a certain range, symmetrically distributed around the average height, with a few people who are relatively very short and very tall.

As shown, not all distributions are symmetric. Skewed distributions have a long tail of bins with few people in them. For example, in the population of interest, if most people are of average height, but there is also one person in each of the shorter categories of height, then the distribution would be skewed to the left. If there is one person in each of the taller categories of height, then the distribution would be skewed to the right. Distributions can also appear to be made of two underlying populations and so are "bimodal." For example, in a population of men and women, the distribution of heights would likely be bimodal, because the subpopulation of men's heights would have a normal distribution with a peak that was taller than the peak for the subpopulation of women's heights.

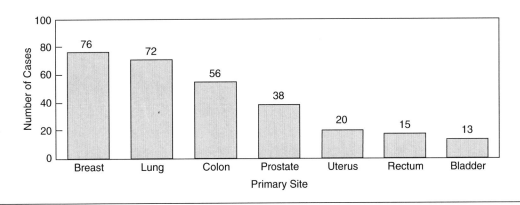

Figure 24-2. The Frequency Distribution of Categorical Data Using a Bar Chart

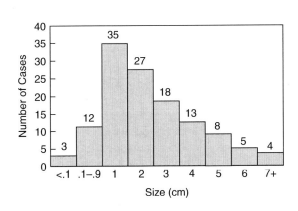

Figure 24-3. The Frequency Distribution of Continuous Data Using a Histogram

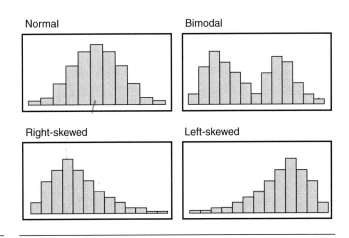

Figure 24-4. Common Shapes of Frequency Distributions: Normal, Bimodal, and Skewed

Describing Data with Statistics

One can describe the distribution of continuous data with the frequency distributions just described or with statistics such as range of the data; measures of central tendency such as the median, mean, and mode; and measures of the variation or spread of the data like the variance and standard deviation. To explore these statistics, we use the sample data in the Appendix, which gives the ages at diagnosis for 12 children with acute lymphocytic leukemia (ALL). Measures of central tendency can be calculated by hand, as we are going to demonstrate here, or the data can be entered into a spreadsheet program such as Microsoft Excel.

The **range** refers to the minimum and maximum values observed from continuous data, or sometimes the difference between the minimum and maximum. For example, the range of the age of diagnosis in the ALL data set is 1 to 8 years old, or the difference between these two numbers: 7 years.

The **mode** is the most frequently occurring value in a data set. In the ALL example, the most common age of diagnosis is 6 years old. When two values are common, the distribution is called a *bimodal distribution.*

The **median** is the middle value. If there is an even number of observations in the data when the data are ordered from the lowest to the highest value, as is the case in the ALL example, then there is no middle value. The median in this situation is the average of the two middle values. To calculate the median age of diagnosis in the ALL data set, first sort the data from the minimum to the maximum value. Here, the two middle values are 4 and 5, so the average is: $(4 + 5)/2 = 4.5$. Therefore, half of the ALL subjects in this sample were diagnosed before age 4.5, and half were diagnosed after age 4.5.

The **mean** is the average. The mean is calculated by summing all of the numbers we wish to find the average of and then dividing this sum by the number of values we have added. In the ALL example, the sum of all of the ages of diagnosis is 53. There are 12 observations, and so the mean age at diagnosis is $53 \div 12 = 4.4$. Thus, on average, the children in this sample were diagnosed at 4.4 years old. When a distribution is skewed, as shown in Figure 24-4, the statistic most apt to change is the mean, which is usually pulled toward the tail.

The distribution of data is described by the shape of the frequency distribution, by measures of central tendency, and by the **variance** or the spread of the data. That is, the data might be clustered close to the mean or spread very far apart. Calculate the variance as follows: First, calculate the difference between each observation and the mean of all of the observations; then square this quantity to make the differences positive; then sum all of these values and divide by the number of observations − 1. Because the variance is a squared quantity, it is often easier to interpret the square root of the variance, called the **standard deviation**. In Table 24-1 below, the value of the standard deviation for the children with ALL has been calculated.

| Table 24-1 | Age at Diagnosis of Childhood Acute Lymphocytic Leukemia (data from Appendix): Calculation of Variance and Standard Deviation |

Case No. (i)	Age (years) (X_i)	Mean (X)	Difference Between Age and Mean Age ($X_i − X$)	Difference Squared ($X_i − X)^2$
1	2		−2.4	5.8
2	5		0.6	0.3
3	6		1.6	2.5
4	4		−0.4	0.2
5	3		−1.4	2.0
6	1	4.4	−3.4	11.7
7	6		1.6	2.5
8	4		−0.4	0.2
9	3		−1.4	2.0
10	8		3.6	12.8
11	6		1.6	2.5
12	5		0.6	0.3

$$Variance = \sigma^2 = \frac{\sum\limits_{i=1}^{n} (X_i - \overline{X})^2}{n - 1} = \frac{42.9}{11}$$

$$Standard\ Deviation = \sigma = \sqrt{\sigma^2} = \sqrt{3.9} = 1.9$$

The reason for the subtraction of 1 in the denominator of the variance formula is based on the individual values that are "free to vary" once the sum and the number of observations is specified. That is, if one knows that eight numbers sum to 64, then if seven of those numbers are known and sum to 54, the eighth number must be 10—it is not free to vary. This concept is called *degrees of freedom.*

Now that we have touched on standard deviation, let us look again at the normal distribution shown in Figure 24-4 and again in Figure 24-5. If data are truly normally distributed, then 68% of the observations will have a value that is within one standard deviation from the mean value, and 27% of the observations will have a value between one and two standard deviations from the mean value. Therefore, 95% (68% + 27%) of the observations in a sample that is normally distributed will lie within two standard deviations from the mean. The probability is low, then (less than 5%), of seeing an observation with a value more than

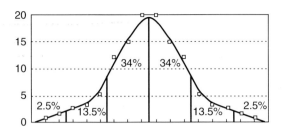

Figure 24-5. Diagram of the Areas under the Normal Curve

Table 24-2	Possible Outcomes When Making a Decision about the True Population Based on a Sample of Data

		Truth	
		H_o	H_a
Decision	H_o	good	Type II error: beta
	H_a	Type I error: alpha	good

[handwritten annotations: "Treatment might appear effective but is not truth is not" pointing to alpha cell; "More acceptable no change" at right]

two standard deviations away from the mean if our data are normally distributed. This concept is the basis for interpreting the results of statistical tests.

Hypothesis Testing

So far, we have discussed statistics, such as the mean and standard deviation, which are used to describe the distribution of data. Statistical tests are used to compare these descriptive values between two populations or samples, to determine whether the populations differ in a meaningful way. That is, the mean age of diagnosis of ALL for boys might be different than the mean age of diagnosis of ALL for girls, and even if there is a numerical difference between these groups, this difference may or may not be meaningful.

Before comparing two groups like this, we must first state our hypothesis. Traditionally, one states the **null hypothesis** (represented in notation as H_o) that there is *no* difference between groups. Therefore, in research, the aim is to *reject* the null hypothesis that the two groups are *not* different, in favor of accepting an **alternative hypothesis (H_a)** that there *is* a meaningful difference between the two groups. Remember that we generally only work with samples of data from the population (i.e., we generally cannot study all children who have ever been diagnosed with ALL); thus, there is a true reality out there that we will never fully know. Instead, we will make a decision about the population based on our sample. The relationship between our hypothesis and "truth" are presented in Table 24-2.

If the two samples we are testing are not different, we reject the alternative hypothesis and "do not reject" the null hypothesis, and if the two populations from which we chose the samples truly are not meaningfully different, then we chose well. Likewise, if the two samples we are testing *are* very different, we reject the null hypothesis and accept the alternative hypothesis, and if the two populations from which we chose the samples truly are meaningfully different, then we also chose well. However, our samples may not represent the true populations from which they were chosen; thus, we could reject the null hypothesis (thinking our samples are very different) when, in fact, the null hypothesis is true (our populations are, in fact, very similar) and thus commit a **type I error**. This is also called the **alpha error**,

and it is the one most dreaded because in a clinical trial, a treatment might appear to be effective when, in fact, it is not (or may even be harmful). It is for this reason that the driving force in most medical research is to have the chances of committing a type I error to be less than 5%.

We could also "fail to reject" the null hypothesis (thinking our samples are very similar) when, indeed, the alternative hypothesis is true (our populations are, in fact, very different) and thus commit a **type II error**. This is also called the **beta error**. In medical research, this error is more acceptable because it would result in no change from the current practice, and thus has less chance (usually) of increased harm for the patient. When designing a study, the acceptable level of beta error is required to calculate the sample size required. Measured as 1 − beta, the **power** of a study refers to the power to find a difference between groups, when it truly exists.

Statistical Tests

A statistical test can be used to determine whether the difference between two groups is more than what would be expected by chance alone; in other words: "Is the difference statistically significant?" To choose the proper statistical test, first ask whether the statistic to be compared is categorical or continuous. For continuous outcomes (such as height or blood pressure), then either correlation, a *t*-test, an **analysis of variance (ANOVA)**, or a regression model will be needed. If the outcome is categorical, then either a chi-square or a logistic regression model will be needed. Each of these tests is described in more detail later.

Correlation is used to analyze how one continuous variable varies with another continuous variable. For example, do taller people tend to weigh more? Do older people tend to have higher blood pressure? Correlations are often graphed with one variable on the *x*-axis and the other on the *y*-axis. The test itself calculates an *r* (or **rho**) statistic, which varies from −1.0 to +1.0. Data with an *r* near −1.0 are negatively or inversely correlated, which means the values for one variable increase when the value for the other declines. Data with an *r* near +1.0 are positively or directly correlated, which means the values for one variable increase when the value for the other increases. An example of positively correlated variables is height and weight: taller people tend to weigh more. A zero value for *r* means the two variables are not correlated with one another. One form of correlation (Pearson's) uses the actual values of the two variables, whereas another form (Spearman's) uses the order of the two variables when they have been ranked. This use of a rank value rather than the actual value is especially useful for skewed distributions or distributions that are not distributed normally. Tests that assume the data are distributed normally are called **parametric** tests; tests that do not assume the data are distributed normally are called **nonparametric** tests.

The **t-test**, sometimes referred to as Student's *t*, is used to compare the means from two samples to determine whether they are statistically significantly different. The *t*-test is favored when the size of each sample is at least 30 observations; at this point, the distribution of data tends to approach a normal distribution. The result of the *t*-test is a *t*-statistic and a *p*-value. The **p-value** indicates the probability that the two samples are similar. When the *p*-value is less than 0.05—that is, when there is less than a 5% probability that two samples are different due to chance alone—then, in general, the samples can be considered statistically significantly different. For example, the mean age at diagnosis among girls with ALL in the sample data given in the Appendix is 5.7; the mean age at diagnosis among boys with ALL in this sample is 4.0. If we perform a *t*-test in Microsoft Excel or other statistical software, $p = 0.22$. This *p* value is not less than 0.05; therefore, even though girls and boys in this sample did have a slightly different mean age at diagnosis of ALL, this difference was not statistically significant. The **Wilcoxon–Mann–Whitney** test is the nonparametric form of the *t*-test.

Another variation of the *t*-test is called the **paired t-test**. For this test, rather than just comparing the means between two samples, each observation from one sample is matched, or paired, with an observation in the other sample on other characteristics so that the two groups are as similar as possible. For example, participants might be matched on sex and year of birth, so that any differences of age at diagnosis that are observed will not be because of sex or year of birth differences. The **Wilcoxon signed rank** test is the nonparametric form of the paired *t*-test.

The ANOVA test is used to compare means like the *t*-test, but more than two groups can be compared. For example, if we wanted to compare the mean age of diagnosis of ALL in the example data set between races (white, black, or other), we could use ANOVA. **Regression** analysis is similar to ANOVA in that we are comparing the mean of a continuous variable between two or more groups. With both ANOVA and regression, we can "adjust" for other differences between these groups at the same time. For example, if we want to know whether girls or boys in our sample are diagnosed with ALL at an earlier age, but we want to know whether the differences in age

$$\chi^2 = \Sigma \; \frac{[(Observed) - (Expected)]^2}{Expected} = \Sigma \; \frac{[O - E]^2}{E}$$

Figure 24-6. Formula for the Chi-Square Test Statistic

at diagnosis are due to other factors beyond race or state of residence, then we can adjust for race and state of residence in a regression model. ANOVA models adjust only for categorical variables, whereas regression models can be used to adjust for continuous variables.

Turning now to comparing a categorical outcome between two samples, we begin with the **chi-square** test, written in as χ^2. The formula for chi-squared is given in Figure 24-6, or a chi-square can be calculated in a spreadsheet program such as Microsoft Excel or other statistical software.

For this sample calculation, consider the sex distribution for the childhood leukemia cases: 9 male and 3 female cases. If we were to compare our sample with the overall sex distribution in the United States (note: these data are contrived for this example), we would have expected to see 8 male and 4 female cases. This gives a $\chi^2 = [(9 - 8)^2/8] + [(3 - 4)^2/4] = 0.38$, which corresponds with a *p*-value greater than 0.05 (the *p*-value corresponding to chi-square values can be found from chi-square distribution tables or by calculating the chi-square in a spreadsheet program such as Microsoft Excel). Therefore, the sex distribution in our sample is different than the distribution we might expect, but not statistically significantly different. The matched form of the chi-square test is the McNemar chi-square. And if we want to compare two groups while adjusting for several other factors, logistic regression can be used; this requires statistical software to perform.

Epidemiology

Epidemiology is the study of the distribution and determinants of disease in human populations, and as such is the basic science of public health. There are three basic elements for disease to occur: the **agent** (the actual biologic cause of the disease process, e.g., a bacterium), the **host** (a person who is at risk for the disease), and the **environment** (the place where the agent and the host encounter one another). If one of these factors is eliminated, then disease can be prevented. A simplified example is: Although mosquitoes are not the cause of malaria, they are part of the environment (they are the vector) that exposes people to the protist that does cause malaria in humans. If mosquitoes could be eliminated, malaria might be prevented. With cancer risk, the disease process often seems much more complicated than this concept implies. Nonetheless, one can identify examples of prevention based on eliminating exposure to a suspected carcinogen (such as smoking) as a form of changing the environment.

Types of Prevention

Prevention has many aspects, depending on what one is aiming to prevent: **primary** prevention begins before the biological onset of disease, and includes lifestyle and behavior modification such as smoking cessation or vaccinations, as well as occupational and environmental regulations the prevent hazardous exposures; **secondary** prevention begins after possible biological onset of disease, but before symptoms of the disease present, and mainly includes screening, such as mammograms; **tertiary** prevention begins after a disease is diagnosed and includes preventing the disease from becoming more severe, such as treatment and palliative care.

Epidemiologic Reasoning

To identify a means of disease prevention, an epidemiologist first considers measures of disease frequency in human populations, then develops a hypothesis of which exposures might lead to increased risk for disease, then develops a study to test this hypothesis. Different epidemiologic study designs are described later. After the data from these studies are gathered, then the statistics described in the first half of this chapter can be used to describe the distribution of exposures and outcomes in the study population, ultimately leading to an understanding of what preventive measures might be most effective.

Measures of Disease Frequency

Prevalence measures the proportion of a given population who is alive and has the condition of interest at a given time. Prevalence is a good measure to understand total burden of a disease on a population.

$$\text{Prevalence} = \frac{\text{Number of cases alive at a point in time}}{\text{Number of people in the population at that time}}$$

The incidence of disease, or the proportion of *new* cases in a population at risk, is often of more interest for public health, as it captures the rate at which new cases develop. There are two main forms of incidence rates: cumulative incidence and the incidence rate.

Cumulative incidence (or just **incidence**), like prevalence, is a simple proportion, but with only new, not existing cases in the numerator. In addition, the denominator includes not the whole population but only those at risk for the disease. For example, the cumulative incidence of uterine cancer in a population should not include men in the denominator, nor should it include women without a uterus, because they are not at risk for uterine cancer. Cumulative incidence also contains an element of time—new cases that developed over a period of time—whereas prevalence is usually measured at one point in time. Be-

cause most diseases, like cancer, are rare, cumulative incidence is often expressed per 100,000 people rather than as a percentage. For example, if there were 93 new cases of cancer in 1995 for Town A (population 25,791), the reported incidence rate would be $(93/25,791) \times 100,000 = 360.6/100,000$. The cancer incidence for Town A would be reported as "360.6 per one hundred thousand population, in 1995." Please note the three elements: number of new events (numerator), population at risk (denominator), and the time period of reference.

$$\text{Cumulative incidence} = \frac{\text{Number of new cases over a period of time}}{\text{Number of people initially at risk in the population}}$$

The **incidence rate** is a more precise measure of incidence because it captures person-time at risk in the denominator rather than number of people. The example in Figure 24-7 illustrates why this difference can be important.

$$\text{Incidence rate} = \frac{\text{Number of new cases over a period of time}}{\text{Person-time at risk in the population}}$$

The example presents 10 individuals followed over a year. Subjects 8 and 9 have the condition of interest before the beginning of follow-up, and Subjects 1, 2, 3, and 10 develop the condition over the course of the year. Subjects 4 and 5 are alive and disease-free at last contact, but they are lost to follow-up midstudy. The prevalence rate includes all new *and existing* cases in the population; thus, prevalence = 6/10 = 60%. The cumulative incidence and incidence rate include only new cases. Thus, Subjects 8 and 9 are not included in the numerator; they are also not at risk for the disease, so they are not included in the denominator either. Thus, cumulative incidence = 4/8 = 50%. However, consider Subjects 4 and 5 again; they may have been diagnosed with the condition, but because they were lost to follow-up, we do not know their fate. The incidence rate takes this "censoring" into account, and thus creates a more precise measure of incidence. To calculate the person-time at risk for the population in this example, add together the 6 months at risk for Subject 1, 8 months at risk for Subject 2, 12 months for Subjects 3, 6, and 7, 3 months for individual 4, and 1 month for individuals 5 and 10; this equals 55 months at risk for this population, and thus an incidence rate of 4/55, or 7 per 100 person-months. The denominator of incidence rates, then, is not number of people but rather person-time at risk. Note mortality rates are just like incidence rates where the condition measured is death:

$$\text{Mortality rate} = \frac{\text{Number of deaths over a period of time}}{\text{Person-time at risk in the population}}$$

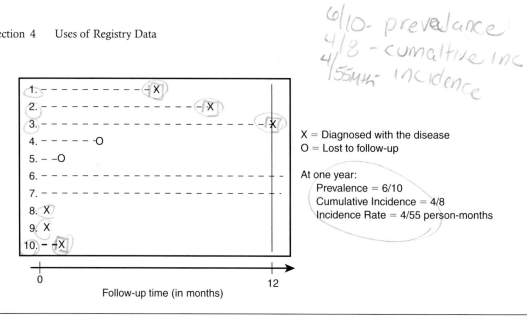

6/10- prevalance
4/8 - cumaltive inc
4/55mth- incidence

X = Diagnosed with the disease
O = Lost to follow-up

At one year:
   Prevalence = 6/10
   Cumulative Incidence = 4/8
   Incidence Rate = 4/55 person-months

0 ——— Follow-up time (in months) ——— 12

Figure 24-7. Calculation of Prevalence, Cumulative Incidence, and Incidence Rate in a Sample of 10 People

Measures of Excess Risk

Once we have measured the risk (e.g., the incidence or mortality) in a population, then we are often interested in whether this risk is in excess of what is expected. For example, if we have an incidence rate for prostate cancer in a study population of 128 per 100,000 person-years, is this higher or lower than one would expect? If this rate is age-adjusted to the 2000 U.S. standard population, then this could be compared with the estimated U.S. age-adjusted incidence rate 158 per 100,000 men in 2009.[1] Then the **observed-to-expected** ratio (or **standardized incidence ratio** [SIR]) of these rates is 128/158 = 0.81, so that our population does appear to have a 19% lower risk for prostate cancer than the United States as a whole. The SIR is more properly calculated for each age category and sex, but as a rough comparison, observed-to-expected rates can be very useful.

$$\text{SIR} = \frac{\text{number of observed cases}}{\text{number of expected cases}}$$

The SIR is used to approximate the main measure of excess risk in epidemiologic studies: the relative risk (or risk ratio or RR). The RR is simply the ratio of the incidence of disease in the exposed to the incidence in the unexposed:

$$\text{RR} = \frac{\text{Incidence in the exposed}}{\text{Incidence in the unexposed}}$$

Note that this can be the ratio of cumulative incidences or incidence rates. A good example of a relative risk is given in Jemal and colleagues'[1] study of cancer mortality rates by education, race, and sex in the United States in 2001. (Remember that mortality rates are just incidence rates of death.) Among white non-Hispanics, the age-adjusted mortality rate for lung cancer for people with less than 12 years of education was 87.3 per 100,000; the age-adjusted mortal-

ity rate for lung cancer for people with at least 16 years of education was 13.7 per 100,000. The relative risk, then, was 87.3/13.7 = 6.4. Thus, people "exposed" to less education in the United States are at four to six times greater risk for dying of lung cancer than people with more education.

Epidemiologic Study Designs

There are two main study designs in epidemiology: the cohort study and the case–control study. We touch on each of these here.

Cohort Study

The **cohort study** identifies a group (or cohort) of people who do not have the outcome of interest and then follows them over time to measure the rate at which they develop the outcome. For example, we might be interested in whether workers in textile factories are at increased risk for lung diseases, so we could identify a group of textile factory workers who do not already have lung disease and follow them over 10 or 20 years to see who develops the condition. We can then compare people with different exposures in the factory, people of different ages or sex, or other characteristics to determine who is at greatest risk for lung disease. Community-based disease registries are also examples of cohort studies, often called *surveillance studies;* with this approach, all persons in the population are studied, and exposure status is determined after the disease has occurred. There are also surveillance efforts based expressly on exposure (such as patients taking a certain drug or who have a certain disease) with more traditional follow-up of subjects.[2]

Cohort studies can be either **prospective**, as in the textile factory study described earlier, where members of the cohort are identified before the outcome occurs, or **retrospective**, where the cohort is identified after the outcome occurs. When performing a retrospective cohort study, however, the cohort should still be determined by the exposure, not by the outcome. To perform a retrospective cohort study to examine whether textile workers are at increased risk for lung disease, we would first need to identify people who worked in a textile factory at some point in the last 20 years and then determine who developed lung disease over that period. An example of a retrospective cohort (or historical cohort) study is a study by the Centers for Disease Control and Prevention of military personnel exposed to Agent Orange in the Vietnam War.[3]

Randomized, controlled trials (RCTs), as discussed in Chapter 40, are a form of cohort study. In this case, the cohort members are randomly assigned to be exposed (to a drug, for example) or not (such as to a placebo). Exposures in epidemiology studies, such as smoking status, sex, or occupation, usually cannot be randomly assigned because it would be impossible or unethical to do so. RCTs, however, are considered the best study design to use when possible because randomly assigning the exposure likely randomizes any bias that would be present in an observational cohort study, where people select exposures and usually do so for a reason.

One of the main benefits of cohort studies is that incidence rates can be calculated directly in a cohort study, because person-time at risk is known, and thus relative risks can be directly calculated as well. In addition, several outcomes of interest can be studied at once. The main disadvantage of cohort studies is that they can take a long time, especially for delayed or rare outcomes such as cancer, and thus can be prohibitively expensive.

Case–Control Study

In a **case–control study**, people with the disease of interest are identified, then people without the disease (controls) are identified in the population from which the cases arose, and the exposures in these groups are compared to determine an association between exposure and outcome. Because the exposures and diseases have already occurred, case–control studies are by nature retrospective. However, in a retrospective cohort study, study subjects are selected based on some exposure and then their disease status is determined; in a case–control study, study subjects are selected based on their disease status and then their exposures are determined. A casefinding system is usually needed for identifying all eligible cases from a defined population from which controls can then be sampled.

The main advantage of a case–control study is that rare or delayed outcomes can be studied more efficiently. In addition, several exposures of interest can be studied at the same time. One disadvantage of the case–control study is that selection of proper controls can be difficult. Ideally, controls should be selected from the population from which the case arose, so that all the controls may have the same risk for development of the disease despite some exposure revealed through the study. Another disadvantage of the case–control study is that person-time at risk cannot be measured, and thus we cannot directly estimate the incidence or prevalence of the outcome in exposed and nonexposed individuals. The relative risk can still be approximated in a case–control study, however, by calculating the odds ratio.

The **odds ratio** is defined as the odds of the exposure in persons with the outcome divided by the odds of exposure in those who do not have the outcome. A common way to calculate the odds ratio is to first display the number of study subjects in each exposure-disease category in a 2×2 table such as this one:

	Outcome	No outcome	
Exposed	A	B	Odds ratio = a*d or
Unexposed	C	D	a/c b*c b/d

Following is an example of calculating the odds ratio (to approximate the relative risk) in a case–control study of cancer in a community where some areas are exposed to hazardous waste: $(a \times d) \div (c \times b)$

	Cancer	No cancer	
Exposed to hazardous waste	24	12	Odds ratio = (24 × 43)/
Unexposed	29	43	(29 × 12) = 2.97

Cross-sectional Study

The final study design covered here is called the **cross-sectional study**. In this study design, the exposure and outcome for each study subject is determined at the same time—there is no follow-up time between exposure and outcome as in the cohort study. The main disadvantage of this study design is that we cannot determine whether the exposure preceded the outcome. If the exposure is known to precede the outcome (such as sex or genotype), then a cross-sectional study can provide a quick and relatively inexpensive way to measure the prevalence of an exposure or outcome.

Bias

All epidemiologic research struggles against systematic errors (bias). The principal sources of bias are misclassification, selection, and confounding.

Misclassification bias occurs when subjects are assigned as exposed or unexposed incorrectly, or are categorized as a case or a control incorrectly. This can happen when people misremember or do not want to admit to past exposures. Cancer patients may recall earlier exposures in more detail than control subjects because of contemplating the cause of their disease. There are several ways to minimize misclassification bias. For example, when interviewing subjects about past medications, images of the medication containers or pills themselves at the time of interview can help people recall their past exposures more accurately.

Misclassification bias usually weakens the relative risk in a study, so a true association might be missed. Sometimes, however, misclassification can have an unpredictable effect on the measure of excess risk in a study, leading to false conclusions that are difficult to assess.

Selection bias occurs when all of the subjects in a population do not have the same opportunity to be included in a study, so that the control subjects who are selected for a study have a different distribution of exposure than that of the population from which the cases were chosen. A classic example of selection bias, called *Berkson's bias,* occurs when study subjects are selected from hospitalized patients. People in the hospital are not representative of the general population; therefore, the exposure level in the control group will likely be overestimated compared with the general population from which the cases arose. Selection bias can also occur, for example, if only people with telephones are able to be contacted for recruitment, or if people of low literacy or who are not English speaking cannot respond. These biases are often addressed in epidemiologic studies by the use of sampling strategies, or restricting study subjects to particular case and control groups.

Confounding occurs when there is a factor that is associated with both the exposure and the outcome, and thus interferes with measuring the true association between the exposure and outcome. For example, a researcher might find that incidence rates of lung cancer are much greater in coffee drinkers than in non-coffee drinkers. However, smoking is associated with lung cancer, and coffee drinkers tend to smoke more than non-coffee drinkers. Therefore, smoking confounds the relationship between coffee drinking and lung cancer, and must be accounted for in any analysis.

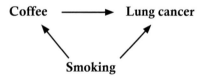

Confounding can be accounted for by restricting the study population (in our example, possibly choosing only nonsmokers), by matching cases and control subjects on potential confounders (such as age, sex, and smoking status), or by stratifying by or adjusting for potential confounders in the analysis.

As another example, consider the incidence rate of prostate cancer in our study population was greater than the incidence rate of prostate cancer in the United States. To compare these two rates, however, we had to adjust for age. Age is a potential confounder because it could be associated with both the exposure (the region) and the outcome (prostate cancer). That is, if the people in our study population tended to be much older than the U.S. population as a whole, then we would expect to see a greater rate of prostate cancer in our study population solely because of age and not the exposure under study. By adjusting both rates to account for age, if we see an increased rate of prostate cancer in our study population, then we can be more confident it is due to some factor other than age.

Screening

Screening is a fundamental aspect of public health as it provides early detection of a disease, before symptoms appear, when preventive measures might be most effective. Unfortunately, screening tests do not perfectly distinguish between people with and without a disease. Therefore, epidemiologists compare screening tests using the measures sensitivity, specificity, positive predictive value, and negative predictive value, as listed in Table 24-3. The letters a, b, c, and d represent the number of people who have the disease (+) or do not have the disease (−) according to the screening test and according to a theoretical "truth" representing whether someone actually has the disease.

An excellent screening test should have sensitivity and specificity greater than 90%. However, as only one test result may be used for determining disease status, the increase in sensitivity is usually compensated for by a decline in specificity, and vice versa. In clinical settings, then, multiple tests are usually used to improve the accurate prediction of disease status.

In today's setting of healthcare concerns, another consideration is the cost of confirmatory tests. Also, in circumstances where some risk is associated with follow-up of a positive test, the **positive predictive value** is a measure to be considered. Simply, this is the percentage of all persons tested as having the disease who will actually be found to have the disease (e.g., for whom the cost and risk of follow-up studies would have been justified).

As an example of the implications of the positive predictive value, and the subtlety of prevalence data, consider a setting with 1,000 cases of a disease that truly exist in a community where 100,000 persons are to be tested. With a sensitivity and specificity of 90%, the test would correctly identify 900 of the cases (90% of 1,000) but erroneously classify 9,900 truly well persons as being ill (10% of 99,000). This would mean that 10,800 persons would have to have follow-

Table 24-3	Diagram of Screening Results		
		Truth	
		+	**−**
Test	**+**	a	b False-positive
	−	c False-negative	d

Sensitivity = a/a+c   Specificity = d/b+d

Positive predictive value = a/a+b

Negative predictive value = d/c+d

up tests for the disease. However, for only 8.3% (900/10,800) would these studies be justified. Such ineffectiveness for cost would likely not be acceptable. For the persons bearing the costs or risks of follow-up studies, not to mention the emotions of being told they had a particular disease, this low positive predictive value could be unacceptable as well.

This concludes the overview of epidemiologic principles. Because of its relevance to the cancer registry field, a brief narrative on cancer biology and cancer epidemiology follows.

Cancer Epidemiology in the United States

Cancer is an ancient term arising from the visual impression of a surgeon that a tumor appeared like a crab with legs extending into the surrounding tissue. The more appropriate term for the diseases we collectively refer to as "cancer" is *malignant neoplasm*. A neoplasm is a new growth. It is the malignancy of cancer that is the salient characteristic to define the disease. Malignancy refers to a tumor's ability to spread throughout the body from the site of origin. This process of spreading is called *metastasis*.

It has long been recognized that the process of carcinogenesis occurred at a cellular level. A two-step process has been proposed for carcinogenesis: **Initiation** means the transformation of a cell to one that has the potential for malignant growth. A later event causes a cell to grow rapidly, to metastasize as a result of uncontrolled growth; the latter distinct event is termed **promotion**. Initiation and promotion may be too simplistic for actual carcinogenesis.

Recent discoveries of oncogenes and a better knowledge of the process of cellular growth regulation have enhanced the general understanding of carcinogenesis. Likely, carcinogenesis requires a series of cellular-level events to transpire, some of which may require a specific sequence to be effective. Often, nutritional factors interact with these genetic events to provide a favorable potential for growth. Cells have many means to repair genetic damage. However, these repair capabilities vary in human populations. Also varying between people is the ability to detoxify chemicals that enter the body. These individual differences represent forms of personal susceptibility.

For the purpose of cancer epidemiology studies, it is necessary to recognize the genetic-level nature of carcinogenesis and to appreciate the interplay of multiple forces to achieve carcinogenesis. Some carcinogens are considered **sufficient** causes of cancer, meaning they can produce carcinogenesis without interaction with other agents (e.g., ionizing radiation). Some agents are **necessary** carcinogens, meaning that a particular cancer cannot occur without this agent being present (e.g., Epstein–Barr virus in Hodgkin's disease).

Cancer is a historic disease, having been observed in ancient Egypt and Greece. Even dinosaur skeletons have been discovered with cancers. However, cancer emerged as a major public health concern in the middle of the twentieth century. The emergence of cancer as a leading cause of death is closely linked to the eradication of infectious diseases as major causes of death and the extension of life expectancy (Table 24-4). Heart disease, cancer, and stroke are all diseases of aging, and as life expectancy increased, these causes of death increased as well, by attrition of the acute causes of death. Soon cancer is expected to become the leading cause of death in the United States and the dominant basis for hospital admission.

It is instructive to note that these data also offer a perspective of cancer in the world as well. The pattern of cancer for 1930–1935 is much like that of the developing world today, that is, stomach and uterine cancer predominate. As countries become more industrialized, their cancer pattern shifts to be more like the developed world. These changes, as well as studies of cancer patterns among migrants, are some

Table 24-4	Ten Leading Causes of Death in the United States

1910	1950	1990	2006
Influenza	Heart disease	Heart disease	Heart disease
Tuberculosis	Cancer	Cancer	Cancer
Diarrhea/Enteritis	Stroke	Stroke	Stroke
Heart disease	Accidents	Accidents	Chronic lower respiratory diseases
Stroke	Disease of infancy	Influenza	Accidents
Nephritis	Influenza	Diabetes	Diabetes
Accidents	Arteriosclerosis	Cirrhosis	Alzheimer disease
Cancer	Diabetes	Arteriosclerosis	Influenza
Disease of infancy	Birth defects	Suicide	Kidney disease
Diphtheria	Cirrhosis	Disease of infancy	Suicide

of the strongest evidence for the assertion that "most cancers arise from environmental sources." However, the "environment" that statement refers to includes diet and lifestyle.

When one speaks of the "big" cancers, this refers to the common cancers. Lung cancer is the "biggest" cancer in terms of lives taken. However, do not think only in terms of mortality, one must also consider incidence as well (see Table 24-5). Prostate cancer is the most common cancer among men, but lung cancer takes many more lives. A similar relation exists for breast cancer and lung cancer in women.

Following is a review of the general epidemiology of several cancers.

- *Lung cancer:* This is the leading cause of cancer death in men and women. Increased risk is strongly associated with cigarette smoking, either direct or passive exposure. Occupational exposures include arsenic, organic chemicals, asbestos, and ionizing radiation exposures, for example, radon gas. These occupational risks are increased for smokers. Vitamin A deficiency is also a suspected risk factor.
- *Prostate cancer:* This is the leading cancer diagnosed in men; it is primarily a disease of older age (>65 years), and blacks are at particularly high risk. Familial association and risk from dietary fat are suspected. Cadmium is a potential occupational risk.
- *Breast cancer:* This is the most common cancer in women and primarily a postmenopausal disease (e.g., age > 50 years). Increased risk is associated with fam-

Table 24-5	Ten Leading Cancer Types for Estimated New Cancer Cases and Deaths, by Sex, United States, 2009

Males		Females	
Prostate	156.9	Breast	122.9
Lung & bronchus	76.2	Lung & bronchus	52.4
Colon & rectum	55.8	Colon & rectum	41.7
Urinary bladder	37.2	Uterine corpus	23.5
Melanoma of the skin	25.6	Non-Hodgkin lymphoma	16.5
Non-Hodgkin lymphoma	23.6	Melanoma of the skin	16.2
Kidney & renal pelvis	19.2	Thyroid	15.2
Leukemia	15.8	Ovary	12.9
Oral cavity & pharynx	15.4	Pancreas	10.5
Pancreas	13.3	Kidney & renal pelvis	9.9
All sites	538.9	All sites	408.0

Incidence rates per 100,000

Males		Females	
Lung & bronchus	68.8	Lung & bronchus	40.6
Prostate	24.7	Breast	24.0
Colon & rectum	21.2	Colon & rectum	14.9
Pancreas	12.3	Pancreas	9.4
Leukemia	9.7	Ovary	8.6
Non-Hodgkin lymphoma	8.7	Non-Hodgkin lymphoma	5.5
Esophagus	7.8	Leukemia	5.4
Liver & intrahepatic bile duct	7.7	Uterine corpus	4.1
Urinary bladder	7.5	Brain & other nervous system	3.5
All sites	225.4	All sites	155.4

Mortality rates per 100,000

Altekruse SF, Kosary CL, Krapcho M, Neyman N, Aminou R, Waldron W, Ruhl J, Howlader N, Tatalovich Z, Cho H, Mariotto A, Eisner MP, Lewis DR, Cronin K, Chen HS, Feuer EJ, Stinchcomb DG, Edwards BK (eds). SEER Cancer Statistics Review, 1975-2007, National Cancer Institute. Bethesda, MD, http://seer.cancer.gov/csr/1975_2007/, based on November 2009 SEER data submission, posted to the SEER web site, 2010.

ily history and no childbearing before age 30. A role for dietary fat is suspected.

- *Colorectal cancer:* This is the third leading cause of cancer death in both men and women, and is associated with a low fiber and/or high fat diet, history of polyps, and inflammatory bowel disease.
- *Uterine cancer:* Cervical cancer is generally a disease of young women, associated with the human papillomavirus, a sexually transmitted disease. Endometrial cancer is a disease of older women, associated with infertility, estrogen therapy, and obesity.
- *Oral cancer:* More common in men, oral cancer is associated with cigarette, cigar, and pipe smoking, smokeless tobacco use, and alcohol consumption.
- *Bladder cancer:* More common in whites and men, bladder cancer is associated with smoking. Workers in dye, leather, and rubber occupations are at risk.
- *Pancreatic cancer:* The rates for pancreatic cancer are greater for blacks, men, and persons older than 65. Smoking is a recognized risk factor; dietary fat, chronic infections, diabetes, and cirrhosis are suspected risks.
- *Skin cancer:* Common skin cancers occur in half of all people; a 98% survival rate, however, has led to these cancers being excluded from most statistical reports. Melanoma is the most common lethal form of skin cancer. Fair complexion is a strong risk factor, as is excessive sunlight exposure. Coal tar, pitch or creosote, arsenic, and radium are occupational risks.
- *Leukemia:* This is a disease of children and older adults. Certain genetic risks are known (e.g., Down syndrome), as are viral agents (human T-cell leuke-

mia virus type 1 [HTLV-1]). Occupational risks are ionizing radiation and benzene.

- *Ovarian Cancer:* A disease of older women (>60 years) and ones who have never borne children. Risk is increased by a history of breast, colorectal, and endometrial cancer.
- *Brain cancer:* Increasing occurrence in recent years, suspected risks with job-related aromatic hydrocarbon exposures and nonionizing radiation.
- *Lymphoma:* Lymphoma rates have been increasing. A mixed group of diseases with many suspected risk factors including agricultural chemicals, viruses, and childhood exposures.
- *Stomach cancer:* This is a leading cancer in developing countries, associated with nitrates in food.
- *Liver cancer:* This is a leading cancer in developing countries, associated with hepatitis B infection, cirrhosis, and occupational, aromatic hydrocarbon exposures.

Cancer is certainly difficult to study, especially from a population-based perspective—numbers of cases are small and the exposure issues are complex. In addition, there is the time scale of cancer. The interval from the induction of disease until it is clinically detected is termed **latency**. For most cancers, latency is believed to be 10 to 20 years. An old adage is that "common things happen commonly and rare things happen rarely." Lifestyle is the most common risk factor for cancer.[1] Lifestyle includes diet, tobacco use, alcohol consumption, sun exposure, and personal sexual history. As these are the common risk factors, it is not surprising that the cancers associated with these common factors are likewise the more frequently occurring ones. This recognition of the "rare" cancers as ones that may represent environmental risks leads to the concept of so-called sentinel events. These

| Appendix | Sample Data of Childhood Leukemia Surival |

Case No.	Age at Diagnosis (years)	Race	Sex	Date of Leukemia Diagnosis	Date of Last Contact	Status at Last Contact	Years
1	2	B	M	Nov-90	Sep-93	D	2.8
2	5	O	M	Mar-92	Jan-94	L	1.8
3	6	W	M	Apr-93	Dec-95	D	2.7
4	4	W	F	Aug-93	Aug-96	A	3.0
5	3	B	M	May-94	Oct-96	D	2.4
6	1	W	M	Sep-94	Sep-97	A	3.0
7	6	B	M	Jan-95	Feb-98	L	3.1
8	4	O	M	Aug-95	Aug-98	A	3.0
9	3	B	M	May-96	Aug-99	A	3.3
10	8	W	F	Jul-97	Oct-98	D	1.3
11	6	W	M	May-98	Jun-99	D	1.1
12	5	O	F	May-96	Feb-99	A	2.8

These data are contrived.
A, alive; B, black; D, deceased; F, female; L, lost to follow-up; M, male; O, other; W, white.

are circumstances where the recognition of an unusual pattern in even a few, rare cancers can be informative.[4]

References

1. Jemal, A., Siegel, R., Ward, E., Hao, Y., Xu, J., Thun, M. J. "Cancer Statistics, 2009." *CA Cancer Journal for Clinicians* 2009;59(4):225–249.
2. Thacker, S. B., Berkelman, R. L. "Public Health Surveillance in the United States," *Epidemiologic Reviews,* 1988;(10):164–190.
3. Centers for Disease Control and Prevention. "Comparison of Serum Levels of 2,3,7,8-Tetrachlorodibenzo-p-Dioxin with Indirect Estimates of Agent Orange Exposure Among Vietnam Veterans." The Centers of Disease Control, Veterans Health Study (pp. 1–172). Atlanta: U.S. Department of Health and Human Services, Centers for Disease Control and Prevention, September 1989.
4. Doll, R., Peto, R. *The Causes of Cancer: Quantitative Estimates of Avoidable Risks of Cancer in the United States Today.* New York: Oxford University Press, 1981.

Suggested Readings

Calle, E. E. "Criteria for Selection of Decedent Versus Living Controls in a Mortality Case-Control Study," *American Journal of Epidemiology,* 1984;120:635–642.

Centers for Disease Control and Prevention. "A National Program of Cancer Registries: At a Glance, 1994-1995." Atlanta: U.S. Department of Health and Human Resources, 1995.

Hanchette CL, Schwartz GG. "Geographic patterns of prostate cancer mortality. Evidence for a protective effect of ultraviolet radiation." Cancer. 1992 Dec 15;70(12): 2861-9.

Gehlbach, Stephen. *Interpreting the Medical Literature: Practical Epidemiology for Clinicians,* 5th ed. New York: McGraw-Hill, 2006.

Gordis, Leon. *Epidemiology,* 3rd ed. Philadelphia: Elsevier Saunders, 2004.

Howe, H. L., Lehnerr, M., Qualls, R. Y. "Using Central Cancer Registry Data to Monitor Progress in Early Detection of Breast and Cervical Cancer (Illinois, United States)," *Cancer Causes and Control,* 1995;6(2):155–163.

Hully, S. B., Cummings, S. R., Browner, W. S., Grady, D., Hearst, N., Newman, T. B. *Designing Clinical Research: An Epidemiological Approach,* 2nd ed. New York: Lippincott Williams & Wilkins, 2001.

Koepsell, Thomas D., Weiss, Noel S. *Epidemiologic Methods: Studying the Occurrence of Illness.* New York: Oxford University Press, 2003.

Last, John M. *A Dictionary of Epidemiology.* New York: Oxford University Press, 1995.

Miller, R. W. "Area Wide Chemical Contamination: Lessons from Case Histories," *Journal of the American Medical Association,* 1981;245:1548–1551.

Rothman, Kenneth J., Greenland, Sander, Lash, Timothy L. *Modern Epidemiology,* 3rd ed. Philadelphia: Lippincott Williams & Wilkins, 2008.

Rutstein, D. D., Berenburg, W., Chalmers, T. C., Child, C. C., Fishman, A. P., Perrin, E. B. "Measuring the Quality of Medical Care: A Clinical Approach," *New England Journal of Medicine,* 1976;294:582–588.

chapter 25

Survival Analysis

Nadia Howlader, MS
Kathleen A. Cronin, PhD
Brenda K. Edwards, PhD
Carol L. Kosary, MA

Cancer survival is an important measure for progress in the fight against cancer and is used to estimate patient prognosis, improvements in cancer care, and disparities between subgroups in the population. However, survival analysis techniques are one of the least understood measures in a hospital cancer registry. This is because it is a specialized topic and often covered in more advanced level statistics course work.

In this chapter, different approaches to calculate survival that are commonly used for measuring cancer prognosis are presented, and guidance on how the measures should be interpreted in practice is given. The concepts will be demonstrated with practical examples using population-based cancer registry data from the Surveillance, Epidemiology, and End Results (SEER) Program.[1]

Survival Measures

Survival measure are often expressed as the proportion of patients alive at some point subsequent to the diagnosis of their cancer, or represented as the probability of a group of patients "surviving" a specified amount of time (e.g., 3, 5, or 20 years).

There are several possible outcomes or *events* after a cancer diagnosis (Figure 25-1). Thus, there are various ways that survival can be measured. The choice of measurement depends on the research question or *event of interest*. The *event of interest* is the outcome being measured; it may be death due to any cause or death related to a specific cause of interest such as the cancer under study. When a patient is no longer followed *(loss to follow-up)* because of the end of the follow-up period, a patient is no longer able to be contacted for follow-up information, or dies from a cause that is not the event of interest, they are no longer at risk and considered to be *censored* at the point that they are no longer followed. Censored patients contribute to the analysis only up to the time they are censored.

Two standard measures[2-4] of survival are as follows:

Observed all-cause survival: Observed survival is an estimate of the probability of surviving *all causes of death*. In other words, both *cancer and other causes deaths* (i.e., Patients 1 and 2 in Figure 25-1) are contributing *events* to the survival estimation. Patients 3 and 4 in Figure 25-1 are censored.

Net (cancer-specific) survival: This is the hypothetical probability of surviving cancer in the absence of other causes of death. Therefore, unlike the observed all-cause survival, only *cancer deaths* are contributing *events* to the net survival estimation. In Figure 25-1, Patient 1 would be an event and Patients 2, 3, and 4 would be censored. This is a measure that is not influenced by changes in mortality from other causes. Therefore, it provides a useful measure for tracking survival across time and for comparisons between populations with different life expectancies.

Net survival can be estimated by the following approaches: (1) *relative* survival and (2) *cause-specific* survival. Figure 25-2 attempts to illustrate the basic concepts behind these two approaches:

Relative survival: This is the ratio of the proportion of observed survivors in a cohort of cancer patients to the proportion of expected survivors in a comparable set of cancer-free individuals. *Expected survival* for the cohort is based on life tables for the U.S. population matched to the cohort on race, sex, age, and date of diagnosis.

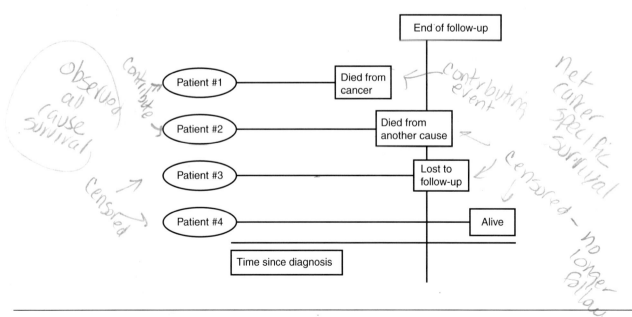

Figure 25-1. Possible Outcomes after Cancer Diagnosis

Relative Survival	Cause-Specific Survival
Observed Survival $\div$ Expected survival of the general population matched to the cancer patient	Specify underlying cause of death from death certificate for each cancer patient

Figure 25-2. Concept behind Net Survival Estimation: Relative and Cause-Specific Survival

Cause-specific survival: This is a net survival measure representing survival of a specified cause of death (COD) in the absence of other causes of death. Estimates are calculated by specifying the COD for each patient. Individuals who die of the cause of interest are classified as events, and individuals who die of other causes are considered to be *censored*.

Example of Different Survival Measures

Observed All-Cause Survival

An observed survival rate is a measure of survival of a patient group for a specific period after diagnosis. In computing the observed survival rate, deaths from other causes are treated the same way as deaths from cancer. Therefore, an observed survival rate should be interpreted as the likelihood of surviving *all causes of death* for a certain time after cancer diagnosis, not the likelihood of surviving that *cancer*.

Table 25-1 presents a life table for calculating a 5-year observed survival rate for patients with breast cancer. The life table shows, for each monthly interval starting from diagnosis, the probability of surviving *all causes of death* in each month interval up to 60 months, that is, 5 years (not all data are shown in Table 25-1). From this table, a number of statistics can be derived, for example, 1-, 3-, or 5-year survival rates. A few things also to note are:

1. Start with a total number of patients alive at the beginning of their diagnosis (N = 314,500), but each subsequent interval is based on number of patients who are *alive* at the beginning of that particular interval of time (column B).
2. For each time interval (column A), calculate an *interval* (column E) and a *cumulative* (column F) survival probability. The survival probability of interest is generally the *cumulative survival probability* (column F).
3. Cumulative survival probability (column F) is equal to the *interval survival rate* for that given interval mul-

tiplied by the *cumulative survival rate* (column E) from the *previous interval*. For example, cumulative survival probability between 59 and <60 (i.e., 5-year) months is: 0.9970*0.8050 = 0.8030, or 80.30%.
4. Standard error presented in column G captures variability of estimated *cumulative* survival rate at each interval. Generally, survival rate with lower standard error are more reliable. Standard errors are also required for generation of a confidence interval, which provides a lower and upper boundary for the estimated survival rate.

Figure 25-3 presents a summary of the life table showing 1-, 2-, 3-, 4-, and 5-year observed survival rate for female patients with breast cancer. Survival rate ranges from 95.7% at Year 1 to 80.3% at Year 5. The confidence intervals (see table adjacent to Figure 25-3) are fairly close to the survival rate, which means that we could be 95% confident that the estimated rate is likely to be within the lower and upper bounds of the confidence interval.

Relative Survival

When someone is more interested in excess mortality associated with a cancer diagnosis, it is better to use *relative survival*, which filters out the effect of mortality from other causes than the disease. Relative survival is calculated by dividing the overall *all-cause* survival after diagnosis of a cancer by the survival as observed in a similar population (e.g., U.S. general population) match on age, sex, race, and so forth. Relative survival has been typically used with cancer registry data because it does not need to rely on the accuracy of the reported COD from death certificates.

Figure 25-4 shows observed, expected, and relative survival rates for female patients with breast cancer. To calculate, for example, 3-year relative survival rate, we will divide 3-year observed rate (87.4%) by 3-year expected rate (94.2%) and that will yield a relative survival rate of 92.8%. The 5-year survival rate here presents an adjusted survival rate that does not take into account causes of death other than *breast cancer deaths*.

There is a second approach for estimating net survival, known as the *cause-specific* survival, which represents survival of a specified COD. Estimates are calculated by specifying the COD, and individuals who die of causes other than the specified cause are considered to be censored. Cause-specific survival is used with caution with cancer registry data as the COD information is obtained from death certificates, and as a result, attribution of a single COD may be difficult and misattribution may occur. For example, a death may be attributed to the site of metastasis instead of the primary site. SEER Program recently developed an algorithm and systematically evaluated each COD to accurately capture death related to a specific cancer. For more information regarding the algorithm, go to the SEER Program Web site.[5] Figure 25-5 shows relative and cause-specific survival for female patients with breast cancer. Survival rates produced by these two approaches

| Table 25-1 | Life Table for Observed Survival Calculation in Patients with Breast Cancer Diagnosed between 1999 and 2006 and Followed through 2007 in SEER-17 Registries |

Month	Interval	Alive at Start (N)	Died (n)	Lost to Follow-up (n)	Observed Survival Interval (%)	Observed Survival Cumulative (%)	Standard Error for Cumulative Rate
	A	B	C	D	E	F	G
1	<1 months	314,500	1,221	0	99.60	99.60	0.011
2	1 to <2 months	313,279	1,769	368	99.40	99.00	0.017
3	2 to <3 months	311,142	1,302	206	99.60	98.60	0.020
	.	.	.	.	.	.	.
	.	.	.	.	.	.	.
10	9 to <10 months	302,072	1,001	220	99.70	96.30	0.033
11	10 to <11 months	300,851	985	209	99.70	96.00	0.034
12	11 to <12 months	299,657	1,095	172	99.60	95.70	0.036
	.	.	.	.	.	.	.
	.	.	.	.	.	.	.
23	22 to <23 months	254,793	951	3,020	99.60	91.80	0.049
24	23 to <24 months	250,822	924	3,266	99.60	91.50	0.050
	.	.	.	.	.	.	.
	.	.	.	.	.	.	.
36	35 to <36 months	204,052	796	3,200	99.60	87.40	0.062
	.	.	.	.	.	.	.
48	47 to <48 months	160,626	581	2,740	99.60	83.70	0.072
	.	.	.	.	.	.	.
59	58 to <59 months	124,524	437	2,497	99.60	80.50	0.081
60	59 to <60 months	121,590	420	2,967	99.70	80.30	0.082

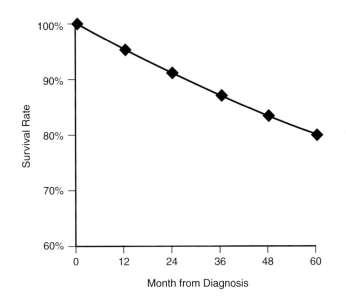

Month from Diagnosis	Observed Survival Rate	95% Confidence Interval	
		Lower Limit	Upper Limit
12	95.7%	95.6%	95.7%
24	91.5%	91.4%	91.6%
36	87.4%	87.3%	87.5%
48	83.7%	83.6%	83.8%
60	80.3%	80.1%	80.4%

Figure 25-3. Observed Survival Rates for Female Patients with Breast Cancer Diagnosed between 1999 and 2006 and Followed through 2007, SEER-17 Registries

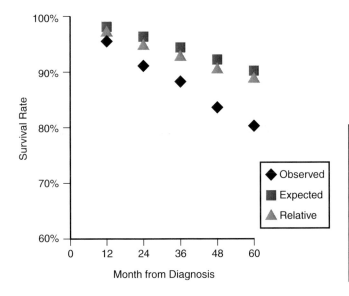

Month from Diagnosis	Survival Rate		
	Observed	Expected	Relative
12	95.7%	98.1%	97.5%
24	91.5%	96.2%	95.1%
36	87.4%	94.2%	92.8%
48	83.7%	92.2%	90.8%
60	80.3%	90.2%	89.0%

Figure 25-4. Observed, Expected, and Relative Survival Rates for Female Patients with Breast Cancer Diagnosed between 1999 and 2006 and followed through 2007, SEER-17 Registries

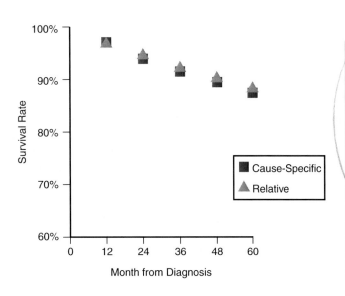

Figure 25-5. Relative and Cause-Specific Survival Rates for Female Patients with Breast Cancer Diagnosed between 1999 and 2006 and Followed through 2007, SEER-17 Registries

	IF GOAL	THEN
1	Describe the observed mortality patterns in the cohort of patients	Overall survival
2	Have reliable cause of death information (e.g., clinical trials)	Cause-specific survival
3	Unreliable information on cause of death but has accurate expected other cause mortality from general population for the cohort	Relative survival

Figure 25-6. Scenarios for Choosing Appropriate Survival Measure

are quite similar. This is because both are measuring the same quantity; that is, they are producing excess mortality associated with a cancer diagnosis, which filtered out the effect of mortality from other causes than breast cancer.

Conclusion

In summary, there are different methods for survival analysis. The choice of a specific method depends on the purpose of the study (Figure 25-6). If one is interested in a survival experience actually experienced by a cancer cohort, observed all-cause survival is the most appropriate choice. However, observed survival rates underestimate survival from cancer because the approach treats deaths from all causes equally. Two net methods that measure the excess mortality associated with a cancer diagnosis are available to correct for this underestimation. If a registry has complete and reliable causes of death information, then *cause-specific survival* can be estimated. But often cancer registry COD information data are not very good[6]; in that case, an indirect way to obtain survival that does not rely on COD is *relative survival*. Use of these approaches, each in appro-

priate circumstances, should enable production of accurate and informative survival statistics.

References

1. National Cancer Institute, Surveillance, Epidemiology and End Results Web site: http://seer.cancer.gov/
2. National Cancer Institute. "Measures of Cancer Survival." Available at: http://srab.cancer.gov/survival/measures.html. Accessed May 21, 2010.
3. Begg, C. B., Schrag, D. "Attribution of deaths following cancer treatment," *Journal of the National Cancer Institute,* 2002;94(14):1044–1045.
4. Ederer, F., Axtell, L. M., Cutler, S. J. "The Relative Survival Rate: A Statistical Methodology," *National Cancer Institute Monograph,* 1961;6:101–121.
5. National Cancer Institute, Surveillance, Epidemiology and End Results. "SEER Cause-Specific Death Classification." Available at: http://seer.cancer.gov/causespecific/index.html. Accessed May 21, 2010
6. Rosenberg, H. M., Maurer, J. D., Sorlie, P. D., et al. "Quality of Death Rates by Race and Hispanic Origin: A Summary of Current Research, 1999," *Vital and Health Statistics Series 2,* 1999;(128):1–13.

chapter 26

Clinical Practice Guidelines

Linda L. Jund, BS, CTR

In researching the literature, care guidelines are most frequently referred to as "clinical practice guidelines" (CPG) or "patient care guidelines" that provide a general template for quality, cost-effective management of patients.

The standard definition of CPG is that of Field and Lohr (1990)[1]: "Systematically developed statements to assist practitioner and patient decisions about appropriate health care for specific clinical circumstances."

CPG are nationally standardized recommendations for health care developed by a formal process that incorporates the best scientific evidence of effectiveness with expert opinion.

CPG are different than clinical protocols; they are less specific. A clinical trial protocol is a document that describes every detail about the research study being conducted including what types of people may participate in the trial; the schedule of tests, procedures, medications, and dosages; and the length of the study. While in a clinical trial, participants following a protocol are seen regularly by the research staff to monitor their health and to determine the safety and effectiveness of their treatment and to answer specific research questions.

They also differ from health care standards in that they are not applied rigidly and followed in virtually all cases. Practice guidelines are designed to be flexible, depending on patient needs. They are intended to support the decision-making process in patient care. Decisions about the appropriateness of guidelines and their application to individual patients should be made by the patient's physician, who is in the best position to know all factors related to his or her patient's care.

The primary purpose of CPG is to improve the quality of care by translating new research findings into clinical practice. Dedication to evidence-based medicine supports healthcare organization in their efforts to provide quality care by reducing the underuse, overuse, and misuse of medical resources. Other purposes of CPG include:

- To describe appropriate care based on the best available scientific evidence and broad consensus
- To reduce inappropriate variation in practice
- To provide a more rational basis for referral
- To provide a focus for continuing education
- To promote efficient use of resources
- To act as a focus for quality control, including audit
- To highlight shortcomings of existing literature and suggest appropriate future research

How Clinical Practice Guidelines Are Developed

CPG are developed by a formal process that incorporates the best scientific evidence of effectiveness with expert opinion. Guidelines should be developed within a structured and coordinated approach by a credible professional organization. Many guidelines include narrative reviews based on the literature but rely heavily on consensus to derive the final product. Extreme care must be taken to develop these guidelines without the perception of commercial or personal bias. The process to develop CPG is difficult, time-consuming, and expensive. With the support of federal agencies and professional societies, many expert guidelines have been developed over the years for cancer and many other disease sites.

Because of the rapid flow of scientific information, especially in oncology, new evidence can emerge and clinical best practice (standard of care) can change; therefore, guidelines need to be updated as new evidence is available.

Evidence-Based Medicine

Evidence-based medicine came to the forefront in the early 1990s. The term and concept originated at McMaster University. It has been defined as "the integration of best research evidence with the clinical expertise and patient values" (Sackett, 2000). The movement toward evidence-based medicine has been gaining ground quickly over the years, motivated by clinicians, politicians, and management concerned about the quality, consistency, and costs of providing health care. CPG, based on standardized best practice, have been shown to be capable of supporting improvements in quality and consistency in health care.

Organizations Involved with Developing Cancer Clinical Practice Guidelines

Many national oncology-related organizations are involved in developing care guidelines and consensus statements. The most comprehensive and most frequently updated and used CPG available in any area of medicine are the National Comprehensive Cancer Network (NCCN) guidelines.

National Comprehensive Cancer Network

In 1995, the NCCN began a program to develop a comprehensive set of diagnostic, treatment, and supportive care guidelines. The NCCN guidelines, developed as algorithms, cover 97% of the tumors seen in oncology practices, as well as managing the major symptoms experienced by patients with cancer. The NCCN guidelines were developed and are updated by their individual panels of numerous clinicians and oncology researchers, from their member institutions and affiliates. The NCCN guidelines are made up of recommendations based on the best evidence available at the time they are derived, but they are continuously updated and revised to reflect new data and new clinical information. The NCCN's disease-management guidelines are stage specific, covering workup through treatment and follow-up, as well as supportive care. These guidelines are available for consumers, as well as the healthcare providers. (For more information regarding NCCN guidelines, visit their Web site: www.nccn.org.)

American Society of Clinical Oncology

Rigorous training, clinical experience, exchange of information among practitioners, and familiarity with the medical literature are not enough to ensure that physicians will do the right thing for their patients. Therefore, American Society of Clinical Oncology (ASCO) began developing guidelines in 1993 for the purpose of improving the quality of care by helping oncologist make choices on treatment, prevention, support care, and follow-up practices that were in line with best available evidence from oncology research. CPG are available on the ASCO Web site, giving physicians immediate access to serve as reminders about the most up-to-date care of their patients.

ASCO guidelines are focused on a single question or a group of questions around an important topic. ASCO expert panels identify and develop practice recommendations for specific areas of cancer care that would benefit from the availability of practice guidelines such as chemotherapy for Stage IV non–small-cell lung cancer. Topics for guidelines are selected on the basis of significant clinical or economic importance; presence of variations in patterns of, or access to care; availability of suitable data; and ethical considerations. (For more information regarding ACSO guidelines, visit the ASCO Web site: www.asco.org.)

Oncology Nursing Society

The Oncology Nursing Society (ONS) has created guidelines related to nursing care in symptom management and other areas to assist nurses in making proper decisions and helping to educate and manage their patients.

The ONS PEP® (Putting Evidence into Practice) resources are designed to provide evidence-based interventions for patient care and teaching. Interventions can be incorporated into telephone triage, policies and procedures, quality/performance improvement activities, and standards of care and order sets. Information from the ONS PEP® resources can be integrated into orientation, educational programs, and nursing grand rounds.

ONS PEP® topics in symptom management are available for many areas including anxiety, pain, nausea and vomiting, and fatigue for cancer patients. Each outcome, or topic area, provides the levels of evidence for all of the interventions identified. Information is organized according to the categories of levels of evidence as to effectiveness and benefits balanced with harmful effects. Interventions recommended for practice are those for which effectiveness has been demonstrated by strong evidence from rigorously designed studies, meta-analysis, or systematic reviews, and for which expectation of harm is small compared with the benefits. In addition, interventions likely to be effective are those for which effectiveness has been demonstrated from a single rigorously conducted controlled trial, consistent supportive evidence from well-designed controlled trials using small samples, or guidelines developed from evidence and supported by expert opinion. (For more information, visit the ONS Web site: www.ons.org.)

Other Organizations

Numerous other organizations have developed care guidelines for cancer patients. Information regarding these care guidelines or consensus statements from various organizations can be found at the following Web sites:

- Cancer Care Guidelines Repository: www.facs.org/cancer/coc/cocpracguide.html
  The American College of Surgeons Commission on Cancer (CoC) Web site contains a Cancer Care Guidelines Repository that includes guidelines in relation to screening, genetics, counseling, early diagnosis, and prevention strategies, as well as treatment and follow-up of the cancer patient. Their index provides a list of organizations affiliated with the CoC and the cancer care guidelines offered. Inclusion of a care guideline on the CoC Web site does not constitute a guarantee or endorsement of the guidelines by the CoC.
- National Guideline Clearinghouse (NGC): www.guideline.gov
  NGC is a public resource for evidence-based CPG. The NGC is an initiative of the Agency for Healthcare Research and Quality (AHRQ), U.S. Department of Health and Human Services. NGC was originally created by AHRQ in partnership with the American Medical Association and the American Association of Health Plans (now America's Health Insurance Plans). The NGC offers syntheses of selected guidelines that cover similar topic areas, and expert commentary on issues of interest and importance to the clinical guideline community. You can use the NGC Browse feature to search for cancer guidelines. For example, a detailed search by the keyword "colon cancer," sorted by publication date and "Guideline Category" of Management, can be refined by several options including publication date, sex, age of target population, care needs (screening, end of life, etc.) and domain (effectiveness, efficiency, patient-centeredness, safety, timeliness).

Utilizing Guidelines to Monitor and Improve the Quality of Care

With the huge worldwide investment in biomedical research, there are many advances in healthcare knowledge each year, especially in oncology. Translating research into clinical practice has always been slow, taking more than 20 years for even the most important advances to be widely integrated into clinical practice. Many factors are to blame for this dilemma in research transfer, but progress is being made recently mostly because of health informatics systems both for offering electronic care guidelines and measurement data for monitoring the quality of care provided.

Promoting the use of care guidelines has become the focus of many national organizations. The CoC, ACSO, NCCN and others have taken the leadership role by acknowledging shortcomings and providing tools, such as guidelines, to help improve care.

Various certification or accreditation programs require effective use of evidence-based CPG to manage and optimize care.

- *The Joint Commission* has the expectation that healthcare organizations utilize CPG. The Joint Commission's Disease-Specific Care Certification Program launched in 2002 requires that CPG are selected, implemented, and fully integrated into the program. Their certification evaluation process will include assessing the organization's method of delivering clinical care for all appropriate patients according to the CPG. The method must identify outcome performance measures to monitor on an ongoing basis, and the data collected on the performance measures must be used for performance improvement. A **performance measure** is a set of technical specifications that define how to calculate a "rate" for some important indicator of quality. Using these measures, one can determine what their rate is and how they compare with others (benchmarking).

- *The CoC* requires the use of CPG in their Cancer Program accreditation program because they have determined that patient management and treatment guidelines used in treatment decisions promote an organized approach to providing quality care. They first supported the use of the College of American Pathologist (CAP) cancer protocols on eligible pathology reports to include all scientifically validated data elements outlined on the surgical case summary checklist of the CAP publication "Reporting on Cancer Specimens." The guidelines required by the CoC have evolved over the years and now require approved CoC-accredited programs to utilize treatment guidelines developed by nationally recognized organizations such as the NCCN or ASCO. The CoC encourages the use of guidelines when discussing treatment options at Cancer Conferences (Tumor Board) and in conducting retrospective quality studies. The Cancer Committee leadership at the facility is charged with ongoing monitoring of the use of guidelines in treatment decisions and the outcomes of patient care.

Care Guidelines are also being used to pave the way to pay for performance. Pay for performance is an emerging movement in health insurance (initially in Britain and United States) in which providers under this arrangement are rewarded for meeting pre-established targets for delivery of healthcare services. This is a fundamental change from fee-for-service payment. Also known as "P4P" or "value-based purchasing," this payment model rewards physicians, hospitals, medical groups, and other healthcare providers for meeting certain performance measures for quality and efficiency. Disincentives, such as eliminating payments for negative consequences of care (medical errors) or increased costs, have also been proposed. In the developed nations, the rapidly aging population and increasing healthcare costs have recently brought P4P to the forefront of health policy discussions. Pilot studies under way in several large healthcare systems have shown modest improvements in specific outcomes and increased efficiency, but no cost savings because of added administrative requirements. Statements by professional medical societies generally support incentive programs to increase the quality of health care, but express concern with the validity of quality indicators, patient and physician autonomy and privacy, and increased administrative burdens.

CPG are viewed as credible sources of data for what might be considered effective care. However, the literature reviewed states that CPG are primarily designed as tools to broadly inform patient care, rather than to be used as a roadmap for the treatment of a specific patient. CPG have a stated goal to improve quality of care, but many believe that there is significant variability in how quality is defined, and that CPG commonly lack validated quality indicators when used for pay for performance.

Measuring and Reporting on Health Care Quality to the National Cancer Data Base and Others

Healthcare organizations around the world are motivated to deliver the best quality care possible to their members and patients, but they need effective tools to help them achieve this goal.

There are many different approaches to assessing healthcare quality: satisfaction surveys, audits, and clinical performance measurement, to name a few. Many organizations use approaches in a range of accreditation, certification, recognition, and performance measurement programs for different types of organizations, medical groups, and even individual physicians. Gathering and providing quality information is vital to consumers, employers, health plans, hospitals, and doctors so that they can make important healthcare decisions.

The first step in assessing quality of care is establishing what aspects of care are connected to optimal outcomes. Large, carefully designed clinical trials are usually necessary to establish which specific processes of care or treatments are effective, and CPG are developed utilizing evidence-based medicine with clinical expertise. Other types of research in health services also help in defining high-quality care.

Next, observations of current medical practice reveal the extent to which effective care is given or whether CPG were utilized. Measures of quality may assess structural aspects of the healthcare delivery system, process of care, or outcomes of care (e.g., survival, quality of life). Each of these dimensions of quality could be assessed to provide information on quality care.

Developing a measure is a multistep process. It involves identifying the clinical area to evaluate; conducting an extensive literature review; developing the measure with the appropriate expert panel of physicians and others; inspection by various stakeholders; and performing a field test that looks at feasibility, reliability, and validity.

Nationally recognized quality measures have been developed over the years and are available from many organizations including the Hospital Quality Alliance (HQA), National Committee for Quality Assurance (NCQA), and the Joint Commission.

- Hospital Quality Alliance (HQA): www.hospital qualityalliance.org
  In December 2002, the organizations representing America's hospitals joined with consumer representatives, physician and nursing organizations, employers and payers, oversight organizations, and government agencies to launch the HQA. The HQA is a national public-private collaboration that is committed to making meaningful, relevant, and easily understood information about hospital performance accessible to the public and to informing and encouraging efforts to improve quality.

  The HQA believes that the availability and use of clinical quality, patient experience, equity, efficiency, and pricing information will spur positive changes in healthcare delivery. A cornerstone of their collaboration is Hospital Compare (www.hospitalcompare.hhs .gov), which publicly reports hospital performance in a consistent, unified manner to ensure the availability of credible information about the care delivered in the nation's hospitals.
- National Committee for Quality Assurance Healthcare Effectiveness Data and Information Set (NCQA-HEDIS): www.ncqa.org

The NCQA is a private, not-for-profit organization dedicated to improving healthcare quality. Since its founding in 1990, NCQA has been a central figure in driving improvement throughout the healthcare system, helping to elevate the issue of healthcare quality to the top of the national agenda. NCQA has helped to build consensus around important healthcare quality issues by working with large employers, policy makers, doctors, patients, and health plans to decide what's important, how to measure it, and how to promote improvement. Organizations participating must pass a rigorous, comprehensive review and must annually report on their performance. The HEDIS is a tool used by more than 90% of America's health plans to measure performance on important dimensions of care and service.

- The Joint Commission: www.jointcommission.org/ PerformanceMeasurement
  The Joint Commission is a recognized international leader with a long-proven ability to identify, test, and specify standardized performance measures. It engages in cutting edge performance measurement research and development activities, and has established successful, ongoing, collaborative relationships with key performance measurement entities. The Joint Commission presides over a growing, national, comparative performance measurement database that can inform internal healthcare organization quality improvement activities, external accountability, pay for performance programs, and advance research.
- National Quality Measures Clearinghouse (NQMC): www.qualitymeasures.ahrq.gov
  NQMC, sponsored by the AHRQ, U.S. Department of Health and Human Services, is a database and Web site for information on specific evidence-based healthcare quality measures and measure sets. The NQMC mission is to provide practitioners, healthcare providers, health plans, integrated delivery systems, purchasers, and others an accessible mechanism for obtaining detailed information on quality measures, and to further their dissemination, implementation, and use to inform health care decisions. NQMC builds on AHRQ's previous initiatives in quality measurement, including the Computerized Needs-Oriented Quality Measurement Evaluation System (CONQUEST), the Expansion of Quality of Care Measures (Q-SPAN) project, and the Quality Measurement Network (QMNet) project.

Quality Measures for Cancer Care

Despite the considerable advances in the diagnosis, treatment, and palliation of life-threatening cancers, some patients will receive suboptimal care that leads to the loss of years of life, decreased quality of life, and the placing of an unnecessarily increased burden on their families and communities. A significant first step to improve these deficiencies would be consensus on a standardized set of performance measures to assess the quality of cancer care. Implementation of consensus standards for cancer care would provide critical information for both public accountability and internal quality.

The National Cancer Institute has made improving the quality of cancer care a major priority (see the Nation's Investment in Cancer Research). An important element of this priority area is identifying, developing, applying, and evaluating quality-of-care measures. The centerpiece of the effort to identify a core set of quality measures is the Cancer Quality of Care Measures Project. In this project, NCI is collaborating with other federal agencies, a number of private sector organizations, and the nonprofit National Quality Forum (NQF) to identify evidence-based quality measures for diagnosing and treating certain major types of cancer.

The NQF has brought together payers, consumers, researchers, and clinicians to disseminate performance measures. This private, nonprofit membership organization was created in 1999 to develop and implement a national strategy for healthcare quality measurement and reporting. Its mission is to improve the quality of American health care by setting national priorities and goals for performance improvement, endorsing national consensus standards for measuring and publicly reporting on performance, and promoting the attainment of national goals through education and outreach programs. (See their Phase I and II projects.)

The two-phase Cancer Care project began in 2002 when NQF convened a steering committee to address cancer care quality measures. The committee recommended seven priority areas for initial attention on identifying a core set of cancer care quality measures: access to care/critical trials/cultural competence; diagnosis and treatment of breast cancer; diagnosis and treatment of colorectal cancer; communication and coordination of care, including information technology issues; prevention/screening; diagnosis and treatment of prostate cancer; and symptom management/end-of-life care. While the committee's work resulted in no formally endorsed measures, its efforts led to the Cancer Care Phase II project.

The NQF Cancer Care Phase II project started in August 2004 was a continuation of the work begun in Cancer Care Phase I. In 2008, NQF endorsed 19 performance measures for gauging the quality of cancer care in the areas of breast cancer, colorectal cancer, symptom management, and end-of-life care. These performance measures for cancer care are at the institutional level (e.g., hospitals, health plans) but not at the individual level.

Measures for Breast and Colorectal Cancer

The public/private partnership led by the NQF brought together payers, consumers, researchers, and clinicians to disseminate performance measures for breast and colorectal cancer. The CoC has been actively engaged in this process. The *e-QuIPs* for breast and colorectal cancers were first released in 2006/2007 in anticipation of the NQF's endorsement of a number of specific measures to assist CoC-approved cancer programs in preparing for the implementation of these quality-focused measures. Through a parallel process, the ASCO and the NCCN developed a similar set of measures for breast and colorectal cancer. Facilitated by the NQF, the CoC, ASCO, and NCCN agreed to synchronize their developed measures to ensure that a unified set were put forth to the public. Breast and colon cancer quality measures include the following:

- Radiation therapy is administered within 1 year (365 days) of diagnosis for women younger than 70 receiving breast-conserving surgery for breast cancer.
- Combination chemotherapy is considered or administered within 4 months (120 days) of diagnosis for women younger than 70 with American Joint Committee on Cancer (AJCC) T1cN0M0, or Stage II or III hormone-receptor–negative breast cancer.
- Tamoxifen *or* third-generation aromatase inhibitor is considered or administered within 1 year (365 days) of diagnosis for women with AJCC T1cN0M0, or Stage II or III hormone-receptor–positive breast cancer.
- Adjuvant chemotherapy is considered or administered within 4 months (120 days) of diagnosis for patients younger than 80 with AJCC Stage III (lymph-node–positive) colon cancer.

The full specifications for the breast and colorectal quality of cancer measures can be found on the CoC Web site (www.facs.org/cancer/qualitymeasures.html).

Measurement Data Collection and Analysis

Providing high-quality care to cancer patients is paramount, but obtaining reliable data about the care provided can be a challenge. Standardized data collection for quality measures is vital for meaningful analysis. Once the measurement data are collected, evaluation of the data are necessary to identify variances from CPG or other quality measures. Internally, this analysis is performed by the Cancer Committee in CoC-approved cancer programs. Data submitted to national organizations can be used for benchmarking to other organizations.

Sources of Measurement Data and National Benchmarking: NCDB and CP3R

For years, the only reliable data collection source was the hospital's Cancer Registry. The Cancer Registry can provide measurement data to assess how CPG are being followed or to monitor other aspects of care. However, a shortcoming with the registry data for use as a quality monitoring system is the time delays. Abstracting the data normally is between 5 and 6 months from the date first seen at the facility. To remedy this issue for the future, registries need to move toward real-time reporting to allow quick analysis of efficiency, variance, and quality.

In CoC-approved facilities, the Cancer Registry data are submitted annually to the National Cancer Data Base (NCDB). The NCDB maintains a number of Web-based benchmarking applications that have been developed to promote access to NCDB data by the general public, researchers, and clinicians. The NCDB Benchmark Reports have been released in two formats: one designed explicitly to facilitate public use; a second for use by CoC-approved cancer programs as a tool by which to evaluate and compare the cancer care delivered to patients diagnosed and/or treated at their facility versus state, regional, and national levels.

The CoC's Cancer Program Practice Profile Reports (CP3R) provide feedback to the CoC-accredited cancer programs on their performance to the breast and colorectal cancer quality measures. The CP3R(v2) for breast and colorectal cancer is directed toward assuring the completeness of data is recorded in each cancer program's Cancer Registry. Once the data are complete, it can then facilitate accurate comparisons of clinical performance among CoC-accredited cancer programs. Beginning in 2009, CoC Accreditation Standard 4.6 required the cancer committee, or equivalent body, to review and monitor the reported quality of care provided to patients with breast and colorectal cancer at their facility using the CP3R(v2) reporting tool. CoC-accredited cancer programs are expected to use these reports to guide cancer committee efforts in their assessment and examination of data accuracy and completeness.

Other Sources of Measurement Data and National Benchmarking

Although the cancer registry database is a useful tool to provide data for measuring compliance to many patient care guidelines and other quality measures, other sources of data and reporting tools have been developed by other professional organizations to capture data for monitoring.

Medical Oncologists participating in ASCO's Quality Oncology Practice Initiative (QOPI®) submit practice performance data for self-assessment and quality improvement. The process used for improving cancer care includes measurement, feedback, and improvement tools for hematology-oncology practices.

Radiation oncologists can participate in the quality improvement program developed by the American Society of Therapeutic Radiology and Oncology (ASTRO). ASTRO's Performance Assessment for the Advancement of Radiation Oncology Treatment program (PAAROT) includes a process for data collection, reporting, and comparison with peers. It involves periodic chart review and reporting on technical and outcomes measures, which are compared with a national database of peer responses, expert consensus, and evidence-based guidelines and national benchmarks. Since its launch in 2008, more than 400 radiation oncologists have taken part in ASTRO's quality improvement program.

Summary

The CPG can be an important tool used to support the decision-making process in patient care and in translating new research findings into clinical practice. CPG, based on standardized best practice, have been shown to be capable of supporting improvements in quality and consistency in health care. Many national oncology-related organizations are involved in developing cancer care guidelines, but the most comprehensive and most frequently updated and utilized are the NCCN guidelines.

Promoting the use of CPG has become the focus of many national organizations including the Joint Commission and the CoC, both of which require utilization of CPG for certification or accreditation. CPG are viewed as credible sources for developing quality measures of care. Although the CPG are being used increasingly to set practice standards and in pay for performance, we need to reinforce the guidelines are not for "cookbook medicine"; they cannot replace individual clinical expertise, nor can they function in the absence of patient-specific information regarding comorbid disease, individual preferences, and available resources.

Establishing meaningful quality measures has been slow, but progress has been made. The public/private partnership led by the NQF brought together payers, consumers, researchers, and clinicians to disseminate performance measures for breast and colorectal cancer. With the rapidly changing healthcare environment, performance measurement must be expanded in a national collaborative effort. To facilitate achievement of the Cancer Registry as a useful tool in collecting and providing quality measurement data, we must find ways to produce complete, accurate, and timely data that can be monitored internally and externally for evaluating quality cancer care.

In CoC-accredited cancer programs, the Cancer Registry data are submitted to the NCDB. The CoC's CP3R provides feedback to the CoC-accredited cancer programs on their performance to the breast and colorectal cancers quality measures. Participation in other quality improvement programs such as ASCO's QOPI® can provide other sources of measurement data for national benchmarking and comparison with CPG.

Reference

1. IOM. *Clinical Practice Guidelines: Directions for a New Program* (p. 38). M.J. Field and K.N. Lohr, eds. Washington, D.C.: National Academy Press, 1990.

chapter 27

Uses of Central Cancer Registry Data

Tom C. Tucker, PhD, MPH

Jaclyn K. Nee, MPH

Previous chapters have described the use of hospital-based cancer registry data[s1]. These include the creation of management reports (see Chapter 22), calculating statistics (see Chapter 24), evaluation of hospital-based survival rates (see Chapter 25), and determining the degree to which hospital patients are treated according to patient care guidelines (see Chapter 26). This chapter focuses on the use of central cancer registry data. Central cancer registry data are different from hospital cancer registry data in that the central cancer registry data represent the cancer experience of the whole population, whereas hospital cancer registry data represent the cancer experience of only those patients who were diagnosed or treated at that hospital. In other words, it would not be possible to calculate a cancer incidence rate for an entire state or even a subsection of a state using the data from a single hospital because not all of the cancer patients were seen at that hospital. In contrast, the hospital registry data are an excellent source of information on the quality and effectiveness of cancer care at that institution. Thus, this chapter focuses on how central cancer registry data are used to understand cancer in whole or defined populations.

Before data from a central cancer registry can truly reflect the burden of disease in a population, it must be complete, accurate, and collected in a timely manner. However, population-based data are of little or no value unless they are used for cancer research or cancer control. The ultimate value of central cancer registries lies not in the complete and accurate collection of data about cancer cases, but rather in the degree to which this information is used and useful. It can be argued that when complete and accurate information contained in a central cancer registry is not used for cancer research or cancer control, the process of organizing, implementing, and operating a central cancer registry is less than justified.

There are two primary uses of central cancer registry data: The first is for population-based research and the second is for cancer control.

Using Central Cancer Registry Data for Research

Central cancer registry data have been used for population-based research for many years. However, in recent years, there has been increased interest in using central cancer registry data to understand issues of external validity.[1] Traditionally, randomized trials have been considered the "gold standard" of science for determining whether one treatment or intervention is better than another. These studies provide excellent internal validity.[1] In other words, randomizing patients to a standard treatment or a new experimental treatment provides a framework that allows researchers to determine whether the new experimental

treatment is better than the current standard of care. Similarly, randomizing eligible subjects to one of two different cancer control intervention strategies provides a framework that allows researchers to determine which strategy is most effective. Although randomized trials have strong internal validity, they do not provide strong external validity. The results from randomized trials that show one treatment or intervention being more effective than another almost never show the same effectiveness when they are applied to an entire population. One reason for this is that the people who participate in randomized trials are not the same as those who do not participate in randomized trials.[2] Thus, in 2004, the U.S. Food and Drug Administration began requiring large population-based studies after randomized clinical trials to determine how well new treatments worked when they were made available to entire populations.[3] At the same time, and for similar reasons, cancer control researchers began to do population-based studies of interventions that were shown to be efficacious in randomized trials. These changes have contributed to an increased demand for and use of central cancer registry data for cancer control research.

Definition of Population-Based Cancer Prevention and Control Research

The National Cancer Institute (NCI) has defined cancer prevention and control research as "the conduct of basic and applied research in the behavioral, social, and population sciences to create or enhance interventions that, independently or in combination with biomedical approaches, reduce cancer risk, incidence, morbidity and mortality."[4]

There are many examples of using central cancer registry data for cancer prevention and control research. These can be grouped into the following categories:

1. Primary prevention and chemoprevention research[5]
2. Biomarkers, screening, and early detection studies[6]
3. Patterns of care research (sometimes referred to as outcomes or population-based treatment research)[7]
4. Survivorship research[8]

Each of these four categories can be and are examined from a number of perspectives. For example, disparities in receiving access to primary prevention programs, screening, treatment, and survivorship can be studied. Disparities also can be explained by a number of dimensions (i.e., age, sex, race/ethnicity, place, etc.).[9–12] Central cancer registry data have been and continue to be used in studies related to all of these categories, perspectives, and dimensions. However, two new and emerging areas of research that are now using central cancer registry data include policy research and gene/environment interaction studies.

Changes in policy such as laws that prohibit or restrict smoking in public places or laws that increase the tax on cigarettes have been shown through population-based studies to have a strong impact on smoking.[13,14] By using central cancer registry data, changes in the lung cancer incidence rates can be monitored after the implementation of new policies that restrict smoking.

Gene-environment interaction studies are important to understand how environmental exposures contribute to the onset of cancer. However, these studies have historically been difficult to do. More recently, central cancer registry data have been used to make these studies possible. One example is a population-based colon cancer case–control study that is exploring how exposure to arsenic (and other metals) works either through oxidative stress or DNA damage to result in colon cancer. This study used the central cancer registry to identify and recruit all of the colon cancer cases that were then matched to control subjects by age, sex, and place (county of residence).[15] Identifying biologic or genetic factors that are present more frequently among the cases who have high exposure to arsenic compared with the control subjects who have high exposure provides a structure for identifying biologic factors that are associated with the onset of cancer.

The list of studies using central cancer registry data that have been done and have been essential to understanding cancer and cancer control is far too numerous to list here. However, it is important to note that central cancer registry data has been essential to all of these research efforts, and without the central cancer registry data, none of these studies would have been possible.

Using Central Cancer Registry Data for Cancer Control

Although the use of central cancer registry data for research has been essential for advancing our understanding of cancer, the use of central cancer registry data for cancer control is equally important. The following section explores the definition of cancer control, provides a model for using central cancer registry data to target and evaluate cancer control activities, discusses limitations associated with using central cancer registry data for cancer control, and provides an example of how central cancer registry data can be combined with other sources of data to target and evaluate cancer control programs.

Definition of Cancer Control

The term *cancer control* has become increasingly popular since the passage of the U.S. National Cancer Act in 1971 and the establishment of a Division of Cancer Prevention and Control (DCPC) within the NCI. Both the concept of cancer control and its definition have evolved since that time. The DCPC has defined *cancer control* as "the reduction of cancer incidence, mortality, and morbidity through an orderly sequence from research on interventions and

their impact in defined populations to the broad systematic application of the research results."[16] This definition combines cancer control and cancer control research.

Stjernsward and Parkin define *cancer control* as having the following six phases:

"(1) primary prevention. Actions taken to reduce human exposure to agents that may cause cancer or to reduce genetic predisposition to cancer;

(2) screening. Actions directed towards asymptomatic people with the objective of identifying those at high risk of development of symptomatic cancer (e.g. genetically susceptible, possess a precancerous lesion or in situ cancer, possess an early invasive cancer) for whom some program of continuing screening, diagnosis, and/or therapy may reduce the subsequent morbidity or mortality from cancer;

(3) early diagnosis. Actions taken to increase the probability that a person with a symptomatic cancer will have that cancer diagnosed at a stage when treatment is likely to result in a cure;

(4) treatment. Actions taken in a patient with a diagnosed cancer which have a cure of the cancer as their objective;

(5) palliative care. Actions taken in a patient who has cancer that cannot be cured, which have continuing maximization of the patient's physical, mental, and social well-being as their objective."[17]

More recently, the Centers for Disease Control and Prevention (CDC) has defined *comprehensive cancer control* as "an integrated and coordinated approach to reducing cancer incidence, morbidity, and mortality through prevention (primary prevention), early detection (secondary prevention), treatment, rehabilitation and palliation."[18] The CDC definition incorporates the basic concepts originally laid out by Stjernsward and Parkin.

A working definition that combines the elements from all three of these contributions to the concept of cancer control is as follows:

> *The use of evidence-based prevention, early detection, diagnosis, treatment, and continuing care intervention strategies to reduce cancer incidence, morbidity, and mortality in defined populations.*

This definition of cancer control is represented in Figure 27-1.

Figure 27-1 suggests that the opportunities for cancer control can occur along the continuum from good health through the development and clinical manifestation of cancer to the treatment and continuing care of patients with cancer.

The ultimate goal of cancer control activities is to prevent the carcinogenic process from developing. This is often referred to as *primary prevention*.[19] Activities directed toward persuading people not to smoke or helping smokers

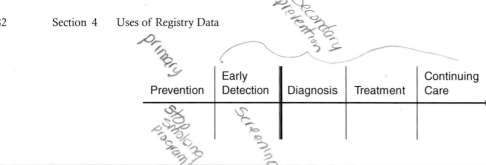

Figure 27-1. Phases of Cancer Control

quit are examples of primary prevention because, if successful, these cancer control activities are likely to result in a reduction in the incidence (occurrence) of lung cancer.

Unfortunately, primary prevention for many types of cancer is not yet possible. However, significant reductions in both morbidity and mortality can be obtained through early detection and prompt treatment. Cancer control activities that result in a cure, in slowing disease progression, in preventing complications, and/or in limiting disability are referred to as *secondary prevention*.[19] Screening programs designed to identify breast cancer at an early, more curable stage are examples of cancer control programs aimed at secondary prevention. Screening for two types of cancer (colorectal and cervical) can contribute to both primary prevention, by finding precancerous disease and removing it before the cancer occurs, and secondary prevention, by finding early-stage cancer for which treatments are more effective.

Cancer control activities focused on prevention or early detection (those to the left of the bold vertical line in Figure 27-1) are usually directed at lay populations. Those activities that effectively motivate individuals in a population to reduce their risk behavior or to present themselves at appropriate healthcare facilities for screening/early detection procedures should result in either primary or secondary prevention. In this regard, healthcare providers have an important role in reminding and encouraging the public to participate in cancer risk reduction activities and in screening programs.

If cancer control programs result in the early detection of disease, but patients are not diagnosed and treated appropriately, we still do not achieve our cancer control objectives. Cancer control activities directed at improving diagnosis, treatment, and/or continuing care (those to the right of the bold vertical line in Figure 27-1) are directed primarily at healthcare providers. Because their ability to manage most cancers effectively is largely dependent on finding the disease at an early stage, emphasis has been placed on improving our detection and diagnosis capability so treatment can be instituted when it is most effective (i.e., for early-stage disease).[20] However, effective treatment at any stage can potentially reduce morbidity or mortality rates, or both. Thus, most cancer control programs are also concerned with ensuring that patients in any stage of cancer have access to state-of-the art care. The importance of these activities was emphasized in the 1999 Institute of Medicine report on "Ensuring Quality Cancer Care."[21]

In 2009, an estimated 1,479,350 new cases of cancer (exclusive of carcinoma in situ and nonmelanomatous skin cancers) were diagnosed. In this same year, approximately 562,340 patients died of cancer. The American Cancer Society estimates that nearly 150,000 lives could be saved annually through effective cancer control efforts directed at primary prevention, and more than 100,000 lives could be saved annually through effective cancer control efforts aimed at early detection and prompt treatment.[22] Thus, cancer control, defined as "the use of evidence-based prevention, early detection, diagnosis, treatment, and continuing care intervention strategies to reduce cancer incidence, morbidity, and mortality in defined populations," is an important healthcare activity.

What is striking and important about this definition of cancer control is its implications for the use of central cancer registry data at all phases of the cancer control continuum. Muir et al.[23] state, "The cancer registry is an essential part of any rational programme of cancer control." If we do not know how often each type of cancer occurs within a specific population, how do we know where to focus our efforts and prioritize the use of our limited cancer control resources? How will we know that our primary prevention efforts have had any effect if we do not know how often the disease was diagnosed before and after our intervention efforts? How can we determine whether cases are being found earlier in a population if we do not know the proportion with early- and late-stage diagnoses before and after our intervention?

In other words, the concept of measuring where specific cancers occur, in whom these diseases occur, the stage at the time of diagnosis, and whether any changes in cancer rates take place over time, is inherent in the definition of *cancer control*.

It is, in fact, difficult to imagine any effective cancer control efforts that do not rely on some type of data collection and analysis. Without the type of information contained in most central cancer registries, how could we know which types of people (men, women; older, younger; black, white; etc.) are a greater risk for specific types of cancer, and how would we know which geographic areas have greater rates of cancer or greater rates of cancer diagnosed at later stages? It is the central cancer registry that provides the mechanism for answering these and related questions.

Thus, the population-based central cancer registry is an integral part of the cancer control process. It provides the means to target our limited cancer control resources at the groups within the population that are at greatest risk for specific types of cancer and allows us to focus on particular geographic areas. At the same time, central cancer registries provide the mechanism for evaluating the effectiveness of our cancer control activities. In essence, the central cancer registry represents the eyes of our cancer control program. Without these eyes, it would not be possible to see our cancer control problems, and we could not see the impact of our cancer control activities.

A Model for Cancer Control

The central cancer registry is clearly an essential component of any cancer control program. When the registry (the "eyes" of the cancer control program) and the organizations from the community that can plan and implement appropriate interventions (the "hands" of the cancer control program) are combined, they form a complete system for cancer control. This model is illustrated in Figure 27-2.

The model has four essential steps. First, incidence data from the central cancer registry together with demographic data, risk factor data, and mortality data, are used to identify variations in the burden of cancer by geography and by characteristic of person. In other words, for cancers where a proven intervention exists, data from the central cancer registry can be used to identify geographic areas with higher than normal incidence rates. Data from the central cancer registry can also be used to identify geographic areas that have a larger than expected proportion of patients diagnosed with advanced (late-stage) disease. These analyses help to identify which areas and which groups are in greatest need for intervention programs.

The second step requires that information about the burden of cancer in specific geographic areas be presented to organizations that can appropriately plan and implement intervention programs. These organizations should include individuals who can identify the target populations that are at greatest risk and develop intervention strategies that are sensitive to the culture, language, and literacy of the selected target population(s).

The third step is the implementation of the intervention plan. The intervention plan is of no value and cannot have an impact unless it is effectively implemented. Like the process of planning the intervention, the implementation of the plan must also be sensitive to the culture, language, and literacy of the target population. Having local people and community organizations actively participate in selecting the target population, designing the intervention, and implementing the intervention helps to ensure sensitivity to language, culture, and literacy issues.

Finally, incidence data from the central cancer registry, together with risk factor data and mortality data, are used to determine whether the cancer control interventions have been successful. The importance of evaluating the impact of an intervention cannot be overstated. Without this step, it is unclear whether the efforts have had any meaningful impact. When data about the effectiveness of cancer control interventions are taken back to the organizations that implemented the intervention, it forms a self-correcting system. In other words, the interventions can be modified if they are not effective; if they have been effective, new cancer control programs can be selected.

The four steps depicted in Figure 27-2 can be summarized as follows:

1. Identify the burden of cancer in geographic areas and by characteristic of person (Measure).
2. Share this information with community organizations so they can select target populations and plan appropriate intervention programs (Plan).
3. Implement the intervention plan (Act).
4. Measure whether the desired changes occurred (Measure).

It should be clear from this discussion that central cancer registries are an essential component of any meaningful cancer control program. However, there are important limitations associated with using data from central cancer registries for cancer control. The next section in this chapter discusses some of these limitations.

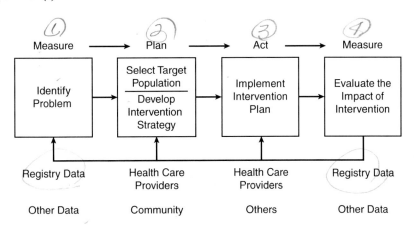

Figure 27-2. Model for Cancer Control

Limitations

Screening Effect

Care must be used when comparing the incidence rates for specific cancers that are sensitive to screening. It is always possible that aggressive screening practices were implemented in one area and not in another. For example, if one county has implemented an effective breast cancer screening program using mammography and another county has not effectively promoted the use of mammography screening, the county with the effective screening program will have a greater breast cancer incidence rate compared with the county that did not promote breast cancer screening. The difference in these two breast cancer rates is a result of screening for the disease in one population and not in the other. This difference is referred to as the *screening effect*.

Data from a central cancer registry can be used to identify areas (populations) that are not adequately screened. This can be done by calculating the cancer incidence rates for early- and late-stage disease separately in each area (population) to be compared. Areas that have high rates of both early- and late-stage disease may have recently implemented a screening program. In other words, when you look for the disease, you find new cases of both early- and late-stage disease. In contrast, areas that have low rates of early-stage disease and high rates of late-stage disease are thought to have minimal or inadequate screening.

Small Numbers

Cancer is clearly a significant health issue. However, specific cancers in small populations can be viewed as rare events. When a small number of cancer cases occur in a population, incidence rates calculated using these cases are considered unstable. In other words, incidence rates calculated using a few cases can vary greatly from one year to the next. For example, if a community of 1 million people had 1,000 new primary cases of lung cancer, the crude lung cancer incidence rate would be $1,000/1,000,000 \times 100,000$, or 100 lung cancer cases per 100,000 population. In contrast, if a community of 1,000 had only two new primary lung cancer cases, the crude lung cancer incidence rate would be twice that of the community with 1 million population ($2/1,000 \times 100,000$, or 200 lung cancer cases per 100,000 population). Notably, this difference in rates is accounted for by only one case. If the community with 1,000 population had experienced only one new primary case of lung cancer, their lung cancer incidence rate would be exactly the same as the community with 1 million population. On the other hand, if the smaller community had three primary lung cancer cases, their rate would be three times that for the community with 1 million. In general, cancer incidence rates calculated with less than 16 incident cases are considered unstable.[24]

Identifying Specific Populations at Risk

Cancer control programs often want to know whether the cancer incidence rates for specific racial or ethnic groups are different. This is important because it allows cancer control programs to focus their limited resources on the groups that are at greatest risk. Central cancer registries are usually able to identify the number of new primary cancer cases by race or ethnicity (the numerator). Unfortunately, it is increasingly difficult to determine the number of people living in the population who are of a specific race or ethnic group (the denominator). In the United States, the census is taken once every 10 years. Estimates of changes in the population are made for the years in between each census. Ethnic groups that may have significant numbers of undocumented individuals are particularly difficult to identify. Thus, the numbers in many of these groups are substantially undercounted, and the estimates may be inaccurate. In addition, the U.S. Census before 2000 asked individuals to identify the racial or ethnic group they most identified with. However, in the 2000 U.S. Census, individuals were given the opportunity to check multiple racial or ethnic groups that they believed they were part of.[25] Thus, some individuals were identified as being part of more than one racial or ethnic group. This has made it difficult to correctly determine the number of people in a specific racial or ethnic group living in a defined geographic area. It is not possible to accurately calculate the incidence rate (risk) of cancer for any of these special populations without knowing the number of people who are part of each special population living in a specific area.

Nature and Complexity of Cancer

Cancer is not one disease. Rather, the word *cancer* represents a group of different diseases that are classified together. These diseases are characterized by abnormal (uncontrolled) cell growth that can spread to other parts of the body and, if unchecked, can lead to death. Unlike infectious diseases, which are generally caused by a single pathogen (bacterium or virus), cancers have multiple factors that can lead to the onset of disease. Furthermore, these factors are different for each specific type of cancer. Factors that lead to the onset of cancer can be grouped into three broad categories: genetic, environmental, and lifestyle. A genetic predisposition to develop cancer is inherited. Environmental factors that increase one's risk for development of a specific cancer are exposures to elements that are exogenous (outside of our control). Lifestyle factors that increase our risk of cancer are those behaviors over which we have some control (smoking, diet, exercise, etc.)

Most of the audiences that cancer control programs are aimed toward do not understand the complex nature of the diseases that are classified together under the label *cancer*. Furthermore, individuals who develop cancer do not want their disease to be a consequence of their behaviors (lifestyle) or their genetics. Rather, individuals who have cancer often believe (or want to believe) that the cause of their cancer is exposure to something in the environment. However, there is substantial evidence that the onset of most cancers can be attributed to lifestyle behaviors or lifestyle behaviors in combination with a genetic predisposition for the disease and/or environmental exposures.[26] When data from the central cancer registry are used to help community organizations identify the specific cancers that present the greatest risk for their community, it is important to carefully and clearly describe known risk factors. If community organizations are not aware of known risk factors, they may attempt to develop interventions that are not appropriately focused.

A Process for Using Data for Cancer Control in Kentucky

The Kentucky Cancer Registry (KCR) is the official population-based central cancer registry for the Commonwealth of Kentucky. The registry is part of a comprehensive, statewide cancer control program. The 120 counties in the state are grouped into 15 area development districts (ADDs). District cancer councils have been formed in each of the ADDs. The cancer councils include public health workers, American Cancer Society staff, healthcare providers, cancer patients, and other interested individuals from the community. In addition, special efforts have been made to include individuals on the cancer councils who represent vulnerable, at-risk populations such as those with low literacy or limited resources. Once a year, data from the KCR are combined with census data, Behavioral Risk Factor Surveillance System (BRFSS) data, and mortality data to create an index of the burden of cancer for each of the major cancers for which evidence-based intervention strategies are available (lung, breast, and colorectal). These data are combined at the ADD level and presented to each district cancer council. The district cancer councils use this information to determine what type of cancer control interventions might be most effective or needed and which specific groups of individuals the interventions should be targeted toward.

This process is a working example of the model for cancer control presented earlier in this chapter. In Kentucky, the focus has been on three major cancers (lung, breast, and colorectal). These three cancers represent 45% of all new cancers diagnosed annually in Kentucky, and there are evidence-based cancer control intervention strategies for each of these cancers. The four data sources (U.S. Census data, BRFSS data, central cancer registry data, and vital records mortality data) were selected because they are available in nearly all of the states and territories. Thus, this model can easily be replicated in other areas. The specific variables collected from these sources include the percentage of people in each ADD below the U.S. poverty level and the percentage of those age 25 or older in each ADD with a high-school education (U.S. Census), screening rates and smoking rates (BRFSS), age-adjusted incidence rates and the proportion of people in each ADD diagnosed with late-stage disease (central cancer registry data), and age-adjusted mortality rates (vital records mortality data).

Figure 27-3 shows how the sources of data are related and why combining these data sources can be useful in determining the burden of cancer. The logic model states that demographic characteristics of a population (literacy and poverty) contribute to risk behaviors (either smoking or not getting screened). These risk behaviors, in turn, contribute to the incidence of cancer or the stage at diagnosis, or both. Finally, the incidence and stage at diagnosis contribute to mortality from the disease.

The logic model and the relations between the data sources can be further explained by examining lung cancer in the 15 ADDs in Kentucky. Figure 27-4 shows the percentage of the population living below the poverty level, the percentage of the population with a high-school education, the percentage of people in the population who are current smokers, the lung cancer incidence rate, the proportion of the lung cancer patients diagnosed with late-stage disease,

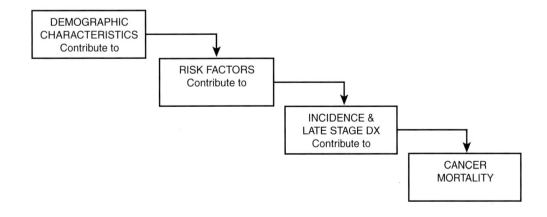

Figure 27-3. Logic Model for Combining Multiple Data Sources

Area Development District	Under Poverty Level (%)	High School + Education (%)	Current Smoker (%)	Age-Adjusted Incidence		Late Stage Incidence (%)	Age-Adjusted Mortality	
				N	Adj. Rate		N	Adj. Rate
US	12.4	80.4	23.1	107922	59	82.5	788812	54.1
KENTUCKY	15.8	74.1	30.1	21568	101.3	80.6	16701	78.89
BARREN RIVER	16.7	70.3	31.9	1358	99.24	78.2	1106	81.13
BIG SANDY	27.9	59.6	35.1	1031	123.57	81.1	794	96.3
BLUEGRASS	13.1	79.0	27.5	3192	95.88	80.9	2479	75.2
BUFFALO TRACE	19.6	66.6	33.5	314	100.6	83.2	239	76.85
CUMBERLAND VALLEY	29.1	58.0	34.8	1444	114.5	79.4	1135	90.48
FIVCO	18.8	71.2	32.7	846	104.83	81.6	674	84.21
GATEWAY	21.2	65.0	32.4	382	95.81	83.6	295	74.45
GREEN RIVER	13.7	77.1	30.5	1146	99.1	80.1	924	79.93
KENTUCKY RIVER	31.0	56.0	35.3	843	131.7	85.4	698	110.95
KIPDA	11.5	81.3	27.9	4575	100.17	80.2	3445	75.8
LAKE CUMBERLAND	23.0	61.3	31	1221	103.48	77.4	946	80.06
LINCOLN TRAIL	12.9	76.1	30.8	1101	90.99	79.4	798	67.18
NORTHERN KENTUCKY	9.0	80.6	28.5	1883	102.17	81.6	1444	79.04
PENNYRILE	15.9	71.7	31.6	1132	97.39	82.1	892	76.45
PURCHASE	15.0	77.1	28.9	1100	91.12	82.5	832	68.3

Figure 27-4. Data from Each Source by Area Development District Compared with the State and the United States

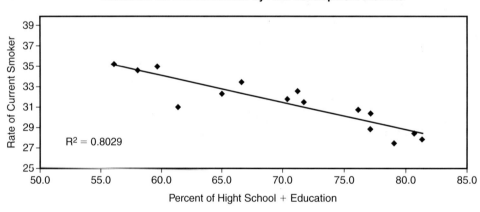

Education vs. Current Smoker by Area Development Districts

$R^2 = 0.8029$

Figure 27-5. Relation between Demographic Characteristic and Risk Behavior

and the lung cancer mortality rate for the United States, Kentucky, and each ADD. These data are for the 5-year period from 2001 to 2005.

All of the data for each variable are included in the table in Figure 27-4. However, for these data to be more useful, they need to be converted into information that can be used by the district cancer councils to better understand the burden of lung cancer in their ADD. The relation between the proportion of the population of people in each ADD with a high-school degree (education) and the proportion of people in each ADD who smoke (risk behavior) is illustrated in the following regression model (Figure

27-5). As the percentage of those who have a high-school education increases, the percentage of those who smoke decreases. In other words, the ADDs with the greatest rates of smoking have the lowest percentages of people with a high-school education. The correlation between education and the smoking rate is nearly 80.3%.

The relation between risk behavior (smoking) and the incidence of lung cancer is shown in Figure 27-6. As the rate of smoking increases in each ADD, the lung cancer incidence rates also increase.

Finally, Figure 27-7 illustrates the relation between the lung cancer incidence rate in each ADD and the lung can-

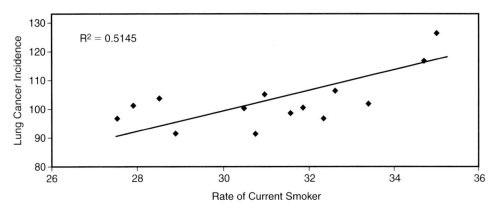

Figure 27-6. Relation between Risk Behavior and Lung Cancer Incidence

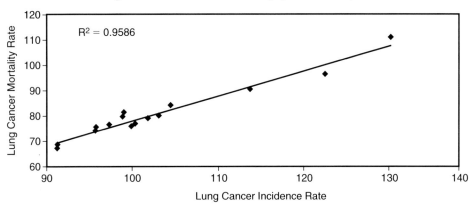

Figure 27-7. Relation between Lung Cancer Incidence and Mortality

cer mortality rate in each ADD. As the incidence rate of lung cancer increases, so does the lung cancer mortality rate. The correlation between incidence and mortality of lung cancer is almost 96%.

Because the data are highly correlated, the sources of data can be combined to create an index of the lung cancer burden in each of the ADDs. The index is created using a simple rank-sum technique. Each ADD is ranked from 1 to 15 for each of the 4 data items (education, smoking, lung cancer incidence, and lung cancer mortality). A 1 (the lowest rank) is assigned to the ADDs with the lowest percentage of those with a high-school education, the greatest percentage of current smokers, the greatest lung cancer incidence rate, and the greatest lung cancer mortality rate. Conversely, a 15 (the highest rank) is assigned to the ADDs with the greatest percentage of those with a high-school education, the lowest percentage of current smokers, the lowest lung cancer incidence rate and the lowest lung cancer mortality rate. Once all 15 ADDs have been ranked for each of the 4 data sources, an overall rank or index is created by summing the 4 ranks assigned for each ADD. The ADDs that have the lowest

overall rank have the highest burden of lung cancer and are in greatest need for an intervention program, whereas the ADDs with the highest overall rank have the lowest burden of lung cancer relative to the other ADDs. The 15 ADDs in Kentucky are categorized into three groups (high burden, medium burden, and lower burden). Each group contains five ADDs. Figure 27-8 illustrates the rank-sum technique used to describe the burden of lung cancer in Kentucky.

The cancer control process used in Kentucky has resulted in a number of successful cancer control intervention programs. The following example is a description of one of these successes.

Example

Near the end of 2001, it was noted that only about one third (34.7%) of the people age 50 or older in Kentucky had ever received a sigmoidoscopy or colonoscopy examination. It was also noted that the incidence rate for colorectal cancer was greater in Kentucky compared with the United States,

Area Development District	High School Ed. +		Current Smoker		Age-Adjusted Incidence		Age Adjusted Mortality		Overall Rank
	%	Rank	%	Rank	Rate	Rank	Rate	Rank	
KENTUCKY RIVER	56.0	1	35.3	1	131.7	1	110.95	1	4
BIG SANDY	59.6	3	35.1	2	123.57	2	96.3	2	9
CUMBERLAND VALLEY	58.0	2	34.8	3	114.5	3	90.48	3	11
FIVCO	71.2	8	32.7	5	104.83	4	84.21	4	21
LAKE CUMBERLAND	61.3	4	31	9	103.48	5	80.06	5	23
BUFFALO TRACE	66.6	6	33.5	4	100.6	7	76.85	7	24
BARREN RIVER	70.3	7	31.9	7	99.24	9	81.13	9	32
GATEWAY	65.0	5	32.4	6	95.81	13	74.45	13	37
NORTHERN KENTUCKY	80.6	14	28.5	13	102.17	6	79.04	6	39
PENNYRILE	71.7	9	31.6	8	97.39	11	76.45	11	39
GREEN RIVER	77.1	11	30.5	11	99.1	10	79.93	10	42
KIPDA	81.3	15	27.9	14	100.17	8	75.8	8	45
LINCOLN TRAIL	76.1	10	30.8	10	90.99	15	67.18	15	50
BLUEGRASS	79.0	13	27.5	15	95.88	12	75.2	12	52
PURCHASE	77.1	12	28.9	12	91.12	14	68.3	14	52

Figure 27-8. The Lung Cancer Burden in Kentucky by Area Development District. Source: Kentucky Cancer Registry

and some ADDs had extremely high colorectal cancer incidence rates. In addition, the proportion of colorectal cancer patients diagnosed with late-stage disease (Surveillance, Epidemiology, and End Results Summary Stages, regional and distant) and the colorectal cancer mortality rates were much greater in Kentucky as compared with the United States. Using the process described earlier in this chapter, the KCR combined data from the U.S. Census, BRFSS, central cancer registry, and vital records. The results of this analysis were presented to each district cancer council.

Between 2001 and 2007, all 15 of the district cancer councils designed and implemented cancer control intervention strategies aimed at improving the proportion of Kentucky residents age 50 or older who ever had a screening sigmoidoscopy or colonoscopy. The Kentucky Cancer Program received funding from the Appalachian Regional Commission to conduct forums on best practices for screening for colorectal cancer, and each district cancer council in the Appalachian region of Kentucky held a special meeting focused on strategies for improving colorectal cancer screening. Based on data provided by KCR, the Comprehensive Cancer Control Program Steering Committee for Kentucky modified the state cancer plan to strengthen the focus on colorectal cancer. The Steering Committee also initiated two successful policy initiatives. The first initiative resulted in a bill passed by the state General Assembly in 2006 that required all health insurers in Kentucky to cover the cost of screening colonoscopy procedures for age-eligible patients. The second initiative resulted in a bill passed by the state legislature in 2007 to establish a program for screening age-eligible patients who are uninsured and to educate the public about the importance of being screened for colorectal cancer.

Although this is not a formal study, it is possible to use the data sources previously discussed to describe changes that have occurred since the more intensified focus on colorectal cancer was initiated. In the 7 years after implementation of the intensified focus on colorectal cancer screening, the proportion of the age-eligible population in Kentucky who have ever had a sigmoidoscopy or colonoscopy has nearly doubled from 34.7% in 1999 to 63.7% in 2008 (see Figure 27-9). [27]

A recent large, population-based, randomized trial in Europe found that screening age-eligible people in a population with sigmoidoscopy or colonoscopy will both reduce the incidence of colorectal cancer by finding precancerous disease and removing it before it becomes cancer, and reduce the mortality rate from colorectal cancer by finding the cancer at an early stage when the treatments are more effective.[28]

The incidence rates for colorectal cancer in Kentucky were increasing in the 3 years preceding the implementation of the intensified colorectal cancer screening initiative. However, the incidence rates for colorectal cancer in Kentucky have decreased every single year since the initiative was implemented (see Figure 27-10). In fact, the incidence rates for colorectal cancer in Kentucky are significantly lower ($p < 0.05$) in the most current 2 years (2005 and 2006) compared with any of the 3 years preceding implementation of the initiative.

The mortality rate for colorectal cancer in Kentucky has also significantly decreased ($p < 0.05$) after implementation of the intensified program to increase colorectal cancer screening (see Figure 27-11). As expected, the mortality rates did not change in the first few years after implementation of the intensified colorectal cancer screening program because many of the people dying in those first few years after the

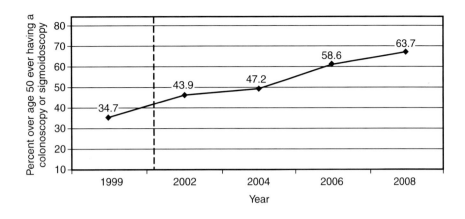

Figure 27-9. Percentage Older than 50 Ever Having Had a Colonoscopy or Sigmoidoscopy.
Source: Data from Centers for Disease Control and Prevention; Graph from Kentucky Cancer Registry

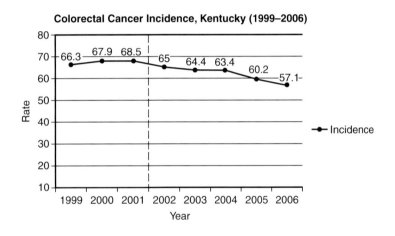

Figure 27-10. Colorectal Cancer Incidence in Kentucky. Source: Kentucky Cancer Registry

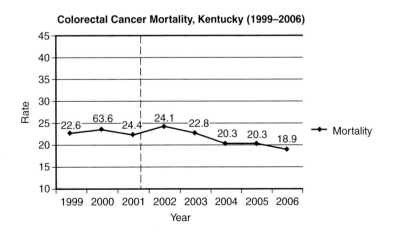

Figure 27-11. Colorectal Cancer Mortality in Kentucky. Source: Kentucky Cancer Registry

implementation of the intensified program were diagnosed before the intervention program was implemented. However, the colorectal cancer mortality rates in 2005, 2006, and 2007 are significantly lower ($p < 0.05$) than the mortality rate for any of the 3 years preceding implementation of the intensified effort.

This is clearly not a causal study, and no inferences can be drawn. However, from a programmatic perspective, the population-based changes that the intervention was aimed at did, in fact, occur. In other words, colorectal cancer screening increased dramatically, whereas both colorectal cancer incidence and mortality decreased significantly.

Summary and Conclusions

Some limitations are associated with using central cancer registry data for cancer control. However, the central cancer registry is a fundamental component of any meaningful cancer control program. When data from the central cancer registry are used by organizations that can plan and implement appropriate intervention programs, a complete system for cancer control is formed. Without the central cancer registry, it would not be possible for organizations to direct their limited cancer control resources at the areas of greatest need, and it would not be possible to evaluate the impact of their cancer control interventions.

References

1. Gordis, L. *Epidemiology*. Philadelphia: Saunders Elsevier, 2009.
2. Ford, J. G., Howerton, M. W., Lai, G. Y., et al. "Barriers to Recruiting Underrepresented Populations to Cancer Clinical Trials: A Systematic Review," *Cancer,* 2008;112(2):228–242.
3. U.S. Food and Drug Administration. "Postmarketing Surveillance Programs." Available at: www.fda.gov/Drugs/GuidanceComplianceRegulatoryInformation/Surveillance. Accessed May 5, 2010.
4. National Cancer Institute. "Division of Extramural Activities." Available at: www.deainfo.nci.nih.gov/Advisory/BSA/bsa_program/bsacacntrlmin.htm. Accessed May 5, 2010.
5. Pieretti, M., Hopenhayn-Rich, Cm., Khattar, N. H., et al. "Heterogeneity of Ovarian Cancer: Relationships Among Histological Group, Stage of Disease, Tumor Markers, Patient Characteristics, and Survival," *Cancer Investigation,* 2002;20(1):11–23.
6. Huang, B., Dignan, M., Han, D., et al. "Does Distance Matter? Distance to Mammography Facilities and Stage at Diagnosis of Breast Cancer in Kentucky," *Journal of Rural Health* 2009;25(4):366–371.
7. Pagano, E., Filippini, C., Di Cuonzo, D., et al. "Factors Affecting Pattern of Care and Survival in a Population-Based Cohort of Non-Small Lung Cancer Incident Cases," *Cancer Epidemiology* 2010;34:483–489.
8. Coker, A. L., DeSimone, C. P., Eggleston, K. S., et al. "Smoking and Survival Among Kentucky Women Diagnosed with Invasive Cervical Cancer: 1995-2005," *Gynecologic Oncology,* 2009;122(2):365–369.
9. Schonberg, M. A., Marcantonio, E. R., Li, D., et al. "Breast Cancer among the Oldest Old: Tumor Characteristics, Treatment Choices, and Survival," *Journal of Clinical Oncology,* 2010;28(12):2038–2045.
10. Paulson, E. C., Wirtall, C., Armstron, K., et al. "Gender Influences Treatment and Survival in Colorectal Cancer Surgery," *Diseases of the Colon and Rectum,* 2009;52(12):1991–1993.
11. Kim, S., Dolecek, T. A., Davis, F. G. "Racial Differences in Stage at Diagnosis and Survival from Epithelial Ovarian Cancer: A Fundamental Cause of Disease Approach," *Social Science & Medicine,* 2010;71:274–281.
12. Schroen, A. T., Brenin, D. R., Kelly, M. D., et al. "Impact of Patient Distance to Radiation Therapy on Mastectomy Use in Early-Stage Breast Cancer Patients," *Journal of Clinical Oncology,* 2005;23(28):7074–7080.
13. Hahn EJ, Rayens MK, Langley RE, et al. "Time Since Smoke-Free Law and Smoking Cessation Behaviors," *Nicotine & Tobacco Research,* 2009;11(8):1011–1015.
14. Centers for Disease Control and Prevention. "State Cigarette Excise Taxes—United States, 2009," *MMWR Morbidity and Mortality Weekly Report,* 2010;59(13):385–388.
15. Li, L., Plummer, S. J., Thompson, C. L., et al. "A Common 8q24 Variant and the Risk of Colon Cancer: A Population-Based Case-Control Study," *Cancer Epidemiology Biomarkers & Prevention,* 2008;17(2):339–342.
16. National Cancer Institute. "Definition of Cancer Control." Available at: www.cancer.gov. Accessed May 20, 2010.
17. Armstrong, B. "The Role of the Cancer Registry in Cancer Control," *Cancer Causes and Control,* 1992;3:569–579.
18. Centers for Disease Control and Prevention. "Definition of Comprehensive Cancer Control." Available at: www.cdc.gov. Accessed May 5, 2010.
19. Timmreck, T. C. *An Introduction to Epidemiology.* Boston: Jones and Bartlett, 1998.
20. Greenwald, H. *Who Survives Cancer?* Berkley: University of California Press, 1992.
21. Hewitt, M., Simone, J. *Ensuring Quality Cancer Care.* Washington, DC: National Academy Press, 1999.
22. American Cancer Society. *Cancer Facts and Figures 2009.* Atlanta: American Cancer Society, 2006.
23. Muir, C. S., Demaret, E., Boyle, P. *The Cancer Registry in Cancer Control* (pp. 13–26). Lyon, France: Institutional Agency for Research of Cancer, 1985.
24. Ellison, J. H., Wu, X. C., McLaughlin, C. C., et al. *Cancer in North America, 1999-2003, Volume One: Incidence.* Springfield, IL: North American Association of Central Cancer Registries, 2006.
25. Crieco, E. M., Cassidy, R. C. *Overview of Race and Hispanic Origin, Census Brief.* Washington, DC: U.S. Department of Commerce, U.S. Census Bureau, March 2001.
26. "Harvard Report on Cancer Prevention. Volume 1: Causes of Human Cancer," *Cancer Causes & Control,* 1996;7(Suppl 1): S3–S59.
27. Centers for Disease Control and Prevention. "Behavioral Risk Factor Surveillance System." Available at: http://www.cdc.gov/brfss/. Accessed May 8, 2010.
28. Atkins, W. S., Edwards, R., Kralj-Hans, I., et al. "Once-Only Flexible Sigmoidoscopy Screening in Prevention of Colorectal Cancer: A Multicentre Randomised Controlled Trial," *Lancet,* 2010;375(9726):1624–1633.

Standard Setters and Professional Organizations

Linda Mulvihill
Section Editor—Textbook

Melissa Pearson
Section Editor—Review Guide

North American Association of Central Cancer Registries, Inc.

Betsy A. Kohler, MPH, CTR

History of NAACCR

Central cancer registries collect cancer data on defined populations in a defined time period. They differ from hospital cancer registries because they are population based, covering the entire population of a given geographic area such as a country, state, province, or county. Population-based registries strive to collect information on every cancer case in the defined population to describe the cancer burden. The data are used to calculate cancer incidence rates and, in some cases, prevalence and survival. Collecting complete high-quality, timely, and accurate cancer data is essential for central cancer registries.

The state of Connecticut began collecting cancer incidence data in the 1930s, and a handful of areas across the United States followed suit. In 1973, the National Cancer Institute (NCI) Surveillance, Epidemiology, and End Results (SEER) Program began collecting a uniform dataset from the states of Connecticut, Iowa, New Mexico, Utah, and Hawaii, and the metropolitan areas of Detroit and San Francisco-Oakland.[1] Over time, the SEER Program expanded to collect information on a broader population and in different geographic areas. It was not until the late 1970s and early 1980s that many states began to collect cancer incidence data on a statewide basis. The SEER Program had become a world-renowned leader in the collection of cancer surveillance data, and many states tried to adopt the SEER methodology of collecting and coding cancer incidence data. However, many states adapted and changed coding rules to meet their individual needs, or adapted and used the data collection rules used by hospitals following the American College of Surgeons (ACoS) protocols. States implemented systems that, at a minimum, were able to produce basic surveillance statistics on newly diagnosed cancer patients for the state as a whole, and often for regions within the state (e.g., counties). However, data were not comparable with other states and geographic regions because a common set of rules was not being used by all states. As the number of state cancer registries grew, the cancer incidence data collection practices became increasingly disparate.

The NCI began to explore ways to support the new registries and to maximize the usefulness of the data collected across geopolitical boundaries. In 1987, Drs. Charles Smart and Edward Sondik of NCI convened a meeting with representatives from the ACoS, the American Cancer Society (ACS), and the American Association of Cancer Institutes (AACI) to discuss how these organizations could benefit from, and assist in, the collection of population-based cancer registry data. Plans were formed to establish an independent association to develop national cancer data standards and to serve all population-based cancer registries in the United States. The American Association of Central Cancer Registries (AACCR) was envisioned as a collaborative umbrella organization for cancer registries, governmental agencies, professional associations, and private groups in the United States interested in enhancing the quality and use of cancer registry data.

In March 1988, the ACoS invited representatives from all existing central cancer registries in the United States to an organizational meeting of the AACCR. AACCR was originally modeled after the International Association of Cancer Registries (IACR), with a secretariat and support services provided by NCI. State registries saw value and opportunity in sharing methods, procedures, and resource materials, and ultimately in improving the information derived from cancer incidence data throughout the United States. A president and five representatives at-large were elected to establish bylaws and standing rules for the association. The National Tumor Registrars Association (now the National Cancer Registrars Association [NCRA]) and the Association of Community Cancer Centers (ACCC) joined the four original organizations (ACS, ACoS, AACI, and NCI) as the founding and sponsoring members of AACCR. The bylaws and standing rules were formally adopted in April 1989 at the second meeting of AACCR held in Chicago. In 1992, AACCR became incorporated in the state of California as AACCR, Inc., a nonprofit organization with 501(c)(3) status. In 1994, the association officially changed its name to the North American Association of Central Cancer Registries, Inc. (NAACCR) to better reflect its broadening membership among the provincial and territorial registries in Canada.

During the 1990s, NAACCR obtained support from CDC and NCI to provide educational services, develop uniform data standards, aggregate data, certify registries, and encourage and support data use. In May 1999, an executive director was hired and an executive office was opened in Springfield, Illinois. By 2002, NAACCR had sufficient infrastructure for the Executive Office to assume the duties of the Secretariat. An elected Board of Directors governs NAACCR, which consists of the President, President-elect [or Past-president], Treasurer, six Representatives-at-Large, one Sponsoring Member Organization representative, and the Executive Director, as an *ex officio* member. All board members serve a 2-year term, except the President-elect and the Past-president, who serve for one year. The bylaws and standing rules define NAACCR structure and the governance of the association.

Mission

NAACCR is a professional organization that develops and promotes uniform data standards for cancer registration; provides education and training; certifies population-based registries; aggregates and publishes data from central cancer registries; and promotes the use of cancer surveillance data and systems for cancer control and epidemiologic research, public health programs, and patient care to reduce the burden of cancer in North America.*

Membership

All population-based central cancer registries in the United States and Canada are NAACCR members. Membership consists primarily of population-based cancer registries, although four membership categories are available: full, sponsor, sustaining, and individual. Full member organizations are central registries that are, or have the potential to become, population-based registries. Sponsoring members are national organizations involved in cancer control, prevention, or research. Sustaining members are organizations interested in promoting the purposes of the association. Individual members are persons who are not currently working in a member organization, but who have demonstrated career and professional commitments and interests that are consistent with or complementary to NAACCR.

NAACCR Committees

The Board of Directors, with input from the Sponsoring Member Organizations, defines the major goals of NAACCR. The standing committees develop and execute specific objectives. The work of the organization is conducted primarily through an extensive committee structure including 11 standing committees, various subcommittees, ad hoc committees, work groups, special task forces, and research groups. Figure 28-1 summarizes the organizational relationship of the Board of Directors, sponsoring members, standing committees, and the executive office. The activities of the standing committees, which are defined by the standing rules, are as follows:

- *Bylaws:* receives and reviews all proposed amendments to the bylaws

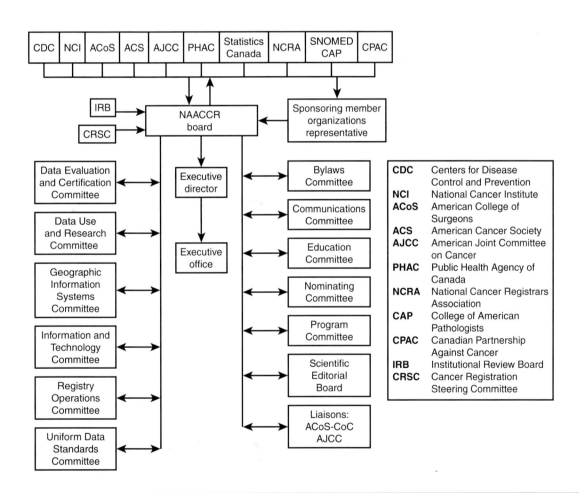

Figure 28-1. North American Association of Central Cancer Registries (NAACCR, Inc.) Organization Relationship 2009–2010. ACS, American Cancer Society; ACoS, American College of Surgeons; AJCC, American Joint Committee on Cancer; CAP, College of American Pathologists; CDC, Centers for Disease Control and Prevention; CPAC, Canadian Partnership Against Cancer; CRSC, Cancer Registration Steering Committee; IRB, institutional review board; NCI, National Cancer Institute; NCRA, National Cancer Registrars Association; PHAC, Public Health Agency of Canada. From NAACCR. Copyright © 2010 by NAACCR. Reprinted with permission.

- *Communications:* compiles and releases the NAACCR newsletter and press releases, runs press conferences, and oversees and directs the Web site content
- *Data evaluation and certification:* evaluates member data submissions and determines and evaluates parameters to identify and assess high-quality data for various data uses, including objective certification standards; implements and oversees an annual process to evaluate data collected by central cancer registries; and conducts an annual recognition of those registries meeting certification standards
- *Data use and research:* prepares publications of cancer incidence and mortality based on data submitted by member registries, provides recommendations on data use, release and confidentiality, oversees the NAACCR research program, develops a research agenda for the Association, and conducts abstract reviews for the scientific program of the annual conference
- *Education:* determines the educational needs of the association and proposes methods to meet the needs
- *Information and technology:* develops the format for data exchange among members and the standards to ensure the security and accuracy of transmitted data
- *Membership:* reviews and approves applications for membership
- *Nominating:* secures candidates for the office of President-Elect, Treasurer, and Representatives-at-Large, and Sponsoring Member Organization representative
- *Program:* plans the technical program for the annual conference
- *Registry Operations:* discusses methodologic issues relevant to policies, procedures, and operational methods of a central cancer registry, and provides models and guidelines for their implementation
- *Uniform Data Standards:* provides a formal mechanism for reviewing and recommending proposed changes in data codes or the addition of new data items and data edits submitted by NAACCR members to ensure that data remain comparable among all cancer registries, both population and hospital based

Major NAACCR Activities

The activities of the organization are tied to its goals, objectives, and ultimately its mission statement. The major groups of activities are:

1. **Provide consensus standards for coding, editing, and data exchange, and promote best practices for the collection and use of cancer and patient information. Coordinate the implementation of standards to promote continuity in data collection and exchange, and analysis.** Initially, NAACCR sought to standardize data definitions, variables, codes, and exchange formats to provide all registries with guidelines and tools to enable collaboration and information exchange, and to maximize data comparability. The first data standards volume appeared in February 1994 and "document(ed) the achievements of a process of collaboration, consensus-building, and compromise among all of the major organizations involved in setting standards for cancer registries, including NAACCR, the American College of Surgeons, the Centers for Disease Control and Prevention, the National Cancer Institute, and the National Cancer Registrar's Association. It represent(ed) the status of agreed-upon data items and codes as of January 1994 and highlights areas where more work is needed."[2] Since that time, all North American cancer registries have adopted NAACCR standardized record layouts, data definitions, and codes. NAACCR now works to promote the interoperability of these standards with other data systems to maximize the use of electronic data exchange. As new data items are introduced, new standards are developed through our committee structure and implementation guidelines are provided to facilitate adoption. NAACCR members also develop operational guidelines to assist central registries. The guidelines balance a single best practice approach with an awareness of the variety of organizations, structures, laws, and administrative codes that contribute to each registry's uniqueness. The Procedure Guidelines for Registry Operations are a compendium of procedures for specific registry operations written by work groups of volunteers.

2. **Train and educate registry staff.** NAACCR is dedicated to identifying and addressing the educational needs of the cancer surveillance community and providing high-quality and timely educational programs. A variety of education and training opportunities are offered each year covering fundamentals of cancer registry operations, data processing and electronic data management tools, and advanced courses that address topical issues. A full spectrum of educational media and venues are utilized to reach the broad audience interested in cancer surveillance. In addition, NAACCR supports a Mentor Fellowship Program for one-on-one training opportunities that supports travel costs for a mentor or a trainee to obtain individualized training on specific registry operation issues.

3. **Certify registries that meet national data quality standards for producing accurate cancer statistics.** In 1997, NAACCR instituted a review of member registries for their ability to produce complete, accurate, and timely cancer incidence information. Certification criteria were established by NAACCR member registries following four principles: the criteria needed to be objective; the criteria should focus on the product not the processes of cancer registries; the results could be used by registries to make improvements; and certification should be the basis for recognizing registries

that have demonstrated excellence in the areas of completeness, timeliness, and accuracy. The criteria were defined with the belief that all NAACCR members should be able to obtain these standards, and meeting the criteria is essential for producing high-quality cancer incidence data that can be aggregated and compared across jurisdictions. The certification criteria are as follows:

Criteria	Gold	Silver
Completeness of case ascertainment	95%	90%
Completeness of information		
Missing/unknown age at diagnosis	≤2%	≤3%
Missing/unknown sex	≤2%	≤3%
Missing/unknown race	≤3%	≤5%
Missing/unknown state/ county/province	≤2%	≤3%
Death certificate only cases	≤3%	≤5%
Duplicate primary cases	≤1/1,000	≤2/1,000
Passing EDITS	100%	97%
Timeliness (data submitted within 23 months of diagnosis)	Yes	Yes

In 2009, NAACCR evaluated 2006 cancer incidence data from 73 population-based cancer registries that were evaluated as part of the certification program. Of these registries, 47 U.S. registries were certified as Gold and 5 were certified as Silver. In Canada, six provincial and territorial registries were certified as Gold.

4. **Evaluate and publish data from member registries.** The American Association of Central Cancer Registries (AACCR, now NAACCR) was the first organization outside of the SEER Program to aggregate cancer incidence data across the United States. It is necessary to ensure that the data are comparable to aggregate data across geopolitical boundaries. That is, the data must be:
- Collected using a universal case definition (reportability) standard
- Collected using uniform rules and standards
- Coded to a common set of rules
- Assessed for completeness within a given area
- Of similar quality
- From the same time period
- Adjusted to a common standard

The SEER Program had contractual relationships with all of its registries, which allowed for these conditions to be met by participating SEER registries. The SEER Program had standardized reportability lists, data collection rules and procedures, and a common code set. In addition, SEER applied a common set of edits to data from the SEER registries, thereby ensuring a standard level of data quality was met.

NAACCR, however, covered a much broader range of central cancer registries. Many of these registries had adopted the SEER rules and codes, and incorporated them into their own procedures in their entirety, but more commonly, central registries adopted some SEER practices and adapted others to suit their individualized needs. Other central registries had their own set of rules and codes. In addition, contributing hospital registries often followed the ACoS guidelines. Because the various organizations used their data for different purposes, some data elements had different meanings, depending on the organization using the data. The systems were not always in agreement. The Commission on Cancer and SEER began working together in the early 1980s to make the codes and definitions in their manuals consistent, but much work was needed to build consensus on these or other standards and incorporate them into central cancer registry operations across the United States.

Therefore, before NAACCR could attempt to aggregate data from different state registries, NAACCR needed to establish a common set of definitions, rules, and procedures to ensure comparability of data. This process brought together representatives from cancer registries across the country to address all of the issues central to the collection of high-quality cancer incidence data. Under the NAACCR committee structure, different groups tackled different problems such as determining a reportable list, adopting a system to define multiple primaries, ensuring that standardized codes and definitions were in place, developing methods to transmit files electronically, developing methods to exchange data between states, and developing standardized edits to ensure data quality. Committee membership included all of the major standard-setting organizations, representation from registry software vendors, and central registries. The NAACCR committee structure provides a national forum to discuss data issues and reach consensus on data standards.

The first aggregate data published by NAACCR appeared in April 1992. *Cancer Incidence in the U.S.A., 1988: American Association of Central Cancer Registries*[3] included data from 25 population-based registries and information on more than 350,000 cases. These registries self-reported as having complete incidence data, but no external standard was applied. Indicators of completeness and quality were calculated, but no data were excluded from the first publications based on not meeting quality or completeness standards.

The data aggregation process evolved over time, adapting as NAACCR and others developed tools to better assess cancer data provided by each registry. Higher standards of data quality were sought to make the aggregated data more reliable and representative of the United States, Canada, and North America. The certification criteria became integral evaluating the fitness of data for use in NAACCR publications (now called *Cancer in North America,* or *CINA*) and for research purposes.

NAACCR first published combined incidence data for the United States and Canada in 1994 in *Cancer in North America 1988–1990.*[4] This publication marked the first time that states and provinces could compare their data with a national standard derived from the same data collection system. The original inclusion criteria for that publication were "combined rates include data from all central registries within its borders that reported cases for 1988-1990, reported a case ascertainment of at least 90 percent completeness, and met at least two of the following three criteria; conduct death certificate clearance procedures, report case ascertainment completeness at 91 percent or higher, and report unresolved duplicates less than 2 percent."[4] In addition, the 1988–1990 publication presented data on all races combined for five male cancer sites and six female cancer sites. A total of 24 U.S. registries and 10 Canadian registries submitted data for that year.[4] Total U.S. cases for the 1988–1990 data publication were 1,016,211, and Canadian cases totaled 298,471.[4]

In contrast, the latest CINA publication, using 2006 data, included 48 U.S. registries with a total of 6,047,783 cases and 6 Canadian registries with 169,837 cases.[5] Eligibility for inclusion in the combined rates has become more stringent over time, and registries must be certified by NAACCR at the Gold or Silver level to have their data included. The 48 registries used in the combined rates cover 86% of the U.S. white population, 83% of the U.S. black population, 92% of the U.S. Hispanic population, 93% of the U.S. Asian Pacific Islander population, and 78% of the U.S. American Indian/Alaskan Native population.

Mortality data were first published in 1995 in CINA covering the period 1989 to 1993. Because of the standardized nature of mortality data, virtually every state and province was represented. Data are presented by race and sex in the United States, and by sex for Canada. State- and provincial-specific data are presented in conjunction with data for the United States and Canada.

Data files are submitted voluntarily and evaluated for completeness and quality using standard methods and metrics. Individualized feedback is provided to all registries on common data quality issues and those that are unique to any registry. When requested, NAACCR staff will work with registries to explain results and to identify operations or methods that could enhance their data in future years.

5. **Promote the use of registry data.** Data quality, including validity, reliability, and completeness, has improved dramatically since 1987 through the efforts of NAACCR, federal programs in the United States and Canada, and extensive training. The maps in Figure 28-2 clearly show that North America is producing high-quality cancer surveillance data. Core to the mission of NAACCR is the promotion of data use that will lead to the better understanding of the cancer burden in North America. Annually, NAACCR produces several products from the data submitted, evaluated, and aggregated by the Data Evaluation and Certification Committee. In addition to *Cancer in North America (CINA),* as described earlier, NAACCR also produces *CINA+ Online,* an interactive, flexible query system on the NAACCR Web site. This online data resource can be accessed by the public for specific cancer information by year, geography, sex, race, cancer type, and age, and by any combination of these variables. Registries may opt to be included in this database when they meet NAACCR high-quality data standards. Data are updated annually with the most recent 5-year interval.

In addition, a data file for researchers is available for NAACCR members who submit a brief research protocol that is evaluated by peers. This analytic file is known as *CINA Deluxe.* NAACCR also organizes special research groups, inviting interested persons to collaborate in producing a set of research and surveillance papers on a particular topic.

Resources and Support for Activities

Since 1987, NAACCR has provided valuable services and resources to central cancer registries and the entire cancer surveillance community. Relying on the outstanding volunteerism from this community and willingness to work collaboratively on mutual areas of interest, NAACCR has grown and has been able to realize its mission. Cancer surveillance personnel from across North America contribute knowledge and expertise for the benefit of all registries. These efforts strengthen the North American infrastructure in standards development, training, and data aggregation, evaluation, and publication. This participation has had a significant impact on the success of the organization. Although active member participation is a hallmark of NAACCR's success, NAACCR has also been successful in obtaining grants, contracts, and other awards that support many cancer surveillance activities. Member dues represent a very small proportion of the resources available for NAACCR activities. Sponsoring member organizations support the organization through dues, in-kind contributions, and support of specific activities. Sponsoring member organizations provide substantial financial support to developing and maintaining the infrastructure, services, and resources that NAACCR provides to the cancer surveillance community.

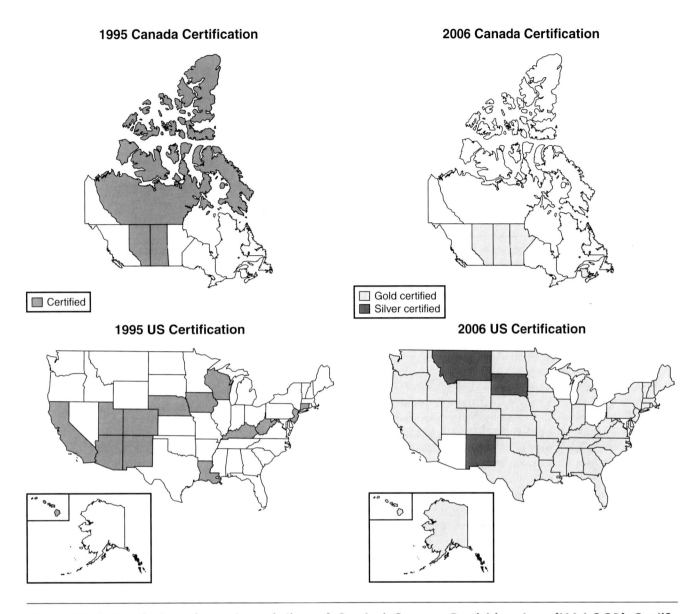

1995 Canada Certification

2006 Canada Certification

Certified

Gold certified
Silver certified

1995 US Certification

2006 US Certification

Figure 28-2. North American Association of Central Cancer Registries, Inc. (NAACCR) Certification for 1995 and 2006. From NAACCR. Copyright © 1995, 2006 by NAACCR. Reprinted with permission.

References

1. Surveillance, Epidemiology, and End Results Program. U.S. Department of Health and Human Services, National Institutes of Health, National Cancer Institute. NIH Publication No. 05-4772, September 2005.
2. Howe, H. L., editor. *Cancer Incidence in North America, 1988-1990.* Springfield, IL: North American Association of Central Cancer Registries, April 1994.
3. *Cancer Incidence in the U.S.A., 1988: American Association of Central Cancer Registries.* American Association of Central Cancer Registries, April 1992.
4. Howe, H. L., editor. *Cancer Incidence in North America, 1988-1990.* American Association of Central Cancer Registries, April 1994.
5. Copeland, G., Lake, A., Firth, R., Lehnherr, M., Bayakly, R., Wu, X. C., Stroup, A., Russell, C., Schymura, M., Hofferkamp, J., Kohler, B., editors. *Cancer in North America: 2002-2006. Volume One: Combined Cancer Incidence for the United States and Canada.* Springfield, IL: North American Association of Central Cancer Registries, Inc., June 2009.

chapter 29

Cancer Registries in Canada

Maureen MacIntyre, BSN, MHSA

Mary Jane King, MPH, CTR

Elaine Hamlyn, CTR

One of the earliest population-based cancer registries in North America was developed by the province of Saskatchewan in 1932 as an integral part of a new, comprehensive cancer-control program.[1,2] Within 40 years, the remaining provinces and territories established registries, bringing Canada to a point of complete population coverage by the mid-1970s. The foundation created by the provinces and territories provided the impetus for an integrated, national-level cancer registry that was developed in partnership with the federal government, starting with the 1969 incidence year.[2]

The intervening 70 plus years since the first cancer registry opened its doors in Canada have been marked by periods of relatively limited change, interspersed with cycles of innovation and transformation (e.g., introduction of automated cancer registration by Ontario in the early 1980s).[3] This chapter provides an overview of the existing cancer registry infrastructure at both provincial/territorial (P/T) and national levels, provides some Canadian context as it relates to cancer burden and registry operations, and also describes some of the key stakeholder organizations that influence registry and surveillance activities.

Canadian Context

Cancer registries, like most health-related programs, operate within a geopolitical context. Various characteristics of any country or jurisdiction, such as demographics, geography, and healthcare system, can all influence cancer registration and surveillance. Examples of opportunities that arise from these features in Canada include the facilitation of case ascertainment through the availability of standardized, unique P/T personal health insurance lifetime identifiers, as well as the highly centralized delivery of key cancer treatment modalities such as radiotherapy.[4] Equally important are the challenges and unique aspects of Canada that must be factored into registry operations. Geographic diversity, lack of uniformity in reporting legislation, and the absence of system-wide, hospital-based cancer registrars fall into this realm.[4,5]

Geography and Demographics

Canada is the second largest country in the world, with a landmass of more than 9 million square kilometers. Bordered on its southern edge by a number of American states, the country meets Alaska in the northwest, stretches into the far north regions of Nunavut to Cape Columbia, and reaches its most easterly point at Cape Spear, Newfoundland.[6]

Composed of 10 provinces and 3 territories, the smallest Canadian jurisdiction is Prince Edward Island, which represents less than 1% of the nation's landmass, compared with the territory of Nunavut at almost 22%.[7]

Data from the last census conducted in 2006 places the total Canadian population at just more than 31.6 million

(comparable with the state of California), approximately a 5% increase from the previous 2001 count.[8] The most recent estimates for 2010 show continued growth in recent years to 33.9 million. Additional 2006 information reports population density for Canada as a whole at 3.5 individuals per square kilometer, with ranges between less than 0.1 in the northern Territories and 23.9 per square kilometer in Prince Edward Island. Total population counts range from a low of 29,400 in Nunavut to a high of 12.1 million in Ontario (see Table 29-1).[8] Ontario, together with the adjacent province of Quebec, represent close to 60% of the Canadian population and combine to heavily influence national cancer trends. The sparse population in many areas of the country certainly impacts the delivery of health care and can make the collection of cancer data challenging.

Recent immigrants from other countries accounted for just more than 3% of the 2006 Census respondents. If all individuals ever reporting immigrant status are examined, then the total within this category as of 2006 is close to 19% of the Canadian population. Persons from Europe and Asia/Middle East represented the largest segments within the immigrant category.[9] Together with the diversity that results from immigration, Canada is home to a significant aboriginal population (North American Indian, Métis, and

Table 29-1	Canadian Provinces and Territories: Total Population and Cancer Registry Startup[2,7]	
Province/ Territory	Population 2006 Census	Initial Cancer Registry Accession Year
Newfoundland and Labrador	505,469	1955
Prince Edward Island	135,851	1969
Nova Scotia	913,462	1964
New Brunswick	729,997	1952
Quebec	7,546,131	1975
Ontario	12,160,282	1964
Manitoba	1,148,401	1937
Saskatchewan	968,157	1932
Alberta	3,290,350	1941
British Columbia	4,113,487	1932
Northwest Territories	41,464	1950
Nunavut*	29,474	1999*
Yukon	30,372	1969

*Nunavut was designated as an official federal territory in 1999, formed from a split of the existing Northwest Territories.

Inuit). Approximately 4% of the full Canadian population identifies as aboriginal in the 2006 Census, with some P/T proportions being much higher (e.g., Nunavut, 84%; Northwest Territories, 50%; Manitoba, 15%).[10] Clearly, Canada is becoming a more culturally diverse population, and it will be important to understand how these factors may influence cancer-control efforts.

Canada's population is rapidly aging because of declining fertility rates and increasing life expectancy, although the effect of aging varies between regions. According to the 2006 Census, the proportion of people aged 65 and older ranged from 2.7% in Nunavut to 15.4% in Saskatchewan. The median age of the Canadian population increased from 35.5 to 39.5 years between the 1999 and 2006 Census periods, whereas life expectancy increased to 76.7 and 82.0 years for men and women, respectively.[8,10] In addition, the 2006 Census highlighted that the 65+ age group had increased to its greatest level ever at 13.7% of the total population, whereas the under 15 age group was at 17.7%, its lowest point ever reported. In recognition of these trends, the 2008 *Canadian Cancer Statistics* publication noted that population size and age structure shifts have been major determinants of the increasing cancer burden in this country.[11] The influence of these trends will continue to be felt for many years.

Government and Health Care

In 2010, Canada celebrated its 143rd anniversary of confederation. A democratic, federal state with a defined constitution, Canada is a bilingual country, counting both English and French as official languages at the federal level. Several provinces including Quebec and New Brunswick also recognize this bilingual distinction. On a practical level, from a national cancer registry perspective, this means materials to support registry operations and statistical reports must be translated into both languages. Under the constitution, a variety of powers and responsibilities have been assigned to the federal government with distinct areas such as healthcare delivery allocated to the P/T level.[12,13]

Canadians enjoy the benefits of a publically funded healthcare system that allows access to "medically necessary hospital and physician care" without direct payment. The system of Medicare originated in Saskatchewan in 1947 and was gradually adopted across the country by 1968.[14] Financial support for the system comes largely through P/T and national taxation. Access by provinces and territories to federal tax dollars occurs through various transfer payment programs and requires adherence to conditions such as those articulated in the *Canada Health Act*.[15] Maintenance of universal access to insured services and portability within the country are examples of these requirements.

Starting in the early 1990s, provinces and territories have administered access to insured services through an individually assigned, unique, lifetime health card number (HCN) specifically for their jurisdiction. If a person moves from one province or territory to another, they are assigned a new number in the new jurisdiction after a defined waiting period. Implementation of HCN systems has been invaluable to a wide variety of health surveillance activities including cancer registration, because they facilitate unique patient identification and record linkage activities. Looking forward, the HCN will also be an important asset in the ongoing development of electronic health records (EHRs).

The public nature of the Canadian healthcare system has generally led to a more streamlined delivery approach, with a focus on centralized services. Expensive and technologically intensive modalities such as radiation treatment for cancer are available only in selected locations. Although there has been recent expansion of radiation treatment services to address growing populations and lengthening wait times for treatment, there are only about 40 locations in the entire country where this service is provided.[5] Programs are often located at a comprehensive cancer center in conjunction with other specialized treatments. Although some cancer surgery and chemotherapy are less centralized, relative to the United States, fewer facilities and organizations are involved and, therefore, less points of contact for data collection. Most provinces also have some type of cancer-control program that deals with standard setting, monitoring, and other elements of system coordination.

A publicly funded healthcare model does limit the private component of healthcare delivery in Canada. It is estimated that approximately 70% of healthcare services are provided via the public system with the remaining 30% addressed through private segments.[16] Growing fiscal pressures within the public system will continue to shift the definition of what is funded. The cancer surveillance system must be aware of this evolution and adapt accordingly to ensure completeness of casefinding and data collection.

Registry Operations

In Canada, cancer registry operations take place on two distinct but connected levels. The foundation for most registry activity is at the P/T level, which supports a second layer in the form of the national Canadian Cancer Registry (CCR). Outlines of historical and current registry operations are provided here for both the P/T and CCR systems.

Provincial/Territorial Systems

Cancer registries have operated since 1935 in both Saskatchewan and British Columbia (see Table 29-1), and represent some of the oldest registries in North America.[2] All 13 provinces and territories have a population-based cancer registry, although there is substantial variation in operations across the country.[17] Two main reasons drive this variation: population size and funding. According to the 2006 population figures reported in Table 29-1, 8 of the 13 P/T registries cover less than a 1 million population. Although small populations present some opportunities to streamline operations, it can be challenging to maintain standards and build a sustainable, critical program mass. In Canada, because health care is primarily a P/T responsibility, funding for cancer registries is provided almost totally by the local jurisdiction. No federal funding programs exist to support routine P/T cancer registry operations. Most cancer registries are the responsibility of a provincial cancer agency or Department of Health, and the level of funding and recognition they are provided can reflect the ongoing challenges facing P/T budgets. In recent years, the three territories that represent the smallest registries have all developed a partnership arrangement with an adjoining province to carry out registry operations.[4,17–19] Over the years it is clear that some P/Ts have had greater degrees of success ensuring adequate funding for their programs.

Additional characteristics of Canadian P/T cancer registries include:

- Legislative and regulatory oversight varies for each registry. For example, in Nova Scotia, cancer is a reportable disease under the provincial *Health Act,* whereas other P/Ts have no explicit reporting requirement. Since 2000, provinces and territories are also dealing with impacts resulting from the adoption of Personal Health Information legislation aimed at improving privacy and data confidentiality practices.[20,21] This places additional requirements and, in some cases, restrictions on access to data required for registry operations.

- Registry information systems have historically varied across the country and, in most cases, were locally developed applications. Rapidly changing registry data standards and the move to increase Canadian data collection in recent years (e.g., stage data) have placed many of these systems under pressure. This has been recognized by many jurisdictions and stakeholders as a limitation for growth in Canadian cancer surveillance.[18,19,22] A renewed focus on cancer control at the national level has led to some federal funding being made available for registry improvements such as systems development. In the 2008-2010 time period, at least four provinces selected U.S. based vendors to provide registry system solutions while others initiated major upgrades to existing systems .[23]

- Cancer data abstraction in Canada has typically been highly centralized. With the exception of Quebec and selected components of the Ontario registry system (e.g., the Princess Margaret Hospital),[24] the use of hospital-based cancer registrars is limited. Most abstracting is done directly at the cancer center or P/T registry. Cancer registries have been closely connected to provincial cancer treatment centers, and many have direct flows of data from centers to registries and, in some cases, may even share data systems (e.g., Newfoundland, Nova Scotia).

- P/T registries typically use trained health information professional staff to support cancer reporting. Canada does not have an independent cancer registrar certifi-

cation, and many Canadian registrars participate in the American-based certification program.

- A number of standardized healthcare administrative data sets exist that can be used to support casefinding and overall data collection with P/T registries. The national Discharge Abstracting System (DAD) and the National Ambulatory Care Reporting System (NACRS) are two examples. Both systems follow *International Classification of Diseases, Tenth Revision* (ICD-10) standards for diagnosis and additional Canadian conventions for intervention reporting.[4,17]

- In addition to administrative data sets, P/T registries use other common casefinding sources such as pathology departments, laboratory services and specialized cancer treatment services. The Ontario Cancer Registry has been a North American leader in the adoption of electronic pathology reporting starting in the 1980s.[3]

- As of 2010, P/T level mortality data are used in each jurisdiction to assist with casefinding and death clearance.

When looking across the range of P/T registry operations, some limitations in registry operations do exist that affect overall surveillance capacity and reporting. One key area of note is the lack of standardized collection for ethnicity data. At this point, it is not possible to produce race-specific cancer burden data for Canada. Variability has also occurred in data collection parameters over time. Most P/T registries were initially focused on population-based case coverage but did not collect a wide range of data for every case. A notable gap has been in the area of stage data collection that was not a required standard in many jurisdictions. For those that did collect stage, it was often for selected case series and did not follow a national standard because one was not in place before 2004. Significant effort has taken place in the last few years to expand data collection, particularly in the area of staging information. Treatment data will likely be a future focus.

National Registry

The first year of cancer incidence data collection in Canada was 1969.[2] Early development of P/T registries across the country formed a strong foundation for the establishment of a standardized national registry system. Surveillance was acknowledged as a vital component of any national cancer-control initiatives that would support a future reduction in the burden of cancer on Canadians. The need to continually evolve and develop the national registry system has been recognized, and many changes have taken place in the years since the first data cycle was reported.

In the first version of national registry operations, the system was referred to as the National Cancer Incidence Reporting System, which was housed at the Dominion Bureau of Statistics, a predecessor organization to Statistics Canada. The National Cancer Incidence Reporting System was an event-based data collection system covering the period 1969–1991, with a standard set of requirements for the P/T agencies that supplied data.[1,2,4] By the late 1980s, stakeholders recognized the need to make substantial changes to the structure of the system. The second generation of the national system came into operation for the 1992 incidence year with a shift to a person-oriented database that continues today as the CCR under the responsibility of Statistics Canada.[4]

The location of the CCR at Statistics Canada has allowed for the enhancement of Canada's cancer surveillance system through ongoing linkages with national mortality data also managed by this federal agency. Routine internal linkages also take place to resolve duplicates. Annual calls for data require the submission of specific personal identifiers on case records to minimize the risk for duplicate reporting. During data quality edit cycles, each registry will receive a list of potential duplicates and must work with any other registry identified as having the same case to resolve the primary owner and allow the case to be appropriately ascertained into the CCR. At the completion of the annual call for data, each registry receives a file from Statistics Canada with the national CCR ID number appended to all newly accepted records. This ID is used to submit any future updates to these existing cases. The current submission deadline for the annual CCR data cycle is 14 months after the end of an accession year. The CCR will contain an estimated 2.5 million records once the 2010 call for data is processed.[25] Detailed documentation on the CCR is accessible through the Statistics Canada Web site (www.statcan.gc.ca/pub/82-225-x/82-225-x2007010-eng.htm).

Management of the CCR takes place through an oversight group involving representatives from each P/T registry and core staff from Statistics Canada. This group, which also includes representatives from several other key national stakeholder organizations, is known as the Canadian Council of Cancer Registries (CCCR). This group recommends new data standards and key operational changes for the CCR.

Data flows between the P/T registries and Statistics Canada are governed by legal agreements signed with each province. An overview of the national system is provided in Figure 29-1. Participation in this national cancer-control effort has always been voluntary, but the overall public health benefit is well understood and accepted by all parties involved, and currently, all P/Ts are submitting data. The voluntary nature of the system and absence of sanctions for nonreporting can certainly impact the adoption of standards. For example, the 2004 agreement to utilize the Collaborative Stage framework to support stage data collection did not establish a hard deadline for implementation. As a result, Manitoba is currently the only province submitting stage data for all cases, whereas others have moved more slowly and tended to adopt by individual disease sites.[26] It will take several more years before stage data are available at the national level for all newly diagnosed incident cases.

Starting in 2005, the CCR has undergone further changes that can be considered the third generation of national cancer registration in Canada. These changes have expanded the record layout to include the Collaborative Stage, Version 1 framework and addressed the adoption of other standards including the 2007 Surveillance, Epidemiology, and End Results multiple primary rules. A new platform for the database was also implemented. This remodeling of the registry system will position the CCR to further expand the data set should more standard changes take place in the future (e.g. adoption of treatment data collection).

In 1995, Canada became a formal part of the North American Association of Central Cancer Registries (NAACCR).[4] This partnership has been essential to enhancing data standards, improving quality assessment

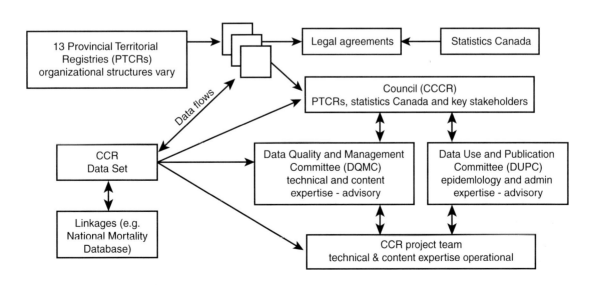

Figure 29-1. Overview of Canada's National Cancer Registry System Structure

of registry data, and the overall evolution of cancer registration in Canada. NAACCR executive members now attend the CCCR annual meetings to ensure clear lines of communication and identify opportunities for further partnership. Many P/T registry members participate in NAACCR committees, and most registries participate in the NAACCR registry certification program. In 2004, the CCCR started work with NAACCR staff to incorporate CCR data standards into NAACCR documentation and outline Canadian registry standards as they compare with other North American standard setters.[27]

Key Partners and Initiatives

Use of registry data by both internal and external users is a major indication of success. Cancer registries must be recognized by key partners for the valuable information they can provide to the cancer-control community. In Canada, registry success and development have been linked with several organizations that have maintained long-term relationships with the CCR and P/T registries, providing both direct and indirect support for cancer surveillance. Since 2006 a renewed focus on cancer surveillance has taken place as a result of a newly defined agency (Canadian Partnership Against Cancer [CPAC]) directed at national cancer-control strategy development. Brief overviews are provided in this section on several of the key partners and initiatives that are currently shaping the future of cancer surveillance in Canada.

Public Health Agency of Canada

The Public Health Agency of Canada (PHAC) is a federal government organization charged with protecting the health and safety of Canadians, including specific target areas such as disease surveillance.[28] A long-term arrangement, supported by legal agreements between Statistics Canada, PHAC, and individual P/T registries, allows an annual copy of the CCR data set to be forwarded each year to PHAC for special analyses and project work including statistical methodology development. PHAC also provides one-time resources for meetings or defined projects to improve surveillance infrastructure. PHAC has also developed online resources to provide public and professional access to cancer and other statistics in various tabular, chart, and map formats.[29]

Canadian Institute for Health Information

The Canadian Institute for Health Information (CIHI) is an independent, nonprofit, national organization that works to provide standardized, high-quality health information for improving the health of Canadians. CIHI accomplishes its work by partnering with federal and P/T governments and other healthcare organizations to identify standards for the collection of health information in Canada and to monitor the quality of data collected.[30] Data are collected at the P/T healthcare organization level and routinely submitted to national databases for storage and analysis. Many P/T cancer registries utilize these standardized data sets such as the Discharge Abstracting System and National Ambulatory Care Reporting System for casefinding and supplementing treatment and follow-up data collection.

Canada Health Infoway

In the same manner that CIHI provides direction on data standards, Canada Health Infoway (CHI) is also a nonprofit organization aimed at working with all levels of government and healthcare organizations and technology providers to promote the use of EHRs in Canada. CHI contributes to the identification of potential technology solutions and best practices, as well as the establishment of important infrastructure components such as data transmission standards.[31]

P/T registries, in particular, are becoming aware that EHR-based solutions must be part of the future vision for cancer surveillance. Cancer registries are, for the most part, secondary users of data, most of which are collected at the point of care. It will be important that the needs of cancer data users are heard at the right forums and incorporated into EHR development from the outset. This is new territory for many cancer registry professionals, but in Canada, recent Canadian initiatives such as synoptic reporting related to cancer (e.g., pathology and surgery) are helping raise the profile of cancer information needs to groups such as CHI.

Canadian Cancer Society

The Canadian Cancer Society (CCS) is one of the oldest cancer stakeholder organizations in Canada and serves to coordinate the activities of the many volunteers, as well as cancer patients, families, and survivors who want to make a difference in how cancer affects this country. CCS is a national group supported by a network of community-based volunteers dedicated to reducing the burden of cancer and improving the quality of life for those living with cancer. CCS works in the areas of fund-raising, advocacy, prevention, information, and support, as well as research.[32] This organization was one of the first to truly recognize the value of making cancer statistical data available to a wide audience.

CCS provides a secretariat and resources to coordinate the annual publication of *Canadian Cancer Statistics*. Working in collaboration with an oversight committee that includes representatives from Statistics Canada, PHAC, and P/T registries, as well as epidemiology and clinical oncology professionals, the CCR data are reviewed and analyzed to produce a high-quality annual publication focused on incidence, mortality, survival, and projection statistics.[11,32] Special topics are also addressed in each publication to highlight emerging trends or topical areas of interest. Published since 1987, Canadian Cancer Statistics represents one of the most important, well recognized, and consistent uses of cancer surveillance data in Canada.

Canadian Partnership Against Cancer

Starting in the late 1990s and spanning close to a 10-year period, many stakeholders within the cancer community, ranging from public advocacy groups, government agencies such as PHAC, Health Canada, and Statistics Canada, as well as many groups from within the cancer professional community (e.g., cancer agencies, healthcare providers), engaged in a vigorous dialogue on the need for a national approach for cancer control. The resulting plan known as the Canadian Strategy for Cancer Control was translated into a business case, which was submitted to the federal government in 2005, requesting national funding to support the implementation of the strategy.[33] After much deliberation, an initial allocation of 250 million dollars over 5 years was provided by the federal government via the Ministry of Health to move forward with the strategy. Canadian Partnership Against Cancer is the organization that has been created to implement the vision for national cancer control.[34]

CPAC is just more than halfway through its initial 5-year mandate. It works collaboratively with a wide range of stakeholder organizations and interested parties across the country to address key areas of focus that have been identified as critical for cancer control. Examples of focus areas include screening, primary prevention, research, quality and standards, as well as surveillance. This concerted emphasis on surveillance has led to an informed priority-setting exercise on the topic. Results of that discussion included recognition of the value of cancer registration at both P/T and national levels, and a need to strengthen and enhance existing systems.

Three priority areas have been identified within the surveillance pillar for this initial 5-year mandate:

- Expansion of core surveillance data collection, particularly in the area of stage data
- Improving analytic capacity in the surveillance community
- Increasing access to and use of registry data

Each priority area has been translated into action plans, and funding has been allocated to support implementation. Access to this type of support and funding has been met with enthusiasm within the surveillance community and is certainly presenting both opportunities and challenges as new program work gets under way.

Although many activities have been started, two are having immediate and tangible impacts on registry operations. The first is the National Staging Initiative, which is providing funding support to individual P/T registries to enhance their ability to collect stage data. This effort was a clear recognition of the slow progress being made within P/T registries to achieve population-based cancer stage data collection. To access this funding, stream registries must commit to collecting population-based stage data for the four main cancers by the 2010 incidence year and as much as possible utilize electronic synoptic pathology reporting to support this collection. Jurisdictions such as Ontario who were already working to implement full synoptic pathology reporting using defined data fields in compliance with known standards have been able to provide leadership and direction to others through this initiative.[3,35]

The second program has been the Surveillance & Epidemiology Networks, which issued a call for proposals aimed at establishing interprovincial teams of epidemiology and analytic staff to address a specific area of cancer surveillance.[34] This program addresses the priority related to developing analytic capacity. Teams have received multi-year funding and are working on various cancer data analyses and products, as well as targeting the development of agreed-on methods and tools to support data analysis.

To date, CPAC has provided strong support for cancer registration and surveillance in Canada. It is hoped that successes during the initial 5-year funding period and lessons learned will lead to a further extension of the organization's mandate.

Summary

Cancer surveillance in Canada is experiencing a positive period of growth. The recent development of a national cancer-control program through CPAC has highlighted the value of surveillance and cancer registries. New resources are available to assist registries to expand data collection and improve infrastructure. Increased awareness of the valuable work carried out by other North American registry standard setters has allowed Canada to improve its systems and approaches to registry operations. Canadians have also played leadership roles in identifying processes and tools such as electronic pathology and surgical reporting to enhance cancer information. This type of innovation will be of increasing importance to registries in the future as they seek to expand data collection and introduce greater operational efficiencies. Opportunities also exist to partner and establish new relationships with key Canadian organizations involved in the development of global health information standards and EHR systems. Registry and surveillance professionals are optimistic that this renewed focus on cancer information will continue.

References

1. Parkin, D. M., Whelan, S. L., Ferlay, J., Raymond, L., Young, J., editors. *Cancer Incidence in Five Continents,* Vol. VII. Lyon, France: International Agency for Research on Cancer, 1997.
2. Band, P., Gaudette, L., Hill, G., Holowaty, E., Hutchcroft, S., Johnston, G., Makomaski Illing, E., Mao, Y., Semenciw, R. *The Making of the Canadian Cancer Registry: Cancer Incidence in Canada and Its Regions 1969-1988.* Ottawa, Ontario, Canada: Minister of Supply and Services Canada, 1993.

3. King, M. J. 2010. *Electronic Reporting at the Ontario Cancer Registry.* Summary Working Document.

4. Menck, H., Deapen, D., Phillips, J. L., Tucker, T, editors. *Central Cancer Registries, Design, Management and Use,* 2nd ed. Dubuque, IA: Kendall/Hunt Publishing Co., 2007.

5. Cowan, D., Robson, D. *National Cancer Stage Facilitation Report (Draft).* Toronto, Ontario, Canada: Canadian Association of Provincial Cancer Agencies, July 2005.

6. Natural Resources Canada. *The Atlas of Canada.* Ottawa: Earth Sciences Sector, Government of Canada, 2004.

7. Health Statistics Division, Statistics Canada. *Census, 2006 Census Release Topics, Population and Dwelling Counts: Statistics Canada.* Available at: www12.statcan.ca/census/2006/rt-td/pd-pl-eng.cfm. http://www12.statcan.ca/census-recensement/2006/dp-pd/hlt/97-550/Index.cfm?TPL=P1C&Page=RETR&LANG=Eng&T=101. Accessed May 14, 2010.

8. Health Statistics Division, Statistics Canada. *Census, 2006 Census: Analysis Series: Statistics Canada.* Available at: www12.statcan.ca/census-recensement/2006/as-sa/97-551/pl-eng.cfm. Accessed May 18, 2010.

9. Health Statistics Division, Statistics Canada. *Census, 2006 Census: Data Products, Topic Based Tabulations, Citizenship, Immigrant Status and Period of Immigration: Statistics Canada.* Available at: www12.statcan.gc.ca/census-recensement/2006/dp-pd/tbt/Rp-eng.cfm?LANG=E&APATH=3&DETAIL=0&DIM=0&FL=A&FREE=0&GC=0&GID=0&GK=0&GRP=1&PID=89424&PRID=0&PTYPE=88971,97154&S=0&SHOWALL=0&SUB=722&Temporal=2006&THEME=72&VID=0&VNAMEE=&VNAMEF=. Accessed May 14, 2010.

10. Health Statistics Division, Statistics Canada. *Census, 2006 Census: Data Products, Geography Selection, Selected Trend Data for Canada, 1996, 2001 and 2006 Censuses.* Available at: www12.statcan.ca/census-recensement/2006/dp-pd/92-596/P1-2.cfm?Lang=eng&T=PR&PRCODE=01&GEOCODE=01&GEOLVL=PR&TID=0 Accessed May 14, 2010.

11. Canadian Cancer Society/National Cancer Institute of Canada Steering Committee: *Canadian Cancer Statistics 2008.* Toronto, Ontario, Canada: Canadian Cancer Society, 2008.

12. Forsey, E. *How Canadians Govern Themselves,* 7th ed. Ottawa, Ontario, Canada: Library of Parliament, 2010.

13. *Canadian Charter of Rights and Freedoms: Schedule B Constitution Act, 1982, Part I,* March 29, 1982. Available at: laws.justice.gc.ca/en/charter/index.html.Accessed May 18, 2010.

14. Makin, K., Sallot, J., Seguin, R., Simpson, J. "The New Face of Medicare," *The Globe and Mail,* June 10, 2005, Section A:1 (cols. 1-4).

15. Department of Justice. *Canada Health Act,* ch. C-6, §1; 2004. Available at: laws.justice.gc.ca/eng/C-6/index.html.

16. *Health Care in Canada.* Ottawa, Ontario, Canada: Canadian Institute for Health Information, 2006.

17. Committee on Data Quality and Management. "Analysis of 2001 Impact Assessment Survey." *Proceedings of Canadian Council of Cancer Registries Annual Meeting.* Banff, Alberta, Canada: Health Statistics Division, Statistics Canada, 2002.

18. *Proceedings of Canadian Council of Cancer Registries Annual Meeting.* Ottawa, Ontario, Canada: Health Statistics Division, Statistics Canada, 2009.

19. Health Statistics Division, Statistics Canada. *Canadian Cancer Registry Survey #3207.* Ottawa, Ontario, Canada: Statistics Canada; updated July 11, 2005. Available at: www.statcan.ca/cgi-bin/imdb/p2SV.pl?Function=getSurvey&SDDS=3207&lang=en&db=IMDB&dbg=f&adm=8&dis=2. Accessed August 3, 2005.

20. Von Tigerstrom, B., Deschenes, M., Knoppers, B., Caulfield, T. *Opportunities and Barriers for Access to and Use of Cancer Patient Information for Surveillance Purposes: A Systematic Review of Legislation, Regulations, Policies, and Guidelines.* Sponsored by the Canadian Coalition on Cancer Surveillance, March 2000.

21. Von Tigerstron, B., Ries, N. "Cancer Surveillance in Canada—An Analysis of Legal and Policy Frameworks and Options for Enhancing Surveillance." Sponsored by the Surveillance Action Group, Canadian Partnership Against Cancer, September 2008.

22. *Proceedings of Canadian Council of Cancer Registries Annual Meeting.* Fredericton, New Brunswick, Canada: Health Statistics Division, Statistics Canada, 2008.

23. *Proceedings of Canadian Council of Cancer Registries Annual Meeting.* Saskatoon, Saskatchewan, Canada: Health Statistics Division, Statistics Canada, 2010.

24. Dale, Darlene. Personal Communication, July 30, 2005.

25. Starratt, Karen. Personal Communication, May 14, 2010.

26. Bu, V., MacIntyre, M., Dewar, R., Turner, D., Vriends, K. "Stage Data Collection in Canada; Initial Comparative Results of CSV1 for Nova Scotia, Manitoba and Prince Edward Island 2004-2008," Presented at the NAACCR Annual Meeting; Quebec City, Quebec, Canada, June 2010.

27. Thorton M, O'Connor L, eds. *Standards for Cancer Registries, Volume II: Data Standards and Data Dictionary,* 12th ed., version 12. Springfield, IL: North American Association of Central Cancer Registries, February 2009.

28. Public Health Agency of Canada. Ottawa, Ontario, Canada: Public Health Agency of Canada, 2010. Available at: www.phac-aspc.gc.ca/about_apropos/who-eng.php. Accessed July 26, 2010.

29. Public Health Agency of Canada. "Disease Surveillance On-Line." Ottawa, Ontario, Canada: Public Health Agency of Canada, 2010. Available at: http://dsol-smed.phac-aspc.gc.ca/dsol-smed/cancer/index_e.html. Accessed July 26, 2010.

30. Canadian Institute for Health Information. Ottawa, Ontario, Canada: Health Services Databases, 2010. Available at: http://secure.cihi.ca/cihiweb/dispPage.jsp?cw_page=home_e. Accessed July 26, 2010.

31. Canada Health Infoway. "The Vision: About Infoway." Available at: www.infoway-inforoute.ca/lang-en/about-infoway. Accessed May 17, 2010.

32. Canadian Cancer Society Web site: www.cancer.ca/ccs/internet/niw_splash/0%2C%2C3172%2C00.html.

33. The Canadian Strategy for Cancer Control: A Cancer Plan for Canada, Discussion Paper, Ottawa, Ontario, Canada, July 2006 Available at: www.cancer.ca/Canada-wide/How%20you%20can%20help/Take%20action/Advocacy%20what%20were%20doing/~/media/CCS/Canada%20wide/Files%20List/English%20files%20heading/pdf%20not%20in%20publications%20section/CSCC%20discussion%20paper%20-%20PDF_1404842209.ashx. Accessed May 15, 2010.

34. Canadian Partnership Against Cancer Web site: www.partnershipagainstcancer.ca

35. MacLean, A. *Overview of National Staging Initiative by Province, Written Summary.* Toronto, Ontario, Canada: Canadian Partnership Against Cancer, March 2010.

chapter 30

American College of Surgeons Commission on Cancer

Connie Bura

Historical Overview

The Commission on Cancer (CoC) of the American College of Surgeons (ACoS) is a consortium of professional organizations dedicated to improving survival and quality of life for cancer patients through standard-setting, prevention, research, education, and the monitoring of comprehensive quality care.

The CoC was initially formed in 1922 as the Cancer Campaign Committee. The committee's early efforts focused on the study of the use of radium treatment for uterine cancers. In the 1930s, the commission teamed up with the already established American Cancer Society (ACS) to pursue a cooperative venture concerned with establishing standards for cancer clinics. This era marked the birth of the CoC's Accreditation Program, and the commission has been surveying and accrediting hospital cancer programs now for more than 75 years.

In 1930, the committee was renamed the Committee on the Treatment of Malignant Disease. The first official standards were published that year under the title "An Organization of Service for the Diagnosis and Treatment of Cancer." These standards were focused on the structural aspects of a cancer program and led to an established evaluation process for cancer clinics and their data registries. In 1940, the committee was renamed the Committee on Cancer, and in 1947, a grassroots program to identify a surgeon at the hospital level who would promote and oversee the cancer program and serve as the "clinical champion" was initiated. This Cancer Liaison Program continues today. In 1954, the standards for cancer programs were updated to include mandates for a multidisciplinary cancer committee, tumor boards, and methods of monitoring and reporting end results. The requirements for cancer program accreditation were expanded in 1956 to include a cancer registry, which incorporated diagnostic, staging, treatment, and annual lifetime follow-up for all cancer patients. This established the foundation of the accreditation program of today, which includes the four cornerstones of comprehensive, quality care: the cancer committee, cancer conferences, a cancer registry, and quality improvement program. Since incorporation of the cancer registry standard in the 1950s, the CoC has been a key supporter and strong advocate for the important contributions hospital-based cancer registries make to measuring and impacting the quality of cancer care delivery in the United States. In recognition of the increasingly multidisciplinary nature of cancer care, the membership of the Committee on Cancer was expanded in 1965 to include members from a variety of professional organizations involved in the care of the cancer patient, and the organization was renamed the Commission on Cancer (CoC).

Commission on Cancer: Purpose, Goals, and Structure

The multidisciplinary CoC establishes standards to ensure quality, multidisciplinary, and comprehensive cancer care delivery in healthcare settings; conducts surveys in healthcare settings to assess compliance with those standards; collects standardized data from CoC-accredited healthcare settings to measure cancer care quality; uses data to monitor treatment patterns and outcomes, and enhance cancer control and clinical surveillance activities; and develops effective educational interventions to improve cancer prevention, early detection, cancer care delivery, and outcomes in healthcare settings.

The CoC includes 100 members composed of individuals representing the ACoS and the 48 national, professional organizations that reflect the full spectrum of cancer care. These participating member organizations are listed in Table 30-1. The CoC plays a major role in the development of standards for cancer data collection and for cancer care delivery with a formal process for program monitoring and accreditation. The CoC is active in the education of members of the cancer care team, as well as in the collection and reporting of data to assess national patterns of cancer care and support quality improvement efforts at the facility level. These activities are reflected in the organizational structure, which includes five standing committees and multiple subcommittees (Figure 30-1). CoC members are elected to a 3-year term with eligibility to serve a second term. Committee chairs serve for 3 years, and the chair of the commission serves for 2 years with eligibility to serve a second term.

The CoC Executive Committee conducts the interim business of the commission, and administers the goals and objectives of the CoC as set forth by its mission statement. The committee reviews policies, plans activities, makes recommendations regarding membership, considers actions coming before it, and recommends actions to the membership of the CoC. The Executive Committee is composed of the chair and chair-elect of the CoC, an advisor from the ACoS Board of Regents, the chairs of the five standing committees, and a representative from each of the following organizations: ACS, American College of Radiology, American College of Surgeons Oncology Group, American Joint Committee on Cancer (AJCC), American Society of Clinical Oncology, American Society for Therapeutic Radiology and Oncology, the College of American Pathologists, National Comprehensive Cancer Network, and the Oncology Nursing Society.

The Member Organization Steering Committee directs the activities of the member organization representa-

Table 30-1	Member Organizations of the Commission on Cancer

American Academy of Hospice and Palliative Medicine

American Academy of Pediatrics

American Association for Cancer Education, Inc.

American Cancer Society, Inc.

American College of Obstetricians and Gynecologists

American College of Oncology Administrators

American College of Physicians

American College of Radiology

American College of Surgeons

American College of Surgeons Young Fellows Association

American College of Surgeons Resident and Associate Society

American Dietetic Association, Oncology Nutrition Dietetic Practice Group

American Head and Neck Society

American Hospital Association

American Joint Committee on Cancer

American Medical Association

American Pediatric Surgical Association

American Psychosocial Oncology Society

American Radium Society

American Society of Breast Surgeons

American Society of Clinical Oncology

American Society of Colon and Rectal Surgeons

American Society for Radiation Oncology American Urological Association

Association of American Cancer Institutes

Association of Cancer Executives

Association of Community Cancer Centers

Association of Oncology Social Workers

Canadian Society of Surgical Oncology

Centers for Disease Control, Division of Cancer Prevention and Control

College of American Pathologists

Department of Defense

Department of Veterans Affairs

International Union Against Cancer

Lance Armstrong Foundation

National Cancer Institute Surveillance, Epidemiology, and End Results Program

National Cancer Institute—Outcomes Research Branch

National Cancer Registrars Association, Inc.

National Comprehensive Cancer Network

National Coalition for Cancer Survivorship

National Consortium of Breast Centers

National Society of Genetic Counselors

National Surgical Adjuvant Breast and Bowel Project

North American Association of Central Cancer Registries

Oncology Nursing Society

Society of Gynecologic Oncologists

Society of Nuclear Medicine

Society of Surgical Oncology

Society of Thoracic Surgeons

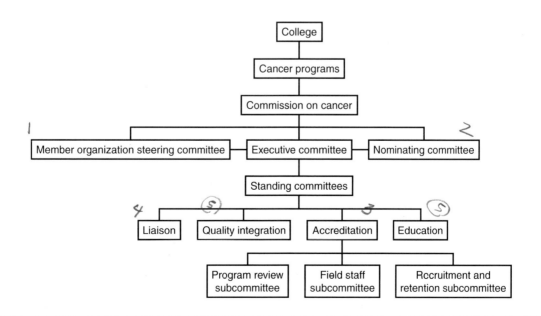

Figure 30-1. Commission on Cancer Structure. From Commission on Cancer. Copyright © 2009 by Commission on Cancer. Reprinted with permission.

tives, and is responsible for developing, implementing and evaluating strategies to support enhanced collaborations and communications with CoC member organizations.

The Nominating Committee is charged with the preparation of a slate of nominees for membership on the CoC. There are three categories of nominees: (1) from the Fellowship of the ACoS, (2) from member organizations who have representation on the CoC, and (3) special members. In addition, the Nominating Committee is charged with preparing a slate of nominees for the role of chair and vice-chair of the standing committees, and the chair and chair-elect of the CoC, and for identifying Executive Committee positions. The Nominating Committee is also charged with evaluating member participation.

The Accreditation Committee encourages hospitals, treatment centers, and other facilities to improve their quality of patient care through various cancer-related programs. Participating programs are concerned with the continuum of cancer care from prevention and early detection, pretreatment evaluation, and staging, to optimal treatment, rehabilitation, surveillance for recurrent disease, support services, and end-of-life or lifelong follow-up care. The Accreditation Committee has three subcommittees: The Program Review Subcommittee is responsible for making accreditation award decisions for programs that do not meet all of the standards; the Field Staff Subcommittee is responsible for the recruitment, training, and evaluation of the cancer program surveyor team, and the Recruitment and Retention Subcommittee is responsible for developing strategies to increase applications by new cancer programs, monitoring program withdrawals, and implementing interventions for program retention.

The Committee on Cancer Liaison directs the activities of the Cancer Liaison Program, which is composed of a network of more than 1,600 volunteer Cancer Liaison Physicians (CLPs) who provide local support for the CoC's programs and activities. The committee also directs the activities of the network's 65 volunteer State Chairs responsible for managing state-based cancer activities and their respective groups of CLPs appointed in local facilities to support the activities of the CoC and ACS. The committee also oversees the implementation of priorities established by the funding agency, the ACS.

The Education Committee directs the activities of the CoC's Education Program by defining and developing programs and products to address the educational needs of the CoC's constituency. As needed, subcommittees may be formed to manage the duties and responsibilities associated with specific educational activities. Activities under the direction of the committee include the development of the CoC's professional education program for the ACoS Clinical Congress, selection of the Keynote Speaker for the CoC Annual Meeting, contributions to the content of the Online Education Portal, and annual planning to address the educational needs of the CoC's constituents.

The Quality Integration Committee is the central advisory panel that guides and assists in the prioritization of work conducted by the National Cancer Data Base (NCDB). The committee is concerned with, and represents, the CoC in matters that address the progress and direction of research and education as it pertains to improving the care of patients with cancer.

Accreditation Program

The Accreditation Committee administers the activities of the Accreditation Program, which is designed to ensure that the structure and processes necessary for quality cancer care are in place. In 2003, the CoC released its current standards for cancer program accreditation. The 36 standards are all mandatory, form the basis for the accreditation award, and are organized into 8 major areas. These standards continue to promote and support the four historic cornerstones of the Accreditation Program: multidisciplinary cancer conferences, a multidisciplinary cancer committee, a program of quality improvement and outcome assessment, and a cancer registry. *Cancer Program Standards 2004* became effective in January 2004 for participating hospital cancer programs. Subsequent revisions have resulted in the current edition: *Cancer Program Standards 2009, Revised Edition.* The standards provide a flexible approach to cancer program management, and take into account the various types and sizes of hospitals, with category-specific requirements defined for many standards. These requirements are designed to recognize the type of facility, services provided, and cases accessioned.

CoC Accreditation provides a framework for cancer program structure and process, includes access to cancer program and data standards; provides for external and internal assessments of the quality of care being provided to cancer patients; allows access to the NCDB to assess and improve care; provides educational tools, resources, and best practices to enhance cancer program performance; and results in promotion and recognition by the public, payers, and government agencies.

The eight areas of program evaluation include institutional and programmatic resources, cancer committee leadership, cancer data management and cancer registry operations, clinical management, research, community outreach, professional education and staff support, and quality improvement. Facilities participating in the CoC Accreditation Program are concerned with the continuum of care from prevention and early detection, pretreatment evaluation, and staging, to optimal treatment, rehabilitation, surveillance for recurrent disease, support services, and end-of-life care. To earn CoC Accreditation, a facility must fulfill the following criteria:

- Meet rigorous quality standards set by the CoC.
- Provide access to the full scope of multidisciplinary services required to screen, diagnose, treat, rehabilitate, and support patients with cancer and their families.

- Make prevention and early detection services available to the community.
- Provide services on-site, by referral, or through coordination with other facilities or local agencies.
- Submit data annually to the NCDB.

Five elements are key to the success of a CoC-accredited cancer program:

- The clinical services provide state-of-the-art pretreatment evaluation, staging, treatment, and clinical follow-up for cancer patients seen at the facility for primary, secondary, tertiary, or quaternary care.
- The cancer committee leads the program through setting goals, monitoring activity, and evaluating patient outcomes and improving care.
- The cancer conferences provide a forum for patient consultation and contribute to physician education.
- The quality improvement program is the mechanism for evaluating and improving patient outcomes.
- The cancer registry and database is the basis for monitoring the quality of care.

CoC Accreditation is granted only to those facilities that have voluntarily committed to provide the best in cancer diagnosis and treatment, and are able to comply with the CoC's established standards. Participation in the Accreditation Program is voluntary. The success of a cancer program depends on the leadership of a multidisciplinary cancer committee. The committee is responsible for planning, initiating, stimulating, and assessing all cancer-related activities at the facility. Because quality of care requires a serious commitment to the necessity and value of the cancer program, facilities are initially surveyed only at the written request of a member of the administrative or professional staff. This request should be made when the cancer committee is confident that the CoC Cancer Program Standards have been met. Before initial survey, the institution must demonstrate 1 year of compliance with the standards, have accrued 2 years of data with 1 year of successful follow-up, and have met the requirements for consideration for accreditation as outlined in the *Cancer Program Standards* manual.

The assessment of cancer programs is conducted by staff-trained, volunteer physician-surveyors and is overseen by the CoC technical staff, and the Program Review and Field Staff Subcommittees of the Accreditation Committee. Each cancer program must undergo a rigorous evaluation and review of its performance and compliance with the CoC standards every 3 years. When the survey visit is scheduled, time must be allotted on the agenda for the surveyor to meet with the administrator, cancer committee chair, cancer registrar, and the CLP, as well as other members of the facility's cancer team. The surveyor reviews documentation of cancer committee meetings, cancer conferences, and quality management processes and improvements. The visit also includes a review of documentation

that supports the cancer program's compliance with the standards, including the electronic CoC Survey Application Record completed by the facility before the survey. At the conclusion of the survey, the surveyor makes recommendations for improving the program that are consistent with current standards.

A quantitative rating system, consistent with that used by the Joint Commission (JC) is in place to ensure objectivity and consistency among reviewers. To ensure consistent interpretation and compliance with the 36 standards, the rating system includes criteria for compliance with each standard, and a compliance rating is assigned by the facility, the surveyor, and the CoC technical staff. Commendation ratings have been established for nine standards (25%). Commendations received for individual standards are acknowledged in the Cancer Program Performance Report that is provided to the program after the survey. A program that receives a commendation rating in all nine defined areas along with a compliance rating for all other (27) standards will earn the "CoC Outstanding Achievement Award." Awards will be granted to each program on completion of the survey and evaluation of compliance with the established criteria. This award will be in place until the next survey. The purpose of the "CoC Outstanding Achievement Award" is to recognize cancer programs that strive for excellence in providing quality care to the cancer patient, motivate other programs to work toward improving their care, foster communication between award recipients and other programs to share best practices, serve as a resource, and act as a "champion" for the CoC Accreditation Program. Cancer programs that achieve this award receive a letter of recognition from the CoC chair addressed to the CEO/administrator, a specially designed press release, marketing information and certificate, CoC publicity via the CoC Flash e-mail newsletter and CoC Web site, and acknowledgment in a public forum including the CoC Annual Meeting.

The Accreditation Committee recognizes that the cancer services available at a facility will vary depending on its size and scope. Therefore, accreditation is given in different categories. Each facility is assigned to a cancer program category by the CoC staff. The type of facility or organization, services provided, and cases accessioned are considered when making category assignments. The CoC has defined nine cancer program categories and describes the requirements for each as they relate to specific standards. A sample of program categories includes those institutions funded by the National Cancer Institute (NCI) as cancer centers, defined as NCI-designated centers; teaching facilities, defined as facilities with at least 4 residency programs; comprehensive community, facilities that see more than 650 analytic cancer cases annually and provide a full range of cancer services; and community hospitals, which see a smaller number of cases annually. The Network Cancer Program category reflects the sharing of cancer treatment and data resources among hospitals in healthcare networks. Additional categories exist that allow participation by facilities that provide only specialized elements of cancer care.

Currently, there are more than 1,450 CoC-accredited cancer programs in the United States and Puerto Rico (Figure 30-2). Of these, 39% are community programs, 35% are comprehensive community programs, and 23% are either NCI-designated or teaching programs. Accredited programs are widely distributed throughout the United States (see Figure 30-2), and a public list is available on the Cancer Programs page of the ACoS Web site (www.facs.org/cancer).

Data from the accreditation process are used to generate Accredited Cancer Program Performance Reports comparable with the hospital performance reports issued by the JC. These reports allow cancer programs to compare their ratings for mandatory standards with accredited programs in their state, their award category, and nationally. The report also facilitates the identification of areas for program improvement.

Today, CoC-accredited cancer programs are credited with diagnosing and treating 71% of all newly diagnosed cancer patients. The Accreditation Program is recognized by other national healthcare organizations, including the JC and Blue Cross Blue Shield Association, as having established performance measures for high-quality cancer care. An accredited cancer program provides a forum for interdisciplinary communication and interaction. It en-

sures that multidisciplinary, integrated, and comprehensive oncology services are being offered to patients, and accreditation demonstrates to the community that the institution is willing to commit the resources necessary to provide the very best cancer care.

CoC-accredited cancer programs benefit from free marketing of their available resources and services, and cancer experience, through the CoC's Hospital Locator Web site. These data are made available to meet the needs of today's consumers by providing useful information to cancer patients and the general public about CoC-accredited cancer programs. These data also assist people in making educated decisions about their options for cancer care based on both the scope of services and the quality of care offered at hospitals accredited by the CoC. The ACS's 24-hour National Cancer Information Center operators (800-ACS-2345) utilize the CoC Hospital Locator to provide targeted referrals to CoC hospitals for resources and services, and the ACS's Web site (www.cancer.org) also links to the CoC Web site and the "Find an Accredited Cancer Program Near You" Hospital Locator (http://www.facs.org/cancerprogram/index.html).

The CoC standards have established the foundation and framework for the coordinated, multidisciplinary delivery of cancer care, and the majority of organized cancer care provided in the United States is based on this framework. The standards and survey processes have routinely been reviewed and revised every 5 to 7 years in an effort

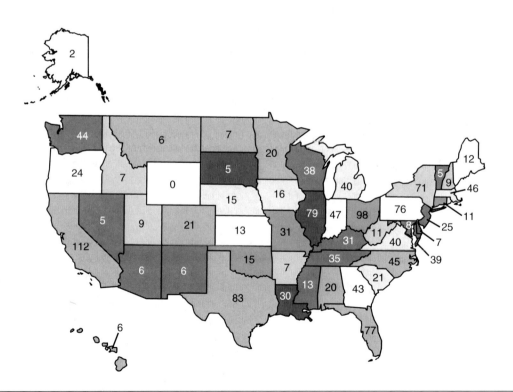

Figure 30-2. Distribution of Commission on Cancer–accredited Cancer Programs by State. From Commission on Cancer. Copyright © 2009 by Commission on Cancer. Reprinted with permission.

to remain relevant and to reflect current cancer care practices. The standards have historically focused on structure and some process; however, outcomes are emerging as an area that requires more focus and integration within the standards. The CoC has continued to remain responsive to participating programs and member organizations when issues relative to difficulty with standards' compliance or issues regarding changes in cancer care have been identified. This responsiveness and flexibility have allowed the CoC to respond to key constituent groups by listening to concerns and effecting change.

The process to review and revise the CoC standards and survey process for cancer program accreditation is currently under way. The goals of the *Cancer Program Standards 2011* project are as follows:

- Modify the current standards to eliminate duplication, establish clear definitions, and define a measurement for each standard.
- Create new standards that focus on improving care for the cancer patient.
- Enhance the survey application process and coordinate changes for the reporting of survey results
- Delineate plans to expand participation in the Accreditation Program.

The overall goal is to develop standards that encompass the entire continuum of care, focus on performance measurement and outcome, and have a direct patient care benefit. Workgroups that include broad representation from all disciplines and organizations committed to improving cancer patient care are engaged in the revision process. The timeline includes release of the standards, pilot testing, and implementation in 2011, with compliance requirements beginning in 2012.

National Cancer Data Base

The NCDB is a nationwide oncology outcomes database for more than 1,450 facilities in the United States and Puerto Rico. The NCDB was founded as a joint project of the CoC and the ACS in 1988. Currently, the NCDB collects data on approximately 71% of all incident cancer diagnoses annually, and includes detailed information on more than 25 million cancer patients in the United States representing 38 different cancer sites. The NCDB has undergone a number of changes since its inception and is now recognized as the world's largest clinical database providing vitally important patterns of care information on which quality improvement can be leveraged at the point of delivery of cancer care in the United States. Information is collected on an annual basis on patient demographics, diagnostic methods, AJCC stage, treatment, and mortality; this allows for the definition of current patterns of care and changes over time. The annual submission of data to the NCDB has been a requirement for accredited cancer programs since 1996. Each year, the NCDB issues a Call for Data to all CoC-accredited cancer programs. Original data collection commenced with 1985 diagnoses and now provides 20 years of follow-up. Relatively uncommon cancers have accumulated in impressive numbers. NCDB data are used as follows:

- To measure treatment patterns and outcomes
- To evaluate hospital provider performance
- To conduct research and develop focused studies to meet the demand for an ongoing assessment of the quality of cancer care
- To assess and validate nationally accepted quality measures for cancer care
- To develop effective resources and tools to improve outcomes at the national, regional, and local levels

Data elements are collected and submitted to the NCDB from CoC-accredited cancer program registries using nationally standardized data item and coding definitions, as defined in the *Facility Oncology Registry Data Standards (FORDS)* manual, and nationally standardized data transmission format specifications coordinated by the North American Association of Central Cancer Registries. This includes patient characteristics, cancer staging and tumor histologic characteristics, type of first course treatment administered, and outcomes information.

The NCDB maintains a number of Web-based tools that have been developed to promote access to the NCDB data. These tools are for use by CoC-accredited cancer programs as a means by which to evaluate and compare the cancer care delivered to patients diagnosed and/or treated at their facility with that provided at state, regional, and national cancer facilities. Included among these reporting applications are the following:

- Benchmark Hospital Comparison Reports allow users access to almost 8.3 million case reports of patients diagnosed between 2000 and 2007, from which reports can be generated showing data reported to the NCDB from the user's own cancer registry; aggregated data by hospital system, state, or region or at the national level; or a comparison of the cases submitted to the NCDB by the user's cancer program and all the other programs identified by the user in the comparative group.
- NCDB Survival Reports, which provide access to AJCC stage-stratified, 5-year observed survival rates for all cancer sites, allow users to generate survival reports filtered by primary site of the cancer, diagnosis period, geographic location of CoC-accredited cancer programs, and cancer program category or corporate affiliation. Users can even generate program-specific results. Computed results are available for cases diagnosed between 1994 and 1997 (AJCC, 4th ed.) or 1998 and 2002 (AJCC, 5th ed.).
- Cancer Program Practice Profile Reports provide CoC-accredited programs with comparative informa-

tion to assess adherence to standard-of-care therapies for breast and colorectal cancers, including measures endorsed by the National Quality Forum (NQF) and developed in collaboration with the American Society of Clinical Oncology and the National Comprehensive Cancer Network.

- The Rapid Quality Reporting System is the most recently launched reporting tool that provides real clinical time assessment of hospital level performance using NQF-endorsed quality-of-cancer care measures for breast and colorectal cancers.

On occasion, hypothesis-based special studies are conducted that allow for the ad hoc collection of specific data to address important cancer problems. Participation by CoC-accredited cancer programs in these studies is mandated by the CoC Cancer Program Standards. Thus, the NCDB collects the traditional dataset (longitudinal) and one-time and ad hoc datasets (cross sectional). The NCDB is also actively engaged in supporting the development of clinical trials through assisting cooperative groups with targeting accruals initiatives.

Data confidentiality is of prime importance, and the NCDB has proactively worked to continually ensure and maintain compliance with the Health Insurance Portability and Accountability Act of 1996, privacy regulations established by the federal government.

The NCDB maintains close working relationships with a number of national cancer surveillance programs, including federal agencies and the ACS. Since its inception, the NCDB has matured as a clinical surveillance mechanism, and a continuous review of NCDB data on patterns of care and outcomes has been maintained. This has included the publication of findings in scientific papers as appropriate, feedback to hospitals in the form of benchmark summary information, and descriptive statistical information. The peer-reviewed publication effort has generated 350 articles since 1990, most frequently concerning patterns of care and outcomes for specific disease sites.

In addition to the tools developed specifically for CoC-accredited cancer programs, the NCDB maintains a Web-based benchmarking application that has been developed to promote access to NCDB data by the general public, researchers, and clinicians. NCDB Public Benchmark Reports include the 11 most commonly diagnosed solid tumors in the United States. Users are provided access to more than 8 million cases from 7 diagnosis years (2000–2007). Users can design queries using data from any one or a combination of three types of hospitals (community, comprehensive community, and academic/teaching facilities) and specify a geographic region or state to narrow the scope of their analysis. As many as three covariates (including patient age, ethnicity, sex, tumor histology, stage, first-course therapy, and type of surgical resection) are available for users to define the type of information they wish to review.

The size and sophistication of the NCDB infrastructure allows data to be collected, aggregated, and used to generate a wide range of reports and peer-reviewed manuscripts. Leveraging its unique relationship with providers through the CoC accreditation program, the database will continue to establish itself as the primary source for developing and implementing quality metrics for cancer care improvement, and to retain and expand broad support within the clinical community. The NCDB is clearly recognized as a valuable resource and one that continues to position itself to maximize its value for both its contributors in CoC-accredited cancer programs and members of the clinical, research, and policy-making communities. (See Chapter 38 for additional information about the NCDB.)

Data Standards

Registry data management is an essential element of each CoC-accredited cancer program. The CoC's data standards ensure consistent and accurate hospital cancer registry data that support the evaluation of patient diagnosis and treatment. All CoC-accredited cancer programs use the data standards defined by the CoC appropriate for the year of diagnosis for that case. Cancer registries may be required to comply with additional mandates pertaining to case and data reporting established by the federal or state government, or by the facility's cancer committee. Following the initial release in 2002, the *FORDS* manual has undergone a series of modifications and revisions. To avoid the need to implement major changes in data annually, the registry community has agreed to the adoption of major changes once every 3 or 4 years. The *FORDS* manual provides definitions and detailed instructions for coding patient diagnosis, treatment, and outcomes. The manual also describes the types of cases that must be abstracted and followed, and explains the relationship among data items. Registry data maintained with standardized quality-control mechanisms support meaningful evaluation and analysis.

To support uniform and consistent interpretation of CoC cancer program and data standards, and promote quality data abstracting, the CoC provides the Web-based Inquiry and Response (I&R) System. Users can access the database online and search by category (AJCC TNM cancer staging, CoC Cancer Program Standards, registry operations, etc.) or by keywords (e.g., "breast," "physician staging"). Users can submit a new question at any time during the search. Members of the I&R Technical Staff Team, composed of certified cancer registrars, are randomly assigned to review, research, and respond to inquiries. Answers that can be supported by reference to CoC publications or other standard sources are entered into the database. More difficult queries and proposed answers are presented at weekly I&R team meetings for discussion and consensus answers. When necessary, questions are referred to external sources. For example, questions regarding histology are referred to the NCI Surveillance, Epidemiology, and End Results (SEER) Program professionals, and questions regarding AJCC staging are referred to physicians who serve as AJCC curators for individual cancer sites. All queries and responses are reviewed for quality before being transferred to the I&R Database on the ACS Web site. A response from the I&R Team is sent to each inquirer. Currently, the database houses more than 5,000 questions and answers. Data from the I&R system are routinely referenced and incorporated into CoC training programs, and are used to identify standards or staging rubrics that lack clarity or consistency for consideration in the development of future versions of CoC data, *Cancer Program Standards* manuals, and the AJCC TNM *Cancer Staging Manual*.

Educational Programs

Each year, the CoC's educational program offers learning opportunities for the cancer registry community, physicians, administrators, and other cancer program team members. Presentations and products reflect the primary initiatives undertaken by the CoC in the areas of data and cancer program standards, and are offered online, through in-person workshops, as webinars, or on CDs or DVDs. In addition, the CoC sponsors symposia and postgraduate courses on cancer care for physician audiences attending the annual ACoS Clinical Congress.

The primary educational vehicle for CoC education is the Online Educational Portal. The CoC strives to meet the educational needs of all members of the cancer care team, as well as organizational administrators and executives. The site is accessible from the CoC Web site (www.facs.org/cancer) and includes a full-page description of each topic, the target audience for each webinar, available educational credits, and other important information describing the scope of the program. Webinars are available in live and archived form. Live webinars are presented via the Internet, with slides and streaming audio, call in for the audio segment, and a live question-and-answer session at the conclusion. On-demand webinars are available within 72 hours after the live presentation and can be viewed 24 hours a day, 7 days a week, to better accommodate busy schedules. All questions and answers discussed during the live call are posted to the on-demand webinars. Slides/notes pages are available for printing for both the live and on-demand webinars.

Cancer Liaison Program

Established in 1963, the Cancer Liaison Program of the CoC was developed as a grassroots network of physician volunteers willing to manage clinically related cancer activities in their local institutions and surrounding communities. Initially, membership was limited to surgeons; however, membership was expanded in the 1970s to reflect the multidisciplinary composition of professionals who care for patients with cancer. Today, 45% of the 1,600 CLPs represent nonsurgical disciplines.

CLPs are volunteer physicians responsible for providing the leadership and direction to establish, maintain, and support their facility's cancer program. They are charged with the task of spearheading CoC activities at the facility and community levels. CLPs are a required component of CoC-accredited cancer programs and serve a 3-year term with eligibility to serve an unlimited number of terms.

CLPs serve a leadership role in their cancer program, support the facility's efforts in complying with and maintaining the CoC's standards, facilitate activities that impact the care of the cancer patients and support the needs of the community, and are dedicated to improving the quality of care delivered to the cancer patient.

Physicians who accept the role as CLP for their facility are required to:

- Interpret and monitor their facility's NCDB data and the facility's plan to use the information to evaluate and improve quality of care.
- Report NCDB data to the cancer committee on a quarterly basis.
- Report on CoC activities to the cancer committee.
- Serve as liaison for their cancer program with the ACS and facilitate development of a collaboration plan.

Criteria are in place for CLP selection and appointment, training and orientation, ongoing educational opportunities, and performance assessment.

CLPs must have a strong commitment to the success of the cancer program and the quality of care provided to patients with cancer, be an active member of the cancer committee, participate in cancer conferences, and have an interest in working with and volunteering for the local ACS on cancer control initiatives. These individuals are appointed by their respective hospital cancer committee's and their term of appointment is for 3 years, with eligibility to serve an unlimited number of 3-year terms based on performance and at the discretion of the cancer committee. Currently, 60% of CLPs are surgeons, with 40% representing other specialties.

Those who provide direction to the CLPs across the country are called State Chairs. The local chapters of the ACoS appoint the 65 CoC State Chair positions. Several states have more than one State Chair to manage the geographic distribution of CLPs; in this case, a State Chair is assigned to a Region or Zone. State Chairs serve a 3-year term and can serve a second term based on evaluation of their performance. The primary areas of responsibility for the 65 States Chairs include communicating regularly with their liaison physicians, coordinating a meeting of the CLPs in their state, promoting participation in CoC and ACS programs at the local level, and participating in collaborative activities in the state. These include serving on the ACoS Chapter Council in their state, working with the division staff of the ACS, serving on the team coordinating the state cancer plan, and making presentations about the CoC and its program at state-based cancer meetings.

The partnership between the ACS and the CoC dates back to 1922, and over the years, collaborations between the ACS and CoC have spread from a national level to state and community partnerships. The ACS-CoC Steering Committee was formed to address the ACS-CoC relationships by engaging in strategy development and educating ACS divisions and ACS field staff working in CoC-accredited cancer programs. Common objectives of the partnership include:

- Expanding cancer awareness/information availability, as well as ACS services delivery at the community level
- Increasing utilization of ACS services and programs at CoC-accredited cancer programs
- Engaging the CLPs in the CoC-accredited cancer programs to support implementation of local prevention and early detection programs and state cancer plans
- Promoting CoC-accredited cancer programs and the quality of care provided at these facilities

This partnership has resulted in publication of a *Commission on Cancer Guidebook* designed to increase the effectiveness of the ACS and CoC collaboration through the cultivation of formal, intentional relationships. The guidelines provide strategies to support the ACS Leadership Roles and CoC priorities. The guidebook is an introductory reference for ACS staff and volunteers who are directly responsible for working with CoC relationships. It provides specific information and instructions about working with facilities and healthcare providers, and defines strategies for preparing for the relationship, building and maintaining the relationship, and evaluating and recognizing the relationship.

Future Directions

Changes in the healthcare environment are driving the increased pressure on providers to engage in performance measurement and reporting. Public accountability has become the rule rather than the exception, and patients have more responsibility and control over their care. Because payers and insurers demand information to monitor and evaluate quality of care, there is a movement toward pay-for-performance, mandated quality measures, and facility report cards.

The CoC is efficiently structured to respond to the changes that impact the ongoing assessment of quality cancer care, and has broadened the level of engagement and collaboration with its 48-member organizations, resulting in increased, multidisciplinary participation in its activities. The CoC has increased responsiveness to internal and external requests from other organizations through the revision of its cancer program and data standards, development of tools promoting access to NCDB data, and educational programs targeted to key constituent groups. The CoC has achieved a high level of program integration by incorporating the NCDB into the accreditation process, and is working to raise awareness among patients, physicians, and health plans of the quality standards for CoC-accredited cancer programs. With the primary focus of measuring quality outcomes, the CoC is positioned to effectively target educational efforts in areas where clinical practice is not compatible with the best available evidence. Physician liaisons are key advocates in helping to initiate change at the local level. The established strengths and infrastructure of the CoC support the schema for an integrated approach to quality improvement. NCDB data will continue to be used to identify variations in care, and the Quality Integration Committee will determine whether there is compelling evidence to support a particular pattern of care. If there is, a focused educational intervention will be undertaken. The Accreditation Committee will determine whether this pattern of care is significant enough to be incorporated as a quality standard for cancer program accreditation. Changes in care as a result of this standard will be monitored with NCDB data.

In conclusion, the CoC is the only program in the United States and Puerto Rico accrediting comprehensive, community-based cancer care and engaging community providers, is the only program collecting and analyzing community-wide cancer treatments and outcomes, and is the only program using national and local data to improve quality.

The CoC is a recognized leader in promoting the delivery of high-quality cancer care. Keys to the CoC's future success in cancer care involve maintaining collaborative relationships with professional organizations, retaining its engagement in the cancer surveillance community, and influencing the national oncology quality agenda. (Further information about the CoC is available from its web site at: www.facs.org/cancer.)

chapter 31

American Joint Committee on Cancer

Karen Pollitt

Historical Overview

The American Joint Committee on Cancer (AJCC) was formally established on January 9, 1959, as the American Joint Committee for Cancer Staging and End Results Reporting (AJC). The driving force behind the organization of this body was a desire to develop a system of clinical staging for cancer that was acceptable to the American medical profession. Formation of the committee was initiated by a joint letter of invitation from the Chairman of the Board of Chancellors of the American College of Radiology and the Chairman of the Board of Regents of the American College of Surgeons (ACoS) to six organizations to participate as cofounders. The six organizations, all accepting the invitation, committed to formulating and publishing systems of classification of cancer, including staging and outcomes reporting, for use by the medical profession for selecting the most effective treatment, determining prognosis, and continuing evaluation of cancer control measures. The founding organizations of the AJCC are the ACoS, the American College of Radiology, the College of American Pathologists (CAP), the American College of Physicians, the American Cancer Society, and the National Cancer Institute (NCI). In 1966, the Cancer Control Program, Division of Chronic Diseases, U.S. Public Health Service, became the seventh organization to join the AJC and remained so for several years.

At the organizational meeting of the AJC, a document entitled "A Statement of Purpose, Rules and Regulations of the Joint Committee on Cancer Staging and End Results Reporting" was adopted.

Since its inception, the AJCC has embraced the Tumor Node Metastasis (TNM) system to describe the anatomic extent of cancer at the time of initial diagnosis and before the application of definitive treatment. In addition, a classification of the stages of cancer was utilized as a guide for treatment and prognosis, and for comparison of the end results of cancer management. In 1976, the AJC sponsored a National Cancer Conference on Classification and Staging. The deliberation at this conference led directly to the development of the first edition of the *Cancer Staging Manual,* which was published in 1977. With the publication of the first edition, the AJC broadened its scope by recognizing its leadership role in the staging of cancer for American physicians and registrars. The second edition of this manual (1983) updated the earlier edition and included additional sites. This edition also served to enhance conformity with the staging espoused by the TNM Committee of the International Union Against Cancer (UICC).

The expanding role of the American Joint Committee in a variety of cancer classifications suggested that the original name was no longer applicable. In June 1980, the new name, the American Joint Committee on Cancer (AJCC), was selected. Since the early 1980s, the close collaboration of the AJCC and the UICC has resulted in uniform and identical definitions and stage groupings of cancers for all anatomic sites so that a universal system is now available. Throughout the development and publication of the seventh edition staging system, the AJCC has worked in concert with TNM Committee of the UICC and other groups with an interest in staging to develop staging classifications based on multiple prognostic factors, supplementary to TNM, which will improve clinical treatment selection and predict survival.[1]

AJCC Structure

The AJCC is composed of 6 founding organizations, 5 sponsoring organizations, and 11 liaison organizations. Membership is reserved for those organizations whose missions or goals are consistent with or complementary to those of the AJCC. These organizations generally demonstrate involvement or activity in one or more of the following areas: cancer epidemiology, patient care, cancer control, cancer registration and surveillance, professional education, research, and biostatistics. Organizations that comprise the sponsoring membership category support the AJCC through the provision of substantial financial resources, either direct or in-kind.

In 2007, a Public Member category was added to the membership of the AJCC. The role of the public member is to provide advice on decisions that affect the work of the AJCC in specialty areas of expertise, such as bioinformatics. Table 31-1 lists the current member organizations and categories.

The ACoS, a Founding Member Organization, serves as the administrative sponsor for the AJCC. The ACoS oversees all administrative functions including the provision of staff support, office space and equipment, meeting arrangements, publications and product development, Information Technology support, and administration of funds from all sources in accordance with committee directives. The AJCC is a program within the Cancer Program of the Division of Research and Optimal Patient Care of the ACoS. The Medical Director of the Commission on Cancer (CoC) functions as the Executive Director of the AJCC. The governance of the AJCC is overseen by designees from the founding and sponsoring member organizations, which comprise the Executive Committee.

The work of the AJCC is undertaken by standing committees. The committee structure is illustrated in Figure 31-1. The purpose and scope of the AJCC committees are as follows:

> **Executive Committee:** The Executive Committee of the AJCC conducts the interim business related to the administrative and professional matters between AJCC annual meetings. The Executive Committee is composed of one member from each Founding and Sponsoring Organization, the chair and the vice-chair, and the executive director. This structure provides opportunities for interested or-

Table 31-1	Current Member Organizations and Categories of the American Joint Committee on Cancer

Founding Organizations (three members each; up to two, 4-year terms)
American Cancer Society
American College of Physicians
American College of Radiology
American College of Surgeons
College of American Pathologists
National Cancer Institute
Sponsoring Organizations (three members each; up to two, 4-year terms)
American Cancer Society
American College of Surgeons
American Society of Clinical Oncology
Centers for Disease Control and Prevention
National Cancer Institute
Liaison Organizations (one member each; up to two, 2-year terms)
American Head and Neck Society
American Society of Colon and Rectal Surgeons
American Society for Therapeutic Radiology
American Urological Association
Canadian Partnership Against Cancer (formerly National Cancer Institute of Canada)
National Cancer Registrars Association
National Comprehensive Cancer Network
North American Association of Central Cancer Registries
Society of Gynecologic Oncologists
Society of Surgical Oncology
Society of Urologic Oncology
Public Members (4-year term)

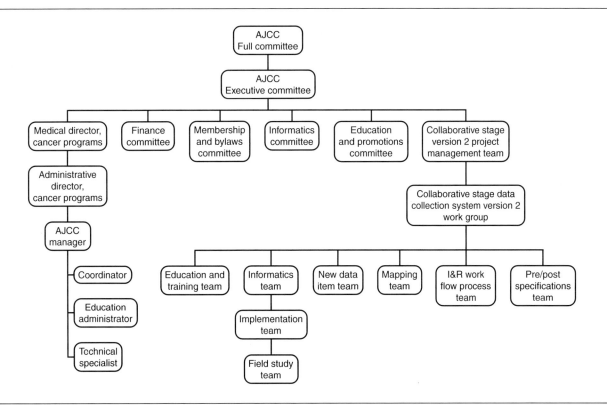

Figure 31-1. AJCC Committe Structure

ganizations to actively contribute to the planning and direction of the AJCC. The Executive Committee selects one representative from each organization to serve. The chair and vice-chair are selected by the Executive Committee from the membership and provide overall leadership for the AJCC. The Executive Director provides scientific and clinical direction, along with financial and administrative oversight.

Education and Promotions Committee: The Education and Promotions Committee is responsible for developing short- and long-term strategies for promoting the AJCC TNM staging system through related products, educational and scientific presentations, journal articles, and other initiatives to increase use of the staging system by all constituents.

Finance Committee: In collaboration with the AJCC staff, the Finance Committee is responsible for monitoring AJCC funds, reviewing and advising on budget considerations, and identifying strategies to expand funding sources to support both short- and long-term activities and initiatives.

Informatics Committee: The Informatics Committee is responsible for contributing to the development and design of AJCC electronic products, investigating and establishing relationships with electronic medical record vendors to promulgate the integration of staging applications, and incorporating AJCC TNM and Collaborative Stage Data into the NCI's Cancer Bioinformatics Grid (caBIG®) and Cancer Data Standards Repository (caDSR) as staging standards.

Membership and Bylaws Committee: The Membership and Bylaws Committee is responsible for identifying potential new members from sponsoring, founding, and liaison organizations, and the oncology community at large, that can provide AJCC with the expertise required to support its mission and objectives, to perform timely and periodic reviews of the bylaws, and to submit recommendations for amendments to the Executive Committee and Full Committee.

Site-Specific Task Forces: In addition to the standing committees of the AJCC, the AJCC has 16 site-specific task forces. Each task force is multidisciplinary with specific representative appointments from the UICC, CAP, and National Cancer Registrars Association (NCRA). In preparation for each new edition of the *AJCC Cancer Staging Manual,* the task forces are convened and charged with the revision and update of their respective site chapter(s) in preparation for publication. They serve as consensus panels to review scholarly material related to cancer staging and make recommendations to the

AJCC regarding potential changes in the staging taxonomy.

The AJCC also maintains active collaborations through formal appointments to key member organizations including the ACoS CoC, the CAP, and the UICC. The AJCC's role within the CoC is to promulgate use of the staging system through integration of staging strategies into the Commission's standards for cancer program accreditation. The AJCC's role on the CAP Cancer Committee facilitates the process for integration of the current staging schema into the CAP cancer protocols that serve as a resource to pathologists in effectively delivering information necessary to provide quality patient care. Finally, as a member of the UICC TNM Process and Prognostic Factors Task Forces, the AJCC evaluates proposals for revisions of TNM, monitors the literature on staging, and promotes the uniformity of the TNM classification between the two organizations.

Strategic Initiatives

In early 2008, the AJCC underwent a strategic planning process. This process was intended to position the AJCC to meet the future needs of the clinical and cancer registration and surveillance communities, and to retain the relevance of cancer staging in patient care. The strategic planning process culminated in a new mission statement, set of objectives, and key strategies to support the objectives and maintain the AJCC's leadership role in cancer staging. The activities of the AJCC are tied to these objectives, and ultimately to its mission statement.

The mission of the AJCC is to provide worldwide leadership in the multidisciplinary development, dissemination, and maintenance of evidence-based systems for the classification and management of cancer in collaboration with organizations dedicated to cancer surveillance and to improving care.

This mission is supported by the following objectives and strategies:

1. *Facilitate a timely and rigorous, evidence-based process to support a biologically relevant system for classification and outcome prediction of cancer that is compatible with systems of cancer population surveillance.*

    Strategies to support this objective include:
    - Monitoring trends in cancer care that impact staging
    - Sponsoring annual forums to understand current and emerging molecular markers and prognostic/predictive tools
    - Identifying strategies/mechanisms for incorporation of such factors into clinical medicine
    - Facilitating the continuous engagement of the site-specific task forces through literature review,

data analysis, and research activities to support the ongoing maintenance of the staging system
- Supporting the ongoing maintenance of the Collaborative Stage Data Collection System

2. *Proactively educate the oncology community through the development and delivery of effective programs and products to guide patient care.*

Strategies to support this objective include the work of the Education and Promotions Committee. These include:

- Development of educational products to support the effective interpretation and utilization of the seventh edition of the *AJCC Cancer Staging Manual,* published in October 2009
- Development of patient education strategies on staging and targeted educational content for non-physician groups (i.e., nurse practitioners, medical studies, etc.)
- Working with the AJCC publisher, Springer, in development, marketing, and distribution of the *AJCC Cancer Staging Manual* and derivative products in support of staging strategies
- Development of a strong Web presence to support and deliver the education and promotion strategies

3. *Promulgate research and serve as the clearinghouse to support the development of clinically relevant predictive tools, prognostic factors, and other indicators that classify and predict cancer.*

Strategies to support this objective involve:

- Establishing the AJCC as a clearinghouse for the dissemination of information and access to existing nomograms and other predictive tools to augment staging
- Defining future opportunities for the AJCC to support research initiatives to develop and evaluate improved staging algorithms for specific cancer sites and types
- Fostering the development of new approaches for and the utilization of datasets to test and validate current or revised staging algorithms

4. *Foster collaborative relationships with AJCC member organizations and organizations with similar objectives in support of systems to diagnose and treat cancer.*

Strategies to support this objective include, in part, the work of the Membership and Bylaws Committee. These include:

- Evaluating the current structure of the AJCC in an effort to optimize member involvement
- Identifying other organizations for involvement
- Assessing relationships with advocacy organizations and cooperatives groups
- Establishing mechanisms to enhance communications with AJCC members and member organizations

In addition, the work of the Finance Committee supports this objective through the following strategies:

- Reviewing and advising on budget considerations
- Identifying strategies to expand funding sources to support both short- and long-term activities and initiatives
- Assisting with grant development and review
- Identifying sources for sponsorship of specific AJCC products or activities

5. *Support and be responsive to public and private efforts to improve care and predict outcomes for patients with cancer.*

Strategies to support this objective include the work of the Informatics Committee. These include:

- Developing and designing AJCC electronic products
- Investigating and establishing relationships with electronic medical record vendors to promulgate the integration of staging applications
- Incorporating AJCC TNM and Collaborative Stage Data into the NCI's caBIG® and caDSR as staging standards

AJCC Cancer Staging Manual

The first *Cancer Staging Manual* was published in 1977 and contained 20 chapters. The first edition stated, "Staging of cancer is not an exact science…Periodically, this manual will be revised so that it reflects the changing state of the art." [2] The intervening years proved that a major challenge to TNM staging is the rapid evolution of cancer biology and the availability of biologic factors that predict cancer outcome and response to treatment with better accuracy than purely anatomically based staging. Beginning with the sixth edition of the *AJCC Cancer Staging Manual,* nonanatomic factors were added to the classifications that modified stage groups. This shift away from purely anatomic information has been extended in the current seventh edition published in October 2009. The seventh edition contains 57 chapters, within which relevant markers that are of such importance that they are required for clinicians to make clear treatment decisions have been included in stage groupings, such as Gleason's score in staging prostate cancer.

Fifty years after the publication of the first edition *Cancer Staging Manual,* the AJCC staging system is now recognized as the worldwide "language of cancer" and the *AJCC Cancer Staging Manual* is in its seventh edition. The development of each edition and the subsequent distribution of educational tools and resources to promulgate use of the staging system by the clinical community is an ongoing activity of the AJCC. Before the next edition of the *AJCC Cancer Staging Manual* is published, and as the era of personalized medicine evolves, the discovery of new markers will make it necessary to include additional markers in staging and will likely require the development of new strategies beyond the current grouping systems. As the

Table 31-2	AJCC Cancer Staging Manual Publication and Effective Dates	
Edition	**Publication Date**	**Effective Dates**
First	1977	1978–1983
Second	1983	1984–1988
Third	1988	1989–1992
Fourth	1992	1993–1997
Fifth	1997	1998–2002
Sixth	2002	2003–2009
Seventh	2009	2010 to present

AJCC continues to work to improve the scientific strength and clinical utility of anatomic staging in the years to come, the importance of anatomic extent of disease (i.e., TNM staging) must remain clear, as it provides the foundation for personalized cancer care.

Currently, the revision cycle for the *AJCC Cancer Staging Manual* is approximately 6 to 8 years, a time frame that provides for accommodation of advances in cancer care whereas allowing cancer registry systems to maintain stable operations (Table 31-2).

Collaborative Stage Data Collection System

The Collaborative Stage Data Collection System is a carefully selected, medically relevant set of data items that describe how far a cancer has spread at the time of diagnosis. It is known to cancer registry professionals as Collaborative Stage, or "CS." CS is sponsored by the AJCC in collaboration with the NCI Surveillance, Epidemiology, and End Results Program (SEER), Centers for Disease Control and Prevention National Program of Cancer Registries (CDC/NPCR), NCRA, North American Association of Central Cancer Registries (NAACCR), ACoS CoC, and the Canadian Cancer Society/National Cancer Institute of Canada (CCS/NCIC).

In 1998, the Collaborative Staging Task Force was formed and convened to address the issue of discrepancies in staging guidelines among the three major staging systems used in the United States. The initial focus of the task force was to develop a translation or other method of conversion between the TNM staging system of the AJCC and the SEER Summary Staging System. Such a translation would eliminate duplicate data collection by cancer registrars reporting to clinical (facility-based) and epidemiologic (central) registries, address the concerns of clinicians for more clinically relevant data, as well as the public health sector's concerns about data reproducibility over time, and provide a higher degree of compatibility between the systems that would expand data-sharing opportunities.[3]

After the release of the CS System in 2004, a series of annual updates or "version releases" were administered. These releases were based on feedback from the user communities resulting in changes that impacted the utilization of the system. In September 2006, the Collaborative Staging Task Force met to conduct a systematic needs assessment of the future requirements and maintenance of the CS System to support the collection of cancer staging and prognostic information, and to begin preparations for the development of CS version 2 in conjunction with the development of the *AJCC Cancer Staging Manual,* Seventh Edition. The needs assessment addressed the enhanced use of state-of-the art informatics programming advances to support the maintenance, validation, and structure of the CS algorithm used to derive stage, appropriate education and training delivery methods, the status of relationships with existing stakeholders, and the process for overall project management. As a result of the needs assessment, a series of work groups were formed to be responsible for ensuring the successful development, implementation, and evaluation of CS version 2, and the ongoing maintenance and management of the CS System. In September 2008, CS was renamed the Collaborative Stage Data Collection System to more accurately depict the major activity of data collection. The AJCC provides the administrative and technical expertise necessary to support the project and workgroup infrastructure.

The need for collection of new predictive and prognostic information contained in the seventh edition of the *AJCC Cancer Staging Manual* and other relevant data items requested by the standard-setting organizations increased the content of the Collaborative Stage Data Collection System and the subsequent number of data items that need to be recorded by the cancer registry community for each cancer patient. Version 2 of the Collaborative Stage Data Collection System was released in January 2010 for implementation with cases diagnosed and treated beginning January 1, 2010.

Other Products and Future Activities

In addition to the *AJCC Cancer Staging Manual* and the Collaborative Stage Data Collection System, AJCC activities fall into two specific areas: (1) promulgation of the use of the current edition of the *AJCC Cancer Staging Manual;* and (2) promotion of activities to support the AJCC's mission to provide worldwide leadership in the multidisciplinary development, dissemination, and maintenance of evidence-based systems for the classification and management of cancer in collaboration with organizations dedicated to cancer surveillance and to improving care.

To support use of the current staging system, the AJCC publishes a suite of companion products to the *AJCC Cancer Staging Manual*. These include the *Cancer Staging Handbook,* the *Cancer Staging Atlas,* and the *e-Staging Tool.* Translations of the AJCC products have been developed in 13 different languages. In addition, program development is ongoing to provide a wide variety of resources and educational tools on general staging rules and principles, as well as the staging systems for specific cancer sites.

Looking to the future, the Molecular Modelers Work Group has been formed and convened to understand the broad spectrum of current and emerging molecular markers and prognostic/predictive tools. This will position the AJCC to serve as a clearinghouse for the promulgation of predictive tools for cancer outcomes and survival, and ultimately to develop a framework/roadmap for future integration of markers into staging.

References

1. Edge, S. B., Byrd, D. R., Compton, C. C., editors. *AJCC Cancer Staging Manual,* 7th ed. (pp. 1–14). New York: Springer, 2010.
2. Beahrs, O. H., Myers, M. H., editors. *AJCC Cancer Staging Manual,* 2nd ed. (p. vii). Philadelphia: J.B. Lipincott Company, 1983.

Collaborative Stage Work Group of the American Joint Committee on Cancer. *Collaborative Stage Data Collection System Coding Instructions, version 02.00.00.*

chapter 32

The Joint Commission (TJC)

Cindy L. Tillman, RHIT, CTR
John W. Tillman, BA, CTR

Mission of The Joint Commission

The mission of The Joint Commission (TJC) is to continuously improve the safety and quality of care provided to the public through the provision of healthcare accreditation and related services that support performance improvement in healthcare organizations.

History of The Joint Commission (TJC)

The conception of TJC began with Dr. Ernest Codman in the early 1900s. Dr. Codman (who also formed the first cancer registry, a bone sarcoma registry at Massachusetts General Hospital) had a simple idea. He believed that every patient's health should be followed long enough to determine whether the treatment had been effective, and if not, why not. Dr. Codman believed corrective action, if necessary, should be taken to ensure that effective treatment was provided. This idea of service to the patient is the backbone of TJC's hospital accreditation program. Dr. Codman shared these ideas with Dr. Edward Martin in 1910,

and together with other physicians, they later founded the American College of Surgeons (ACoS).[1]

In 1912, at the Third Clinical Congress of Surgeons of North America, a proposal was made to establish an ACoS. Part of the proposal was to include a hospital standardization program as part of the ACoS. This was suggested by Dr. Edward Martin and proposed by Dr. Allen Kanauel. Hospital standardization was one of the first activities of the newly formed organization. In October 1917, 300 fellows from the Committees on Standards from every state in the United States and every province in Canada met with 60 leading hospital superintendents to discuss hospital standardization. Today, TJC continues to formulate policy by gathering informed and capable healthcare professionals to deliberate hospital standards.[1] After this Conference on Hospital Standardization, the ACoS formally established the Hospital Standardization Program, which was field tested with poor results. Of the 692 hospitals surveyed in the United States and Canada, only 89 hospitals met the standards, and most of the countries' most prestigious institutions did not qualify. These results further emphasized the need for standardization, and national support grew for the program.[1]

In December 1919, the college's board of regents approved five standards, which became known as the *minimum standard* (Table 32-1). These principles were consid-

Table 32-1	The Minimum Standard

1. That physicians and surgeons privileged to practice in the hospital be organized as a definite group or staff. Such organization has nothing to do with the question as to whether the hospital is 'open' or 'closed,' nor need it affect the various existing types of staff organization. The word STAFF is here defined as the group of doctors who practice in the hospital inclusive of all groups such as the "regular staff," "the visiting staff," and the "associate staff."
2. That membership upon the staff be restricted to physicians and surgeons who are (a) full graduates of medicine in good standing and legally licensed to practice in their respective states or provinces, (b) competent in their respective fields, and (c) worthy in character and in matters of professional ethics; that in this latter connection the practice of the division of fees, under any guise whatever, be prohibited.
3. That the staff initiate and, with the approval of the governing board of the hospital, adopt rules, regulations, and policies governing the professional work of the hospital; that these rules, regulations, and policies specifically provide:
   (a) That staff meetings be held at least once each month. (In large hospitals the departments may choose to meet separately.)
   (b) That the staff review and analyze at regular intervals their clinical experience in the various departments of the hospital, such as medicine, surgery, obstetrics, and the other specialties; the clinical records of patients, free and pay, to be the basis for such review and analyses.
4. That accurate and complete records be written for all patients and filed in an accessible manner in the hospital— a complete case record being one which includes identification data; complaint; personal and family history; history of present illness; physical examination, special examination such as consultations, clinical laboratory, X-ray and other examinations; provisional or working diagnosis; condition on discharge; follow-up and, in case of death, gross and microscopic pathological findings; progress notes; final diagnosis; condition on discharge; follow-up and, in case of death, autopsy findings.
5. That diagnostic and therapeutic facilities under competent supervision be available for the study, diagnosis, and treatment of patients, these to include, at least (a) a clinical laboratory providing chemical, bacteriological, serological, and pathological services; (b) an X-ray department providing radiographic and fluoroscopic services.

Reprinted with permission from the American College of Surgeons. *Bull Am Coll Surg;* 8:4, 1924. Codman, E. A. "Committee for Standardization of Hospitals [of the American College of Surgeons]. Minimum Standard for hospitals."

ered necessary to ensure the proper care of patients in any hospital and were the beginning of the accreditation process as we know it today. The request for accreditation was, and continues to be, considered voluntary.[1]

The ACoS continued to administer the accreditation program until after World War II. It was at this time that the emergence of many medical specialties and the increasing complexity of health care dictated the need to establish an independent, nonprofit association. The ACoS joined with the American College of Physicians, the American Hospital Association, the American Medical Association, and the Canadian Medical Association to form the Joint Commission on Accreditation of Hospitals (JCAH), which actively began issuing accreditation to hospitals in 1953. The Canadian Medical Association formed its own hospital accreditation system in 1959, whereon it withdrew from the JCAH.[1]

The next major milestone in TJC's history was reached in 1966, when the JCAH was faced with competition from state government licensing boards and the federal government's requirements to participate in the Medicare program. The JCAH, concerned that they could become obsolete, changed their focus from ensuring the minimal acceptable level of hospital care to establishing the optimal achievable level of care. This resulted in the publication of the *1970 Accreditation Manual for Hospitals*. What had originated as 5 minimum standards was now a 152-page manual of updated standards.

The 1960s also saw the scope of the accreditation process increase to accredit other healthcare facilities such as psychiatric facilities and long-term care facilities. In the mid-1980s, to accommodate this increased scope, the name of the organization was changed by replacing the word *Hospitals* with *Healthcare Organizations*. The Joint Commission continues to add healthcare facilities to their survey process as they are established.

In 2007, JCAHO changed its name to The Joint Commission (TJC).

Quality Assurance

Quality assurance was a formal approach to one of the original minimum standards. In the 1970s, hospitals were required to regularly review and evaluate their care of patients. However, reviews were informal, may have been biased, and were dependent on a reviewer's ability to judge care. Quality-assurance research led to the development of more structured and objective patient care assessment. Two common principles evolved from this research: objective and valid criteria for measuring quality of care must be established, and review procedures must be systematic.

The audit, which is retrospective, became a recognized tool to assess quality of care. Ongoing monitoring was conducted by required medical staff monitoring through surgical case review (indications and validation of diagnosis), pharmacy and therapeutics review (selection,

distribution and handling, and administering drugs and diagnostic tests), blood usage review (appropriateness of transfusions), and health records review (documentation). Standards were also established for reviews of medical and support staff departments in the areas of safety management, infection control, and utilization. Also, hospitals were asked to consider the results of these retrospective and ongoing audits when verifying credentials and assigning staff privileges to physicians.[1]

Unfortunately, hospitals became overly focused on producing paper trails of formal audits for the sole purpose of passing The Joint Commission's accreditation surveys, instead of focusing on the quality of care they were providing to the patients. In 1979, to counter this unforeseen problem, TJC determined that there should be evidence of a well-defined, organized program to enhance patient care through the ongoing objective assessment of important aspects of patient care and the correction of identified problems. The three parts of the quality-assurance process included implicit peer-based discussions; retrospective, time-limited audits; and ongoing monitoring using well-chosen process and outcome indicators.[1] The Quality Assurance programs then transformed into Performance Improvement programs.

Performance Improvement

Discussion of performance improvement cannot begin without a review of TJC's Agenda for Change, which was launched in 1987. The Agenda for Change was TJC's response to critics who believed that TJC was more concerned with policy documentation and minutiae in hospital manuals than with the actual quality of the care delivered. Critics charged that "good writers fared better than good providers."[2]

This was happening simultaneously with industry's development of total quality management (TQM) and continuous quality improvement (CQI). TQM is an organizational environment in which 100% quality is pursued. Principles include communication, empowerment, participation, continuous improvement, and customer-centered focus. CQI is the uninterrupted process of evaluating outcomes and the processes to achieve the goals of TQM. CQI theorists W. Edwards Deming and Joseph M. Juran stated, "Every process produces information on the basis of which the process can be improved."[3]

Both TQM and CQI "stress the importance of leadership, organizational culture, preeminence of external and internal customers' needs, goal-driven design of new products and services, broad deployment of measurement systems, data-driven performance assessment, and systematic redesign of important organizational functions or processes."[4] As industries developed systems for maintaining and improving the quality of services provided to the public while controlling costs, the public began to demand the same accountability for its health care services. The Joint Commission adopted many of the principles of TQM and CQI in drafting the Agenda for Change.[5]

Agenda for Change

The Agenda for Change was a result of a new movement in health care in the 1980s, which was a response to the dramatic increase in healthcare costs. This movement demanded greater efficiency in the delivery of services and insisted on objective evidence of the effectiveness of care. The public was demanding that the costs and quality of health care be balanced. At this same time, TJC was realizing that their focus should change from examining an institution's capabilities to deliver quality care to monitoring an institution's performance of healthcare delivery and evaluating the actual improvements achieved in the results.

The Agenda for Change was a response to these concerns, and marked the first time that improving performance would be a goal of the accreditation process. The Joint Commission's Agenda for Change has four underlying concepts:

1. Patient outcomes are influenced by all of the activities of a healthcare organization.
2. Continuous improvement in the quality of care should be a priority of healthcare organizations.
3. The Joint Commission should focus on those activities of healthcare organizations that are most important to the quality of care.
4. Traditional assessments of compliance with standards should be complemented by the accredited organization's collection, analysis, and feedback of data that reflect their actual performance in undertaking key activities.[6]

Because one of the goals of the Agenda for Change was to improve outcomes, TJC stopped dictating to hospitals criteria that must be fulfilled. Instead, they expected hospitals to creatively use TJC'S performance expectations to improve patient results. The Joint Commission also began to view the institutions as using a multidisciplinary approach to patient care. "The new survey process moves away from the evaluation of specific departments and services. It focuses on assessing, across an organization, performance of important patient-focused and organizational functions that support quality patient care, rather than evaluating activities that may have been conducted primarily to 'pass' the survey."[7] The Agenda for Change revolutionized TJC's survey process. "Old standards were revised and new standards developed to emphasize evaluation of hospital performance aimed at continuously improving the outcomes of patient care."[7]

The three major initiatives were as follows:

1. Redesign of TJC's standards to stress the entire organization's effectiveness in patient services
2. Redesign of the survey process to provide more interactive consultative services
3. Development of a national performance measurement system, commonly known as the Indicator Measurement System (IMSystem®)[7]

With the goal being to evaluate an organization's performance improvement efforts and results, the survey process now includes a review of hospital documents, an interview with hospital leaders, a review of patient care and administrative units to determine whether practices reflect policies, and a review of the performance improvement activities, with an emphasis on determining multidisciplinary involvement in performance improvement. Then the surveyors report on their findings and recommendations to TJC's staff.[2]

During the interview with hospital leaders, the surveyors seek to ensure that the leaders have developed a performance improvement plan that identifies priorities for improvement, have communicated the plan to staff throughout the organization, have provided a framework for reaching these goals, and have shown that they are teaching and directing the staff. Interviews with staff members and patients in the clinical and administrative areas are used to determine whether all staff members are working together to improve performance in areas identified by the leaders in their performance improvement plan.[2] In the past, the emphasis was on finding individuals whose performance was unsatisfactory, and either correcting that performance or eliminating those individuals. The current focus is on systems, and improvement efforts should now concentrate on fixing and improving systems.

Framework for Improving Performance

A large part of the Agenda for Change consists of the Framework for Improving Performance. The cycle for continuous performance improvement (see Figure 32-1) includes four elements: design, measurement, assessment, and improvement or innovation.[5] A hospital must have a model for performance improvement in use, but it does not necessarily have to use TJC's Framework for Improving Performance. However, in a hospital's performance improvement plan, the model on which it is based must be identified. (A common model used by many hospitals is the *plan, do, check, and act* model, or PDCA.)

Organizations should incorporate the needs and expectations of patients and staff when designing specific objectives for ascertaining quality of care. The procedures that will achieve those objectives are instituted, and data are collected systematically on preselected performance measures (originally called *clinical indicators*). The internal data are then assessed in reference to an external comparative database.

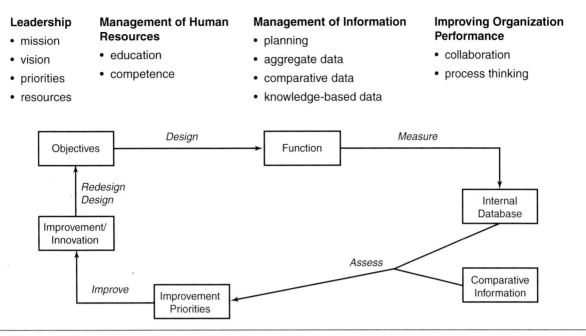

Leadership
- mission
- vision
- priorities
- resources

Management of Human Resources
- education
- competence

Management of Information
- planning
- aggregate data
- comparative data
- knowledge-based data

Improving Organization Performance
- collaboration
- process thinking

Figure 32-1. Critical Aspects of a Healthcare Organization's Internal Environment. Reprinted with permission by the Joint Commission on Accreditation of Healthcare Organizations, *Comprehensive Accreditation Manual for Hospitals*. Chicago: The Commission, 1995, p. 36.

The assessment includes reviewing current data in addition to examining prior patterns of performance. The performance improvement cycle has no beginning or end. It is an ongoing process that may be entered at any point.[7] The accreditation surveyors look for positive responses to three critical questions: Has the organization developed a framework for improving care? Is the cycle being followed well? Is the cycle itself being continuously improved?

Clinical practice guidelines and critical pathways can be used to assess the organization's data. Clinical practice guidelines are outlines of strategies for patient management that describe a range of acceptable ways to diagnose, manage, or prevent specific diseases and conditions. The practice guidelines have been developed by a consensus of experts in the specified field. Critical pathways are descriptions of key elements in the process of care that should be accomplished to achieve maximum quality at minimum cost.

Critical pathways define the optimal sequence and timing of functions performed by physicians, nurses, and other staff for a particular diagnosis. Variations from the guidelines, or from the institution's desired performance targets, create improvement opportunities. These opportunities result in the redesign of an existing function or the innovative design of a new approach to meet or surpass the expectations and needs of the patients.

Deciding what to improve can often be difficult, but priority should be given to problems whose solution will result in the greatest improvement in patient care. High-risk, high-volume, problem-prone areas, in addition to high-impact clinical services (such as surgical procedures) and high-cost functions, should be assigned high priority. Collected data should include measures in both high-priority areas. Likewise, when hospital cancer committee members plan the two evaluation priority studies required yearly by the Commission on Cancer (CoC) of the ACoS, they should also include measures in both high-priority areas. For example, choose one of the top five sites at a hospital to meet the high-volume criteria, or a topic related to either a high-impact clinical service or a high-cost function, or both.

In addition to the performance improvement cycle, TJC developed performance measures and a computerized system to evaluate an organization's performance with more accuracy and consistency than has been possible in the past.

Performance Measurement Systems

According to TJC, a performance measurement system is an inter-related set of outcomes measures, process measures, or both, that supports internal comparisons of organizations' performances over time and external comparisons of performances among organizations at comparable times. Performance measurement activities serve as the basis for internal quality improvement activities in healthcare organizations. Also, The Joint Commission staff will begin to use performance data to focus the accreditation process on clinical care issues and make it more immediately relevant to health professionals."[8]

A performance measure is a quantitative measure of an aspect of patient care that can be used as a guide to monitor and evaluate the quality and appropriateness of healthcare delivery. These measures serve as the data collection components of a performance measurement system. Performance measures are not direct measures of quality but screens or flags in a performance measurement system to indicate which areas require more detailed analysis. The measures should incorporate data on processes or outcomes, using existing data elements whenever possible, with an emphasis on sparse collection of data. Measures should have known reliability and validity.[9]

As part of the Agenda for Change, TJC developed the IMSystem® to provide hospitals with internal and external benchmarking capabilities. Internal benchmarking is the process of reviewing performance on critical measures of patient care quality. External benchmarking is the process of comparing performance on critical measures of patient care quality against others or the "best" in the industry. Internal benchmarks help a hospital improve its own performance over time; external benchmarks help hospitals assess where they are in comparison with other institutions, based on industry standards. By developing a performance measurement system, TJC wanted to measure the results of care (outcomes). Performance measurement data would allow TJC to give hospital-specific information, on request, to the public[2] and to enhance TJC's survey process by allowing intracycle monitoring through this clinical indicator–based performance measurement system.[9]

According to TJC, the original intent of the performance measurement system, when fully implemented, was as follows:

- To continually collect objective performance data from each participating accredited healthcare organization
- To aggregate, risk adjust (as necessary), and analyze performance data
- To provide comparative performance data to participating accredited healthcare organizations for use in internal performance improvement activities
- To identify trends and patterns in the performance of individual participating accredited healthcare organizations that may call for more focused attention by those organizations[7]

The actual performance measures created at TJC were developed in consultation with groups of experts who worked in the field to which each measure pertained and who had been nominated by national organizations and professional societies at the request of TJC. The original 25 performance measures were as follows: 1 to 5 were perioperative indicators, 6 to 10 involved obstetrics, 11 to 15 involved cardiovascular care, 16 to 20 were the on-

cology indicators, and 21 to 25 were the trauma indicators. The oncology performance measures were chosen from the high-volume sites of breast, colon/rectum, and lung cancer. The qualifying patients were inpatients with a diagnosis of one of these cancers. The oncology performance measures were designed to be collected retrospectively, whereas the majority of indicators for the other disciplines were collected both prospectively and retrospectively.

The original five oncology performance measures examined were: (1) the availability of data for diagnosis and staging, (2) the use of staging by managing physicians, (3) the use of tests critical for the prognosis and clinical management of female breast cancer, (4) the effectiveness of preoperative diagnosis and staging for patients with lung cancer, and (5) the comprehensiveness of diagnostic workup of patients with colon cancer.

The Joint Commission's Performance Measurement Initiative was finalized in 1994 with the publication of the final performance measures for their own performance measurement software system called the IMSystem®. However, in 1995, the Performance Measurement Initiative underwent another major change. The Joint Commission announced its intention "to include a group of acceptable measurement systems in its accreditation process under a single performance measurement umbrella. An important objective of this plan was to preserve the element of choice for the accredited organization by allowing it to select the approved measurement system that best met its needs. Within each system, further choice was available to the accredited organization in permitting it to select the specific indicators that were most applicable to the patient care services it provided."[8]

The revised approach was more flexible and complete. It incorporated performance measurement systems developed by other organizations in addition to the IMSystem® developed at TJC. Hospitals were offered a menu of performance measures so that each healthcare organization could choose a performance system relevant to its needs.[10] The Joint Commission did this in response to requests for inclusion of other measures and measurement systems developed by other entities as part of the accreditation process so that hospitals could have a choice as to which system to use for outcome measures.

The revised Performance Measurement Initiative was finalized in 1997, when TJC announced ORYX®: The Next Evolution in Accreditation. ORYX® was the name of TJC's initiative to integrate performance measures into the accreditation process. It was a term different from any other currently used in health care, reflecting the magnitude of the anticipated changes in TJC's accreditation process in the years ahead. Initially, 60 performance measures were accepted, some of which were the performance measures created by TJC for their own system, including the oncology performance measures outlined earlier in this chapter.

In 1997, hospitals were required to notify TJC which two performance measures they would be using. By 1998, hospitals had to be enrolled in at least one performance measurement system chosen from the list of acceptable performance measurement systems. (The IMSystem® was sold in 1998.) Data collection on two measures representing at least 20% of the organization's patient population had to be instituted. The requirement went up incrementally: In 1999, four measures had to be chosen that represented at least 40% of the organization's patient population, and in 2000, six measures, representing 60% of the organization's population, had to be collected and data on these measures submitted to TJC.

The Joint Commission has continuous performance data that will help identify performance trends and provide a database resource. However, it has not yet been determined how indicator rates will affect a hospital's final accreditation status. Some possibilities being considered are that performance improvement data could be used to determine the length of time between surveys, or an organization may be queried as to how the indicator data are being utilized internally to improve performance.

With the advent of the ORYX® initiative, hospitals could choose from more than 200 performance measurement systems that were reviewed by TJC's staff and deemed acceptable. From these acceptable systems, an organization could choose among 8,000 performance measures to fulfill a hospital's internal measurement goals and their TJC ORYX® requirements. While the hospital staff appreciated this flexibility, it became a challenge for TJC staff, as there was a lack of standardization across measurement systems. According to the Specifications Manual for National Hospital Quality Measures: Introductions Version 2.2, "Although many ORYX® measures may appear to be similar, valid comparisons can be made only between health care organizations using the same measures that are designed and collected based on standard specifications. The availability of over 8,000 disparate ORYX® measures may also limit the size of some comparison groups and hinder statistically valid data analyses. To address these challenges, standardized sets of valid, reliable, and evidence-based 'core' measures were implemented by TJC for use within the ORYX initiative." The process to select the Core Performance Measures was similar to the process used to create the ORYX® initiative. In its Specifications Manual for Joint Commission National Quality Core Measures (2010A2), Appendix CTJC, TJC defines a core measure set as a "unique grouping of performance measures carefully selected to provide, when viewed together, a robust picture of the care provided in a given area." Five initial core measurement areas were selected and approved by the Executive Committee of The Joint Commission. These measures are acute myocardial infarction (including coronary artery disease), heart failure, community acquired pneumonia, pregnancy and related conditions (including newborn and maternal care),

and surgical procedures and complications. The last core measure, surgical procedures and complications, will be delayed in their implementation to ensure that duplication of data collection efforts does not occur, because the Centers for Medicare and Medicaid Services (CMS; formerly the Health Care Financing Administration) is also identifying measures related to surgery.

By July 2002, accredited hospitals were expected to begin data collection on at least two measure sets of the ORYX® core performance measures. The various software systems that provided the acceptable measurement systems to hospitals to fulfill their original ORYX® requirements have all been given the computer specifications to enable them to include these core measures into their existing performance measurement software systems. By January 2004, hospitals were to select three core measure sets based on the healthcare services they provide. If the hospital serves patient populations with conditions that correspond with two or more core measure sets, the hospital shall select two of the initial four sets and submit data via their selected measurement system. The hospital will no longer be required to collect and transmit data on their noncore measures.

At the time of surveys, TJC surveyors examine how an organization uses the core measures in their performance improvement activities. Future performance measurement requirements will be modified over time to reflect the application of evolving technologies and care practices. Additional core measure sets will become available based on type of facility, and will be driven by CMS and National Quality Forum as appropriate. The adoption of electronic health records, however, is a prerequisite to TJC's ability to undertake this strategy.

Several mechanisms for the transmission of performance measure data will be available to healthcare organizations in the future. These will include an Extranet-based option, direct receipt of data from CMS, and/or the ability to continue using a listed performance measurement system. It is envisioned that the number of systems supporting the ORYX® initiative in the future will likely decline, but that the quality of service and support will greatly improve as expectations for participation are continuously increased. The ultimate goal is to achieve a standardized core set of measures that provide maximum flexibility and minimum data collection effort for healthcare organizations.

The Joint Commission of Today

The Joint Commission of today includes accreditation programs for ambulatory care, behavioral health care, critical access hospitals, home care, hospitals, laboratory services, long-term care, office-based surgery, and international accreditation. There are multiple certification programs that include advanced certifications for a limited number of diseases and conditions, disease-specific care certifications launched in 2002, healthcare staffing services certification, and international certification. Each of these areas has unique accreditation or certification requirements. National Patient Safety Goals are also an integral part of TJC's scope of activities.

Public reporting of measure data was initiated in 2004 and provides a user-friendly format for accessing organization-specific data for each core measure. This gives the consumer the ability to not only search for accredited healthcare organizations, but to obtain a quality report for the organization indicating whether a specific program is compliant or noncompliant with all applicable standards.

The overall future goal of TJC is to coordinate data demands and prioritization of critical measurement by the various public and private sector entities to minimize data collection burden and eliminate redundancies for healthcare organizations, maximizing the consistency and usefulness of the data. The overall goal is to have future efforts result in demonstrable improvements in healthcare quality and patient safety.

Summary

A thorough understanding of TJC's performance measurement initiatives is critical to the cancer registry profession. The ACoS CoC Accreditations Program surveys institutions for compliance with standards that cover eight areas of the evaluation. They encourage organizations to improve their quality of patient care through various cancer-related programs encompassing prevention, early detection, pretreatment evaluation, staging, optimal treatment, rehabilitation, surveillance for recurrent disease, support services, and end-of-life care. Standards for quality improvement encourage interdepartmental collaboration to enhance patient outcomes and are easier for cancer programs to comply with once they understand the principles of performance improvement outlined by TJC in their survey process.

A department can no longer operate in isolation, but must join the multidisciplinary efforts of hospital-wide performance improvement initiatives. All performance improvement activities completed by the Cancer Committee to fulfill the ACoS standards should be included in the hospital-wide performance improvement activities. Cancer registrars must join these efforts and become recognized as members of the healthcare team.

References

1. Roberts, J. S., Coale, J. G., Redman, R. R. "A History of the Joint Commission on Accreditation of Hospitals." *Journal of the American Medical Association,* 1987;258(7):936–940.
2. Veatch, R. "Hospital Accreditation in 1994: The joint Commission Applies TQM to the Survey Process." *Quality Letter for Healthcare Leaders,* 1994;6(4):3.
3. Berwick, D. M. "Continuous Improvement as an Ideal in Health Care." *New England Journal of Medicine,* 1989;320:54.
4. Anonymous. "A Framework for Improving the Performance of Health Care Organizations." *Joint Commission Perspectives,* 1993;13(6):A2.
5. Schyve, P. M., Kamowski, D. B. "Information Management and Quality Improvement: The Joint Commission's Perspective." *Quality Management in Health Care,* 1994;2(4):54–62.
6. Joint Commission on Accreditation of Healthcare Organizations. "The Joint Commission's Agenda for Change: Stimulating Continuous Improvement in the Quality of Health Care." In *Trauma, Oncology and Cardiovascular Indicators Beta Phase Training Manual and Software User's Guide* (pp. 3-1–3-17). Oakbrook Terrace, IL: The Commission, 1991.
7. Joint Commission on Accreditation of Healthcare Organizations, *Comprehensive Accreditation Manual for Hospitals* (p. 29). Oakbrook Terrace, IL: The Commission, 1995.
8. Brown, A. "Joint Commission Announces Evaluation Framework for Performance Measurement Systems." News release from the Joint Commission on Accreditation of Healthcare Organizations, January 1996.
9. National Cancer Registrars Association, Inc. *NCRA Oncology Indicators Workshop Handouts* (p. 10). Lenexa, KS: The Association, 1992.
10. Seidenfeld, J., Harold, L., Loeb, J. "From the Joint Commission on Accreditation of Healthcare Organizations a New ToolRequest for Indicators." *Journal of the American Medical Association,* 1995;273(9):69.

Surveillance, Epidemiology, and End Results Program

Brenda K. Edwards, PhD

Steven Peace, BS, CTR

Judith Swan, MHS

The Surveillance, Epidemiology, and End Results (SEER) Program of the National Cancer Institute (NCI) is a coordinated system of cancer registries strategically located across the United States charged with providing timely and accurate data on cancer incidence, mortality, treatment, and survival. SEER has a long and distinguished history, tracing its roots back to the establishment of NCI in 1937. Ten percent of NCI's initial funding was allocated to cancer surveillance, and the Ten Cities Survey of that year assessed the magnitude of the national cancer problem by tabulating incidence over multiple locations. Repeat surveys were launched in 1947 and 1969, whereas in 1956, NCI sponsored the End Results Group of hospitals that monitored survival from cancer among their patients. Out of these activities, a committee of experts recommended collecting both incidence and survival data on a continuous basis. The recommendation was codified in the National Cancer Act of 1971, which marked the beginning of the nation's "War on Cancer."

Coverage

SEER provides fundamental data that support scientific and clinical research, inform national health policy decisions, and provide a foundation to health services planning across the United States, a process that is extensive and growing. The SEER registries cover approximately 26% of the U.S. population, with an aggregated database containing more than 5.7 million cancer cases. SEER registries add more than 380,000 cases per year to the database. In addition to capturing data on the anatomic origin of each cancer or primary site, there is information on more than 300 anatomic subsites and 500 histologic subtypes. The SEER Program is the only comprehensive source of population-based data in the United States that includes stage of cancer at the time of diagnosis and survival rates by stage. It is the population-based national source with the longest record of incidence and survival data with a 35-year history in most of its registries. As medicine becomes more personalized, data on biomarkers, genetic variation, and targeted treatments will be more available, and analysis of these, together with SEER longitudinal data, will be in greater demand.

SEER began collecting data on cancer cases on January 1, 1973, in the states of Connecticut, Iowa, New Mexico, Utah, and Hawaii, as well as the metropolitan areas of Detroit and San Francisco-Oakland. In 1974 to 1975, the metropolitan area of Atlanta and the 13-county Seattle-Puget Sound area were added. In 1978, 10 predominantly black rural counties in Georgia were added, followed in 1980 by the addition of American Indians residing in Arizona. Three additional geographic areas participated in the SEER Program before 1990: New Orleans, Louisiana (1974–1977, rejoined 2001), New Jersey (1979–1989, rejoined 2001), and Puerto Rico (1973–1989). The Alaska Native Tumor Registry became an official SEER registry in 1990.

In 1992, the SEER Program responded to the changing demographics of the country by expanding the number and location of SEER registries to increase coverage of minority populations, especially Hispanics, by adding Los Angeles County and four counties in the San Jose-Monterey area south of San Francisco. In 2001, the SEER Program again expanded coverage, adding Kentucky and the remaining counties in California (Greater California); in addition, New Jersey and Louisiana once again became participants. For these four registries, NCI funds are combined with funding from the Centers for Disease Control and Prevention (CDC) through the National Program of Cancer Registries (NPCR) and with funding from the states (Figure 33-1).

One of the most important aspects of the SEER database is its coverage of disparate populations within the United States. SEER coverage includes 23% of African Americans, 40% of Hispanics, 42% of American Indians and Alaska Natives, 53% of Asians, and 70% of Hawaiian/Pacific Islanders. The population covered by SEER is comparable with the general U.S. population with regard to measures of poverty and education, and it tends to be somewhat more urban and has a higher proportion of foreign-born persons (Figure 33-2).

The data source for these statistics is the 2000 U.S. Census. SEER areas included in Figure 33-2 are the states of Connecticut, Hawaii, Iowa, Louisiana, New Jersey, New Mexico, Utah; multicounty areas of Atlanta and rural Georgia, Detroit, San Francisco-Oakland, Seattle-Puget Sound, San Jose-Monterey, Los Angeles County, remaining counties of California; and American Indians/Alaska Natives in Arizona and Alaska.

Data Flow

The SEER Program registries routinely collect data on patient demographics, primary tumor site, tumor morphology and stage at diagnosis, initial course of cancer treatment, and follow-up for vital status. Initially, a registry receives cancer-related data from local sources, including hospital registries, pathology laboratories, and physicians' offices. Data from multiple sources are aggregated to complete a synopsis of the cancer case history regardless of where a patient might receive workup for diagnosis and staging or treatment. SEER also performs active follow-up of patients for vital status through these sources. Additional patient and treatment information and follow-up data are received by linking with databases of other organizations, such as the Social Security Administration, state vital records departments, the National Death Index, and the Centers for Medicare & Medicaid Services. The mortality data reported by SEER are provided by the National Center for Health Statistics. The population data used in calculating cancer rates are obtained periodically from the U.S. Census Bureau.

The SEER Program's 17 cancer registries are responsible for aggregating data from multiple sources, validating

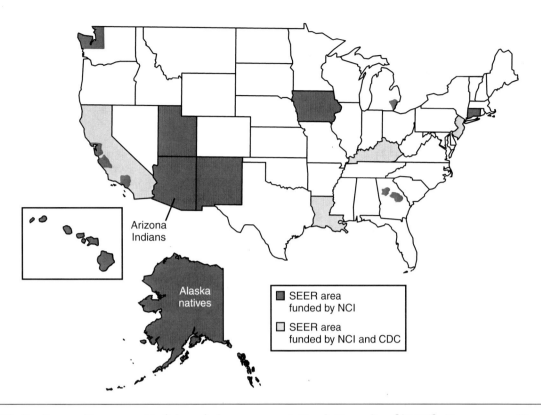

Figure 33-1. Surveillance, Epidemiology, and End Results (SEER) Program Coverage.
CDC, Centers for Disease Control and Prevention; NCI, National Cancer Institute.

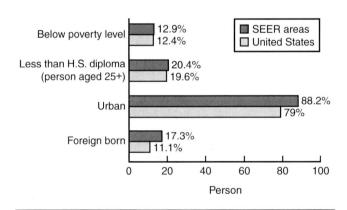

Figure 33-2. Population Characteristics of the Surveillance, Epidemiology, and End Results (SEER) Program and the United States.

data, consolidating records into a "best record," and removing all personal identifiers (e.g., name, Social Security number, address, date of birth). Once this information has been removed, data are sent to SEER annually, where they are stored in a central database. Data submitted in November are complete to January 1 of the preceding year (e.g., data through 2006 is submitted in 2008).

NCI disseminates these data sets to researchers and the general public via fact sheets, reports, public-use data-bases, analytical software (i.e., SEER*Stat or SEER*Prep), and Web sites (e.g., http://www.seer.cancer.gov). NCI provides many online resources related to cancer statistics for both researchers and the general public. As new statistical methods for analyzing the data are developed, the companion software is made available online. The following software tools have been developed for the analysis and reporting of cancer statistics, and several of the applications can be used with SEER*Stat:

- Cancer Survival Analysis (CanSurv): software to analyze population-based survival data
- Complete Prevalence (ComPrev): used to calculate complete prevalence based on limited-duration prevalence statistics
- Probability of Developing or Dying of Cancer (DevCan): used to calculate the lifetime risks for being diagnosed with or dying of cancer
- Joinpoint Regression Program: software for the analysis of trends using joinpoint models, enabling the user to test that an apparent change in trend is statistically significant
- Projected Prevalence (ProjPrev): used to take limited-duration prevalence statistics from SEER*Stat and apply them to a different population
- SEER*Stat Bridge: a plug-in for ArcMap (part of the ESRI ArcGIS Desktop suite) that helps users import data from SEER*Stat to make a map

A recent addition to the SEER Web site is the Health Disparities Calculator (HC*Calc), a statistical software designed to generate multiple summary measures to evaluate and monitor health disparities. HD*Calc was created as an extension of SEER*Stat that allows the user to import SEER Data or other population-based health data such as National Health Interview Survey, California Health Interview Survey, Tobacco Use Supplement to the Current Population Survey, and National Health and Nutrition Examination Survey. An important function of HD*Calc is to facilitate use of a range of HD measures so that researchers can explore their utility in different situations. Cross-sectional and trend data (e.g., cancer rates, survival, stage at diagnosis) categorized by disparity groups (e.g., area socioeconomic status, race/ethnicity, geographic areas) can be used with HD*Calc to generate four absolute and seven relative summary measures of disparity. The application extends the work published in the NCI Surveillance Monograph Series entitled *Methods for Measuring Cancer Disparities,* which evaluates measures of health disparities included in HD*Calc.

Other Features of Surveillance, Epidemiology, and End Results Program Data

The SEER Program has made unique contributions to the field of population surveillance, most notably in the following areas:

- Depth of the database available for research
- Accessibility and usability of public-use data and software
- Leadership in defining data elements and setting data standards
- Innovation in data collection, such as linkages and electronic data capture
- Development of analytical methods for use with population-based data

One reason for the vast usefulness of SEER is the number of data elements collected, which are more comprehensive than for any other national cancer surveillance system. Beyond collecting data on patient demographics, primary tumor site, morphology, stage at diagnosis, and first course of treatment, one of the most important responsibilities of the SEER registries is patient follow-up for vital status. In addition to its own set of data elements, SEER can be linked to other data sources, such as the census and Medicare databases, to enrich the analysis of cancer rates and trends.

Two of the primary objectives of the SEER Program have been to monitor trends in cancer incidence in population groups defined by demographic and geographic characteristics, and to provide continuous information on changes in stage at diagnosis and therapy and consequent changes in survival.[1] Of the SEER registries, nine have annually reported data since 1975, covering the years from 1973 to the most recent year for which data are available. The addition of other registries over the years has provided several groupings of data sources for longitudinal analyses, and a number of SEER monographs (http://seer.cancer.gov/publications) have examined trends in specific breakdowns, including the following titles:

- *Cancer Epidemiology in Older Adolescents and Young Adults 15 to 29 Years of Age, 1975–2000*
- *SEER Survival Monograph: Cancer Survival among Adults: US SEER Program, 1988–2001, Patient and Tumor Characteristics*
- *New Malignancies among Cancer Survivors: SEER Cancer Registries, 1973–2000*

In addition, published reports use SEER data to study the influence of cancer control interventions such as screening or treatment on trends in incidence, mortality, and survival. Examples include an analysis of the relative effects of mammography use and treatment on breast cancer,[2] and the link of prostate-specific antigen testing to prostate cancer trends.[3]

Pooling Data from Multiple Sources

SEER staff work with the North American Association of Central Cancer Registries (NAACCR) to guide all state registries to achieve data content and compatibility acceptable for pooling data and improving national estimates. The SEER team has developed computer applications to unify cancer registration systems, and to analyze and disseminate population-based data. Use of surveillance data for research has been improved through Web-based access to the data and analytic tools, and linking with other national data sources. For example, a Web-based tool for public health officials and policy makers, State Cancer Profiles, provides a user-friendly interface for finding cancer statistics for specific states and counties. This Web site is a joint project between NCI and CDC, and is part of the Cancer Control PLANET Web site, which provides links to comprehensive cancer control resources for public health professionals. Other partnerships are described in the following section as part of the uses of the data.

Leadership in Data Collection

Surveillance, Epidemiology, and End Results Program Data Management System

The SEER Data Management System (SEER*DMS) provides support for all core cancer registry functions: importing data, editing, linkage, consolidation, and reporting. The individual SEER registries actively participated in the requirements analysis and design of SEER*DMS. It was determined that despite the variety, number, and complexity of the registries' processes and corresponding functional requirements, a centrally designed data management system could be used by the various SEER registries. SEER*DMS improves cost efficiency and reduces duplication of effort in terms of system maintenance and administration. Furthermore, the centralized system design and development improves data quality and consistency, increases efficiency, and increases the sharing of knowledge and experience among registries.

Because a project of this magnitude should result in an end product that goes beyond a mere duplication of the systems currently in place, going beyond to also encompass areas where needs exist or new technology can be applied to accomplish increased efficiencies, it was determined that the scope must include the entirety of the business of Central Cancer Registry Operations, not merely the operations of the current systems. The applications, therefore, are business driven, developers user-centric, and requirements include systems, people and manual components, and appropriate technology solutions in all areas. The system is managed and operated by a governing body known as the Change Control Board (CCB), a committee that consists of SEER*DMS project staff and registry representatives. There is also an active SEER*DMS User's Group that focuses on best practices, user issues, and enhancements.

Electronic Pathology Software

Electronic Pathology (E-Path) facilitates the process of efficiently collecting complete and accurate pathology information from hospital-based and free-standing pathology laboratories that report to SEER's centrally based cancer registries. In its basic form, E-Path will report cancers that are diagnosed through histology, which comprise greater than 95% of all cancers. However, the scope of E-Path case finding can be extended by integrating E-Path with other types of electronic records, such as other laboratory results (diagnostic imaging, hematology, etc.) or admission, discharge, and transfer (ADT) information. Cancer registries rely heavily on pathology reports to identify new cases and to determine key characteristics of the cancer required for its classification standards. Utilizing information technology to standardize and automate this process is cost effective, labor saving, and reduces errors when compared with hands-on methods. E-Path utilizes an automated International Classification of Diseases for Oncology, Third Edition (ICD-O-3) coding assistant, in conjunction with natural language processing technology and pathology-specific terminology to automatically identify, index, abstract, and codify potentially reportable cancers from text-based reports. Cases can then be transmitted electronically from the pathology laboratory to the registry, increasing both the timeliness of case reporting and the quality of information being transmitted. E-Path is provided to all the SEER registries and their major reporting laboratories, and has currently been implemented in more than 200 reporting hospitals and laboratories.

Cost Tracking

As part of a multiyear, multiphase evaluation of the SEER Program, NCI is conducting a cost analysis of central registry operations. Whereas SEER registries collect certain core data items (e.g., patient demographics, tumor characteristics, method of diagnosis, and treatment) using a uniform set of definitions established by NCI, registry personnel may collect these data by different methods. SEER registry personnel also may perform activities for local, state, and other federal purposes beyond those specified by SEER Program requirements. Evaluation of central registry resource utilization, outputs, and the relationships between these inputs and outputs will provide both NCI and SEER registry personnel with an opportunity to reach more informed decisions concerning program management, budget, and resource allocation.

In Phase I of the cost analysis study, NCI conducted a feasibility study to clarify the specific types of cost questions that could be answered from central registry accounting and operations data, and to develop and test a data collection and analysis tool in five registries. The results from the feasibility study were used to plan a full-scale cost analysis (Phase II) of all SEER registries. Data obtained will provide a basis on which to examine the total costs of operating the 15 contracts and how these costs vary by category across registries, how different sources of revenue are used by the registries to fund their operations, the relationships between various inputs and the outputs produced by specific registry functions, and the geographic, population, and organizational factors that account for some of the variability in costs across the registries. Throughout both phases, all SEER registries participated in a consensus process to develop the data collection and analysis instrument.

Leadership in Cancer Reporting

Estimation of Prevalence

Prevalence is a statistic of primary interest in public health because it identifies the level of burden of disease or health-related events on the population and healthcare system. Prevalence represents new and preexisting cases alive on a certain date, in contrast with incidence, which reflects new cases of a condition diagnosed during a given period. Prevalence is a function of both the incidence of the disease and survival.

- *Limited-duration prevalence* represents the proportion of people alive on a certain day who had a diagnosis of the disease within the past x years.
- *Complete prevalence* represents the proportion of people alive on a certain day who previously had a diagnosis of the disease, regardless of how long ago the diagnosis was, or if the patient is still under treatment or is considered cured.

NCI statisticians developed a method to estimate prevalence from incidence and follow-up data from the SEER cancer registries. The SEER Cancer Statistics Review includes tables and figures showing complete and limited duration cancer prevalence. Prevalence estimates are presented by cancer site, race, sex, and years since diagnosis. NCI's Office of Cancer Survivorship provides these estimates to the public with additional interpretation and graphical presentation. The software for calculating prevalence is available on the SEER Web site.

Adjustment for Reporting Delay

Timely and accurate calculation of cancer incidence rates is hampered by reporting delay, the time elapsed before a diagnosed cancer case is reported to NCI. Currently, the NCI allows a standard delay of 22 months between the end of the diagnosis year and the time the cancers are first reported to the NCI in November, almost 2 years later. The data are released to the public in the spring of the following year. In each subsequent release of the SEER data, all prior diagnosis years are updated either as new cases are found or as new information is received about previously submitted cases. The submissions for the most recent diagnosis year are, in general, about 2% less than the number of cancers that will be submitted for that year in the future, although this varies by cancer site and other factors. Starting with the April 2009 release of the *Cancer Statistics Review,* SEER is producing delay-adjusted incidence rates based on 13 SEER registries. This differs from previous years when delay adjustment was available only for the oldest nine SEER registries. The formulas for delay adjustment are available on the SEER Web site.

The idea behind modeling reporting delay is to adjust the current case count to account for anticipated future corrections (both additions and deletions) to the data. These adjusted counts and the associated delay model are valuable in more precisely determining current cancer trends, as well as in monitoring the timeliness of data collection—an important aspect of quality control.[4,5] Reporting delay models have been previously used in the reporting of AIDS cases.[6]

Uses of Surveillance, Epidemiology, and End Results Program Data

As a research resource, SEER has been responsible for many findings with remarkable impact on the study of cancer. Since the 1970s SEER has significantly helped to increase the breadth of epidemiologic studies to include environmental exposures, geographic determinants, diet, reproductive factors, physical activity, genetic factors, and biological determinants of disease. A number of efforts have measured the national burden of cancer and evaluated cancer risk factors, such as the studies of estrogen and the risk for endometrial cancer and studies of cancer incidence among immigrant populations.[7–9] SEER's usefulness as a key data source is demonstrated not only by descriptive and correlational studies, but by population-based case–control and cohort studies. Examples include the examination of environmental tobacco smoke (ETS) and lung cancer, on which findings the Environmental Protection Agency (EPA) based its report labeling ETS as a human carcinogen.[10,11] There have been invaluable studies of patterns of care, quality of life, and years of survival. Examination of cancer trends coupled with information on costs or economics and policy has provided critical benchmarks for measuring progress against this disease. In this category are the Prostate Cancer Outcomes Study, the Breast Cancer Surveillance Consortium, and studies of second cancers and cancer prevalence. The many publications from these studies are accessible online through the SEER Bibliography (http://seer.cancer.gov/pubsearch/index.html).

Annual Reports

SEER data are reported annually in April on the program's Web site (http://seer.cancer.gov) in the *SEER Cancer Statistics Review.* In addition, the data are summarized in several joint reports. First issued in 1998, the "Annual Report to the Nation" is a collaboration among NCI's SEER, the American Cancer Society (ACS), CDC, NAACCR, and various external organizations. It provides updated information on cancer rates and trends in the United States. SEER data are also compiled with that of the CDC's NPCR and from Canadian cancer registries for the report from NAACCR,

Cancer in North America. In addition, the U.S. Department of Health and Human Services annually releases *U.S. Cancer Statistics,* containing state-specific cancer rates for the most recent year of complete data.

Public-Use Files and Software

Through its Web site, SEER makes available public-use data, which include SEER incidence and population data associated by age, sex, race, year of diagnosis, and geographic areas (including SEER registry and county). The data file is free, but a signed data agreement is required. For individuals who prefer a quick look-up for cancer rates, the Web application Fast*Stats (http://seer.cancer.gov/faststats) provides statistics that include incidence, mortality, survival and stage, prevalence, and lifetime risk (the probability of developing or dying of cancer), presented as tables and graphs. For a quick look at a statistical summary for major cancer types, fact sheets are available on the SEER home page.

Users who find the choices available in Fast*Stats too limiting can use the Cancer Query System (http://seer.cancer.gov/canques). More complex than Fast*Stats, it provides access to a wider range of statistics. Both Fast*Stats and the Cancer Query System are Web-based applications that enable immediate access to statistics and produce their output in the same format. SEER*Stat (http://seer.cancer.gov/seerstat) is the most powerful and complex mechanism for obtaining cancer statistics that SEER offers. In addition, users who have their own data can use SEER*Prep (http://seer.cancer.gov/seerprep) to convert that data to the SEER*Stat format.

Linkages

SEER registries link to various databases for case finding and follow-up for survival, for example, the Social Security Death Index, National Death Index, and healthcare facility patient encounter and discharge databases.

The SEER Program has been on the forefront of reporting cancer health disparities and working to improve cancer statistics among populations for whom cases may be undercounted. Among American Indian/Alaska Native populations, coverage is incomplete and difficult to piece together to give an overall picture, especially because of regional and tribal differences in lifestyle and health-related factors.[12] Beginning in 2003, NCI funded SEER registries to link their data to the Indian Health Service (IHS) patient registration database, and the linkage is now conducted annually. This effort is aimed at addressing racial misclassification in the cancer registries, and although not perfect, it is a logical step in the process of identifying additional cancer cases among American Indian populations. As a result, the NPCR also links its data with the IHS database.

The SEER-Medicare data (http://healthservices.cancer.gov/seermedicare) reflect the linkage of two large population-based sources of data that provide detailed information about elderly persons with cancer. The linkage combines SEER data on clinical, demographic, and cause-of-death information for persons with cancer and the Medicare claims for covered healthcare services from the time of a person's Medicare eligibility until death. The result is a unique population-based source of information that can be used for an array of epidemiologic and health services research. For example, investigators using this combined data set have conducted studies on patterns of care for persons with cancer before a cancer diagnosis, over the period of initial diagnosis and treatment, and during long-term follow-up. Investigators have also examined the use of cancer tests and procedures and the costs of cancer treatment. The linkage of the SEER-Medicare data is a collaborative effort of NCI, the SEER registries, and the Centers for Medicare and Medicaid Services (CMS). The linkage was first completed in 1991 and has been updated in 1995, 1999, 2003, 2005, and 2009. For each of the linkages, 93% of persons 65 and older in the SEER files were matched to the Medicare enrollment file. NCI and CMS plan to update the SEER-Medicare linkage every 3 years, with Medicare claims for linked cases extracted in the intervening years.[13] The SEER-Medicare linkage has resulted in more than 400 scientific articles.

In a collaboration begun in 1999 with the Census Bureau and other federal agencies, NCI is working to overcome the limited availability of sociodemographic information on death certificates and to obtain self-reported racial/ethnic data. This has involved the extension and expansion of the U.S. National Longitudinal Mortality Study (NLMS) and linkage to the National Death Index. A related project under development will link SEER to the NLMS to add socioeconomic data at the individual level that cannot be obtained from the SEER database itself. Researchers can explore the combined database as a resource for estimation of differentials in cancer incidence, survival, and tumor characteristics according to self-reported race/ethnicity, marital status, education, income, occupation and industry, residence, nativity/immigrant status, smoking status, health status, and availability of health insurance.

Rapid Response Surveillance Studies

The SEER Program provides a mechanism for augmenting data collection beyond the current reporting requirements and established standard data items. Since the 1980s the NCI research program has utilized this flexible mechanism to conduct studies by individual and collaborative groups of SEER investigators. Begun in 1987 as SEER's first "patterns of care study," the studies were expanded in 1992 to a broader range of topics. The Rapid Response Surveillance Studies (http://seer.cancer.gov/rapidresponse) have six categories:

1. Evaluating methodologic issues
2. Evaluating cancer treatment and outcomes

3. Monitoring screening practices
4. Monitoring health behaviors and risk factors
5. Linking databases
6. Improving technical aspects of registry operations

Beyond providing in-depth information related to the quality of cancer registry data and techniques for more efficient registry operations, they are also a research resource for obtaining population-based comparisons for evaluation of biobehavioral and risk factors, screening patterns, and molecular or genetic surveillance to quantify the progress of cancer control at the population level. The mechanism provides for a rapid response to scientific inquiries of high priority, as well as for methodologic development and feasibility studies on which larger initiatives can be built. It is the best mechanism available to mount potentially high-impact studies in priority areas, and it has resulted in exceptional productivity. The continuing goal of Patterns of Care/Quality of Care research is to evaluate the dissemination of cancer therapy into community practice, examine possible determinants of the receipt of cancer therapies, and explain the relationship between cancer treatment and cancer outcomes. In addition, NCI has previously used such data to describe treatment for cancer sites and to compare these descriptions with the guidelines for care.

Residual Tissue Repository Program

The SEER Program provides a unique potential for performing biospecimen studies on a representative sample of cancer cases from a particular geographic area. Established in 2003, the residual tissue repository was initiated to preserve pathology specimens associated with cancer cases in SEER registries that would otherwise be discarded and to use these specimens to test relevant hypotheses. SEER registries are population-based, collecting data on all cancer cases in their geographic area. This differs significantly from hospital-based specimen banks. The representativeness of the specimens available for research and suitable for incorporation into tissue microarrays can be determined. It is also possible to analyze data on cases for which specimens are not obtainable and provide information on biases that may result because of lack of incorporation of some specimens.

Standard Setting

Over the many years the SEER quality-control program has been in place, it has developed the ability to address both long-term issues, such as changes in coding requirements or instructions, and more urgent issues as they arise. It has become a resource for both hospital-based and central cancer registries, and has developed from a monitoring position to continuous quality improvement and training. Training and coding manuals have become available elec-

tronically for downloading on personal computers, and Web-based training modules have been developed, where consistency in coding and data analysis is emphasized (http://training.seer.cancer.gov).

As an example, the third edition of the *International Classification of Diseases for Oncology* (ICD-O-3) (http://seer.cancer.gov/icd-o-3) was published by the World Health Organization after a 2-year effort involving NCI SEER Program staff and other oncology coding experts from England, Singapore, and the International Agency for Research on Cancer (IARC) based in France. ICD-O-3 was implemented in the United States for cases diagnosed after January 1, 2001. In addition to the computer programs, lists, and other items necessary for implementation, NCI's SEER Program staff developed extensive training opportunities. In cooperation with other standard-setting partners, NCI helped to develop documents discussing how the implementation issues should be handled at both the hospital and the central registry levels.

The SEER Extent of Disease coding system formed the basis for the Collaborative Staging (CS) System (www.cancerstaging.org/cstage/manuals.html), implemented in 2004 as part of the effort to simplify and standardize the rules and guidelines for collecting cancer data in the United States. As the name implies, development of this system was a collaborative effort of the many organizations involved with cancer registration. Cancer registrars collect the facts about a cancer case in a structured code, and a set of computer algorithms converts the individual raw case data into a variety of staging systems, including the historical stage used for SEER reporting since 1973, various editions of the TNM system, and even site-specific staging systems such as FIGO or Dukes. The system was updated for a release of version 2 (CSv2) for use beginning in 2010.

SEER registries must adhere to strict standards of data quality to ensure the accuracy and reliability of its data. Since 1973, quality-control efforts have covered the many aspects of registry operations. Validation of data quality is a coordinated process involving audits of completeness and accuracy of coding and abstracting. The audit scores are combined with two other aspects of a registry's performance—the NAACCR certification standards and analysis of the public use data file—to produce a Data Quality Profile (DQP). Examples of data quality goals used for the DQP are less than 1.5% death certificate only cases, greater than 98% estimated completeness, and more than 90% follow-up of patients (95% for those 65 years old). There are also goals for defining site, histology, stage, census tract, and for geocoding. A recent list of requirements for the DQP is included in Table 33-1.

The SEER Quality Improvement (QI) process is decentralized. In addition to the QI staff located in the main office at NCI, the SEER program also utilizes QI staff resident in each of the SEER central registries and outside contractors, all under the direction of the SEER QI Manager. The SEER Program is viewed as the standard for quality among cancer registries around the world. Each SEER Program registry has a contractual obligation to

Table 33-1	Data Quality Profile	

Data Quality Marker	Goal
1. Death certificate only	<1.5% and >0.0%
2. Cause of death missing for patients known to be dead	<2.5%
3. Unknown or ill-defined primary site	<2.5%
4. Nonspecific histology	<2.5%
5. Unknown laterality	<6.0%
6. Unknown historic stage	<10.0%
7. Invalid or missing census tract	<2.0%
8. SEER estimated completeness	≥98.0%
9. Percentage complete as of February 2009	≥95.0%
10. 1-Year reporting delay	<2.5%
11. Follow-up age < 20 years	≥90*; ≥80†
12. Follow-up age 20–64 years	≥90*; ≥80†
13. Follow-up age ≥65 years	≥95*; ≥90†
14. Follow-up all in situs	≥90*; ≥80†

*Contractual standard.
†Minimum acceptable.

Data Quality Marker Not Scored

Data Quality Marker	Goal
A. Geocoding accuracy	≥90% Urban ≥80% Rural

meet specifically defined data quality goals on an ongoing basis. Collaborative efforts with national committees and national data standards contribute to high data quality.

Tools for Cancer Registrars

For cancer registrars, there are online training modules, along with access to complete coding manuals and data collection and reporting tools. SEER guides cancer registrars to improve cancer registry data by providing information, education, and training opportunities through a special section of its Web site. The site assists cancer registrars by presenting the SEER data submission requirements by year, as well as SEER data items; providing the reporting guidelines in the form of updated coding and staging manuals; linking to the current software and services most used by SEER registrars, including the interactive query system and drug database; and giving information on registrar training by SEER and other cancer registration partners. Recent additions to the site include the revisions made in 2008 for the Multiple Primary and Histology Coding Rules, with relevant information and training modules.

Among the most recently updated features of the Web site are:

- The *Hematopoietic and Lymphoid Neoplasm Case Reportability and Coding Manual,* embedded in the Hematopoietic Database, contains reportability instructions and rules for determining the number of primaries, the primary site and histology, and the cell lineage or phenotype. Online training is available.
- SEER*Rx, the Interactive Antineoplastic Drugs Database, developed as a one-step lookup for coding oncology drug and regimen treatment categories in cancer registries. The program is free and can be downloaded from this site. The databases are scheduled to be updated annually.
- SEER Inquiry System (SINQ) is a searchable collection of questions that cancer registrars have had while coding cancer cases.
- Data Documentation and Variable Recodes are resources providing variable definitions and other documentation related to reporting and using SEER data, including site and behavior recodes and the policy for calculating Hispanic mortality, and childhood cancer documentation.

Education and training programs are conducted at various SEER registries and in conjunction with the annual meetings of national professional organizations. These training sessions focus on problem areas identified from the quality-control studies and cover any changes introduced in data collection procedures. Among the offerings, SEER Advanced Topics for Registry Professionals is a training event usually held in conjunction with the National Cancer Registrars Association annual meeting.

Web-based self-instructional training modules available on the SEER Web site include the following:

- Hematopoietic & Lymphoid Neoplasms online training: educational recordings of presentations for the hematopoietic and lymphoid neoplasms project
- Multiple Primary and Histology (MP/H) Coding Rules training: recordings of the online MP/H Coding Rules training sessions
- SEER's training Web site: Web-based training modules for cancer registration and surveillance

The Future of Surveillance, Epidemiology, and End Results

Future priorities for the SEER Program were laid out during a 2-day workshop in late 2009 by a large gathering of experts from NCI and across the country, including SEER investigators, academic researchers, and cancer surveillance partners. Emphasis was placed on preserving and improving the timeliness, quality, and relevance of data; the efficiency and flexibility of processes; visibility of program activities and services; and expansion of data sources and users. Specific focus areas for the workshop included the following:

1. Defining the scope and content of cancer surveillance
2. Increasing the use of integrated health informatics in cancer surveillance
3. Developing analytic methods and models to support surveillance research
4. Understanding differences in risk and prognosis for population subgroups using geography, genetics, race/ethnicity, disparities, and social determinants
5. Disseminating data and analytic results

The workshop participants endorsed the continuation and expansion of SEER's current activities to track changes in cancer trends and support epidemiologic, cellular, and molecular research. Cancer surveillance research opportunities for the next 3 to 7 years were identified in cancer data collection that would be expanded to include detailed patient characteristics, using tools that help refine understanding of population differences, and communicating these statistics to researchers and the public. Statistical methodologies and applications can be applied to further the understanding of risk, prognosis, and population differences. Among the many research opportunities, particular emphasis was placed on the following:

* *Understanding risk of disclosure of identity to ensure patient confidentiality.* Methods will need to be put in place to ensure patient privacy when combining data sources.
* *Small area estimation methods and measures of uncertainty.* Interest in producing estimates for small geographic areas or small subpopulations continues to grow, leading to results with large levels of uncertainly. Understanding the data limitations and communicating the uncertainty is essential to avoid misinterpretation of results.
* *Classification methods to identify cases with similar prognoses.* As biological markers for risk and prognosis continue to be discovered, grouping of patients with similar prognoses will become more complex. It is an important step to estimating survival and other outcomes that are part of personalized medicine.

Specific approaches under consideration for the future include collection of data items for specific purposes; extension of electronic data capture to radiology services and hematology laboratories; building and analyzing multilevel data systems; development and application of analysis tools for new data submissions and incomplete data sets; and application of advanced statistical methods, including classical and Bayesian.

References

1. Hankey, B. F., Ries, L. A., Edwards, B. K. "The Surveillance, Epidemiology, and End Results Program: A National Resource." *Cancer Epidemiology, Biomarkers & Prevention,* 1999;8:1117–1121.
2. Ravdin, P. M., Cronin, K. A., Howlader, N., Berg, C. D., Chlebowski, R. T., Feuer, E. J., Edwards, B. K., Berry, D. A. "The Decrease in Breast-Cancer Incidence in 2003 in the United States. *N Engl J Med,* 2007;356:1670–1674.
3. Etzioni, R., Penson, D. F., Legler, J. M., di Tommaso, D., Boer, R., Gann, P. H., Feuer, E. J. "Overdiagnosis Due to Prostate-Specific Antigen Screening: Lessons from U.S. Prostate Cancer Incidence Trends." *Journal of the National Cancer Institute,* 2002;94(13):981–990.
4. Clegg, L. X., Feuer, E. J., Midthune, D., Fay, M. P., Hankey, B. F. "Impact of Reporting Delay and Reporting Error on Cancer Incidence Rates and Trends." *Journal of the National Cancer Institute,* 2002;94:1537–1545.
5. Midthune, D. N., Fay, M. P., Clegg, L. X., Feuer, E. J. "Modeling Reporting Delays and Reporting Corrections in Cancer Registry Data. *Journal of the American Statistical Association,* 2005;100(469):61–70.
6. Harris, J. E. "Reporting Delays and the Incidence of AIDS." *Journal of the American Statistical Association,* 1990;85: 915–924.
7. Weiss, N. S., Szekely, D. R., English, D. R., Schweid, A. I. "Endometrial Cancer in Relation to Patterns of Menopausal Estrogen Use." *Journal of the American Medical Association,* 1979;242(3):261–264.
8. Kolonel, L. N., Hinds, M. W., Hankin, J. H. "Cancer Patterns among Migrant and Native-Born Japanese in Hawaii in Relation to Smoking, Drinking, and Dietary Habits." In Gelgoin, H. V., et al., editors. *Genetic and Environmental Factors in Experimental and Human Cancer* (pp. 327–340). Tokyo: Japan Sci Soc Press, 1980.
9. Ziegler, R. G., Hoover, R. N., Pike, M. C., Hildesheim, A., Nomura, A. M., West, D. W., Wu-Williams, A. H., Kolonel, L. N., Horn-Ross, P. L., Rosenthal, J. F., et al. "Migration Patterns and Breast Cancer Risk in Asian-American Women." *Journal of the National Cancer Institute,* 1993;85:1819–1827.
10. National Cancer Institute. "Health Effects of Exposure to Environmental Tobacco Smoke" (Smoking and Tobacco Control Monograph No. 10). Bethesda, Md: U.S. Department of Health and Human Services, National Institutes of Health, National Cancer Institute, 1999.
11. U.S. Department of Health and Human Services. "The Health Consequences of Involuntary Smoking: A Report of the Surgeon General" (DHHS Pub. No. [CDC] 87-8398). Bethesda, Md: U.S. Department of Health and Human Services, Public Health Service, Centers for Disease Control, Center for Chronic Disease Prevention and Health Promotion, Office on Smoking and Health, 1986.
12. Swan, J., Edwards, B. K. "Cancer Rates among American Indians and Alaska Natives: Is There a National Perspective?" *Cancer,* 2003;98:1262–1272.
13. Warren, J. L., Klabunde, C. N., Schrag, D., Bach, P. B., Riley GF. "Overview of the SEER-Medicare Data: Content, Research Applications, and Generalizability to the United States Elderly Population." *Medical Care,* 2002;40(8 suppl):3–18.

chapter 34

National Program of Cancer Registries

Fran Michaud, CTR

Reda Wilson, MPH, RHIT, CTR

Population-based cancer registries collect data on all cancer cases in a defined population. This includes data on the occurrence of cancer, primary site, histology, stage at diagnosis, first course of treatment, and vital status.[1] Cancer data are reported to population-based cancer registries from a variety of medical facilities, including hospitals, physicians' offices, radiation facilities, freestanding surgical centers, and pathology laboratories.

Originally, population-based cancer registries were primarily used to describe cancer patterns and trends. More recently, the role of registries has expanded to include the planning and evaluation of cancer control activities.[2] Currently, information derived from cancer registries is critical for directing effective cancer prevention and control programs toward specific geographic areas or populations. These programs focus on preventing behaviors that increase risk for developing cancer (e.g., smoking) and on reducing environmental risk factors (e.g., occupational exposure to known carcinogens).

Cancer registry information is also essential for identifying populations who would benefit from enhanced cancer screening efforts, and for developing and implementing long-term strategies for ensuring access to adequate diagnostic and treatment services. Local-level data motivate action at the community level and provide incentives for community involvement and ownership.[3] Pooled data at the national, regional, and state levels enable federal and state public health professionals to establish, prioritize, and monitor national public health surveillance initiatives, and track progress toward the national goals and objectives set forth in *Healthy People 2010,* the nation's health promotion and disease prevention agenda.[4]

Overview of National Program of Cancer Registries

Citing the need for a national program of cancer registries that would provide the local, state, regional, and national cancer incidence data required for national and state health planning, the U.S. Congress established the National Program of Cancer Registries (NPCR) in 1992 through Public Law (PL) 102-515, the Cancer Registries Amendment Act.[5,6] This law authorized the Centers for Disease Control and Prevention (CDC) to provide funds to states and territories to improve existing cancer registries; to plan and implement registries where they did not exist; to help develop model legislation and regulation for states to enhance the viability of registry operations; to set standards for data completeness, timeliness, and quality; to provide training for registry personnel; and to help establish a computerized reporting and data processing system.

PL 102-515 requires funded states to develop legislation authorizing the establishment of a central cancer registry and provide regulations as specified in the law. These regulations assure the following: case reporting from all facilities and practitioners, access to medical records, reporting of uniform data, protection of patient confidentiality, access to data by researchers, authorization to conduct research, and protection from liability for individuals who abide by the law. PL 102-515 provides the framework for needed legal support for operation of central cancer registries. (The full text of the act is available online at: http://www.cdc.gov/CANCER/NPCR/npcrpdfs/publaw.pdf.)

In 1994, through cooperative agreements, NPCR began providing financial support and technical assistance to state health departments for the operation of statewide, population-based cancer registries. In a cooperative agreement, CDC staff is substantially involved in the program activities, above and beyond routine grant monitoring. State health departments or their authorized designees were eligible for one of two funding categories. The first category of funding supported the operation of existing cancer registries. These "enhancement" programs were required to maintain their current (i.e., at the time of initial CDC funding) level of support and to contribute (i.e., match) one state dollar for every three federal dollars of support received. Matching funds could be in the form of financial or direct (i.e., in-kind) assistance. The second category of funding supported the planning and implementation of a new cancer registry where none previously existed.

After the first program announcement in 1994 and the approval of a congressional appropriation of $16.8 million, 42 states and the District of Columbia were awarded funds (34 enhancement programs and 9 planning programs). In 1997, three additional states and three territories were awarded funds (two enhancement programs and four planning programs). Since 1998, NPCR funds have supported 45 states, the District of Columbia, and three territories (Pacific Islands, Puerto Rico, and the Virgin Islands), covering 96% of the U.S. population (Figure 34-1).

Program contact and other information, including available program highlights for a specific state or territory, are available at the NPCR website (http://www.cdc.gov/cancer/npcr/). Requests for information may be submitted to the Program Consultant assigned to individual states or territories (e-mail: cdcinfo@cdc.gov).

NPCR-funded central cancer registries are required to collect and report information on all state/territory residents who are diagnosed or treated with cancer, including residents who are diagnosed and treated outside of their state/territory of residence.

PL 102-515 defined reportable cancer as "each form of in situ and invasive cancer (with the exception of basal cell and squamous cell carcinoma of the skin and carcinoma in situ of the cervix)."

Data required to be collected include:

• Cancer incidence
• Demographic information

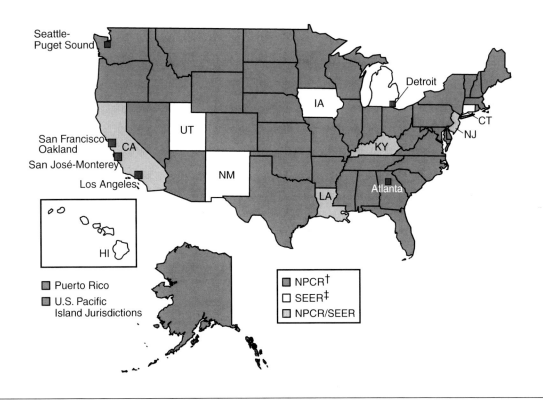

Figure 34-1. Population-based Registries Funded by CDC-NPCR and NCI-SEER

- Administrative information (including date of diagnosis and source of information)
- Pathologic data (including cancer site, stage at diagnosis, and type of treatment)

In response to the need for national population-based incidence data on all central nervous system (CNS) tumors, Congress passed the Benign Brain Tumor Cancer Registries Amendment Act in 2002.[7] This law changed NPCR's definition of reportable tumors to include benign and borderline CNS tumors. Both the National Cancer Institute's (NCI) Surveillance, Epidemiology, and End Results (SEER) Program and the American College of Surgeons (ACoS) Commission on Cancer (CoC) agreed to require reporting of nonmalignant brain tumors, beginning with cases diagnosed on or after January 1, 2004.

In 2000, NPCR-Cancer Surveillance System (NPCR-CSS) was established to receive, evaluate, and disseminate data from participating central cancer registries. NPCR-CSS is designed to provide cancer incidence data to meet CDC's public health surveillance responsibilities and to help monitor progress toward NPCR goals.

CDC-NPCR Organization

CDC includes 11 centers, institutes, and offices that focus on a wide range of public health concerns ranging from environmental health to infectious diseases. Each center has divisions that focus on specific public health areas.

The National Center for Chronic Disease Prevention and Health Promotion (NCCDPHP), with 10 divisions, assists states/District of Columbia/tribes/territories to promote health and well-being through the prevention and control of chronic disease.

The Division of Cancer Prevention and Control (DCPC) is one of these 10 divisions and administers the NPCR, within the Cancer Surveillance Branch (CSB).

The CSB is responsible for program management and capacity building within the participating central cancer registries. CSB surveillance functions include data collection and enhancement, data receipt and evaluation, and data analysis and dissemination. The performance of these functions is distributed among the three structural teams.

CSB is composed of the Office of the Chief and three structural teams: the Operations Research and Technical Assistance Team (ORTAT), the Data Analysis and Support Team (DAST), and the Surveillance Research Team (SRT).

ORTAT functions include:

- Leading program management
- Developing and monitoring program standards
- Performing quality assurance
- Coordinating creation of educational products
- Coordinating the annual NPCR Program Directors meeting

DAST functions include:

- Providing technical, statistical, and data analysis support to CSB and DCPC

- Providing support in the collection, evaluation, and release of data
- Developing and supporting cancer registry software products and Web-based applications
- Promoting electronic reporting of surveillance data to central registries

SRT functions include:

- Describing cancer incidence and mortality at the state, regional, and national levels, and for special populations
- Promoting the use of surveillance data for cancer prevention and control
- Building capacity for NPCR registries to conduct advanced surveillance research and activities

CDC utilizes cooperative agreements to provide support and resources to its public health programs. A Funding Opportunity Announcement published by CDC is used to identify and establish the long-term goals of the National Cancer Prevention and Control Program (NCPCP) through performance measures. A work plan is developed by each program to measure progress in meeting the requirements in the Funding Opportunity Announcement.

The Funding Opportunity Announcement CDC-RFA-DP07-703, released in 2007, incorporated funding guidance for NPCR, National Comprehensive Cancer Control Program (NCCCP), and National Breast and Cervical Cancer Early Detection Program (NBCCEDP). More information about each of these programs can be found at: http://www.cdc.gov/cancer/dcpc/about/programs.htm).

To receive CDC funding, NPCR central cancer registries must engage in a minimum of activities in each of the following areas:

- Operations and Administration
- Data Management
- Data Quality Assurance
- Data Linkages
- Data Submission to NPCR
- Data Use and Collaborative Relationships

Performance is measured by the extent to which the NPCR Central Cancer Registry has met NPCR Program Standards as evidenced by review of the annual NPCR-CSS Data Evaluation Reports; the results of the NPCR Data Completeness and Quality Audit (NPCR DCQA), the NPCR Program Evaluation Instrument (NPCR PEI), progress reports, and site visits.

NPCR Program Standards and Registry Operations

CDC-NPCR publishes the NPCR Program Manual, which brings together all documents and procedures that define NPCR's expectations and provide guidance on specific activities into a single reference document. Detailed information on the current program standards and required registry operations can be found in the NPCR Program Manual (http://www.cdc.gov/cancer/npcr/registry/).

CDC-NPCR also publishes Program Standards to guide priorities and activities of funded programs, provide objective measures of program progress, improve program processes that ultimately affect outcomes, and allow NPCR to set and monitor its own goals and objectives.

All funded programs must meet standards for:

- Legislative Authority
- Administration
- Electronic Data Exchange
- Data Content and Format
- Completeness/Timeliness/Quality
- Quality Assurance
- Data Use and Data Monitoring
- Data Submission
- Collaborative Relationships

In passing the National Cancer Registries Amendment Act (which can be found online at: http://www.cdc.gov/cancer/npcr/npcrpdfs/publaw.pdf), Congress required applicants, under state law, to provide for the authorization of the statewide cancer registry, including promulgation of eight categories of regulations that must include the following:

- Require reporting of newly diagnosed cancer cases by hospitals and other healthcare facilities
- Require reporting of cancer cases by physicians and other healthcare practitioners
- Guarantee access by the statewide cancer registry to all records of medical status of persons with cancer
- Require the use of standardized reporting formats
- Ensure confidentiality of cancer case data
- Allow use of confidential case data by certain researchers
- Authorize the conduct of studies using cancer registry data
- Ensure protection of persons complying with the law from liability

NPCR communicates requirements for data collection to funded registries through Funding Opportunity Announcements and posted data submission requirements for the NPCR-CSS. These standards include reportability or case definition, data item definitions and coding structures, data edits, and data transmission formats.

NPCR collaborates with other national organizations in creating, identifying, and publishing data standards. NPCR specifies the use of NAACCR-defined data layouts for the electronic transmission of cancer information between central registries and from registries to NPCR.

Reportability

Reportability, within the context of a public health surveillance system, defines the disease entities whose occurrences within individual persons must be identified, and about which characteristic data elements must be collected and reported to the designated public health agency.

Reference Date

The reference date is the effective date cancer registration starts in a specified at-risk population or in a specific facility. Each cancer registry establishes a reference date for reportable cases.

Residency

A population-based registry includes all tumors occurring in the at-risk population, and rules must be in place for determining the members of that population. The goal of central registries is to include all cases of disease in state residents diagnosed and treated at facilities within state boundaries. Through data exchange agreements with other states, registries also collect data on state residents diagnosed and treated at facilities outside state boundaries.

Reportable Conditions

PL 102-515 and its amendments identify reportable conditions for NPCR. The *International Classification of Diseases for Oncology,* Third Edition (ICD-O-3) is the standard classification system used to determine reportability.

Data Submission

To meet national cancer prevention and control objectives, fulfill agency responsibilities for public health surveillance and meet CDC missions, comply with congressional mandates, and better meet the needs of state public health departments, CDC established the NPCR-CSS by receiving, assessing, enhancing, aggregating, and disseminating cancer incidence data from the registries funded by NPCR.

NPCR-funded registries annually submit to CDC a cumulative dataset containing all de-duplicated cancer incidence case records diagnosed beginning January 1 of the registry-specific, NPCR reference year. Data are submitted in a standardized format and include selected NPCR-required data elements relating to demographic, tumor, stage-at-diagnosis, and treatment information.

The goal of NPCR-CSS is to allow the analysis of aggregated data from NPCR-funded registries on a regional or national level, as a statistical basis for the planning and implementation of cancer prevention and control initiatives. Analysis of aggregate data provides more accurate and stable estimates of cancer incidence for population groups including racial and ethnic minorities, medically underserved groups, and other subpopulations. Analysis of aggregated data also reveals geographic variability in cancer treatment practices, use of state-of-the-art cancer treatment, and deviations from standards of cancer care.

All data collected and maintained by NPCR-CSS must be managed, presented, published, and released with strict attention to confidentiality and security, consistent with the general principles and guidelines established by CDC for confidential case data[8] and specific restrictions imposed on NPCR-CSS data.[8] Special care must be given to cancer incidence data that are not directly identifiable because geographic and small-cell data may be indirectly identifying when combined with detailed information in case reports, laboratory reports, medical records, or linkage with other data files.[8]

NPCR-CSS has approval for protection under section 308(d) of the Public Health Services (PHS) Act (42 U.S.C. 242m(d)). The 308(d) confidentiality assurance protects identifiable and potentially identifiable information from being used for any purpose other than the purpose for which it was collected (unless the person or establishment from which it was obtained has consented to such use). This assurance protects against disclosures under a court order and provides protections that the Privacy Act of 1974 (5 U.S.C. 552a) does not.

Data and Program Evaluation

Data evaluation, or quality measurement, provides information on areas where additional training and resources are needed, and also serves as documentation of high-quality data that are ready for use in comprehensive cancer control efforts. The NPCR Program Standards enhance the capacity of funded programs and NPCR to achieve a common purpose through cooperative agreements and identify resources provided by NPCR and our partners. The standards enhance the ability to address important issues, allow development of new skills, increase use of cancer surveillance services, add to new knowledge, and enhance the ability to affect public policy.

NPCR evaluates the progress toward meeting these standards through a variety of activities to assess program performance to assure effective and efficient cancer surveillance operations. The purpose of doing evaluations is to promote the most effective use of resources. Data evaluation results are used as a component in NPCR's overall evaluation of central registry program performance. These results are also used to determine registry data eligibility for inclusion in national cancer statistics, publications, and other data use activities.

NPCR-CSS Data Evaluation Reports

One evaluation is produced from the NPCR-CSS annual call for data and reported to each funded program in Data Evaluation Reports. These reports include an estimation of the programs' completeness of case ascertainment and accuracy of certain data items (Standard Status Report 1), results of electronic data and inter-record edits (Submission

Summary Report 2), and results of NPCR Data Quality Indicators (NPCR Data Quality Indicator Report [DQI]). The Standard Status Report 1 evaluates the following five criteria:

- Percent Completeness Adjusted for Duplicates: The percentage of observed to expected, unduplicated cases where the expected cases are estimated by using methods developed by the North American Association of Central Cancer Registries (NAACCR).
- Unresolved Duplicate Rate: Because some cancer patients receive diagnostic or treatment services at more than one reporting facility, cancer registries perform a procedure to identify and resolve duplicate case reporting to ensure that each cancer case is counted only once. Before the submission of data to NPCR-CSS, each registry performs a protocol developed by NAACCR for assessing duplicate cases. This information is reported to CDC at the time of the data submission.
- Percent Death Certificate Only Cases: Another measure of the completeness of case ascertainment is the proportion of cases ascertained solely on the basis of a death certificate, with no other information on the case available after the registry has completed a routine procedure known as "death clearance and follow back."
- Percent Missing Critical Data Elements (Age, Sex, Race and County): This refers to the proportion of cases missing information deemed critical for the reporting of population-based cancer incidence data.
- Percent Passing Edits: Edits test the validity and logic of data components. Edits are applied to single field variables, interfield variables and multiple records (each record denotes a case of cancer in a patient) in those instances when a patient has multiple cancer diagnoses. Inter-record edits are run on the entire data submission from the reference year through the most current 22-month data. There are two types of edits: core edits that are applied to variables deemed necessary for reporting incidence data, and advanced edits that are applied to variables used for advanced surveillance activities such as survival analyses. At this time, it should be noted that there are no standards for advanced edits. Detailed results of these edits are provided in the Submission Summary Report 2.

The Data Evaluation Reports are used to identify cancer registries whose incidence data meet data standards established by NPCR. The Advanced National Data Quality and the National Data Quality standards are applied to data of the diagnosis years being evaluated. The *United States Cancer Statistics (USCS)* publication criteria are a subset of the National Data Quality standard. These criteria are used to identify data for inclusion in the *USCS* report published jointly with the NCI's SEER Program and in collaboration with NAACCR.

As demands for accountability in health care are more widespread today than at any time in the past, the NPCR DQI represents an effort to provide stakeholders with the data needed to make judgments about the quality of data collected by NPCR-funded registries, and to ensure the NPCR-CSS accurately describes the care provided.[9] Poor quality data can mislead important healthcare decision making. The underlying premise of DQI is that registries can improve only what can be measured.

The DQIs are designed to give an idea of the trustworthiness of the cancer registry process and the confidence in which that process is held. In addition, the DQIs identify any points of inaccuracy and variation, assist in explanations, and identify opportunities for elimination or reduction of inaccuracies. The objective is to utilize indicators documenting data quality for continuous quality improvement, and to identify and document training needs.

Each DQI selected has the potential to affect incidence rates and/or the quality of data available for research on topics such as patterns of care, disparities, survival, and health event investigations. NPCR-funded registries are using these DQIs to identify areas for additional training to reporting sources' staff in areas such as the need to review all documentation and case-finding sources, and to central registry staff on standards for data item consolidation, nonhospital case finding, death clearance practices, and using local rules or policies that differ from the national standards. The DQIs provide a method for self-assessment by evaluating each indicator by type of reporting source so that potential patterns are identified and reassessing the indicator each year to monitor progress. DQIs help to determine whether a process is in tune with the identified performance expectations (or Program Standards) and may also serve as a statistical measure or benchmark to facilitate comparison.

NPCR Program Evaluation Instrument

Another evaluation mechanism is the NPCR Program Evaluation Instrument (PEI). The PEI assesses central cancer registry system attributes to determine defensible and consistent progress toward funded programs meeting NPCR Program Standards and toward NPCR meeting its own program goals. System attributes evaluated include[10]:

- Simplicity (the structure and ease of operation)
- Program flexibility
- Data quality activities
- Acceptability (completeness of case ascertainment)
- Activities affecting surveillance sensitivity
- Representativeness (completeness of reporting by all sources)
- Timeliness
- Program stability

The PEI is a series of Web-based questions designed to provide a consistent approach to evaluating NPCR. This eval-

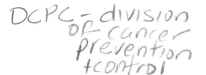
DCPC - division of cancer prevention + control

uation assesses whether the national and program-specific designs and purposes are clear and defensible, whether valid annual and long-term goals are set, and focuses on how well the systems operate to meet its purposes and objectives. The PEI provides NPCR the information needed to focus attention on strategic planning, meaningful performance measures for funded programs and NPCR, and program results. The information also facilitates appropriate technical assistance that can improve data quality, and program efficiency and usefulness.

NPCR Economic Analysis

Evaluating how resources are used in conducting registry operations and what resources will be needed in the future is another area of program evaluation and planning that is being studied by CDC. The NPCR Economic Analysis will utilize a cost allocation tool to collect information on program costs and also allocate these costs to specific activities performed by NPCR registries. Analysis of the cost data will provide critical information to reach informed decision making by assessing the program in relation to the cost expended on registry activities. Registry activities have been identified, and activity-based costs will be collected. This approach allows systematic calculation of all costs related to performing specific activities. Activity-based data collection will allow CDC to perform in-depth evaluation of the NPCR that has not been possible previously using budget information and federal expenditure.

Central Registry Workload Management Study

NPCR is also conducting a workload and time management study to assess the current practices of central cancer registries. The study purpose is to document the staffing requirements, by task, required of central registries. These staffing requirements will then be studied as a function of covariables. The study outcomes will include providing additional data to the NPCR Economic Analysis, Workload Guidelines/Time Standards, and Workload Standards Brochure.

Completeness, Quality, and Timeliness

The importance of high-quality, complete, and timely population-based central cancer registry surveillance data is widely recognized, and these data are essential to achieve the objectives outlined in the Cancer Registries Amendment Act (PL 102-515).[5] NPCR is committed to the continual improvement of surveillance data that can be used in comprehensive cancer control activities. Recognizing that all aspects of a registry's operations impact these attributes, NPCR requires funded registries to comply with established data quality standards as outlined in the NPCR Program Standards[11] and its references.

Quality is defined as an encompassing term comprising utility (usefulness), objectivity (accuracy, clearness, completeness, unbiased), and integrity (security, confidentiality).[12] Through ongoing strategic planning, CDC's DCPC identified assessment and surveillance as an important division attribute. DCPC's overarching assessment and surveillance goal is to provide and promote the use of high-quality data to monitor the cancer burden and guide cancer control planning and policy. Data quality is integral to every step in the development of that data, including creation, collection, maintenance, and dissemination. Before providing and promoting the use of NPCR data, these data must be reviewed and categorized as to their quality, completeness, and suitability. NPCR must ensure that the data accurately represent what they purport to measure in a consistent manner regardless of the data collection methods or sources utilized.

A major evaluation mechanism is the CDC-NPCR Data Completeness and Quality Audits (DCQA). Discrepancies in the completeness and quality of cancer data among states have made analysis of cancer patterns by state and by geographic region difficult. As a consequence, there is an ongoing need to assess the completeness and quality of cancer reporting, case finding, and data abstracting. CDC-NPCR conducts a continuous program of data assessment through the DCQA process auditing programs once every five years. These audits focus on the central cancer registry and evaluate the completeness and data accuracy, including treatment data, of all primary cancer sites as submitted by reporting hospitals. Feedback is provided to the central cancer registries through postaudit debriefing sessions at which time audit results and recommendations are discussed.

For the same reasons that CDC-NPCR conducts data completeness audits of funded central cancer registries, central cancer registries should, in turn, conduct audits of their reporting sources. NPCR Program Standards require central cancer registries to conduct case finding and/or reabstracting audits, based on a sampling of source documents, for each hospital-based reporting facility at least once every 5 years. These audits may include manual review of source documents, as well as data linkages of electronic files from submitting facilities with the central registry database.

Interstate Data Exchange

The model central cancer registry collects complete population-based data for a defined geographic area regardless of where the cases are diagnosed or treated. CDC-funded registries capture information on patients who are not residents of the geographic region and then exchange that information with the resident geographic region. In some instances, data received through interstate data exchange agreements account for approximately 15% of the cases in the central registry's database. Existing state laws, rules, and/or regulations currently allow most NPCR-funded central registries to exchange data with other central cancer registries. The exchange of data among central cancer registries is essential to assure complete and timely data are available to accurately evaluate the burden of cancer at the local, regional, and national levels in support of comprehensive cancer control efforts.

Death Clearance Activities

Death clearance is defined as the process of matching registered deaths in a population against reportable conditions in the central cancer registry database for two purposes: (1) ascertainment of vital status for persons in the registry (death clearance match), and (2) identification of all deaths with a reportable condition mentioned as a cause of death that are not found in the central cancer registry (death clearance follow-back). A Death Certificate Only (DCO) case is a reportable case for which the death certificate is the only source of information. NPCR central registries perform a data linkage with the state's death records at least annually to enhance the completeness and quality of central registry data.

Data Linkages

NPCR encourages, and in some cases, requires, funded programs to perform data linkages to enhance the completeness of central cancer registry data. A required data linkage is with the state program(s) funded by the NBCCEDP. This linkage may identify cancer cases missing in the registry database or discrepancies in diagnostic and treatment information between the NBCCEDP and the central registry database. The NBCCEDP programs are required to collect and report a set of minimal data elements for all client participants. Some of these minimal data elements are provided by the central cancer registry through this linkage.

Data Timeliness

Timely reporting is critical to allow access to the most current information for cancer control efforts. The speed with which central registry data are collected, processed, analyzed, and reported depends on many factors, some of which are within the registry's control and some of which are not.[13]

NPCR Program Standards include completeness requirements by diagnosis year and transmission format to help ensure cancer data are available for use in a timely manner. Because NPCR completeness standards include time requirements, NPCR standards for timeliness are the same as those for completeness.

Education and Training

CDC-NPCR considers education an essential element in achieving data quality, completeness, and timeliness. The content of education programs and products must respond to issues identified in quality assurance activities and be offered continuously in diverse formats and methods of access. CDC-NPCR's objective is to foster the development of a consistent central cancer registry knowledge base so that the goals of NPCR can be met.

Therefore, the objectives of CDC-NPCR's Education and Training program are as follows:

- To provide resources through sponsoring training opportunities, developing materials, and funding registries to participate in educational sessions
- To build the capacity of NPCR registries to provide education within their community of reporting facilities
- To monitor the educational infrastructure for gaps in access to education
- To search for methods and technology to improve access to education for the entire cancer surveillance community

With this education and training effort, CDC ensures that the resulting knowledge base is consistent with national standards, not only in the participating registries but in other central cancer registries as well.

NPCR Education and Training Series

The NPCR Education and Training Series (NETS) modules are a series of educational tools for state trainers to support central cancer registries in their role of providing education to staff and reporters. Each module provides specific instructions for the presenter(s), a comprehensive overview with Power Point slides, complete speaker's notes, case scenarios, and exercises with answer sheets that include the rationale for each answer. The modules cover the entire spectrum of education, from basic incidence reporting to advanced abstracting, and include topics of special interest for central registry staff. (Modules are available online at: http://www.cdc.gov/cancer/npcr/training/.)

Cyber Cancer Registry

The Cyber Cancer Registry is an interactive virtual registry system for developing and assessing the skills of cancer registry personnel. This virtual registry provides new cancer registrars an opportunity to gain hands-on practice in core areas of cancer registry operations. The Cyber Cancer Registry gives immediate feedback to the user through practical exercises and assessments to evaluate the level of competency, track training scores, and provide a certificate of completion for each assessment. Use of the Cyber Cancer

Registry can serve to satisfy part of the clinical practicum for formal education programs approved by the National Cancer Registrars Association (NCRA). (More information on the Cyber Cancer Registry is available online at: http://www.cdc.gov/cancer/npcr/training/ccr.htm.)

Collaborations among the National Cancer Surveillance Partners

Collaboration between CDC-NPCR and national partners includes committee and workgroup participation. The NPCR Scientific Work Group provides guidance to CDC on the evaluation, enhancement, aggregation, and utilization of NPCR data. The NPCR Central Registry Council provides a forum for NPCR-funded registries to provide input prior to major changes in data collection and data submission requirements, program standards, and quality assurance activities. CSB staff serve as subject matter experts on a number of national and international committees and workgroups.

CDC-NPCR collaboration occurs in many forms:

- Providing funding and technical support for studies performed by collaborating agencies
- Recruiting program states for collaborative studies
- Requiring the collection of data items or data linkages to support other agency goals
- Providing technical advice on surveillance issues
- Working with many agencies to effect a major change in surveillance models, coding systems, or rules
- Sponsoring and participating in national organizations
- Publishing data cooperatively with other organizations
- Cosponsoring conferences to define directions for cancer surveillance policies and activities

The CDC-NPCR Web site (http://www.cdc.gov/cancer/npcr/partners.htm) lists DCPC partners and highlights collaborative activities focusing on cancer surveillance issues.

Collaboration among the national cancer surveillance partners has been formalized in the National Coordinating Council for Cancer Surveillance (NCCCS).[14] NCCCS members include the American Cancer Society (ACS), ACoS, American Joint Committee on Cancer (AJCC), CDC, NCI, NCRA, and NAACCR. The mission of NCCCS is to coordinate cancer surveillance activities within the United States through communication and collaboration among major national cancer organizations.

CDC-NPCR also works in collaboration with the Indian Health Service (IHS). "Nationally, American Indian and Alaskan Native (AI/AN) communities have lower rates of cancer. However, in certain regions such as Alaska and the Northern Plains states, AI/AN cancer incidence and mortality rates exceed those for the US general populations. As a response to these disparities, the CDC supports numerous cancer surveillance, prevention and control projects in Indian Country through an Inter-agency agreement between the Indian Health Service (IHS) and the CDC's Division of Cancer Prevention and Control, National Center for Chronic Disease Prevention and Control" (http://www.ihs.gov/epi/index.cfm?module=epi_cancer_main).

Data for Native Americans are included in *USCS* (http://apps.nccd.cdc.gov/uscs/). NPCR requests programs to conduct data linkages between the IHS patient registration database and the central registry databases to improve identification and classification of American Indians and Alaska Natives in the cancer registries.

CDC-NPCR, AJCC, NCRA, SEER, NAACCR, National Cancer Institute of Canada (NCIC), and CoC have come together to develop, produce, and maintain the Collaborative Staging (CS) system, an innovative approach to collecting stage data uniformly in cancer registries throughout the United States and Canada. This system has replaced separate stage data collection by the AJCC's Tumor, Node, Metastasis (TNM) system, the SEER Extent of Disease (EOD) coding scheme, and two versions of a summary staging system used by many state central cancer registries. The CS system collects several discrete data elements related to extent of disease and their determination by clinical or pathologic criteria; these elements are then evaluated by a computer algorithm to derive stage classifications needed for data analysis. The CS system was implemented for cancers diagnosed as of January 1, 2004. (Information on CS is available at the AJCC website at: http://www.cancerstaging.org/cstage/index.html.)

North American Association of Central Cancer Registries

NAACCR is a membership organization that develops and promotes uniform data standards for cancer registration; provides education and training; certifies population-based registries; aggregates and publishes data from central cancer registries; and promotes the use of cancer surveillance data and systems for cancer control and epidemiologic research, public health programs, and patient care to reduce the burden of cancer in North America.

NPCR currently funds NAACCR under CDC's Standards Development and Maintenance for Cancer Surveillance cooperative agreement to provide resources for standard-setting activities related to the operation of population-based cancer registries.

National Cancer Registrars Association

NCRA is a not-for-profit association representing cancer registry professionals and Certified Tumor Registrars (CTRs). NCRA's primary focus is education and certification with the goal to ensure all cancer registry professionals have the required knowledge to be superior in their field. Worldwide, there are more than 4,900 NCRA members and more than 4,500 CTRs. Cancer Registrars capture a complete summary of the history, diagnosis, treatment, and disease status for every cancer patient. Registrars' work leads to better information that is used in the management of cancer and, ultimately, cures.

CDC provides funds to support the NCRA annual conference. This conference advances professional development of cancer registrars by providing an educational opportunity for registrars in hospitals and central registries to increase their knowledge and expand their professional expertise.

International Association of Cancer Registries

The International Association of Cancer Registries (IACR) was founded in 1966 as a professional society dedicated to fostering the aims and activities of cancer registries worldwide. It is primarily for population-based registries, which collect information on the occurrence and outcome of cancer in defined population groups (usually the inhabitants of a city, region, or country). To ensure that cases are properly recorded, and that the statistical data gathered are complete and can be used to make valid comparisons, cancer registries must conform to accepted working practices and standards. The association was created to foster the exchange of information between cancer registries internationally, thus improving quality of data and comparability between registries. The association is a nongovernmental organization that has been in official relations with the World Health Organization since January 1979.

CDC provides funds to support the IACR annual conference. This conference advances professional development by providing an educational opportunity for cancer registrars from international cancer registries to increase their knowledge and expand their professional expertise. Support of this conference is consistent with CDC's mission to support population-based cancer registries worldwide. The IACR is headquartered in Lyon, France.

International Union Against Cancer

The International Union Against Cancer (UICC) is the leading international nongovernmental organization dedicated exclusively to the global control of cancer. Its vision is of a world where cancer is eliminated as a major life-threatening disease for future generations. UICC's mission is to build and lead the global cancer control community engaged in sharing and exchanging knowledge and competence; transferring scientific findings to clinical, patient, and public settings; systematically reducing and eliminating disparities in prevention, early detection, and treat-

ment; and delivering the best possible care to people living with cancer in every part of the world.

Providing National Statistics

CDC and NCI have a joint responsibility for the dissemination of national cancer surveillance statistics. CDC's emphasis is on its responsibilities for public health surveillance, characterizing the cancer burden nationwide and in states, and meeting the needs of state health departments and the nation in developing, implementing, and evaluating effective cancer prevention and control efforts. In 2000, CDC and NCI entered into a Memorandum of Understanding (MOU) to coordinate cancer surveillance activities around a shared vision for a comprehensive, federally integrated national cancer surveillance system. This system builds on and strengthens the existing infrastructure, improves the availability of high-quality data for measuring the nation's cancer burden, and advances the capacity for surveillance research. The scope of this coordinated cancer surveillance system includes coverage of the entire U.S. population with high-quality data to measure cancer risk, health behaviors, incidence, treatment, morbidity, mortality, and other outcomes.

United States Cancer Statistics

The MOU was the genesis for the annual *USCS* report, a joint publication of CDC and NCI, in collaboration with NAACCR.[1] Since 2002, CDC and NCI, in collaboration with NAACCR, have combined their data sources to publish the official annual federal cancer statistics in the *United States Cancer Statistics (USCS): Incidence and Mortality* report. (This report is available online at: http://www.cdc.gov/cancer/npcr/uscs/.) The report includes cancer incidence from registries with high-quality data with the latest report representing 98% of the U.S. population. Cancer mortality statistics in *USCS* are based on information from all death certificates filed in the 50 states and the District of Columbia, and processed at the National Center for Health Statistics (NCHS). For consistency with the cancer incidence data in *USCS,* cancer sites in mortality data are grouped according to the revised SEER recodes dated January 27, 2003. Because NCHS uses different groupings for some sites, the death rates in *USCS* may differ slightly from those published by NCHS.

CDC WONDER: Online Data-Reporting System

CDC has collaborated with NPCR-funded programs to define, test, and release NPCR data in CDC WONDER, an online reporting system hosted at CDC. Launched in early 2006, CDC WONDER allows greater access to

NPCR data than is available through the County Cancer Incidence Dataset. Users can obtain reports containing age-adjusted rates, crude rates, and case counts, requested by state, large metropolitan statistical areas, year of diagnosis, sex, race, and age for both adult and childhood classifications of cancer. This system provides easy access to critical data that can help guide and evaluate interventions focused on cancer prevention and control. (The CDC WONDER Web site is: http://wonder.cdc.gov/cancer.html.)

National and International Data Use

NPCR data are included in national and international compilations of cancer information in addition to *USCS*. NPCR data are also included in national compilations of healthcare information in which cancer care is one of many healthcare issues addressed.

Published by the International Agency for Research on Cancer, *Cancer Incidence in Five Continents* is a recognized reference source on the incidence of cancer in populations around the world and is available online at: www-dep.iarc.fr. The ninth volume includes cancer incidence data from 32 NPCR-funded registries. The aim of the Cancer in Five Continents (CI5) Series, published by IARC, is to assess the incidence of cancer across the globe.

Annual Report to the Nation on the Status of Cancer

CDC, NPCR, and NCHS collaborate with the ACS, NAACCR, and SEER to produce the *Annual Report to the Nation on the Status of Cancer,* first published in 1998. This report includes an update of current trends in cancer incidence and death rates in the United States, and features timely, in-depth analyses of selected topics.[15]

National Healthcare Quality Report

Since 2003, the Agency for Healthcare Research and Quality (AHRQ) has published a *National Healthcare Quality Report (NHQR)*. This report is published on behalf of the U.S. Department of Health and Human Services (HHS) in collaboration with an HHS-wide Interagency Work Group. The NHQR examines and tracks the quality of health care in the United States, using the most scientifically credible measures and data sources available. Measures of healthcare quality address the extent to which providers and hospitals deliver evidence-based care for specific services, as well as the outcomes of care provided. The NPCR is a contributing source of data for the reports.

State Cancer Profiles: Agency for Healthcare Research and Quality *National Healthcare Quality Report*

NPCR data are submitted to several surveillance reports or Web sites, including State Cancer Profiles (SCP), the AHRQ *NHQR,* and CI5. SCP provides statistics for prioritizing national, state, and county cancer control efforts. AHRQ's *NHQR* provides a set of healthcare quality measures across four dimensions of quality—effectiveness, safety, timeliness, and patient centeredness—and, within the effectiveness component, nine clinical condition/care-setting areas including cancer.

Special Studies

NPCR and central registry staff participate in active research and publication in the cancer registry field. These studies may encompass the collection and analysis of additional cancer case data, with publication of findings to the larger registry community.

Patterns of Care Studies

NPCR has funded central registries to conduct studies examining the care provided to cancer patients. The Breast, Colon, Prostate Cancer Data Quality and Patterns of Care Study was designed to assess the quality and completeness of stage at diagnosis, and the treatment data collected by the participating registries. The study goal was to determine the extent to which patients received guidelines-based, stage-specific treatments for localized breast and prostate cancers, and stage III colon cancer. The study design also included participation in the CONCORD Study, a multinational project. The Ovarian Patterns of Care study was designed to evaluate medical record information on ovarian cancer, and the stage and treatment data reported to the registry.

The most recent Patterns of Care study, the Breast and Prostate Cancer Data Quality and Patterns of Care Study, supported enhanced surveillance and operations research to improve the completeness, timeliness, quality, and use of first course of treatment and stage data. The study is expected to describe treatment patterns and determinants of receipt of guideline-concordant treatments for breast cancer and appropriate therapy for prostate cancer. A particular focus is placed on whether disparities in care exist among racial/ethnic and age groups, geographic areas, or socioeconomic levels. The study is evaluating the quality and availability of existing data from a variety of sources, including cancer registries, medical records, and insurance claims, to support such analyses, and will identify ways to strengthen the data infrastructure for cancer care assessment.

Using State and Local Data

Cancer surveillance data are used to identify populations at increased risk for cancer diagnosis, late-stage diagnosis, or less-than-optimal care by race/ethnicity, age, geographic location, and access to care factors. This information is used by comprehensive control programs and other public health organizations to target interventions, as well as to evaluate ongoing activities. In addition, data gained from cancer registries guide the efforts of clinicians, legislatures, and researchers to increase primary and secondary prevention activities, to implement successful interventions, to improve treatment protocols, or to adopt changes in public policy.

A primary goal of NPCR is to provide data to public health planners and others monitoring the burden of disease and planning effective cancer prevention and control programs. Cancer control efforts are best served when data are analyzed, interpreted, and disseminated. Using data will improve the quality and consistency of that data, uncover new areas for analysis, and improve the understanding of the cancer burden in the United States.[16] Following are examples of how cancer registries have utilized data to guide and formulate public health priorities:

> **Increasing primary and secondary prevention activities:** The Colorado Central Cancer Registry noted a greater breast cancer incidence and later stage at diagnosis in a north Denver census tract during one of their routine surveillance activities. They alerted their state counterparts in the NBCCEDP and the National Comprehensive Cancer Comprehensive Program, who worked to increase awareness and services in this geographic area. The Colorado Central Cancer Registry monitored an increase in early-stage breast cancer diagnoses—a marker that primary and secondary prevention activities are successful—over time.
>
> **Implementing a successful intervention by changing public policy:** The Louisiana Tumor Registry collaborated with researchers from the Louisiana State University Health Sciences Center to develop a financial report on colorectal cancer incidence and death rates that was presented to state legislators. The presentation included data on the low-income and uninsured, a proposal for a colorectal cancer screening program, and an evaluation component based on Louisiana Tumor Registry data. State funding was increased to support this new activity, and the Louisiana Tumor Registry will monitor and update legislators to show program outcomes and justify future funding.
>
> **Improving treatment protocols:** The California Cancer Registry initiated a descriptive study to characterize a specific type of breast cancer known as the "triple-negative" (estrogen receptor negative, progesterone receptor negative, and human epidermal growth factor receptor-2 negative) breast cancer. The detailed information about these tumor markers is required by the California Cancer Registry, but is not for state-level cancer registry funded by CDC. The results showed that younger age, African American race/ethnicity, more advanced stage at diagnosis, lack of cell type differentiation, lower socioeconomic status, and shortened survival time were associated with triple-negative breast cancer. This type of breast cancer is not amenable to any form of endocrine therapy, and efforts to develop targeted therapies are under way.

Ongoing Work

Many of the activities described in the previous section are ongoing core activities and are re-evaluated and enhanced to meet the changing needs of the program on an annual basis. Planned enhancements to the core activities and new innovative projects that are envisioned are described below.

- Supporting NPCR registries to provide reporting of sentinel cancers with the focus of informing and driving policy and systems change at the state and local level
- Continuing collaborations with national partner organizations and state registries on publications using registry data, such as the *Annual Report to the Nation on the Status of Cancer* and two supplements to the journal *Cancer.* One supplement focuses on cancers associated with the human papillomavirus. The other supplement focuses on the cancer burden among American Indians and Alaska Natives.
- Assessing the completeness and accuracy of data required to be collected by NPCR registries, including data about race and ethnicity, stage at diagnosis, and treatment
- Continuing studies that focus on the patterns of care for cancer patients
- Supporting ongoing efforts to link registry data with the National Death Index that would allow for cancer surveillance studies on survival and survivorship
- Leading a collaborative effort to develop a model for sending data from clinical electronic health records to hospitals and registries
- Supporting ongoing efforts to test the collection of data in an electronic format using national data transmission standards; one pilot project is testing the reporting of data from a national pathology laboratory to the registries, and another is testing the collection of discrete data items directly from anatomical pathology reports using standardized checklists
- Conducting a multiyear economic analysis of NPCR to compare operating costs for registries that have

achieved standards for high-quality data with costs for registries that have not; the study will examine the costs of performing core surveillance activities, enhancing the infrastructure and operation of NPCR registries, and performing advanced surveillance activities; researchers will determine factors and variables that influence costs, and will develop a resource-allocation model based on cost-effectiveness

Note: Frances Michaud and Reda Wilson are Public Health Advisors for the Centers for Disease Control and Prevention. *The findings and conclusions in this report are those of the authors and do not necessarily represent the official position of the CDC.*

References

1. U.S. Cancer Statistics Working Group. *United States Cancer Statistics: 2004 Incidence and Mortality Web-Based Report Version.* Centers for Disease Control and Prevention, and National Cancer Institute, 2007. Available at: http://www.cdc.gov/cancer/npcr/uscs. Accessed October 2009.
2. Parkin, D. M. "The evolution of the population-based cancer registry." *Nat Rev Cancer,* 2006;6(8):603–612.
3. Black, B. L., Cowens-Alvarado, R., Gershman, S., Weir, H. K. "Using data to motivate action: the need for high quality, an effective presentation, and an action context for decision-making." *Cancer Causes Control,* 2005;16(Suppl 1):15–25.
4. U.S. Department of Health and Human Services. *Healthy People 2010* (2 vols), 2nd ed. Washington, DC: U.S. Government Printing Office, 2000.
5. Public Law 102-515. "Cancer Registries Amendment Act 1992." Available at: http://www.cdc.gov/cancer/npcr/npcrpdfs/publaw.pdf.
6. "State cancer registries: Status of authorizing legislation and enabling regulations—United States, October 1993." *MMWR Morb Mortal Wkly Rep,* 1994;43(4):71, 74–75.
7. Public Law 107-260. "Benign Brain Tumor Cancer Registries Amendment Act 2002." Available at: http://www.cdc.gov/cancer/npcr/pdf/btr/Amendment_Act.pdf Last accessed August 15, 2010.
8. Centers for Disease Control and Prevention. "NPCR-CSS Data Release Policy." Available at: https://www.npcrcss.org/docserver/ Last accessed August 15, 2010.
9. Ledford, K., Cardinez, C., Wilson, R. "NPCR Data Quality Indicators to improve population-based Central Cancer Registry Data." *Journal of Registry Management,* 2006;33(3):113–119.
10. Centers for Disease Control and Prevention. "Updated guidelines for evaluating surveillance systems." *MMWR Morb Mortal Wkly Rep,* 2001;50(RR13).
11. National Program of Cancer Registries Program Standards. Available at: http://www.cdc.gov/cancer/npcr/pdf/program_manual.pdf Last accessed, August 15, 2010.
12. Office of Management of Budget. "Guidelines for ensuring and maximizing the quality, objectivity, utility, and integrity of information disseminated by federal agencies." Available at: http://www.whitehouse.gov/omb/fedreg_reproducible/. Last accessed, August 15, 2010.
13. Hofferkamp, J., editor. *Standards for Cancer Registries, Volume III, Standards for Completeness, Quality, Analysis, and Management of Data.* Springfield, IL: North American Association of Central Cancer Registries, 2008.
14. Swan, J., Wingo, P., Clive, R., et al. "Cancer surveillance in the U.S.: Can we have a national system?" *Cancer,* 1998;83(7):1282–1291.
15. "Annual Report to the Nation on the Status of Cancer, 1975–2005, Featuring Trends in Lung Cancer, Tobacco Use, and Tobacco Control." *JNCI Journal of the National Cancer Institute,* 2008;100(23):1672–1694.
16. Centers for Disease Control and Prevention. "CDC/ATSDR Policy on Releasing and Sharing Data." 2003. Available at: http://www.cdc.gov/od/foia/policies/sharing.htm. Last accessed, August 15, 2010.

chapter 35

National Cancer Registrars Association

Lynda Douglas, CTR

The National Cancer Registrars Association (NCRA) is a not-for-profit association for cancer registry professionals. NCRA's purpose is education and certification (Certified Tumor Registrar). NCRA promotes professional development and education for all CTRs. There are currently more than 4,800 national and international members of NCRA. The NCRA annual budget is approximately 1.9 million dollars.

NCRA Vision and Mission Statements

Vision Statement: Improving lives through quality cancer data management.

Mission Statement: Serve as the premier education, credentialing and advocacy resource for cancer data professionals.

History

The NCRA was chartered in May 1974, and it was incorporated in October 1976. Before that time, registrars worked with little support in the field. Based on what was seen as a real need to expand the profession and commitment to providing adequate education and training for registrars, a dedicated group of cancer registry professionals held the first meeting of the National Tumor Registrars Association (NTRA) in Dallas, Texas, in May 1974. An integral part of that early vision was to develop educational standards for registrars and design a certification process. In 1983, the first credentialing process was implemented, and the credential Certified Tumor Registrar (CTR) was bestowed on those who met the qualifications and passed the credentialing examination. Since that time the association has experienced continued growth and change. In 1992, the association underwent a name change from NTRA to NCRA, and in May 2001, NCRA for the first time hired staff and established its own executive office, becoming self-managed.

NCRA Strategic Management Plan

In the late 1990s, NCRA's leadership made the decision that NCRA needed to change to achieve its mission. The operational structure in place at that time did not support the significant needs of the cancer registry field. NCRA had a wealth of knowledge, information, and commitment from its volunteer members, but remained unable to move forward to advance the field. To maximize the volunteer effort, NCRA moved from a management firm to hiring an Executive Director and paid staff to provide support. To further clarify NCRA's vision, a consultant was contracted to work with NCRA stakeholders to develop a business model, which was implemented in 2003. Through the use of an e-mail survey, the membership at large provided input into the process, and five key areas of focus were identified. These areas include education, administration, certification, communication and advocacy. The following strategies were determined (see Table 35-1) and are referred to as the NCRA Strategic Management Plan:

I. Education/Professional Development

Provide comprehensive educational opportunities that are accessible, cost appropriate, and forward thinking.

II. Credentialing

Advance, administer, and deliver a continually improving credentialing program to meet the needs of the profession.

Table 35-1	NCRA Strategic Objectives				
I. Education/ Professional Development	**II. Credentialing**	**III. Recruitment & Retention**	**IV. Member & Customer Services**	**V. Advocacy**	**VI. Administration & Finance**
1. Develop a comprehensive education plan to meet the changing demands of the profession and the CTR-credentialed individual.	1. Hold credentialing process to the highest standards.	1. Implement recommendations from NCRA's Workforce Study.	1. Establish a communication plan: (a) Increase communication with state and local associations; (b) increase communication and involvement with standards setters; and (c) explore ways to maximize effective communications with NCRA's other audiences.	1. Expand the advocacy process and outcomes mechanism by creating and implementing a process to develop and evaluate NCRA policy statements.	1. Establish a 5-year financial plan and 6-month reserve.

Table 35-1	NCRA Strategic Objectives *(continued)*

I. Education/ Professional Development	II. Credentialing	III. Recruitment & Retention	IV. Member & Customer Services	V. Advocacy	VI. Administration & Finance
2. Deliver *basic* and *advanced* (post-CTR) education opportunities.	2. Evaluate the need for new credentials to support the field.	2. Increase partnerships with peer organizations.	2. Continually evaluate innovative opportunities that would improve the quality, access, and delivery of NCRA published information and materials to membership and the field (includes all products, services, research, and development).	2. Enable member input regarding standard changes—before implementation.	2. Establish a financial growth plan.
3. Expand and enhance formal education opportunities.	3. Evaluate the relevance of the CTR nomenclature, and take appropriate action.	3. Increase and develop the leadership skills and participation of members.	3. Increase members' satisfaction with NCRA benefits and services.	3. Position NCRA as part of the decision-making process.	3. Establish a governance philosophy to function as a "knowledge-based" Board of Directors.
4. Monitor and encourage informatics role in cancer registry profession.	4. Promote credentials offered by NCRA.	4. Monitor and encourage professionalism and skills.	4. Develop and implement a marketing plan.	4. Develop programs to raise awareness and improve image perception of the profession.	4. Ensure adequate human resources: volunteers, staffing, and contract services to support organizational goals.
5. Evaluate, enhance, and deliver the certification maintenance process.					

III. Recruitment and Retention

Expand the workforce of the cancer registry profession by encouraging new people to enter the field and by improving retention of those currently in the field.

IV. Member and Customer Services

Assure satisfaction of internal and external NCRA customers and excellence in communications.

V. Advocacy

Be a strong advocate for our members by actively engaging in processes to network and communicate to effect an opinion.

VI. Administration and Finance

Maintain financial viability with an effective and efficient infrastructure.

Membership

As a multidisciplinary organization, membership is open to all individuals involved in cancer registry activities. The membership year is the calendar year, January 1 through December 31. All memberships are on an individual basis and cannot be transferred from one individual to another. NCRA maintains eight membership categories: Active, Associate, Honorary, Honorary Life, Inactive, International, Student, and Sustaining.

NCRA Membership Categories

Active

An active member is a person whose primary occupation is related to cancer registry work. An active member in good standing shall be entitled to all membership privileges including the right to vote, hold office, and chair or serve on a committee.

Associate

An associate member is anyone who is interested in the purpose of the association who does not meet the qualifications of active membership. An associate member shall not vote, hold office, or chair a committee, but may serve on a committee.

Honorary

Persons other than past presidents who have made a significant contribution to the profession of Cancer Registry Administration or have rendered distinguished service in the profession or its related fields may be elected to honorary membership by a unanimous vote of the corporation's active members present and voting, after recommendation by the Board of Directors. Honorary members shall be exempt from dues. Honorary members shall not vote, hold office, or chair or serve on a committee. Honorary members shall not hold any other class of membership in the corporation.

Honorary Life

Past presidents shall become honorary life members at age 60. They shall retain all privileges of active membership without payment of dues or annual conference registration fees. An honorary life member shall not hold any other class of membership in the corporation.

Inactive

A person who previously qualified as an active member but is no longer in the workforce is eligible to be an inactive member. This category includes retirees, unemployed persons, and persons on extended leave from their jobs. An inactive member shall not vote, hold office, or chair a committee, but may serve on a committee.

International

Any person who is not a resident of the United States, Canada, or Mexico may join as an international member. Persons residing outside of North America are not restricted to this membership classification. International members shall not vote, hold office, or chair a committee, but may serve on a committee.[1]

Student

Any full-time, college-level student interested in NCRA's purpose may join as a student member. A student member shall be eligible for this classification for no more than 5 years from the date the member first joined in this category. A student member shall not vote, hold office, or chair a committee, but may serve on a committee.

Sustaining

Any person, institution, or organization interested in promoting the purpose of the corporation may join as a sustaining member. A sustaining member shall not vote, hold office, or chair or serve on a committee.

Governance

A 12-member volunteer board of directors is elected from the membership to provide governance for NCRA. These include officers who are president, president-elect/secretary, immediate past president, treasurer senior, treasurer junior, professional development board director, recruitment and retention board director, public relations and communications board director, education board director, advocacy and technical practice board director West, advocacy and technical practice board director Midwest, and advocacy and technical practice board director East.

Terms of office are that the president-elect/secretary and treasurer junior are elected for 1 year. When the president-elect/secretary's term expires, the position rolls over to a 1-year term as president. When the current president's term expires, the position rolls over to a 1-year term as immediate past president. When the treasurer junior's term expires, the position rolls over to a 1-year term as treasurer senior. The professional development board director, recruitment and retention board director, public relations and communications board director, education board director, advocacy and technical practice board director West, advocacy and technical practice board director Midwest, and advocacy and technical board director East are elected for 2-year terms.

---

[1]Bylaws of the National Cancer Registrars Association.

Volunteer Activities

NCRA has multiple committees made up of volunteers from the membership to assist in the delivery and management of various association activities. Currently, NCRA has 16 active committees.

Alternative Methods of Earning Continuing Education (CE) Credit Committee: This committee is charged with developing high-quality, meaningful, affordable, and easily accessed education programs for CTRs to earn continuing education credit hours.

Annual Conference Program Committee: This committee prepares and coordinates the educational program for the NCRA annual conference.

Awards: Coordinates the selection and delivery process for the awards program to recognize individuals and their contributions in specific areas. NCRA offers the following awards: Distinguished Member Award, Outstanding New Professional Award, Literary Award, and Education Award.

Continuing Education Program Recognition Committee: This committee evaluates activities for educational value. If the committee determines that an activity provides continuing education, it assigns a clock hour value to the activity (continuing education credit hours [CEs]). This committee also participates in the development and maintenance of a program for CTRs to demonstrate their attainment of credit hours necessary to maintain their certification as established in the Bylaws and Standing Rules of NCRA.

The Connection: NCRA's membership newsletter committee is responsible for publishing *The Connection* quarterly in the spring, summer, fall, and winter.

Education Committee: The Education Committee identifies the educational needs of NCRA, makes recommendations to the Board of Directors, and coordinates existing continuing education programs. The Education Committee is the umbrella committee for all educational activities, and the chair serves on each of the other committees to maintain continuity. The Chair of the Education Committee coordinates with the Formal Education Committee and the Alternative Methods Committee. The committee establishes minimum standards for all NCRA educational presentations.

Educational Materials Committee: Development and marketing of new educational products is the responsibility of this committee. The Educational Materials Committee also assures that current products marketed by NCRA contain up-to-date information.

Ethics Committee: This committee reviews possible violations of the Code of Ethics of NCRA. The committee may recommend action to be taken to the Board of Directors.

Finance Committee: The Finance Committee is a standing Committee of NCRA that is chaired by the Treasurer. This committee maintains the fiscal stability of NCRA by monitoring and directing the flow of NCRA funds.

Formal Education Committee: This committee is charged with reviewing all formal education program applications to verify that these programs meet the Council on Certification's standards for the Certification Eligibility Route related to formal education requirements.

Formal Education Review Committee: NCRA's Formal Education Review Committee is responsible for establishing, maintaining, and applying standards that ensure the quality and continuous improvement of cancer registry education and reflect the evolving practice of Cancer Registry Management.

Governance Planning and Evaluation Committee (GPEC): GPEC offers advice to the President and Board of Directors, monitors the strategic plan, and administers the NCRA annual conference scholarship fund.

Informatics Committee: The Informatics Committee is charged with developing a comprehensive informatics education plan to meet the changing demands of the cancer registry profession. This committee also evaluates and delivers basic and advanced informatics training opportunities.

Journal of Registry Management (JRM): JRM is the official NCRA journal. *JRM* publishes original manuscripts on topics related to management of health data registries and the collection, management, and use of cancer, trauma, AIDS, and other health registry data. All contributed manuscripts are peer-reviewed before publication. The International Standard Serial Numbers (ISSN no.) for *JRM* are 1945-6123 (print) and 1945-6131 (online). *JRM* has been accepted for indexing in MedLine and is searchable through PubMed.

National Cancer Registrars Week (NCRW) Committee: This committee works with NCRA's Executive Office staff to coordinate the publication of all NCRA noneducation promotional materials. This committee develops and maintains an NCRA Store brochure that lists NCRA publications, pamphlets, and other advertising or marketing materials.

They are also charged with organizing the NCRW, which takes place during the second week of April, Monday through Friday.

Nominating Committee: The Nominating Committee is responsible for preparation of the ballots for elected officers and representatives serving on the Council on Certification. This committee has seven members. The committee chair is appointed by the President; the other members are elected and include two members from each of three regions (East, Midwest, and West).

Web Site Committee: This committee oversees NCRA's Web page and Web presence.

Special Interest Groups

Registrars function in varying fields of practice and because of this diversity in membership, NCRA supports special interest groups (SIGs) to provide technical expertise and networking opportunities. The SIG groups include Cancer Program Managers, Central Registries, Federal Registries, Hospital Registries, National Cancer Institute Designated Comprehensive Cancer Centers, Pediatric Registries, and Registry Services (contractors/vendors). The SIGs are given time at the NCRA annual conference to meet, select leadership, and network.

Liaisons

NCRA's liaisons act as a formal interface between partner organizations involved in the cancer registry profession. NCRA has formal liaisons with the *Advance* (Magazine for Health Professionals), the American Joint Committee on Cancer (AJCC), College of American Pathologists (CAP), Commission on Cancer of the American College of Surgeons (CoC/ACoS), National Accreditation Program for Breast Centers (NAPBC), National Coordinating Council for Cancer Surveillance (NCCCS), NCI Surveillance, Epidemiology, and End Results (SEER), and North American Association of Central Cancer Registries (NAACCR). The *Advance* is a publication for health information professionals. AJCC is responsible for publishing and maintaining the *AJCC Cancer Staging Manual* used for staging most cancer cases. CAP sets standards for pathology reporting. COC/ACoS approves hospital cancer programs and is an industry standard-setting organization. NAPBC sets standards for breast cancer treatment. NCCCS is an organization made up of the leaders in cancer standard-setting organizations, and their purpose is to coordinate and facilitate the direction for cancer registry. NCI/SEER is a federal standard-setting organization, as well as a federal funding agent for certain areas of the United States. NAACCR is an organization that is dedicated to creating and maintaining uniform cancer data standards, as well as creating guidelines for registry operations and informatics.

Special appointments may be made to promote NCRA or to represent NCRA members regarding special issues at specific meetings or events of other organizations. These organizations may include American Cancer Society, American Health and Information Management Association, Association of Cancer Executives, Association of Clinical Oncology Administrators, Association of Community Cancer Centers, Joint Commission, and American Society of Clinical Oncologists.

Activities of NCRA

NCRA sponsors an annual conference and regional workshops offering educational sessions designed to improve registrar's knowledge and professional expertise. The annual conference also provides an excellent networking opportunity. The regional workshops assist registrars who cannot attend the annual conference by allowing them to maintain their skills locally. The Advocacy and Technical Practice Board Directors offer a mechanism whereby local and state associations are kept informed of activity on a national level and any local concerns are communicated back to the NCRA board for discussion and action if needed.

Members are given updated information through the quarterly publication of the association newsletter, *The Connection,* and more frequently via NCRA's Web site and broadcast e-mailing. NCRA has seven educational publications in print, and two revisions are under way. The *JRM,* a recognized scientific journal, is published quarterly by NCRA. In addition to registry management and scientific articles, the *JRM* includes another feature to improve data quality. This is the Continuing Education Quiz, which provides an easy way to maintain continuing education credit. *JRM* has been accepted into the PubMed database.

NCRA has an Executive Director and staff in an established corporate office to enhance the significant volunteer effort that has been the true foundation of NCRA since 1974.

Council on Certification

Representatives for the Council on Certification

The CTR remains a standard of quality in the registry profession. The NCRA Council on Certification administers this examination process. The qualifications for candidates who would like to become a CTR have expanded to include a college degree. Candidates must meet eligibility requirements that include a combination of experience in the cancer registry field and educational background. After successfully passing the certification examination, the CTR credential is awarded. These registrars have demonstrated that they have met or exceeded the standard level of experience and knowledge required for effective performance. To maintain the CTR, continuing educational requirements must be met. This requirement provides assurance that the registrar's knowledge and skills are continuously monitored and maintained. Governance of the credentialing process was changed with the establishment of a Council on Certification in 2002.

The Council on Certification is made up of an administrator and up to eight representatives (no less than six). These are elected positions to administer and manage NCRA's certification program.

To be eligible for the office of the Council on Certification Representative, the active CTR certificant shall have a minimum of 3 years' experience as a CTR and shall not hold employment in any educational services related field that provides education to future registrars. Elected members of the Council on Certification serve a term of not more than 2 years and may not serve more than two consecutive terms, and they do not have to hold membership in NCRA.

Terms of office are that the elected administrator of the Council on Certification serves a 3-year term and cannot serve more than two consecutive terms. Representatives for the Council on Certification are elected for a term of 2 or 3 years (positions are staggered) and may not serve more than two consecutive terms. Appointed members of the Council on Certification serve a term of not more that 2 years and may not serve more than two consecutive terms.

CTR Credential

The CTR credential:

- Establishes a standard of knowledge and experience required for professional registry practice
- Is formal recognition for professionals who meet the requirements of the CTR credential
- Assures employers and members of allied health professions that credentialed employees meet standards of cancer registry industry
- Provides recommended or required credential for many employment opportunities
- Is a required staff credential for ACoS-approved cancer programs
- Is a required credential for reporting to some state central registries

Earning and Maintaining the Credential

The CTR credential is earned by successfully completing the CTR examination with a passing score. It is maintained through the accumulation of 20 continuing education hours every 2 years.

Eligibility

NCRA has seven approved programs providing formal education in cancer registry science. Schools with accredited programs sometimes change. The Council on Certification's Web site (http://www.ctrexam.org) provides up-to-date program information.

Candidates must meet all the requirements (experience and education) of ONE of the routes by the application deadline or request NCRA's Council on Certification to review specific eligibility:

> **Route A. Experience:** Successful completion of 160 hours of work practicum in a CTR-staffed Cancer Registry (may be part of a NCRA-approved program curriculum).

AND

Education: *NCRA-Accredited Associate's Degree Program*

OR

Successful completion of an *NCRA-Accredited Formal Education Program* AND successful completion of a minimum of an associate's degree or equivalent (4 semesters/6 quarters).

> **Route B.** Minimum 1-year full-time (12 months or 1,950 hours) or equivalent experience in the Cancer Registry field AND successful completion of a minimum of an associate's degree (or equivalent [4 semesters/6 quarters]) in an approved college-level curriculum in a recognized allied health field as determined by NCRA's Council on Certification.

> **Route C.** Minimum 1-year full-time (12 months or 1,950 hours) or equivalent experience in the Cancer Registry field AND successful completion of a minimum of an associate's degree (or equivalent [4 semesters/6 quarters]) AND license or certification in a recognized allied health field as determined by NCRA's Council on Certification.

> **Route D.** Minimum 1-year full-time (12 months or 1,950 hours) or equivalent experience in the Cancer Registry field AND successful completion of a master's level or higher college-level curriculum in a recognized allied health field.

More information can be found on NCRA Council on Certification's Web site (http://www.ctrexam.org).

NCRA Education Foundation

In 2004, the NCRA Education Foundation was established and granted a 501C3 tax status. This allows the foundation to receive donations that are tax exempt. The foundation's only member is the NCRA. The foundation allows NCRA to receive and expend funds for educational development and products to benefit NCRA members at lower prices (tax exempt). The NCRA Education Foundation has a nine-member Board of Directors. The Board includes the Foundation Chair, Vice Chair, Secretary, Treasurer, and five Directors at Large.

There are five committees in the NCRA Education Foundation: Finance, Fundraising, Nominating, Public Relations & Marketing, and Project Review. The foundation has four goals:

1. Administration and Internal Communications to assure a sound infrastructure to maintain the Foundation
2. Finances to maintain financial stability
3. Public Relations and External Communications to promote the activities and achievements of the foundation

4. Project Development and Fundraising to identify, prioritize, and fund projects consistent with the NCRA Education Foundation mission and vision

Summary

NCRA is the professional association for the entire cancer registry industry. NCRA's considerable strengths include diversity, volunteerism, staff, dedicated members, mentors, financial security, and history that positions the association significantly to attain the goals set out in this aggressive strategic plan. The strength of the association strengthens the members and, in turn, provides them with the skills and tools necessary to continue the fight against cancer.

The Council on Certification (http://www.ctrexam.org/) ensures consistent, professional certification routes and testing. The NCRA Education Foundation (http://www.ncraeducationfoundation.org/index.html) is a separate organization that serves the NCRA members (http://www.ncra-usa.org).

Note: Lynda Douglas is a Public Health Advisor for the Centers for Disease Control and Prevention. *The findings and conclusions in this report are those of the author and do not necessarily represent the official position of the Centers for Disease Control and Prevention.*

Central and Other Registries

Linda Mulvihill
Section Editor—Textbook

Melissa Pearson
Section Editor—Review Guide

chapter 36

Central Cancer Registries

Herman R. Menck, BS, MBA, CPhil, FACE
Kathleen K. Thoburn, CTR
Betsy A. Kohler, MPH, CTR

Central cancer registries have much in common with hospital-based cancer registries. This chapter addresses unique aspects of central registries, including types and administration, data set planning, data collection, computerization, quality management, certification, follow-up, incidence and survival rates, other uses and history of central registries.[1-5] Central registries are by definition multihospital and either population based[6-8] or hospital based (not population based).[9-13] Numerous non-U.S. population-based central registries are also operating.[14-17]

Types of Central Registries

Central registries are definitively described by a combination of primary characteristics including goals and objectives, population coverage, data set used, their data recipient, their organizational setting, and their source of funding.[18-21]

Goals and Objectives

The goals and objectives of registries include various components:

1. Incidence surveillance, such as monitoring incidence rates and trends by age, sex, and race/ethnic group
2. Survival surveillance, such as contributing to the annual Surveillance, Epidemiology, and End Results (SEER) survival statistics[22-24]
3. Analytic research, such as contributing cases to be interviewed for etiologic case–control studies[25]
4. Clinical research, such as contributing cases to clinical trials
5. Patient care surveillance, such as contributing case information to national studies of patterns of care[26,27]
6. Professional education for clinicians and others[28]
7. Enumeration of caseload statistics (for administrative and planning purposes) such as *ACS Cancer Facts and Figures*[29]
8. Community and state outreach, and public policy
9. Evaluation of cancer control initiatives

These goals can be focused at the local (state) level or the national level (through data submittal to a national data collector such as the SEER Program and the National Program for Cancer Registries [NPCR]), or both.[6]

Population Coverage

Most central registries are population based and are regional, state, multistate, provincial, or national. Ambiguity exists in the definition and use of the term *central* cancer registry; some define it as including only population-based registries, whereas others define it as including nonpopulation-based registries such as the National Cancer Data Base (NCDB) or military registries. The most widely used definition refers to population-based registries, which are the main focus of this chapter. The geographic area from which the population source of the central registry is drawn is sometimes referred to as its *catchment area*.

Population-based registries include all cancer cases in a defined geographic area (e.g., the state of Illinois), allowing the calculation of incidence and mortality rates for the geographic area. These rates include all cases diagnosed in the population at risk. The population from which the cases are derived must be explicitly determined from census or related data. Cases reported from multiple hospitals for the same patient and tumor must be consolidated into one record, and counted only once per primary cancer.

Some population-based registries operate at the incidence-only level, whereas others are multipurpose. Incidence-only registries have as their primary goal determination of cancer incidence rates in different groups of people living in their defined geographic area. Various surveillance activities are enabled including the tracking of cancer trends in the population. Necessary requirements include an accurate and complete case count; reasonable timeliness, ranging from 9 to 24 months after the close of the calendar year; quality control of casefinding and abstracting; and data necessary to categorize patients and tumors into groups for which rates are computed. For these registries, generally no treatment data or outcome data are collected. The incidence-only registry provides incidence and trend data for a specific geographic area to assess the burden of cancer in that specific geographic area. For example, it has become common for government health agencies to evaluate cancer clusters and suspected cancer problems related to possible environmental contamination using such registry data. Incidence-only registries may also collect data on healthcare providers and may support cancer research such as case–control studies and cohort linkage studies. They can also be used to predict cancer caseload.

Many population-based registries serve multiple purposes such as combining incidence reporting with survival results, patient care, and various other research and cancer-control activities.[30,31] In recent years, some cancer registries have extended activities to include direct participation in epidemiologic research, evaluation of interventions against cancer at the population level, situation analysis and cancer control planning, coordination of screening, and monitoring the performance of cancer control programs.[32]

Often, the primary objective of a registry supporting epidemiologic research is to notify the study manager of eligible study subjects for survey or questionnaire as quickly as possible.[33] Therefore, the cases must be ascertained rapidly. Sometimes this necessitates the utilization of a diagnostic pathology report preceding the slower, traditional medical record–based process. This is often referred to as rapid case ascertainment. An advantage of research derived from population-based patient rosters is the reduction or avoidance of selection bias in casefinding for both demographic and tumor classification purposes. Incomplete casefinding is undesirable because it compromises the generalization of results.

Some central registries are not population based, but are multihospital registries. Examples of these would be all hospitals using a particular software package or related professional services, or a military registry. Several suppliers of data systems and services pool the data of their client institutions into a single file that can be used for comparative purposes.[9,10] These databases are characterized by the geographic dispersion of their particular clients but are not representative of all patients in the geographic area.

Another example of a nonpopulation-based central registry is formed by all hospitals that choose to participate in the NCDB of the Commission on Cancer (CoC).[11] As of 2009, the NCDB included data reported from more than 1,400 CoC-accredited cancer programs in the United States and Puerto Rico, providing a convenience sample of approximately 70% of U.S. incident (newly diagnosed) cancer cases.[34] The NCDB has a total case file that includes more than 25,000,000 cases accessioned from 1985 through 2008, and is renowned as the largest clinical registry in the world.[34,35] Another example is of a network of all hospitals in one branch of the government.[12]

Some registries operate as central repositories for hospitals from one or more of the military services or the Veterans Administration. An example of one of these military central registries is the Department of Defense (DoD), which uses Automated Central Tumor Registry (ACTUR)[13] as its cancer-reporting software.

Data Sets

Data sets are predominantly influenced by what data are necessary to meet the goals and objectives of the registry, and what available data set standards may prevail. Often, the registry's funding source will specify requirements for the data set. In addition to data collected by hospital-based registries, central registries often supplement the data with information obtained from linkage to other data sources such as vital statistics (annual follow-up) and geographic information from the residence at diagnosis, and will consolidate data from multiple sources to create a single record for a primary cancer.

Data Submittal

Often, population-based central registries submit their data to a larger geographically based data system, so that data can be aggregated for large population groups, often on a national or international level. These national data collections are generally maintained by a primary funding source or sponsoring organization. The National Cancer Institute (NCI) SEER Program, the Centers for Disease Control and Prevention (CDC) NPCR Cancer Surveillance System (NPCR-CSS), the North American Association of Central Cancer Registries (NAACCR), and the International Association of Cancer Registries (IACR) are the largest and most well-established population-based data systems that have multiregional, national, or international coverage, whereas the NCDB's collection of hospital-based data is the largest repository of clinical data on cancer.[11] As of 2010, the SEER Program collected and published cancer incidence and survival data from population-based cancer registries covering approximately 26% of the U.S. population, including 23% of African Americans, 40% of Hispanics, 42% of American Indians and Alaska Natives, 53% of Asians, and 70% of Hawaiian/Pacific Islanders.[36] The NPCR began funding states in 1994, and in 2010 supported central registries representing 96% of the U.S. population.[7,37] Together, NPCR and the NCI SEER Program collect data for the entire U.S. population. Note that a central population-based registry might submit data to more than one data system; for example, a central registry might submit data to SEER, NPCR, and NAACCR.

Organization Setting/Funding Source

A legislative mandate often empowers a central registry to establish and maintain a mechanism for cancer data collection and related surveillance activities, and provides some or all of the necessary funding. The department of health within the state, provincial, or federal government often sponsors central registries. Sometimes they are hosted by a university, a medical or hospital association, a prominent hospital or medical center, or multiple sources.

Administration of Central Registries

The administration of a central registry is a complex matter involving organizational concerns and interrelationships with various outside groups.[33,38]

Legislation, Affiliation, and Governance

Early central registries, which were often based on voluntary participation, were usually started by a core organization, which formed alliances with other interested parties or a consortium of cancer treatment facilities (e.g., Connecticut, Utah, Los Angeles County). Cancer reporting is now required in every state in the United States as a result of federal and state legislative mandates.[39,40] Both voluntary and legislatively mandated registries take time to be implemented. Many of the initial tasks are easier to accomplish with a legislative mandate. The legislative mandate often specifies operational requirements, provides a process for determining compliance, and establishes funding.[38] The legal requirement for reporting (with sanctions for failing to report) and protection from liability for those who report are key factors in enabling a central registry to be truly population based.

Although some registries were started earlier, the pace of registry-enabling legislation increased greatly during the 1990s. SEER and NPCR are the major funding sources for U.S. central cancer registries, and all states now have statewide, population-based central registries as a result of NPCR or SEER funding, or both.[41–42]

In addition to enabling legislation, central registries need the advice and support of a variety of stakeholders, including clinicians from major medical facilities, public health and government officials, epidemiologists, biostatisticians, university and other researchers, local cancer registrar organizations, the CoC, the American Cancer Society, and community special interest groups.[43–44] In many respects, a population-based registry is a public trust, and should encourage and enjoy wide participation.

Many central registries have an advisory committee, an executive committee, or a governing board. The functions and responsibilities of these committees vary from giving advice to setting policies. The members of the advisory committee are usually representatives of the various community and state organizations that have alliances with the central registry.

Participation by clinicians from the local major medical facilities is essential and fosters cooperation. Public health officials welcome the central registry as an aid in understanding cancer burden and in performing other surveillance activities. Central cancer registries serve as a valuable source of useful statistical data for epidemiologists and other health researchers. Participation by key hospital-based registrars whose facilities report to the central registry can keep the governing committee informed of data collection problems encountered at the hospital level. The organization chart of a central registry often reflects two governance groups at the top: both an advisory committee and the hosting organization's line of authority (such as an official from the state health department).

Staffing

Operation of a central cancer registry is labor intensive. Composition and number of staff depend to a large extent on the goals of the registry, the registry's caseload, and the nature of the data collection process.[45–50] The goals of the registry determine what data items are collected, the rapidity of data collection, whether follow-up is conducted, and the uses to which the data are put; all of which influence staffing. The geographic area and population covered by the registry also affects staffing needs. Other factors affecting registry staffing include longevity of the database, managerial and administrative responsibilities, computerization, and cancer program functions.

The scientific or medical director often has budgetary responsibility for the central registry and may serve part time or full time, depending on the size of the registry and the responsibilities entailed. Almost every central registry has a full-time administrative manager or director who is responsible for its day-to-day operation. Most administrative managers have direct casefinding, abstracting, and quality-control experience, and are well connected with local, related professional organizations.

How the processes of quality control, data processing, and statistical analysis are accomplished often depends on the size of a central registry. Large central registries usually have one or more full-time staff for both quality control and data processing. Because of their specialized nature, statistical analyses may be done by experts who are members of another department or organizational entity, in particular, in small and midsize registries. Registries with smaller budgets often use part-time personnel for these functions.

The number of staff needed for quality control depends on the nature of the data collection, the scope of the data set collected, and the quality-control measures used (such as edits, reabstracting, and casefinding). If the data include treatment and stage, more expertise and time are needed to collect and validate the data. Requiring that data collection staff be certified by the National Cancer Registrars Association, Inc. (NCRA), as a Certified Tumor Registrar (CTR), helps to ensure an acceptable level of quality.

A registry's information technology (IT) requirements are determined by the type of computer system used to collect, store, process, and retrieve the data. Computerized systems require software development, maintenance, and support. Development of customized software is time consuming and expensive. Additional functions such as geocoding, death clearance, report generation, and statistical and spatial analyses further define the registry's IT requirements.

Public relations activities and related outreach activities vary from registry to registry. The ability of the registry to work with legislators, the medical community, community interest groups, and concerned citizens is an important responsibility that should not be overlooked. These responsibilities often fall to the medical or administrative director, although some registries have a spokesperson specifically designated for this role.

A past survey of 31 population-based registries included data on the number of full-time equivalent (FTE) employees who were funded and the number of incident cases ascertained annually.[45] Size of caseload for these central registries varied from 1,200 to 83,000 incident cases per year. For these 31 central registries combined, there was a reported average staff ratio of 0.8 FTE employee per 1,000 incident cases. Reflecting different registry goals and methodologies, there was a wide range of staffing ratios, from a low of 2.5 FTE employees for a registry accessioning 20,000 incident cases (0.1 FTE employee per 1,000 cases) to a high of 42.5 FTE employees for 14,000 cases (3.0 FTE employees per 1,000 cases).

Much of registry staffing variation relates to the data collection, coding, and processing methodologies used. Registries collecting already coded and computerized data reported lower staff needs for these processes. A 1985 international report on population-based registries also found wide diversity among registration techniques and staffing patterns.[51] For the 61 registries included, there was an average of 1.0 FTE employee per 1,000 incident cases. Minimal and multipurpose central registries were grouped together in this international survey, following a wide range of data collection, coding, and processing methodologies.

In the U.S. survey, several typical central registry job titles were listed, including Medical or Scientific Director/Epidemiologist, Registry/Project Manager, Office/Accounts Manager, Abstractors, quality control, data processing, statistician, coding/processing, research analyst, data entry, and secretarial/clerical. The types and average number of FTE employees reported are summarized in Table 36-1.

Fifty percent of the reported staffs were either abstractors or coders/processors, and were often CTRs. Although the breadth of necessary staffing for a central registry is well suggested by the survey, caution should be exercised in interpreting these past surveys of earlier central registration characteristics. More recently, central registries are increasingly reliant on IT staff to conduct a large proportion of tasks relating to electronic reporting to, and computerization of, the registry. As a result, a limitation of the staffing numbers and percentages cited in Table 36-1 is the lack of information regarding IT staff.

Table 36-1	Full-Time Equivalent Staffing for Central Registries	
Job Title	Full-Time Equivalent Employees	Percentage
Director	0.6	4
Registry Manager	0.7	5
Office/Accounts Manager	0.4	3
Abstractor	3.7	27
Quality Control	1.2	9
Data Processing	1.1	8
Statistician	0.5	4
Coding/Processing	3.2	23
Research Analyst	0.3	2
Secretarial	1.1	8
Data Entry	0.9	7
Total	13.7	100

Modified from Watkins, S., MacKinnon, J., Price, W. "Budgets and Staffing" (pp. 111–130). In *Central Cancer Registries: Design, Management and Use,* edited by H. R. Menck, C. R. Smart. Langhorne, PA: Harwood Academic Publishers, 1994, by permission.

Budget

Similar to staffing, the most important factors that influence central registry budgets are the registry's annual caseload, the amount and type of data, as well as the number of source reports collected per case, and the data collection methods.[45-53] The legislative mandate itself or the administrative policies that govern the mandate with regard to who must report and how they must report also affects the funding necessary for the registry. For instance, the staffing and salary needs of a registry in a state in which institutions are required to submit data to the central registry are quite different from those of a registry in which the registry's staff are required to obtain the data from the institutions.

Even with the most careful planning, adequate funding for the registry can be difficult to obtain. As with many projects, the budgetary allocation can determine the scope of work rather than the other way around. Ideally, it is wise to develop the registry budget for a 3- or 5-year period. A central registry's budget is not static, nor is its annual caseload; although annual caseload may increase over time, competing public health priorities do not assure stable or increasing registry budgets. If annual increases are not built into the appropriation, the registry will have to absorb the costs of the additional workload that occurs with an increase in the number of cases and increasing demand for expanded data elements. As a result, registries are always striving to improve efficiency and incorporate technology into operations.

The major categories of a central registry's budget include personnel, travel, and IT costs. There must be an adequate number of well-trained personnel in the registry, and the salaries must be competitive. There must be adequate money for travel within the state or region for the conduct of routine business and for professional meetings. In addition, there is a need for adequate funding for out-of-state travel for national professional and educational conferences, and meetings with standard setters and funding agencies. On-site training, quality-control visits, and audits are important and must be conducted regularly. And finally, the data processing budget must be sufficient to achieve the registry's goals. Whether the data processing functions are performed in-house or are contracted out, data must be entered, edited, aggregated, and reported in some form.

The relationship among incident caseload, FTE staffing, and dollar cost as reported by central registries in 1994 is summarized in Table 36-2.[45]

The average staff productivity was found to be 1,251 cases per FTE. There was a wide range of cases per FTE reported, from 192 cases to 6,120 cases per FTE. These wide ranges may reflect differences in productivity and cost-effectiveness, but probably more clearly reflect differences in registry operations, as well as goals and objectives. In a more recent study in 2005, it was found that the average NPCR cost to report a case of cancer decreases as the number of incident cases increases, suggesting an

Table 36-2	Incident Caseload, Full-Time Equivalent Staffing, and Dollar Cost Reported by Several Central Registries	
Incident Cases	**FTE Employees**	**Cases/FTE Employees**
15,300	30	510
52,000	21.3	2,441
3,900	11.7	333
3,608	3.7	975
13,983	42.5	329
28,000	15.0	1,866
16,500	14.9	1,107
15,300	2.5	6,120
3,900	3.2	1,219
37,000	44.2	837
83,000	24.7	3,360
57,000	16.5	3,455
7,000	38.4	192
5,000	5.0	1,000
Average: 24,392	19.5	1,251

FTE, full-time equivalent.

economies-of-scale relationship between these two major factors that is most likely a result of fixed costs, such as administrative and IT support (i.e., the average cost per case will be less when fixed costs are distributed across a greater number of cases).[53] However, the same study reported that the average cost to report a case of cancer increased as the geographic coverage of the registry increased.

Notably, the number of incident cases generated by a central registry is, in general, much less than the number of reported cases processed by the state because of multiple reports of the same tumor from various reporting sources. The number of reports per tumor increases with an increase in electronic reporting to the registry. For example, with the implementation of electronic pathology reporting to a registry, the registry will often receive a pathology report for a tumor before the report of the tumor from the facility of diagnosis and/or treatment, and all reports for the tumor are consolidated to one incident case. In addition, eliminating nonreportable cases that have been reported to a registry also consumes staff time and resources, and these cases do not contribute to the total number of incident cases reported by the registry.

Security/Confidentiality

Central cancer registries are sizable databases that store important confidential information about large numbers of patients with cancer.[54–57] It is essential that specific and precise identifying information be present in the patient record to resolve duplicate (redundant) case reporting. The storage of this confidential information is justified by the breadth and utility of medical research, patient care surveillance, patient follow-up, and other uses made of the data, but a strong imperative regarding patient confidentiality is created.

Complicating the need for confidentiality is the fact that central cancer registries frequently collect information from a number of different physical locations, and transmit/transport that data to a central location where it is stored. Hospital data are taken outside the walls of the hospital itself. Security must involve physical protection of the collected data from the reporting source to the central registry. In the central registry, physical access to paper and electronic records must be controlled. The central registry employees sign a security precaution statement when they are employed at the central registry, and those security statements are reviewed annually.

In general, a registry should ensure that data are available only to those that need to access or use it for a legitimate purpose. Controlling access to cancer registry data is required by various federal agency policies and regulations. In the United States, registries are required to follow policies and procedures for data security established by leading organizations in the central cancer registry and healthcare fields, such as the U.S. Department of Health and Human Services (HHS), SEER, NPCR, and NAACCR.

NAACCR provides central registry guidelines for data security in *Standards for Cancer Registries, Vol. III: Standards for Completeness, Quality, Analysis, and Management of Data,* section 6.4, Information Technology Policies and Procedures.[58] NAACCR guidelines specify that member registries develop written security policies that are distributed to staff and included in staff training. Security policies are to address provision of User IDs and passwords to those accessing registry data; provision of the minimum access to data required for each staff to conduct his or her specific tasks; logging of data accesses, encryption of digital communications, and storage of media containing confidential data; having firewall protection for network servers, workstations, and laptops; having an intrusion detection system in place to prevent unauthorized or malicious accesses; and having data, equipment, and media retention and disposal procedures in place.

The Office for Civil Rights (OCR) enforces the Health Insurance Portability and Accountability Act of 1996 (HIPAA) Privacy Rule, which protects the privacy of individually identifiable health information, and the HIPAA Security Rule, which sets national standards for the security of electronic protected health information.

Security concerns for central cancer registries have changed swiftly as interpretations of the impact of HIPAA have been rolled out. Because of the complex nature of HIPAA, interpretations of its requirements are still being proposed and studied. In a 2001 letter, NAACCR summarized advice for central registries regarding HIPAA[59-60]:

> To summarize, HIPAA has very little impact on cancer reporting to central cancer registries. Specifically, HIPAA provides for the continuation of reporting identifiable data for reportable diseases to public health entities for the purpose of public health surveillance. Additionally, HIPAA does not obstruct any state law that supports or mandates the reporting of disease or injury for public health purposes. Written informed consent from each cancer patient reported to public health entities is not required under HIPAA; rather hospitals must document that reporting has occurred. This can be done simply for all cancer cases since reporting is mandatory for all cases.

To view the entire HIPPA Rule, and for other additional helpful information about how it applies, see the OCR Web site,[61] which includes a helpful Summary of the HIPPA Privacy Rule document. HIPPA included Administrative Simplification provisions that required HHS to adopt national standards for electronic healthcare transactions and code sets, unique health identifiers, and security. In addition, Congress incorporated into HIPAA provisions that mandated the adoption of federal privacy protections for individually identifiable health information.[61]

HHS published a final Privacy Rule in December 2000, which was later modified in August 2002. This rule set national standards for the protection of individually identifiable health information by three types of covered entities: health plans, healthcare clearinghouses, and healthcare providers who conduct the standard healthcare transactions electronically. Compliance with the Privacy Rule was required as of April 14, 2003 (April 14, 2004, for small health plans). HHS published a final Security Rule in February 2003. This rule sets national standards for protecting the confidentiality, integrity, and availability of electronic protected health information. Compliance with the Security Rule was required as of April 20, 2005.[61] Current insights into HIPAA compliance should be gleaned from cancer registry Web sites such as NAACCR, and Web sites specializing in HIPAA itself (such as OCR). Clearly, confidentiality must be a concern to the central cancer registrar.[62]

Ethics

Useful descriptions of ethical concerns for cancer registrars including ethical codes specifically for cancer registrars[63-66] and those for public health concerns in general[67] have been previously described.

Central registries are generally run under review of the institutional review board (IRB) of the hosting organization.[68] If no IRB is maintained by the hosting organization, an IRB of a related organization can sometimes be

Table 36-3	Institutional Review Board Concerns Regarding Central Cancer Registries

1. Uphold confidentiality and privacy of the data
2. Preservation and securing registry records
3. Disclosure of data only to proper authorities

Minimizing Potential Risks/Harms to the Patient

4. Conditions of initial contact with patients
5. Nature of written patient consent for interview, and/or specimen
6. Response to subpoena of registry records

Other Ethical Concerns

7. Maximizing societal benefits (utility) of registration
8. Maintaining public use samples[57]
9. Ensuring equitable distribution of registry benefits
10. Preserving confidential nature of committees
11. Cooperating with other professions and health service entities
12. Increasing profession's body of knowledge
13. Participating in recruitment and setting of a good example
14. Planning appropriate levels of quality management
15. Avoiding conflicts of interest
16. Acting in a professional matter

found. IRB review is concerned with many matters, but ethical concerns garner special attention. The IRB is of fundamental importance in the registry's effort to maintain public trust. It is prudent for the central registry to have written policies that are IRB-approved concerning all possible matters of potential public interest or ethical concern, and that continuing periodic reviews be scheduled. Many registries include IRB review as a part of the funding solicitation process.

Concerns of the IRB typically include privacy and security of the data, which have been previously discussed and are summarized in Table 36-3.

Data Set Planning/ Standards

There is a growing recognition of the need to base cancer control policies on high-quality, detailed, and timely cancer data. As a result, data set planning is an essential task for any cancer registry. When deciding on what information is to be collected by the central registry, consideration should be given to the registry's overall goals and objectives, as well as the eventual intended uses of the data.[4] At a minimum, those data items required by funders of the registry or necessary for data aggregation and calls for data should be collected. In addition, data items necessary for record transmission, and registry database function and maintenance (e.g., confidential patient data items necessary for patient linkage and tumor consolidation, system fields) must be included. Specific data needs of the Department of Health or university responsible for the cancer registry should be considered, as well as those of facilities reporting to the central registry.[4] Other factors to consider when deciding what data items to collect are the availability of the requested information; reliability of the information being requested and the ability to code the information accurately; the continuity of the information being collected over time; compatibility of the data with national standards; and clinical relevance.[4]

Standardization of data collected by cancer registries is a vital factor for surveillance of cancer and allows for comparability of cancer data across geopolitical boundaries.[68–72] Standardized cancer data are necessary to ensure that information on trends in incidence, mortality, and survival is readily available for planning and evaluation; to evaluate that cancer patient care is consistent and conformant with national guidelines; and so that disparities in the provision or outcome of treatment and services can be identified. Whenever possible, the registry should collect standard data elements that already exist and are uniformly defined, rather than redundantly creating or defining new data items.

In the early years of central cancer registration, states often developed their data collection rules, definitions, and response sets without detailed regard to what each other— or hospitals—were collecting. The result was multiple definitions and coding rules for concepts as central to cancer registration as primary site and date of diagnosis. There was also a lack of uniformity in the coding of items that have generally shared definitions. For example, the major categories of sex might be represented by M and F, 1 and 2, or 2 and 1 depending on the registry. These practices led to misinterpretation of codes when data were aggregated.

Several organizations have been historically instrumental in developing the de facto standards for central cancer registry data item specification in the United States. The CoC of the American College of Surgeons (ACoS) first published its recommended data set for cancer registries in 1956, when cancer programs became part of their accreditations process.[73] The 10 Cities Survey, followed by the Third National Cancer Survey and now known as the SEER Program, developed its data set over several decades.[74] In 1979, at a workshop sponsored by the ACoS, a comparison of CoC's, SEER's, and the Comprehensive Cancer Center Patient Data System's data sets, was presented.[75] As more central cancer registries were formed, a need emerged for a uniform data set and standardized data collection rules. In 1987, the first meeting of the American Association of Central Cancer Registries (later NAACCR) was convened, and this voluntary association assumed the primary responsibility of ob-

taining consensus around data standards and establishing a Uniform Data Standards Committee (UDS). In 1992, the CDC NPCR was created as a result of federal legislation that provided funds for the development and enhancement of state central cancer registries, and was recognized as another major standard-setting organization in the United States.[4]

Cancer registration in North America is quite advanced in terms of data standardization. A national minimum data set has been defined for collection of cancer registry data in the United States and Canada, which includes standardized data items, definitions, codes, and coding instructions. All major standard-setting organizations have contributed to the definition of this standard data set, including SEER, NPCR, CoC, the World Health Organization (WHO), and NAACCR.[3,4] Although this minimum data set is contingent on national agreement to collect uniform data, it also allows central registries to collect additional registry-specific data items to meet needs specific to their goals, locale, and registry-specific projects.

By consensus of the cancer registration professional community, NAACCR's UDS maintains responsibility for data set standardization of central cancer registries in North America. The UDS provides a formal means for reviewing and recommending the addition of new data items or proposed changes in data codes for existing data items submitted by standard setters or NAACCR members to ensure comparability of data across North America.[76] Membership of the UDS includes representatives of those organizations that have traditionally been stakeholders in such data set planning. The standardized data set is documented in NAACCR *Standards for Cancer Registries, Vol. II: Data Standards and Data Dictionary* (Volume II),[72] which includes specifications of data items, data item definitions and their codes, and data transmission format.

The UDS works in conjunction with the NAACCR Cancer Registration Steering Committee (CRSC) to ensure coordination among all organizations regarding the development and implementation of standards and data items. In addition, the UDS works with the NAACCR IT Committee, which is responsible for the development of the standard format for data exchange, as well as the development of standards to ensure the security and accuracy of transmitted data.[76]

The process for approval of new data items or changes to existing data items includes extensive review and consideration. If a request for a new data item is made by an NAACCR member, it is first considered by the UDS, which forwards UDS-approved requests to the CRSC. The CRSC considers the utility and feasibility of the proposed data item. If approved by the CRSC, the UDS works to develop data item specifications for final approval. Standard-setting organizations may suggest a new data item directly to CRSC. Once the UDS has approved the addition of a new data item, the specifics are forwarded to the IT Committee for assignment of data item number and position in the record layout, and this information is subsequently formally incorporated into the Volume II document by the Volume II Work Group (a work group of the UDS).[77]

NAACCR publishes Volume II, as well as many other standards including a standard for data transfer between states, and similar transfers.[78] SEER and CoC have continued to maintain separate documentation of what is increasingly becoming a mutually agreeable data set. The CoC current data set definition is given in the CoC *Facility Oncology Registry Data Standards (FORDS) Revised for 2010* manual.[79] The most recent version of SEER's coding manual was published in 2008.[80]

Standard Setters for Central Registries

Standard setters for central registries include a wide range of organizations, notably the CoC, American Joint Committee on Cancer (AJCC), SEER, NPCR, NCRA, NAACCR, and WHO.[81] In addition to these primary standard setters, each of these organizations has liaisons or links to other interested organizations, notably the College of American Pathologists, American Cancer Society, and National Coordinating Council for Cancer Surveillance (NCCCS), which, therefore, have had an indirect influence on cancer registration standards.

Commission on Cancer of the American College of Surgeons

The initiation of standards for cancer registration can be traced to 1921, when Ernest Codman, MD, FACS, established the first cancer registry. This bone sarcoma registry and its inherent data set introduced the role of cancer registry data standards for medical care in hospitals and among clinicians.[82] Building on that beginning, the CoC's activities have included the basic accreditations program of U.S. hospitals,[83–86] various education programs, the Cancer Liaison physician network,[87–89] and the NCDB.[11,90,91]

A hospital cancer registry is a requirement of a CoC-accredited cancer program. Compliance with standards for the organization, function, and data elements, including quality assurance, are mandated. This is the primary building block and financial underpinning of data collection for cancer registration in the United States.

The Cancer Liaison Physicians form a cancer control/communication network of approximately 1,600 surgeons and physicians who are each linked to individual hospitals, and provide oversight for various programs of the hospital cancer program, notably including the cancer registry, as well as the use and quality of the data.

The NCDB, a joint project of the CoC and the American Cancer Society, is a resource for benchmarking patterns of cancer management and outcomes based on data available from hospital-based cancer registries. The data are not population based. The benchmarks assist hospitals in assessing their services, programs, and performance as compared with established guidelines.

American Joint Committee on Cancer

The objectives of the AJCC include the development and publication of schemas or standards to classify cancers, including anatomic staging, multiple prognostic factors, and end results reporting. These coding schemas are designed for use by clinicians for the purpose of treatment selection, estimation of prognosis, and ongoing assessment of cancer control interventions.[92]

In addition, there is a long-established collaboration between the AJCC and the International Union Against Cancer (UICC) T (tumor), N (node), M (metastasis) Staging Committee to ensure that all refinements to the staging schema are consistent and introduced simultaneously to the medical and data management communities.

Surveillance, Epidemiology, and End Results

The NCI SEER Program of the National Institutes of Health (NIH) was established as a population-based registry in accordance with the National Cancer Act of 1971.[6] As of 2010, there were 18 SEER registries. The SEER registries are the source of incidence and mortality rates, survival rates, and prevalence estimates. The SEER Program has played a significant role in formalizing cancer registration systems, coding and definition of data items, abstracting rules, and training. Most central and hospital-based registries can trace some portion of their development, procedural, and reference documentation to the SEER Program. Collaboration between the CoC, NPCR, and the SEER Program has continued to refine and realign registration techniques and requirements to reduce the number and significance of data set variations.

CDC-National Program of Cancer Registries

With the passage of the Cancer Registry Act in 1992, the NPCR was implemented by the CDC.[7] Through this program, the CDC has promoted model state legislation and regulations that make cancer reportable in every state. As of 2010, the NPCR provided funding for central registries in 45 states, the District of Columbia, Puerto Rico, and the U.S. Pacific Island Jurisdictions. The CDC has been the linchpin for the development or expansion of central registries in states not covered by the SEER Program. State registries use their incidence data for planning and resource allocation, determination of the efficacy and need for cancer control initiatives, and for the identification of high-risk populations. Through the CDC, NPCR standards for completeness, timeliness, and quality of data have been developed for state registries.

National Cancer Registrars Association

The NCRA, formerly the National Tumor Registrars Association, was chartered in 1974 "to promote research and education in Cancer Registry administration and practice."[93] NCRA establishes education standards, develops courses of study for registry professionals, disseminates information, and is involved in programs and activities to improve and standardize cancer registration. In 1983, NCRA initiated a cancer registrar certification program. The credentialing of registry professionals has raised the standards of performance and quality of cancer data management. As of 2010, nearly 4,600 CTRs were certified by NCRA.

North American Association of Central Cancer Registries

NAACCR is a collaborative umbrella organization for cancer registries, governmental agencies, professional associations, and individuals interested in enhancing the quality and use of cancer registry data. It is the professional organization representing central registries in North America.[94] The organization has played an important role in organizing the standards of the major standard-setting groups into a common framework and in documenting them. All the major standard setters are represented on NAACCR committees that are charged with the development and maintenance of specific areas of standardization.

National Coordinating Council for Cancer Surveillance

The NCCCS was formed in 1993 in an effort to define the roles of the major organizations involved in cancer surveillance.[95] The council membership includes representatives of the American Cancer Society, ACoS, AJCC, CoC (NCDB), CDC (NPCR), NCI (SEER), NCRA, National Center for Health Statistics, and NAACCR. The NCCCS provides oversight of issues in cancer surveillance, including resolution of data set, staging or reporting inconsistencies, development of cancer surveillance processes, and reduction of duplication among the various databases.

World Health Organization

The standardization of cancer registration for disease classification has been defined by the WHO. Their publication, *International Classifications of Diseases for Oncology (ICD-O)*,[96] was widely accepted as the standard reference for coding cancer topography and morphology. The second edition of the ICD-O[97] was introduced as the standard used by all U.S. cancer registries beginning with malignancies diagnosed on or after January 1, 1992. The current edition in use, the third edition (ICD-O-3), became effective with malignancies diagnosed on or after January 1, 2001.[98]

Collaborative Staging

In 1998, a Collaborative Staging (CS) Task Force was created to address the issue of discrepancies in staging guidelines among the three major cancer staging systems used in the United States: the TNM Stage groupings of the AJCC, the Extent of Disease (EOD) system of the SEER Program, and the SEER Summary Stage System.[99] Sponsored by AJCC in collaboration with SEER, NPCR, CoC, NCRA, NAACCR, and the Canadian Cancer Society/ National Cancer Institute of Canada (CCS/NCIC), the initial focus of the task force was to develop conversion between the TNM staging system of the AJCC and the SEER Summary Staging System. The AJCC maintains overall management of the CS Data Collection System. A Project Management Team including representatives in leadership positions from all of the standard-setting organizations involved in CS was formed in 2007.[100]

It is hoped that CS will eliminate one last area of significant variation in data management standards between different types and networks of cancer registries. A recent study using NCDB data compared the registrar's AJCC stage derived from CS and the physician-assigned AJCC stage. It was found that derived staging by registrars was minimally more complete than physician AJCC staging, and that 78% of cases with required staging had identical stage groups assigned by registrars and physicians.[101] In another recent study accessing the collectability of all of the CS data items introduced with release of version 2 of the CS Data Collection System (CSv2), it was found that the collection of some of these data items posed a challenge, in particular, for registrars that primarily relied on the hospital medical record.[102] However, this study further suggests that with the advent of electronic pathology reporting and electronic health records, the information necessary to code these data items will become more readily available.

Data Set Content

Central cancer registry data sets in North America are highly standardized, but are also a reflection of the type of registry, its sources of information, its funders and supporters, specific needs of the population served, and the intended use of registry data.[69,70,72,78,103] For these reasons, state central registries may require hospitals to provide information that is not required for CoC-accredited programs and, therefore, not published in the *FORDS* or required by SEER or NPCR.[78]

Generally, the types of data collected and maintained by central registries are similar to the types collected by hospitals: patient identification, cancer identification, treatment information, follow-up information, and information that describes the nature and source of the data.

Central registries consolidate information from many sources, including multiple hospitals, physicians' offices and free-standing clinics, pathology laboratories, radiation centers, nursing homes and rehabilitation centers, coroners' offices, and death certificates. To link all of this information correctly requires high-quality patient identification details and the ability to distinguish among slightly disparate descriptions of what may be one or more independent primary cancers. Consequently, central registries collect information from every facility that is required to report the case. Descriptive demographic and cancer information is necessary for nearly every use of central registry data. Individual central registries may require additional information specific to their own circumstances. For example, some states collect tribal membership for Native Americans or generation of immigration in addition to race and place of birth. Other registries may collect information regarding patient exposure to potentially cancer-causing natural or accidental events.

All central cancer registries in North America collect first course of treatment information on all cancers in a standardized format. Central registries whose data are used for some types of investigative research collect far more extensive treatment information for certain types of cases as part of these special studies.

Follow-up activities vary considerably among central registries. Although some may track recurrence and subsequent treatment, the majority do not. Some provide feedback about readmission elsewhere to the hospital responsible for following the analytic case, but many cannot because of state confidentiality restrictions. Central registries perform death clearance to identify patients in the database who have died, to gather additional information such as cause of death or place of birth if it was not already recorded, and to identify cancer deaths that may not have been reported by any other source. Some states use additional sources of information to determine whether patients otherwise lost to follow-up may still be alive, such as matches to drivers' licenses or Medicare rolls.

Because central registries collect coded information from such a wide variety of sources, and because much of the data use depends on many years of data collection, central registries have a particular need for the kinds of data items that describe the nature of the data. For example, they need to know the type of facility that originated the report, its identity, when the report was submitted, and the coding system version in use for the various items collected (e.g., treatment coding system). They may also document items that represent data processing steps, including the date the report was reported, and date the edited report was entered into the full database.

The coding system versions bear special mention because they necessarily are provided by the facilities that report data to the central registry. A "current coding system" version data item describes the coding system currently used to code a specific data item. It is necessary to interpret the meaning of the code itself. The "original coding system" version item describes the response categories available to the coder when the data item was originally abstracted and coded. It is used principally in data analysis

and is, therefore, fundamental to the operations of central registries. In facility registries, these items can be handled largely behind the scenes by the software, but the registrar may need to enter version information when it changes.

Today, one of the principal requirements in selecting a data set is standardization of the definitions, coding rules, and response sets used. As mentioned earlier, all central registries in the United States conform to the NAACCR standards as defined in Volume II. Standardization of coding rules and methods of data collection allow for the aggregation and comparison of data across jurisdictions. The standard documented by NAACCR includes the requirements and recommendations for collection and transmission of each standard data item required by each standard setter including:

1. Minimum data elements required for data exchange
2. NPCR requirements/recommendations
3. CoC requirement/recommendations
4. SEER requirements[72]

The NAACCR-recommended data elements have been developed to carefully balance the needs and necessary data collection of the hospital-based registry with those of the central registry. Data set collection requirements is one of several ways in which hospital registries and central registries are closely interdependent. The basic data items needed by central cancer registries are similar but not identical to those of hospital registries and include those listed in Table 36-4.

In addition to Volume II,[72] NAACCR has also developed a standard to assist in the interstate transfer of data between registries,[78] e-path reporting,[103] completeness and quality,[72] and recommendations to assist in the use of Health Level Seven (HL-7).[104-106]

Table 36-4	Basic Data Items for Central Cancer Registries

Patient identification and demographics

Cancer identification

Hospital-specific (admission dates, class, and analytic status) data

Stage and prognostic factors

Treatment: first course and subsequent

Follow-up

Death

Edit overrides

System administration (case completed, changed)

Patient, hospital, and physician

Narrative text

Case Ascertainment

Reportable List

A central registry's rules for reportability usually include a reportable list, reference date, and rules for residency, multiple primaries, analytic cases, ambiguous terms, and diagnostic confirmation.[107–110]

The reportable list should include all diagnoses that are to be reported and specify which diagnoses are not reportable. The reportable lists for central registries are closely interrelated with the reportable lists of reporting facilities in their reporting area, as well as the requirements for national data collection. Reportable cases for central registries usually include all diseases with a behavior code of 2 (in situ) or 3 (invasive) as identified in the current edition of the *International Classification of Diseases for Oncology (ICD-O-3).*[98] The SEER Program's reportable list includes all such cases except for the cases listed in Table 36-5. A federal law has been recently passed requiring the reportability of benign central nervous system (brain) tumors.[108] These standards are specified in the NAACCR standards document.[72]

Ambiguous Terminology

A patient has cancer when a recognized medical practitioner states that the patient does. However, there may be times when the diagnosis is vague or inconclusive, such as "probable carcinoma of the lung." Rules have been defined to indicate whether terms should be considered diagnostic of cancer for the registry's purposes. As stated in the SEER manual,[80] the terms that are considered diagnostic of cancer are "apparent(ly)," "appears," "comparable with," "compatible with," "consistent with," "favor(s)," "malignant appearing," "most likely," "presumed," "probable," "suspect(ed)," "suspicious (for)," and "typical of."

Reference Date

Central registries adopt and publish their reference (starting) date, usually January 1 of a given year, from which their coverage begins. All cases diagnosed among area residents on or after the reference date must be included. For population-based central registries, it is required that all cases of cancer occurring in the population residing in the reporting area be entered into the registry, regardless of the place of diagnosis or treatment. Procedures must be in place to achieve the most complete coverage possible.

Residency

All cancers diagnosed in persons who are residents of the population-based reporting area at the time of diagnosis are reportable. Central registries generally include nonresidents who were seen within the catchment area to facilitate sharing of data with registries in neighboring areas, to simplify death clearance, and to allow preparation of individual hospital reports that include all of the hospital's cases. Standardized rules should also be in place for handling part-year residents (such as retiree "snow birds"), military personnel, college students, undocumented aliens, or any other group whose residency status might be ambiguous. Whenever possible, rules for determining residency should be comparable with rules used by the Bureau of the Census in determining place of residence, so that numerator definitions will be the same as the definitions for the population at risk when incidence rates are calculated.

Multiple Primaries

Rules for collecting information on multiple primary cancers in the same patient differ somewhat internationally. Notably, rules from SEER[111] and International Agency for Research on Cancer (IARC)[71] are somewhat different. In the United States, central and hospital-based registries follow the definitions developed by the SEER Program, which are published in the Multiple Primary and Histology Coding Rules manual, effective with cases diagnosed 2007 and later.[111] These definitions include rules for determining primary site and multiple and subsequent primaries.

Analytic Cases (Class of Case)

Class of case is a data item and concept used by hospital-based registries to denote whether the case was diagnosed and/or treated at the reference hospital, or has received treatment previously elsewhere. The concept of "analytic" refers to whether the case belongs in a particular analysis cohort. Generally, central registries are interested in all cases of reportable tumors and malignancies within their

Table 36-5	Nonreportable Cases for the Surveillance, Epidemiology, and End Results Program of the National Cancer Institute

Malignant neoplasms, NOS (morphology codes 8000-8004) of the skin (C44._)

Epithelial carcinomas (8010-8045) of the skin (C44._)

Papillary and squamous cell carcinomas (8050-8082) of the skin (C44._)

Basal cell carcinomas (8090-8110) of any site except the genital sites—vagina (C52.9), labium majus, (C51.0), labium minus (C51.1), clitoris (C51.2), vulva (C51.8-C51.9), prepuce (C60.0), penis (C60.9), and scrotum (C63.2)

catchment area, no matter at which hospital or other facility they were first diagnosed or treated.

Diagnostic Confirmation

In the past, some central registries elected to register only pathologically confirmed cases. Central registries generally adopt explicit rules for hospitals that report to them to deal with clinically confirmed cases and other special circumstances, such as whether a hospital should report cancers in patients who are diagnosed in the emergency department only, dead on arrival at the hospital, seen for consultation only, evaluated for cancer but who have no active disease at the time of admission, or seen for treatment but who are transient in the area and only referred for care while passing through or visiting. A list of nonreportable cases is often specified by central registries.

Casefinding (Source of Cases)

The principal source of most cases for a central registry is the hospital, but nonhospital sources are becoming increasingly important. The most common sources are listed in Table 36-6.[109,110,112,113] The registry can identify potential sources of cases by contacting the state government agencies that license healthcare facilities and practitioners, by contacting professional societies and trade associations, and by referring to telephone directories.

Hospital Registry Sources

Hospital registries have not always emphasized certain data items that are crucial to a central registry, such as determination of the patient's residency at the time of diagnosis, and hospitals may not be abstracting all cases of interest to the central registry, for example, consultations only, pathology only, nonanalytic cases, or carcinoma in situ of the cervix, so requirements must be carefully spelled out.

Because the criteria for which cases are abstracted may differ between the central registry and reporting facilities, it is important that the central registry's abstracting requirements be clearly defined. For example, as mentioned earlier, the CoC does not require that hospitals abstract so-called nonanalytic cases; that is, those cases that were diagnosed and received their entire first course of treatment before admission to the reporting hospital. Central registries, however, often require abstracts on nonanalytic cases that are incidence cases for the registry's coverage area.

The CoC does not require abstraction of carcinoma in situ of the cervix, but some central registries may collect these cases. On the other hand, the cancer committee or other group may require that the hospital registry collect certain types of cases not required by the CoC or the central registry. The central registry must decide whether to accept these cases if they are submitted by hospitals, and work with them to obtain all necessary cancer reports, even if they are not required by the hospital, to comply with state and federal laws.

Regular monitoring of completeness of casefinding and abstracting is an essential component of a central registry's quality-control plan. Monthly monitoring enables the registry to quickly identify problems and have sufficient lead time to take corrective action.

Data transmission to the central registry is primarily achieved through electronic submission. NAACCR has adopted a standardized format for data exchange, intended as a "second language" that many systems use to share data with each other.[78] Sometimes, a mail-in reporting option is developed for use by small rural hospitals, but confidentiality concerns can limit mail reporting. Many registries have some type of Internet-based, FTP, or encrypted e-mail mechanism available to their reporting sources, so that data may be securely uploaded to the registry in electronic format.

Nonhospital Registry Sources

For hospitals without cancer registries, as well as for nonhospital sources such as clinics, physicians' offices, pathology laboratories, nursing homes, and any other potential sources of cases, the central registry cannot rely on abstracts prepared by a hospital cancer registrar. Central registries must work with these individual facilities to promote standardized electronic reporting wherever possible. To the extent that hospitals do not automatically ascertain all

Table 36-6	Common Casefinding Sources

Hospital Sources

Pathology reports: histology, autopsy, cytology, and hematology reports

Health records reports: disease index and daily discharges

Radiation therapy reports: radiation therapy log and treatment summaries

Diagnostic radiology reports: nuclear medicine logs and reports, ultrasound

Outpatient records

Surgery reports

Nonhospital Sources

Outpatient centers

Independent pathology laboratories

Radiation and surgery centers

Physicians' offices, such as oncologists' and dermatologists' offices

Managed care organizations

Hospices and nursing homes

Bureau of Vital Statistics, and coroners' offices for death records

Out-of-state facilities

Prisons

cases the central registry requires, the central registry must perform extra casefinding. An alternative successful practice uses "circuit riders," or abstractors who are employed by the central registry, to visit reporting facilities and perform casefinding and abstracting of data in the field.

Out-of-Region Cases

Registries have used various methods to obtain reports on their resident cases that have been diagnosed or treated outside the catchment area. First, referral patterns must be determined. When central registries exist in neighboring areas, formal agreements for exchange of data can be implemented.

Timeliness of Reporting

SEER central registries are required to provide complete counts of new cases for a calendar year within 20 months of the end of that calendar year. CDC NPCR Program Standards require that 90% of expected cases be included in the registry within 12 months of the close of the diagnosis year, and 95% of expected cases should be included within 24 months of the close of the diagnosis year.

Rapid reporting is a consideration when cases are needed for epidemiologic protocols, research, or tumor board presentations at hospitals. Using this method, cases are usually identified within 15 to 30 days after diagnosis or hospital admission. For example, the New Hampshire State Cancer Registry requires baseline data on patient, diagnostic, and other information to be reported within 15 days. The complete information on the patient must be subsequently reported within 180 days. This allows cases to be identified rapidly at the central registry for inclusion in research studies, but allows more time for the hospital registrars to complete abstracts. The disadvantages of this method include provision of incomplete information to the central registry, requiring the hospital staff to pull the medical record more than once, and possible duplication in case reporting.

If time is a less important criterion, cases may be reported within 3 to 6 months from admission to the hospital. For hospitals participating in the accreditations program of the CoC, the maximum allowable delay in abstracting is 6 months calculated from the date of first contact to the time that the data are available for analysis.

E-path Reporting

Cancer registration is characterized by pathologic confirmation of diagnoses; thus, pathology reports serve as a basis for the great majority of cancer case ascertainment. Increasingly, high-volume pathology laboratories, both independent and hospital based, manage their specimen flow, reporting, and billing in electronic form.[114]

The need for rapid case ascertainment and a desire for easier, efficient, and more complete reporting from pathol-

ogy laboratories independent from hospitals have contributed to the increased reliance on e-path reporting. The term *e-path* reporting was first used to connote the concept of automation of cancer casefinding from independent pathology laboratories.[103] Since that time, the major components of e-path reporting—casefinding and electronic transmission to a central registry—have become more broadly described, and e-path reporting from hospital-based pathology laboratories has been implemented, as well as independent pathology laboratories.[33,115,116]

The majority of pathology reports at most pathology laboratories are not cancer related. The emerging importance of the HIPAA and other security concerns may favor automated review of pathology reports within a secure environment. Avoidance of manual review of these noncancer cases may be viewed as enhancing protection of confidentiality and, therefore, patient satisfaction. Also, automated pathologic casefinding offers cost savings over manual methods, thereby freeing cancer registrars for other key registry functions.

The benefits of e-path reporting can include automated, complete, and rapid casefinding; transmission and central registry storage requiring little human intervention; receipt of the complete pathology report in digitized form, with HL-7 or other data transmission standards compatibility; improved HIPAA compliance (including encryption, authentication, and identification, and complete audit trails for all transactions); reduction of human visual review of noncancer pathology reports; and decreased pathology hard copy ground transfer.

The automatic nature of this casefinding may potentially obviate the need for routine manual pathology review by central or hospital registry staff. Labor savings of approximately 0.2 FTE for every 1,000 incident cases have been estimated.[33,48] However, preliminary screening of electronic pathology reports does not eliminate the need for visual review of submitted pathology reports to verify reportability and process as new or secondary reports.

Electronic casefinding without transmission generally includes several discrete steps: (1) extraction of the pathology report from a Laboratory Information System (LIS), (2) opening of a casefinding dictionary, (3) encoding the various sections of the pathology report into numeric codes, (4) applying specified case selection criteria, (5) parsing of the selected pathology reports to HL-7 if desired, and (6) writing of the selected pathology reports to a CD-ROM, or other electronic media.

The casefinding dictionary typically includes a list of search terms that appear on reportable cancer pathology reports (e.g., invasive carcinoma, lymphoma). A list of such terms is maintained on the NAACCR Web site. The term list is programmed to perform like a human screener: the text of the entire pathology report is scanned for reportable terms that are indicative of cancer. The presence of any one of these terms in the pathology report qualifies the report as potentially reportable. Pathology reports that contain none of these words are considered negative for cancer, or alternatively, some form of algorithm is used to find negated terms. Screening sensitivities of near 100% with specificity of 75% have been reported.[33]

In addition to electronic casefinding, external electronic transmission typically includes: (1) queuing messages to send; (2) establishing an IP circuit; (3) exchanging of encryption keys between computers over the Internet; (4) encrypting the pathology report message; (5) sending the encrypted message over the Internet (the sending computer and receiving computer are typically separated from the Internet by firewalls; (6) receiving the message; (7) decrypting the message; (8) electronic storage of the pathology report in central registry files, including, in some cases, mapping to the standard NAACCR file format and codes; and (9) quality control of the electronic casefinding and transmission process.

The design of a particular casefinding process and the enabling software depends on whether electronic transmission is needed and whether it will occur before standard casefinding or after. Casefinding systems without external transmission are considerably easier to implement but are not as automatic. The total preplanning effort for e-path implementation, which is, in essence, an automation task, takes time. Important stakeholders including IT, IRB, and pathology laboratory personnel must be identified and involved. This preplanning includes various site assessment and preparation tasks, including LIS file formatting and interface, hardware assessment, and firewall and security protocol planning.

E-path software is typically installed on a PC or server on location at the laboratories. The installation process can be straightforward, and the software can possibly share the resources of a single PC or server. Like other evolutionary steps in cancer registration automation and computerization, the progress of e-path reporting may depend on the availability of cost-effective and transportable e-path software systems. Cooperation of the reporting organization is essential for a successful e-path installation. For registries desiring rapid case ascertainment, as well as the many other benefits of e-path reporting, the investment in development, time, and money is worthwhile.

Death Clearance

Death clearance in a population-based cancer registry occurs at least once a year and includes two processes.[118–123] The first process is to link all death records from the state's vital statistics office to registry records to identify patients in the registry database who have died, providing essential follow-up information for the registry. This linkage produces three outcomes: positive matches, possible matches, and nonmatches. The possible matches are manually reviewed to determine whether they are indeed matches.

Death clearance requires that the registry work closely with its state's vital statistics office. Routine linkage of

death records updates the vital status of the matched cases already in the database. In population-based registries that conduct active patient follow-up, the frequent passive death-record linkage prevents the generation of unnecessary active follow-up inquiries.

Vital status, date of death, cause of death, and other related follow-up information are added to the database for those cases that are matches. The death record information is compared with the registry files and consolidated or updated when possible (e.g., patient name, including maiden name, Social Security number or national identification number, race, Hispanic surname or ethnicity, birth date, birthplace). For matched deaths with cancer as a cause of death, it is also important to identify discrepancies between the cancer cause-of-death codes and the diagnosis codes in the registry database to determine if there are unreported primaries.

The second process of death clearance in a population-based cancer registry is the identification of death records that mention cancer as one of the causes of death but do not link with previously registered cases. These cases require follow-back to determine their reportability. For an unmatched cancer death that occurs in a facility that reports to the registry, the presumption is that the case was missed in routine reporting, and a request is made for an abstract to be completed. For cancer deaths that did not occur in reporting hospitals, follow-back must be made to the certifying physician, nursing care facility, or coroner requesting an abstract, or at least minimal history information. After all follow-back sources have been exhausted and no other information on the case is available, the case is entered or retained on the registry's database as a death certificate only case.[120,121] Information on conducting death clearance is discussed in detail in NAACCR's Death Clearance Manual.[122] The percentage of death certificate only cases included in a central registry's Call for Data submission data file is used as a data evaluation standard for the NPCR CSS, the U.S. Cancer Statistics publication, and NAACCR Gold and Silver registry certification.

Abstracting

The abstracting process for central registries is similar to that done by hospital-based registries. However, some differences pertain.[110,123–126]

Hospitals with Cancer Registries

Most central cancer registries utilize abstracts prepared at the data source, by hospital cancer registries. There are multiple advantages to doing so, including reliance on on-site trained hospital abstractors who can transmit a complete and edited abstract electronically to the central registry, which then concentrates on consolidation and quality control rather than primary data abstraction. This method works best when the central registry can standardize the data set and format that the hospitals are using to report cases to the central registry.

When hospital abstracts are utilized, the central registry must plan for a system of quality control. Resources that would otherwise go into case abstraction can be used for abstract review, audits, and training of hospital personnel. Hospital cancer registries benefit from having their data incorporated into a central registry, as they have the potential of receiving compatible relevant comparison data. The quality of their data will improve through the quality control and training activities of the central registry.

One disadvantage of use of hospital abstracts is that the central registry has less direct control over the quality and timeliness of the data than they would have if they collected it directly themselves. Any potential problems should be addressed in the registry's planning stages, in any mandatory reporting legislation, and in the budgeting process, with the importance of standardization and a quality-control component being recognized from the beginning. For example, standards for timeliness of reporting can be written into mandatory reporting legislation, and even a requirement that hospitals use CTRs can be made.

Hospitals without Cancer Registries

For hospitals without cancer registries, as well as for nonhospital sources such as clinics, offices of physicians, pathology laboratories, nursing homes, and any other potential sources of cases, the central registry cannot always rely on abstracts prepared by a hospital cancer registrar, although some central registries require electronic abstracted case reporting from these sources.

The use of "circuit riders" has been mentioned earlier. Although this method is costly, the central registry can more easily control qualifications, training, and continuity of staff. Alternatively, the central registry can minimize costs by utilizing electronic reporting of casefinding source documents, particularly pathology reports and disease indices, for these facilities. This enables the central registry to perform casefinding procedures centrally.

Physician Reporting

Requirements for physician reporting vary by locale. Most central registries have active physician reporting mandated by state law. Central registries have developed physician query systems to query physicians on cases identified by sources that are not subsequently reported.

Format of Reporting

The advantages of requiring standardized machine-readable reporting from hospital or nonhospital sources are overwhelming from the central registry's point of view. They are summarized in Table 36-7.

Table 36-7	Advantages of Computer-Readable Abstracts

1. Timely, higher quality data available sooner
2. Elimination of separate key entry of cases
3. Possibility of performing extensive data editing via computer at the time the case is being abstracted and the medical record is at hand for making corrections
4. Ease of uploading to the registry's main computer file without the need for extensive conversions or pre-editing, allowing for speedy linkage and retrieval of reported records
5. Decreased time spent in visual editing or quality control, because data items can be presented in identical order, are always legible, can be decoded into English, and checks for validity of codes and consistency among items can be performed via computer before visual editing is begun
6. Facilitates consolidation of cases

Data transmission to the central registry can be via diskette, Internet based, FTP, or encrypted e-mail mechanism. Central registries exchange data electronically via the NAACCR data exchange format. Registries need to be aware of the manner in which hospital-based registry software vendors handle changes to coding schemes. Central registries may choose to assign a vendor-liaison role to one of its staff; this individual would be responsible for communicating the central registry reporting and data editing requirements to the various cancer abstracting software vendors that service facilities reporting to the central registry. Software vendors are often amenable to customizing requirements and edits to meet the central registry reporting of their customers.

Abstractors can be provided with portable computers and standardized software for auditing, casefinding, and abstracting in the field. In California, a "mail-in" reporting option was developed for use by small rural hospitals. Hospitals with 50 or fewer beds, without registries, and that were located in isolated areas at least 1 hour's travel from another hospital were offered the option of having their own staff perform casefinding, with subsequent photocopying of pertinent parts of the medical record that are sent into the central registry where abstraction by central registry employees is conducted. The central registry audits the hospital's casefinding to ensure that all cases are being submitted. The photocopied records are retained for a short time to allow for quality control and then destroyed.

Reports from Outside the Area

Registries have used various methods to obtain reports on their resident cases that have been diagnosed or treated outside the catchment area. First, referral patterns must be determined so that the registry can identify areas or facilities where significant numbers of their residents are seen. Formal interstate data exchange agreements must be implemented to allow sharing of resident case reports between state registries. It is important to be aware of idiosyncrasies that can be introduced into the data when including reports from another registry. Special attention to state-specific fields will improve the quality of the imported data.

NAACCR's Registry Operations committee has generated detailed guidelines for interstate data exchange, which include recommendations for evaluating the impact of completeness, timeliness, and data quality of exchanged data; media and format to be used for data exchange; confidentiality issues related to case sharing; and case-sharing agreements.[127] These guidelines also include a helpful data exchange checklist for outgoing case sharing with other central cancer registries. In addition, NAACCR has developed a National Data Exchange Agreement that will allow states to exchange data with all cosigners of the agreement.

Abstracting Requirements

Another issue to consider is whether there should be a reduced abstract or data set required by nonhospital reporting sources, such as free-standing cancer centers. A "treatment-only" abstract can be more efficient for the reporting facility, whereas any proliferation of standards will increase the complexity of the central registry's system.

Federal facilities in the central registry's area of coverage may be unwilling or unable to meet any mandatory reporting standards, although they will probably be willing to provide cases in their own format if they already have registries, or to provide the central registry access to records for the central registry's circuit riders to abstract at the central registry's expense.

For military facilities the ACTUR was established in 1986 to satisfy DoD and ACoS requirements for a comprehensive cancer data reporting system. ACTUR was developed as part of the Defense Enrollment Eligibility Reporting System (DEERS) to facilitate interhospital usage by military beneficiaries, promote the cost savings associated with a single interhospital system, and provide the ability to produce automated reports and studies on a DoD-wide basis.[128] For reporting from military facilities, the central registry should explore obtaining machine-readable records from the DEERS-ACTUR system.[13]

Monitoring of Status of Facilities and Completeness of Reporting

Regular monitoring of completeness of casefinding and abstracting is an essential component of a central registry's quality-control program. Central registries must have complete reporting because statistics generated based on incomplete data may result in misleading cancer rates, inaccurate trends, and an underestimation of the cancer burden for the registry's catchment area. NAACCR has published a training module on management reports for central cancer registries.[129]

Central registry monitoring of facility case completeness should be performed on an ongoing basis. Frequent monitoring, at least monthly, enables the registry to quickly identify problems and have sufficient lead time to take corrective action. Management reports can be built into the registry's computer system so that reports are automatically generated. The registry will want to monitor progress of all of the activities it is performing itself, as well as progress of data collection being performed by reporting sources such as hospital registries. The central registry should expect to process one-twelfth of its annual caseload each month. Types of reports that can prove useful for monitoring are summarized in Table 36-8.

Table 36-8	Suggested Reports for Monitoring Casefinding, Abstracting, and Processing Status

1. Status reports of review of each casefinding source within a facility
2. Status reports of progress in screening each type of pathology report within a facility, showing dates and report numbers screened
3. Progress reports on follow-back to physicians' offices of cases identified in pathology laboratories; this can be reviewed by primary site and diagnosis year
4. Reports comparing counts of cases by facility by diagnosis month for the current year against a base year, or average across years; these reports can also be prepared for selected sites of cancer, especially those that are likely to be diagnosed in outpatient settings
5. Percentage histologically confirmed by facility and for the registry as a whole, by month or year; this may identify facilities or time periods where some casefinding sources have not been reviewed
6. Reports including frequency distributions of missing and unknown values submitted for key data items, as well as unspecific values (such as ICD-O-3 topography to C80.9, C76_, or morphology of 8000, 8010, or 8800)
7. Distribution by diagnosis year and month of cases submitted during a given month; a high number of incidence cases abstracted in the current month for a previous year may indicate a deficiency in an area of casefinding; the deficiency can indicate either under-reporting or over-reporting for that previous year
8. Reports including the number and percentage of nonreportable or duplicate cases submitted

Computerization

Like staffing, planning for computerization is centrally important to the overall functioning of the registry. It affects almost every aspect of registry operation, and almost always involves highly technical characteristics requiring specialized expertise. Those responsible for computerization of central registries face a series of decisions or concerns.[51,130–132] The computer system and its components are generally chosen closely based on the goals and objectives of the registry. For example, Will online data entry and retrieval be required? Will the registry be a data user itself, or prepare files for use by external biostatisticians, epidemiologists, or others? Is the central registry information system also to subsume the goals of the hospital cancer programs? What hardware, operating system, and software are most compatible with meeting the registry's goals?

Computer System Planning

In the United States, it has become common for central registries to receive electronic submissions in NAACCR file format from contributing hospitals. Thus, the central registry computer system should be conceived of as an integrated central and hospital registry information system.[117] Each hospital's computer should be capable of operating on its own to meet its hospital registry demands, and of transferring or transmitting its data to the central registry. In some states, hospitals report to regional registries that, in turn, report to the state and national registry, creating four levels of integration. Thus, there can be hospital registry systems, networks of hospitals reporting to a central registry, and networks of central registries reporting to a state or national registry.

Make-or-Buy Decision

Several predesigned systems are available to central registries.[132–136] The central registry must weigh advantages and disadvantages of designing, converting, or buying a system.

Three major constraints faced when designing a new system are its potential cost, development schedule, and design risk. For these reasons and others, importing or converting a predesigned system is often seriously considered. The most effective way to look into acquiring a registry information system would be by observing them in operation in functioning registries.

Several circumstances limit transportability of central registry systems. Predefined hardware restraints, data requirements, governance relationships, and the telecommunications mode on which a given system is based may not be amenable to the needs of a new central registry. Few systems are designed with transportability and universality in mind. More frequently, they are customized for each new user. Some central registry systems have been successfully transported from one central registry to another, with varying degrees of redesign performed by the new registry user.

Conversely, to a large extent, the computer needs of a hospital registry are often largely met by a vendor or a related central registry with an off-the-shelf system.[132,137–140]

Data Editing

Most central registries perform both manual and computerized data editing. Computerized edits typically check for completion of all required fields, allowable range, allowable values, and interfield consistency (such as primary site consistent with sex).[117,141] They can test for invalid entries, such as an unusual site-histology combination, or flag unusual entries for review. For some data quality edits, it is necessary for the central registry computer system to be able to override the edit error. This increases the complexity of the data system and its usage. Central registry data editing also includes inter-record editing across records for the same patient, as well as cross-checking reports about a patient reported from more than one facility. This also adds to the complexity of use of the system. It is in the central registry's interest that comprehensive data-editing routines are built-in upfront into the software of those hospitals that contribute data.

NAACCR for central registries and the CoC for hospital-based registries have standardized data editing.[142,143] NAACCR has also issued instructions,[144,145] downloadable metafiles,[146,147] and narrative descriptions. SEER has also published on the subject of data edits.[148] The NPCR distributes software free of charge that is used to improve data quality and standardize data item validity checks, create and maintain data edit checks, maintain standard definitions, and run edit sets against data to produce edit error reports for data correction.[134]

In the United States, the running of edits is performed at all levels of data processing and reporting. Reporting facilities use edits for evaluation of data quality before submission to a central registry or standard-setting organization, correcting edit errors reported to them by their central registry or standard setter, and for abstracting, usually via interactive data validation within their abstracting software. Central cancer registries run a wide variety of edits on incoming data submissions to assess for accuracy and completeness and to identify training needs, another set of different edits after data consolidation, and Call for Data edits before submission to standard-setting organizations.

Standard setters run edits on central registry and reporting hospital submissions to enforce national data standards, assess data quality and completeness, and provide feedback to central registries and reporting hospitals. On receipt of data for a Call for Data, all major standard setters in the United States (SEER, NPCR, NAACCR, and CoC/NCDB) evaluate submitted data for data quality via the running of edits. The percentage of cases passing certain core edits included in a central registry's Call for Data submission data file is used as a data evaluation standard for the NPCR-CSS, the U.S. Cancer Statistics publication, and NAACCR Gold and Silver registry certification. Computerized data edits should be used in combination with other quality-control techniques.

Data Conversion

Because data sets change over time, conversion of past records to current standards is necessary. Every effort is made to minimize changes as much as possible. Nonetheless, important standards such as ICD-O and the AJCC and CS do change as medicine advances and other changes occur.

For data analysis purposes, it is important that all of the years of data in the registry's analytic file be maintained in uniform coding. It is sometimes easier to collect and computerize new cases, an immense task in itself, than it is to handle conversion of past files to current standards. SEER has published certain conversion protocols in the form of computer programs and text documents,[149] and NPCR maintains a conversion utility program that converts records in older NAACCR file formats to the latest NAACCR file format.[134]

Electronic Data Interchange/ Data Communications

Electronic data interchange (EDI) refers to the linking of computers via telephone lines or other communication methods. EDI is also sometimes referred to as teleprocessing, data communications, and electric commerce. More recently, "e" is added to a wide range of functions to denote electronic Internet methods (e.g., e-commerce). The registry world has been transformed by the Internet, including e-mail, search engines, and many other facilities.[150,151]

EDI may include a simple transfer of data from one computer to another, or may involve two-way exchange of data or interactive use of one computer and its files by a second, remote computer. For those information systems that include and link the central registry and participating hospital registries, EDI with encryption is frequently a necessary requirement. The establishment of a link between a hospital computer and the central registry system is not necessarily a simple or automatic procedure, and sometimes entails consultation between IT personnel at the hospital and IT personnel at the central registry. Once effective telecommunication has been established, it often works quite reliably. Such telecommunications require that the central registry either maintain a 7-day, 24-hour capability to handle several linkages at once, or that some process for scheduling of calls be instituted.

EDI can be both the means by which the hospital reports their data and the means by which the central registry provides follow-up information to hospitals. At its best, EDI can save critical time spent on routine registry functions.

Geocoding

Central cancer registries code the residence at diagnosis to the most specific level possible. For the study of cancer clusters or for other surveillance purposes, it is often desirable to determine the small geographic area, such as the census tract, where the patient resides. Most central registries in the United States use commercial software to geocode the address to the census block or latitude/longitude codes, or both.[152] When geocoding, it is necessary for the user to enter the patient's address explicitly in terms of zip code, street name, street title (Drive, Street, Blvd., and so on), and street direction. Geocoding programs require a large reference file of street names and related information for the specific geographic area concerned, and are therefore quite specialized and complex. In general, when geocoding is performed on a real set of addresses, only 70% or 80% are geocodable at the census tract level. The remaining 20% to 30% are resolved manually by registry personnel. Geocoded residence at diagnosis is used in a variety of analyses including access to care studies, stage at diagnosis, linking with other socioeconomic status variables, environmental and cancer cluster studies, and public health resource allocation studies.

Record Linkage

An important function of central registries is the ability to combine information from several sources on the same patient or record linkage.[153] Central registries perform linkage for several reasons: casefinding, linking in new patient reports to the registry database, duplicate detection, passively obtaining follow-up information, improving information on a case, analytic purposes, and conducting special studies (e.g., linkage of the registry database with an HIV database to ascertain how many individuals with HIV also have cancer).

When new reports of cancer are being added to the central registry database, it is vital that the record be accurately linked to patients and tumors already registered in the registry database. If a new patient record, or a new tumor record for an existing patient, is erroneously added to the database as a new case because of inaccurate linkage processes, duplicate records will be generated, and incidence counts and rates will be misleadingly high. Likewise, if an incoming record is erroneously linked to existing data, incidence counts and rates may be artificially decreased.

Before performing any linkage of registry data, the data items to be used in the linkage process should be evaluated for their quality, coding conventions (e.g., race), and standardization (e.g., address).[154] Checks for consistency in coding conventions and standardization between the two data sources being linked is essential or false-positive or false-negative matches will occur. If the same code has different meanings or if the code representing the same information differs between the two data sources, then matches based on that code will be inaccurate.

Record linkage generally involves two steps: blocking and then matching. Blocking is an initial linkage step that reduces the number of record comparisons between data sources when matching takes place. Basically, blocking entails exact matching between the two data sources on key data items, creating smaller "blocks" of data that are more likely to match. Matching is subsequently performed only within the identified blocks. Blocking removes very unlikely matches before the actual matching process and can save valuable time and computing resources. Common blocking data items are patient first and last name, Social Security number, and date of birth.[155,156]

Common matching data items are patient name (first, middle, and last), sex, Social Security number, date of birth, and race. Matching can be achieved via deterministic or probabilistic approach. Deterministic linkage entails comparing data items between two records where the two records are considered a match only if the values on the matching items are identical. The result is either a match or a nonmatch. Because data sources commonly include variations in data or missing data between the data items being linked, the deterministic approach tends to miss a significant number of true matches. However, deterministic linkage can be augmented by matching on partial fields (e.g., the year component of date of birth rather than the entire data item); performing multiple passes of linkage using different combinations of data items; applying a phonetic system to name-matching data items to reduce the number of matches missed because of variations in spelling, typographic errors, and misspellings; or using an algorithm based on the results from the matching of multiple data items.[58] In addition, deterministic linkage can be easily incorporated into a cancer registry data system.

Probabilistic linkage involves estimating the probability that two records represent the same person; a linkage score is calculated that indicates how likely it is that a certain pair of records is a positive match. The overall linkage score is basically the sum of the scores generated from matching on individual data items. Partial matching of data items is taken into account and the score assigned to matching of individual data items is both item specific (a match on a specific data item such as birth date weighs more than a match on a less specific data item such as sex) and value specific (a match on a rare value for a data item weighs more than a match on a common value, e.g., "Janiqua" vs. "Jane").[155,156]

Although probabilistic linkage is generally recommended for external linkages, deterministic linkage may be more practical to implement for patient linkage within a cancer registry system. However, central cancer registries can achieve efficient and accurate linkage of incoming records using deterministic or probabilistic linkage, or both.[58]

In addition to geocoding and patient linkage, common types of record linkage that a central registry may need to perform include:

- Linking duplicate reports about the same patient in a list of case reports
- Linking of the registry's cases with out-of-state reports
- Linking cancer registry cases to reports of death in death certificate files
- Linking cancer registry cases to cohort lists from special studies[157,158]

Some registries use record linkage for a broad set of other reasons, including linking their cancer patient file with groups of environmentally exposed workers or linking them to Department of Motor Vehicle records to determine whether the patient is still driving and, therefore, alive (see Follow-up Methods and Evaluation section later in this chapter).

It is not unusual for central registries to receive duplicate reports on 20% or more of their cases. Therefore, resolution of the possible duplicates becomes one of crucial importance to incidence rate calculation. Deduplication is a special type of record linkage where records in the same file are blocked, compared, and scored against each other, and high-scoring pairs are potential duplicates. Deduplication of the registry database is a fundamental requirement for accuracy and validity of counts in the cancer registry, and should be performed at both the patient and tumor level. The NPCR and NAACCR standard for duplicates in a central registry are to maintain less than or equal to 0.1% (≤1 per 1,000 cases) duplicates in the registry. Any central registry in the United States that is not detecting numerous duplicate reports most likely has a troublesome quality-control problem.

Various data linkage programs are available for central registries to use. Some programs are online and interactive, with provision for indicating which computer-selected matches are correct or incorrect as matching proceeds. Others use batch linkages. A low-cost alternative to commercially available software is Link Plus, a stand-alone, probabilistic record linkage program available free of charge from the CDC-NPCR.[134] Link Plus was designed specifically for cancer registry linkages, accepts NAACCR-formatted files, fixed width, and delimited files, and can be used to detect duplicates within a registry or to link cancer registry files with other data files. Link Plus is used extensively within the cancer registration community and across a diversity of research disciplines.[159–164]

Computerized Death Clearance

Death clearance activities have been described earlier in this chapter. Central registries use death certificates both as casefinding sources and as sources for date and cause of death for cases already on record. Death certificates may be available in electronic form, both as individual images and annual files. Central registries should link with vital statistics files at least annually.

Customized Output Programs

A primary purpose of central registries is to actively use the data obtained for epidemiologic and other purposes. A wide range of computer output programs is needed for this. Each use of a central registry's data may entail one or more types of output program.

The most basic type of output preparation is some form of patient record selection. These lists may be produced in hard copy or in the form of a subfile. For many needs, a list of the identified patients is the required output, for example, a list of patients due for follow-up. Patient record selection capabilities are typically built into commercial database systems, but registries that have designed their own file management system must program their own patient record selection or subfile extraction, or both. Lists are used for editing, record linkage, and many other purposes. A sort capability is often built into list-generating programs.

The next level of output for central registries is based on counts of cases meeting specific criteria in the form of frequency distributions and cross-tabulations. A generalized program of counting and cross-classifying (e.g., comparing age with primary site) is commonly needed. These counting and cross-classifying programs often must also be able to group the individual data values into categories (such as from single years of age into 5-year age groups).

Many registries have customized programs for generating follow-up letters. Typically, these programs act on a selected subfile of patient names produced by the list or subfile generator.

Other necessary programs include those for incidence, mortality, and survival rate calculation. Calculation of age-specific and age-adjusted incidence and mortality require population at-risk data for the geographic area and subpopulations being covered. Notable among these are SEER*Stat and SEER*Prep for use on SEER and related databases; central registries can create a database of data from their registry and load it into the SEER*Stat program for analysis.[165–167]

Survival analysis programs, which use actuarial (lifetable) methodology and may provide an age-adjustment (relative), are among the more complicated output programs that are used by central registries. The quality of survival analysis is dependent on good follow-up information. Other special purpose analysis programs are available.

Quality Control/ Management of Central Registries

A major requirement for central registries is to maintain a level of quality that supports the uses the registry plans to make of its data.[168–177] The primary quality-control concerns of central registries involve two straightforward questions: (1) How complete is case ascertainment? and (2) How complete and accurate are the data that are collected? Data collection, however, is not the only registry activity in need of monitoring. Every aspect of the registry should be considered. Data processing and computer program development can be important contributors to quality. Additional quality concerns should also include timeliness and accuracy of coding and analysis. Several topics in quality control for central registries that have been previously discussed include data editing and detection of unwanted duplicate case reports.

Feedback, communication, and training are also necessary features of a comprehensive quality-control program. The results of quality-control activities should be communicated effectively to data producers, registry managers, and end users. Front-line abstractors should be aware of the results of their efforts and may be in a favored position to identify the causes of special variations or problems.

The design of an appropriate quality-control program must be based on a balance of costs and anticipated benefits. The objectives of a particular registry may influence, to some extent, the specifics of a central registry's approach to quality control. The quality challenge and the potential sources of error that registries face have been previously described, including casefinding (missing cases), abstracting error, coding error, address uncertainties, undetected duplicates, and population-at-risk uncertainties.[178–180]

Quality-Control Methods

Various facets of quality review are performed by central registries including:

1. Visual review
2. Case completeness, reabstracting and recoding audits and studies
3. Rejection standards
4. Computerized edit checks
5. Process monitoring
6. Record consolidation quality control
7. Death certificate follow-back
8. Designed experiments
9. Education and training
10. Directly measuring quality

Many registries, using several of these quality activities, seek to achieve registry certification.

Visual Review

Visual review is the form of quality control most visible to hospital registrars. It involves record-by-record evaluation by visual review. In visual review, an inspector examines a sample of abstracts (sometimes all abstracts) for errors. Discrepancies are identified and corrected. Acceptable abstracts are passed along for further processing. Visual review is time intensive. Problems discovered in visual review are generally resolved before the case can be added to the central registry database.

Sometimes all abstracts in a batch must be resolved before any records in the batch can be accepted to guard against systematic problems, some of which may not be detected by the review procedure if the procedure checks only certain records or only certain instances of inconsistencies.

Because acceptance-sampling procedures for visual review evaluate the individual report record, and often result in the need to query the registrar who originally recorded the information, it is most efficient to conduct the review as close to the time the data are entered into the original database as possible.

Case Completeness, Reabstracting, Recoding Audits and Studies

Data completeness and accuracy must be monitored at the level of the reporting facility where the data originates to fully evaluate both the completeness and quality of the data in the central registry.[181,182] One routine data quality assurance activity is the auditing of facilities reporting to the central registry. Audits of facilities reporting to the central registries are an important tool to monitor and improve quality, and to inform educational efforts.

Typically, casefinding completeness, data item completeness, and data item accuracy are audited. SEER and NPCR routinely conduct audits of central registries via audit of the facilities reporting to the registries. For example, NPCR Program Standards state that NPCR central registries must have an overall program of quality assurance that includes conducting casefinding and/or reabstracting audits from a sampling of source documents for each hospital-based reporting facility at least once every 5 years. Although these audits may include external audits, such as those conducted by NPCR and SEER, to fully meet this standard, in general, registries must independently conduct audits of their reporting facilities. Audit results can help inform any abstracting rejection criteria, as discussed later. Audits of reporting facilities commonly include the three following types of audits: casefinding audits, reabstraction audits, and recoding audits.

Casefinding Audits

To monitor case completeness of reporting facilities, central registries can carry out casefinding audits of their reporting facilities. Casefinding audits involve independently identifying all cases diagnosed and/or treated at a facility that are eligible for reporting to the central registry, usually for a sample time period. Auditors examine various casefinding data sources in the audited facility that cover the audited time period, including medical records disease indices (MRDI), pathology reports (including nongynecologic cytology, bone marrow, and autopsy), radiation therapy logs, cytology reports, autopsy records, and other sources. Reportable tumors for the specified time period are identified via the review of the casefinding sources and then matched against a list of tumors that have been reported by the facility to the central registry. Tumors that are identified at audit but do not match to the list of reported tumors (nonmatches, missed, or unreported tumors) are then reconciled with the facil-

ity. After reconciliation efforts, the number of tumors that matched expressed as a percentage of all tumors identified at audit provides an estimate of case completeness for the audited facility.

NAACCR, NPCR, and SEER have sponsored such audits. In general, all potential sources for the time period must be visited, and this effort is time intensive and requires preplanning.[183]

Reabstraction Audits

To monitor data quality and to ensure that the actual patient experience reported by the facility is represented in the central registry database, central registries should perform reabstraction audits. Reabstraction audits identify specific problem areas in need of improvement. Reabstraction audits include independently reabstracting a sample of case records reported by the facility from the actual source patient medical records and comparing the reabstracted data with the data already in the registry.[181-183] The goal of a reabstraction audit is to describe the level of agreement between the data reabstracted from the source records and the data in the central registry. For each reabstracted data item, the auditor's codes are compared with the codes originally reported by the facility to identify and classify discrepancies. If the codes do not match, the discrepancy may be classified as a major or minor discrepancy based on definitions set up in advance of the audit. Discrepancies that are identified at audit are then reconciled with the facility. After reconciliation efforts, the number of tumors for which agreement was found for a particular data item expressed as a percentage of the total number of tumors reabstracted for that data item provides an estimate of the data accuracy for the audited facility.

Recoding Audits

Central registries also perform recoding audits. Recoding audits involve independently recoding particular data items from abstracted text that was submitted to the central registry by the reporting facility, rather than reviewing actual source documents. The goal of a recoding audit is to describe the level of agreement between the data recoded from the submitted text and the data in the central registry. For each recoded data item, the auditor's codes are compared with the codes originally reported by the facility to identify and classify discrepancies. As with reabstraction audits, if original and audited codes do not match, discrepancies may be classified as major or minor discrepancies based on definitions established before the audit. Discrepancies that are identified at audit are then reconciled with the facility. After reconciliation efforts, the number of tumors for which agreement was found for a particular data item expressed as a percentage of the total number of tumors recoded for that data item provides an estimate of the data accuracy for the audited facility.

In addition to formal audits, recoding and reabstracting studies can be conducted to assess reproducibility (agreement among data collectors) and validity (agreement with source documents). The objective of a typical reabstracting study is to characterize the degree of agreement between data already in the registry and data reabstracted from source records by a different expert cancer registrar.

Rejection Standards

All central cancer registries are forced to walk a fine line between data quality and case completeness when addressing the quality of cancer reports received from reporting facilities. If a central registry accepts all submitted records regardless of the quality of the data they contain, this may result in the registry having greater case completeness but poorer data quality. Furthermore, if a central registry allows errant data to be submitted, then the errors must be identified and cleaned at the central registry level before submission to standard-setting organizations, and there is no assurance that the errant information will be corrected in the submitting facility's database. However, if a central registry rejects a record because of poor data quality, then the registry takes the risk for that record not being resubmitted, thereby affecting the registry's case completeness. Ideally, data cleaning should occur at the level of the submitting facility at the time of initial abstraction. However, as reporting facilities may use a variety of different software to abstract and submit their data, it is difficult for a central registry to uniformly approach this issue from within abstraction software.

Central registries may implement a variety of rejection standards. They may choose to run data quality edits on submission of a file of abstracts (see later) and may choose to apply some type of error percentage threshold for file rejection (i.e., if the submitted file contains more than a specified percentage of edit errors overall, then entire file is rejected), or they may choose to reject individually errant abstracts. In addition to edit errors, the central registry may choose to run other checks on the data, for example, assessing for overuse of edit overrides being set, or too many unknown, missing, or unspecific values for particular data items in the submitted records. Registries may also choose to perform a visual check on the abstracted text that was submitted and reject because of insufficient textual information. Some registries reject nonreportable records, or records that are submitted before some specified amount of time (i.e., "early reportables") after diagnosis to ensure that records contain complete treatment information.

Regardless of the rejection criteria that the registry decides to implement, if rejecting any records, a robust system of follow-up should be in place to ensure resubmission of rejected records to the central registry.

Computerized Edit Checks

Automated edit checks that are designed by central registries and incorporated into the facility registry software are especially well suited to that goal.[141–149] The adoption by central registries of standard data items and coding rules has facilitated development of standard edits maintained by NAACCR with input from the standard-setting organizations.[184] Central registries can use the CDC-designed EDITS software to tailor selection of those edits to fit their data sets and can add edits for items unique to their own uses.[134] They can be used for all records for a selected period or on a sample to establish that the new staff member or procedure being reviewed is functioning as expected.

Data edits are used to eliminate gross inconsistencies but cannot guarantee correctness. Edit checking typically includes checking for allowable codes, range checks, interterm checks, inter-record checks, and sometimes interdatabase checks. Edit checks are cost-effective and, therefore, should be applied to 100% of cases.

Process Monitoring

Process monitoring involves the tracking of statistical indicators over time to detect changes indicative of a need for intervention.[169] The indicators themselves can be familiar measures: percentage of records with edit errors, time lag between hospital admission and submission of the record to the central registry, number of cases submitted every month, percentage unknown for specific items, and so on. They also can be measures specific to the operations of the central registry: percentage of records processed that linked to records already in the data set, or time between receipt of the report and its availability to users in the central registry database. The important point is that process monitoring requires statistical evaluation to determine when the natural variability of these measures moves significantly outside its normal range of variation. When that happens, the central registry will apply its own procedures to identify the probable cause of the change and determine whether or what kind of response is called for. The response may be anything from training, to clarification of a coding rule, to ascertaining that a facility changed its services resulting in a change in the number of types of cases submitted.

The comparison baseline for process monitoring is often set based on historical data. This historical data method compares the number of cases expected (based on previous years or on standard incidence rates) with those observed.

Record Consolidation Quality Control

Emphasis up until this point has primarily been placed on timeliness, quality, and completeness of data submitted to the central registry. However, once data arrive at the central registry, records must be further processed before incorporation into the central registry database. Although some proportion of patient linkage, tumor consolidation, and data item consolidation may take place automatically within the central registry system, there will always be a proportion of records that must be manually reviewed and guided through these processes. The majority of central registries employ central registry staff who have the following responsibilities: guiding the patient linkage process for incoming reports with questionable matches to existing patients on the central registry database; manual geocoding efforts; reviewing submitted abstracts for selected code accuracy and agreement with submitted text; manual tumor consolidation to ascertain if multiple primaries exist across multiple source reports; and data item consolidation if multiple sources reported information regarding the same tumor.

Before any record consolidation processing, it is important that the source data to be consolidated be edited to ensure the validity of submitted codes (see earlier Computerized Edit Checks section). If invalid codes are submitted for record consolidation, this will hinder the record consolidation process and may result in inappropriate consolidation of information in the central registry.

Just as reporting facility abstractors, and the data that they produce, must be assessed for potential coding issues, so must the work of central registry staff. Systematic error on the part of a central registry coder can have a serious effect on the quality of the registry data, in particular, for patients with multiple primary tumors or a very large number of reporting sources. Central registries take a variety of approaches to quality control of the record consolidation process. The most common activity would be the running of data quality and inter-record edits after record consolidation has been completed. Although the source data being presented for consolidation may not contain any errors, quite often central registry coders will correct information on the source record or consolidate information from different source records and potentially generate new edit errors in the process. In addition, routine deduplication of the registry database on both a patient and tumor level, as discussed earlier, can provide important feedback regarding record consolidation conducted at the central registry.

One of the most effective quality-control activities for record consolidation is to provide continual feedback and education to the central registry coder on an ongoing basis. This may be achieved in a number of ways. The central registry may require that all or a certain percentage of their central coders be CTRs. The central registry may designate staff to oversee the central registry coding and editing efforts. These individuals may perform reconsolidation of samples of records reviewed and consolidated by central registry staff to identify any potential issues in the visual review or consolidation process, and then meet with each individual on a regular basis to go over any identified issues. A running log of all issues identified, together with questions that come up and their resolutions, is also a helpful mechanism to keep central registry staff informed, in particular, about new data items or consolidation rules.

Central registries may also choose to implement a partner-based visual review system among their staff in which staff review all or a sample of each other's work on a routine basis. The rotation of partners ensures that each person has a chance to review the work of others and

prevents any bias that may occur. The registry may have routine internal data quality review meetings or training sessions at which issues are discussed and consensus regarding difficult coding rules may be defined. In addition, the central registry should have their staff attend external training opportunities, such as educational conferences, online courses, and Webinars.

Another routine quality-control activity is to develop, maintain, and continually build on a set of coding and record consolidation tests with the results of each staff compared with already existing gold standard results, allowing for uniform and fair assessment of staff performance. The NPCR, in conjunction with NCRA, has recently developed an interactive, virtual registry system for developing and assessing the skills of cancer registry personnel called the Cyber Cancer Registry.[170] The Cyber Cancer Registry application is Web based, and uses real, deidentified medical records to provide a simulated registry experience including activities of various levels of difficulty with which to practice coding and editing skills, and gives immediate feedback that evaluates competency, tracks training scores, and provides certificates of completion.[170]

Death Certificate Follow-Back

The surest method to check on potential missing cases is to review all death certificates for the reporting period, and thereafter search for mention of cancer that may not have been previously reported.[120,185] The absence of many new cases found first at death certification is the most rigorous and independent indicator that cancer diagnoses are not being missed in the catchment area.

The death certificate method uses the percentage of cases reported by death certificate only as a measure of incompleteness. Also, the ratio of cancer deaths in a period to incident cancer cases in the same period is compared with ratios from other population-based registries. A central registry can determine any pattern of missing cases by following back the death certificate to determine where the cancer diagnosis was made and why it was missed.

Designed (Special) Experiments

Designed experiments are most expensive and time-consuming to central registries, and may not have the same direct effect on current data quality obtained from acceptance sampling or process monitoring.[169] However, they are the often the most effective method of evaluating the effects of current processes or directing possible changes in procedures. For example, a central registry might use a designed experiment to evaluate the effects of adding a new report source—for example, physicians who review patient slides in-office instead of sending them to a pathology laboratory—in terms of case coverage and costs.

Measuring Quality/Certification

Another method of quality management, which overlaps with some of those already mentioned, is the direct measurement of the accuracy and completeness of the registry's data. Some of these measures may be used as criteria in the certification of registries.[186,187] Several methods have been used to assess completeness of registration including reabstracting, recoding, and sample casefinding studies (audits). NAACCR provides two levels of certification ("Gold" and "Silver") based on characteristics of the central registry data[188–192] (see NAACCR Certification of Central Registries section later in this chapter).

Using the Data

Epidemiologists and other analysts often find that using the data and thinking seriously about the findings and their implications leads to useful insights into possible data quality issues or shortcomings of the data, especially where the data's robustness may be questionable. For example, new data edits can be suggested by use of the data that may lead to previously unidentified data errors. Population-based rates reflect not only inaccuracies in the cancer data collected, but uncertainties regarding the populations at risk used in calculations. Census enumerations are estimates subject to survey error.

Education/Training

Specialized training for central cancer registry staff is available in several formats and in a variety of formats. Textbooks for central registries have been published,[1,2,4] as well as a series of self-instructional manuals.[193] SEER and NPCR provide training for central registry personnel for the registries they fund.[194–196] The NAACCR training program includes Web-based and live workshops and conferences in cancer registry operations and cancer surveillance for cancer registry professionals, as well as opportunities at its annual conference.[197] In addition, central registries recruit experienced cancer registrars and encourage their staff to obtain certification as cancer registrars.

Central registries often provide regional training for hospital registrars and other interested parties in their region.[198] In addition, other educational opportunities are available for central registry staff.[199–205]

Quality Assurance Summary

In summary, automated edit checks have the additional advantage of being fast and inexpensive to apply to all records. Visual review, reabstracting, and recoding are expensive and time consuming, and are most productive when used under targeted circumstances. For example, they can be used to identify problems faced by new personnel, or raised by new or modified data items or coding procedures, new software, or expansion of collection to types of cases formerly not collected. Identification of duplicate reports is important and can be challenging in highly mobile populations or in databases where case identifiers are based on self-reported information such as name and birth date.

Analyzing and publishing studies using central registry data can provide important quality-control feedback to the registry. Periodic publication of a central registry's data should follow a consistent format and use accepted statistical procedures to be useful and reliable. Standardization of methodology can assist in that effort. Quality-control tools develop "data on data quality," an essential component of a comprehensive quality-control program. Continual education of both facility and central level staff is crucial. In addition, achieving and maintaining registry certification is a good way for registries to obtain an external and objective measure of their data quality, completeness, and timeliness, in comparison with other registries.

Follow-up Methods and Evaluation

Purpose of Follow-up

The primary purpose of patient follow-up for the central cancer registry is to evaluate the survival of groups of patients according to various parameters such as demographic characteristics, primary site, stage of disease, and first course of treatment.[206]

The central registry and the hospital registry can help each other with follow-up activities. The hospital registrar may send follow-up information to the central registry. The central cancer registry may facilitate hospital follow-up by providing information and services, for example, sending follow-up lists to hospitals and physicians, sharing follow-up information, contacting patients, and utilizing follow-up methods that may not be available to hospitals or physicians.

Because the central registry has population-based composite data from all sources, it can calculate population-based survival statistics. Hospitals may compare their data with the population-based statistics. Finally, the central registry may validate diagnoses or changes in diagnoses that may not have been reported to the hospital.[207]

Active versus Passive Follow-up

The central cancer registry may use active or passive follow-up methods. Active follow-up refers to someone, usually a physician's office or cancer registrar, initiating direct contact with patients. From a central registry perspective, active follow-up may also include contacts made by hospital registrars with physicians' offices.

There are primarily four active follow-up methods used by some central registries, although most now use automated or passive methods of follow-up, or a combination of active and passive follow-up. First, a list of patients due for follow-up can be sent directly to the reporting facility or physician responsible for patient care. Second, patients due for follow-up may be directly contacted by central registry staff, but any such contacts should be made with the full knowledge of the hospital and the governing IRB. Third, central registries may conduct research programs, and results of patient contacts that ascertain survival can be reported to the central registry. Finally, some central cancer registries conduct active follow-up with specific patient populations that are difficult to follow using traditional passive methods. For example, childhood cancer cases are often difficult to track over time using passive methods because of name changes and mobility. Therefore, sometimes children are targeted for active follow-up.

Passive follow-up refers to methods that do not require registry contact with hospitals, physicians, or individual cancer patients. Passive methods are used primarily to determine the patient's vital status and current date last seen alive or date of death. These methods usually involve computerized searches of existing nonregistry files that may contain the cancer patient's name and the follow-up information, or information from which vital status can be derived (e.g., driver's license or tax files). There are many possible passive follow-up methods; some of these are listed in Table 36-9.

Passive methods are inexpensive to use and are time efficient. Methods vary in efficiency and cost-effectiveness depending on the completeness and accuracy of the identifying information and fields used for data linkage. Most methods require complex computer programs, but over the years, central registries have developed expertise in this area. Confidentiality must be protected when electronic media with identifying information of cancer patients are provided to an agency external to the registry for linkage. It should be noted that if quality-of-life data are needed, passive methods will not provide the desired information.

Generally, a successful follow-up program in a central registry uses both active and passive follow-up methods. It is not clear what bias exists if only one or a limited number of methods are used. Regardless of methods successful registries aim for a low lost to follow-up percentage. In calculating survival statistics, there are no guidelines regarding the percentage that can be lost before the assumptions are violated regarding life-table and other methodologies. However, it is important that those lost to follow-up are not different from the rest of the cases being followed.[208] Unfortunately, those that are lost to follow-up may be different. They may have different ages, social class, and stage of disease than those who are successfully followed. The kinds of cases lost to follow-up may also be biased with regard to the follow-up methods used.

Patient follow-up can be complex and costly,[209] so hospital and central registries should work together. Cooperation leads to efficiency, accuracy, and high follow-up rates, thus improving patient care and also the accuracy of survival statistics.

Services Provided to Hospital-Based Registries by Central Registries

A central registry relies heavily on information obtained from hospitals and other reporting facilities. A significant burden of collecting cancer incidence data falls to the hospital registrar. It is important for central registries to be aware of challenges faced by reporting facilities, and to do what it can to minimize duplication of work related to reporting of cancer to the central registry. There are many useful services that a central registry can provide to hospitals in order to encourage their cooperation, including those listed in Table 36-10.

Table 36-9	Passive Follow-up Methods Used by Central Registries

Linkage with state death certificate files

Linkage with state motor vehicles records or tax files

Linkage to National Death Index

Linkage to state health files such as Medicare

Linkage to national health records, such as the Center for Medicare and Medicaid Services

Review of records of local election boards

Linkage with hospital discharge summaries

Review of resident lists in geographic areas

Linkage to rosters of health plans (HMOs)

Table 36-10	Services Provided to Hospitals by Central Registries

Feedback on death certificates

Backup of computerized data (in the event of individual computer or system crashes)

Edits and quality checks of data

Assistance in computerizing the hospital registry (providing a backlog of the cases already stored in the central registry and providing workshops and other training)

Providing participating hospitals with the latest information on all of their patients who have been admitted to other hospitals to determine the total treatment received from all sources

Ensuring that only one follow-up letter is generated no matter where the patient was accessioned

However, some state mandates do not allow the sharing of such information, especially if it was obtained from a facility other than the reporting facility.

Calculation and Assessment of Incidence Rates

Definition of an Incidence Rate

One of the primary and unique functions of a population-based registry is to measure the amount or rate of disease in a known geographic area or population. The most commonly used measure of cancer in a population is the incidence rate (IR), defined as the measurement of disease frequency over a specified period of time.[1,210,211] Researchers also use it to determine the burden of disease in a population and how the risk of disease varies in different subgroups of the population. The definition of an incidence rate is shown in Figure 36-1.

The numerator includes only newly diagnosed cases during a given time period. The denominator includes only individuals in the same population who are "at risk" for the disease during the same time period. For instance, the incidence rate of prostate cancer in Iowa would only include men in the numerator and denominator. The populations used in incidence rates are generally multiplied by a factor such as 100,000, to create rates expressed in whole numbers, which are easier to use than decimal numbers.

An annual incidence rate is an incidence rate calculated for a one-year period. If the incidence information is combined for several years, an average annual incidence rate can be calculated by dividing the sum of the numerators by the sum of the denominators. This is frequently done to increase the stability offered in several years of data compared to a single year.

Incidence rates are commonly calculated as crude rates, age-specific rates, and age-adjusted rates. Rates that are calculated for a total population (e.g. all ages combined) are called crude rates.

Another measure of disease is prevalence, which includes the total number of cases with a disease at a particular point in time. Unlike prevalence, incidence is not influenced by differences in the survival of cases. Prevalence is a useful measurement, however, for health care planning purposes, but can be difficult to measure.

Age-Specific Incidence Rates (ASIR)

Rates that are calculated for subgroups of the population, such as age-group, are called specific rates. Rates for specific age groups are referred to as age-specific rates, and rates for a given cancer site are termed site-specific rates. Rates are further generally calculated separately for men and women (sex-specific) because combining genders hides information.

Age-Adjusted Incidence Rates (AAIR)

A method used to compare rates in different populations or areas that may have different age distributions is to calculate an overall rate and adjust it for age. These rates are known as age-adjusted incidence rates (AAIR's), or sometimes as standardized rates. Three methods are commonly used to age-adjust rates: cumulative incidence, direct standardization, and indirect standardization. Only direct standardization is discussed here.

With direct standardization, we answer the question "What are the rates in a standard population if the age-specific rates in population A and population B were both to occur in the standard population?" In this way, AAIR's can be calculated that are directly comparable across different populations because they are derived using the same standard population reference.

Table 36-11 presents an example of the calculation of age-adjusted incidence rates for Asian/Other and Hispanic women in California by the direct method using the 1970 U.S. population as the standard or reference population. The 1970 U.S. standard population, which totals 1,000,000, is shown in column 1. The age-specific incidence rates for breast cancer in Asian/Other women, as calculated in Table 36-6, are listed in column 2. These rates are then multiplied and then divided by 1,000,000, giving a product, shown in column 3. The sum of these products across all age groups is 60.77, the age-adjusted incidence rate for breast cancer in Asian/Other women for 1988-1992, using the 1970 U.S. standard population. Similar calculations are given for Hispanic women in columns 4 and 5 with an age-adjusted rate of 69.75.

The rate for breast cancer, age-adjusted to the 1970 U.S. standard population, is 60.77 per 100,000 per year for Asian/Other women and 69.75 per 100,000 per year for Hispanic women. This implies that, if the 1970 U.S. population had the same age-specific rates as Asian/Other women and as Hispanic women, there would be an average of 61 cases among Asian/Other women and 70 cases among Hispanic women per 100,000 women in California for each year from 1988 to 1992.

Number of new cases of disease for N during a specified time period

$$IR = \frac{}{P} = \frac{}{\text{Number of people at risk in the population during the same time period}}$$

Figure 36-1. Definition of a Crude Incidence Rate (IR)

396   Section 6   Central and Other Registries

Table 36-11	Example of Calculation of an Annual Age-Specific Incidence Rates (ASIR) and Age-Adjusted Incidence (AAIR'S) Rates for Asian/Other and Hispanic Women in California by the Direct Method Using the 1970 US Standard Population. Female Breast Cancer, Asian/Other and Hispanics Age-Specific Incidence

		Asian/Others		Hispanics	
	1970 U.S. Standard Population	Average Annual ASIR per 100,000	Age-Specific Product	Average Annual ASIR per 100,000	Age-Specific Product
Age Group	(1)	(2)	$(3)=(I) \times (2)/1,000,000$	(4)	$(5)=(1) \times (4)/1,000,000$
0-4	84,416	0.0	0.00	0.0	0.00
5-9	98,204	0.0	0.00	0.0	0.00
10-14	102,304	0.0	0.00	0.0	0.00
15-19	93,845	0.2	0.02	0.0	0.00
20-24	80,S61	2.2	0.18	1.0	0.08
25-29	66,320	5.9	0.39	5.7	0.38
30-34	56,249	20.6	1.16	1.5	1.77
35-39	54,656	50.4	2.75	47.6	2.60
40-44	58,958	91.6	5.40	81.4	4.80
45-49	59,622	149.4	8.91	129.8	7.74
50-54	54,643	155.0	8.47	150.7	8.23
55-59	49,077	157.5	7.73	186.5	9.15
60-64	42,403	154.1	6.53	196.6	8.34
65-69	34,406	196.4	6.76	255.5	8.79
70-74	26,789	188.1	5.04	281.1	7.53
75-79	18,871	220.2	4.16	271.5	5.12
80-84	11,241	163.9	1.84	300.3	3.38
85+	7,435	191.7	1.43	247.8	1.84
	1,000,000		60.77		69.75

Rates, California 1988-1992. From California Cancer Registry, Cancer Incidence and Mortality in California by Detailed Race/Ethnicity, 1988-1992. April 1995.27 (215). Copyright © 1992 by California Cancer Registry. Reprinted with permission.

Note that the age-adjusted rate for Hispanic women is higher than that for Asian/Other women. Comparison of the crude rates would have shown the opposite conclusion: an incidence of 56 per 100,000 for Asian/Other women compared with 43 per 100,000 for Hispanic women. Comparing crude rates leads to an erroneous conclusion as a result of the age difference of the two populations (the average age of Hispanic women is much lower than that of Asian/Other women in California).

Choosing a standard population is a matter of judgment. A standard commonly used internationally is the world population. In the past, the 1970 U.S. population, and populations of the country, state, or other geographic location being studied were frequently used. In 1999, the 2000 U.S. standard population was adopted as the stan-

dard.[213] It is generally preferable for the age distribution of the standard population to be similar to the age distributions of the study populations. A comparison of the 1970 and 2000 standards are given in Table 36-12. The 2000 standard population reflects the aging of the US population. Since cancer is age-progressive, this increased weighting of the older age-specific cancer rates will increase age-standardized rates.

Other risk measures are used in population-based epidemiology, including proportional methodologies.[214] Proportional methodologies are useful where populations-at-risk are not available for the subgroups of interest. An example would be the proportional incidence rate (PIR) of lung cancer among spray painters. The PIR would be the proportion of spray painters with lung cancer (cases/

Table 36-12	Standard US Populations, 1970 and 2000	
Age Group	1970	2000
0-4	84,416	69,135
5-9	98,204	72,533
10-14	102,304	73,032
15-19	93,845	72,169
20-24	80,S61	66,478
25-29	66,320	64,529
30-34	56,249	71,044
35-39	54,656	80,762
40-44	58,958	81,851
45-49	59,622	72,118
50-54	54,643	62,716
55-59	49,077	48,454
60-64	42,403	38,793
65-69	34,406	34,264
70-74	26,789	31,733
75-79	18,871	26,999
80-84	11,241	17,842
85+	7,435	15,508
	1,000,000	1,000,000

all spray painters) divided by the proportion of all other workers with lung cancer (possibly age-adjusted). The appropriateness of proportional methodology depends heavily on the homogeneity of the reference group; in this case all workers who are not spray painters. Age-adjustment can be performed as appropriate.

Calculation and Assessment of Survival Rates

Survival-rate calculations in the hospital setting were described earlier in this textbook and elsewhere.[215–218] The observed survival rate is the proportion of persons in a defined population who remain alive during a specified time interval. The beginning of the surveillance period is usually defined by a particular event, such as cancer diagnosis, exposure to a carcinogen, or the beginning of treatment. The surveillance period generally ends at death, although the same methods can be used to evaluate other endpoints, such as cancer recurrence.

Several forms of survival analysis are discussed earlier in this textbook, including the direct method and the life-table (actuarial, cohort) method; often referred to as observed survival rates. The direct observed survival method requires that all subjects be available for survival throughout the complete interval of interest. The life-table ob-

served survival method allows including subjects who may have been lost to follow-up, or may be alive after several years of observation. Survival rates can be expressed as a ratio such as 0.917, or as a percent, 91.7%.

The relative survival rate is "the ratio of the observed survival rate in the study population to the expected survival rate in the subset of the general population with the same characteristics as the study population."[215] The relative survival rate is the observed survival rate, adjusted because some of the subjects can be expected to die from causes of death other than that under study. Age-sex-race/ethnic specific tables of life probability are generally used to calculate this adjustment. The five-year observed survival rate for breast cancer summarizes how many of the observed breast cancer patients can be expected to die from all causes of death. The five-year relative survival rate of the breast cancer patients defined as the percent that will die from breast cancer alone. Observed and relative survival rates can differ materially and clarity of definition when presenting data is important.

The cancer survival rate is also sometimes confused with the cancer mortality rate, which is the rate at which persons in the general population die of cancer during the time period of interest. The mortality rate provides a measure of the risk of death attributable to a disease in a population, whereas the survival rate is determined by following a specific group of people with the disease until death. The survival rate is interpreted as the risk of dying among people who have the disease. Hospitals calculate survival rates for their patients, but if such rates are desired for an entire population, they must be calculated by central registries.

Uses of Cancer Registry Data

Cancer registries are a rich source of information for a wide variety of surveillance and other important public heath purposes.[219–224] There are several categories into which these uses can be summarized, but no rubric seems completely inclusive.

Cancer Case Statistics

Population-based cancer registries provide the baseline information defining the burden of new (incident) cancers in catchment areas. Multihospital central registries that are not also population-based provide similar baseline information for hospital cohorts.[11] Surveillance includes what types of cancers are being diagnosed (patient age, gender and race/ethnicity) and where they are diagnosed. Frequency estimates of prevalent patients are made from the incident counts. Several of the standard setters provide population-based statistics, including IARC, SEER, NPCR, NAACCR, and the American Cancer Society.[15,22,225–228]

Incidence/Prevalence Surveillance (Descriptive Epidemiology)

In addition to these frequencies counts (statistics), central registries provide incidence rates by age group, gender and race/ethnicity. A comparative analysis of such rates is often referred to as descriptive epidemiology.[229-240] Essentially all population-based registries annually publish a report of case frequencies and incidence rates. Depending on the analytic resources of each central registry, a broad range of incidence and prevalence surveillance including time trends is maintained. In some cases analysts of central registry data also perform corresponding mortality surveillance, with the data for such efforts coming from health department death statistics not central registries.

Patterns of disease occurrence can be studied to identify groups who are experiencing different rates of cancer than others. These comparisons are used to generate hypotheses to explain rate disparities and causes, which may lead to analytical studies to test these hypotheses or to develop cancer control programs to reduce the risk in the high-risk groups.

Examples of descriptive data include documentation of the higher rate of prostate cancer in African-American men as compared to white men, lower lung cancer rates in Utah (with a large Mormon population that does not smoke cigarettes) than the rest of the United States, and the rapid rise in diagnosed breast cancer beginning in the 1980s (due to the increased use of screening mammography for earlier detection). One of the most interesting examples has been the comparison of cancer rates in immigrants, between their native and host countries. These studies have shown that many cancers increase or decrease in immigrants to reflect the rates in the host countries. For example, breast cancer rates in Japanese women are low, but they increase in Japanese women immigrating to the United States.

In addition to the basic case frequencies and incidence, central cancer registries can also provide baseline information about the distribution of cancer by stage of disease. For example, areas with increased late stage cancer at diagnosis can be determined to identify area where cancer screening should be increased. Studies have been conducted of late stage breast cancer, in regards to location of mammography facilities and other determinants of screening behavior.[241]

Cancer Cluster Surveillance

Reported cancer clusters can become of great public and media concern. Neighborhood groups, real estate interests, industry groups, occupation groups, school groups, and a variety of other interest groups periodically become strongly interested in one or another reported cancer hot spots. In many cases, analysis of clusters along with surveillance of incidence trends are the twin pillars of the original cancer registry justification and funding. Analysis of clusters in time and space is a difficult and demanding task.[242-245] Presentation of this information to the interested parties can also be

demanding and time-intensive. Essential to cancer cluster analysis is that all cases be included with accurate diagnostic criteria and dates of diagnosis. The population-based central registry is the only available source of such information.[6-8]

Cancer Mapping

An important element among the tools of cancer surveillance is cancer mapping. The pictorial presentation of color-coded data is an intuitively clear method of analyzing and presenting spatial information. For example, color-coded county maps may be used to show early versus advanced stage diagnosis of breast cancer.

Geographic Information Systems (GIS)

GIS offer interesting potential for analysis of cancer and population-related data.[246-248] Although cancer mapping has long been used in cancer epidemiology, the GIS offer more sophisticated tools than county mapping and color-coding.

Ecologic or Correlation Studies

Another common form of cancer surveillance is to study whether cancer incidence or mortality rates in a population are correlated with some other factor measured in the population, for example, dietary fat. If incidence is the measure of interest, then the population-based registry is the source of these data. These studies correlate the amount of change in the factor of interest compared to changes in the cancer rate. One way this can be demonstrated is to plot cancer rates for different areas on the vertical axis of a graph and the corresponding factor of interest for each country on the horizontal axis.[249,250]

A correlation statistic can be calculated, 1.0 indicating perfect correlation and 0.0 indicating no correlation. For example, when colon cancer rates and dietary fat consumed for many countries are plotted, there is a very high correlation between these factors. One limitation of these studies is that they may show that variables are correlated, but there is no way to determine whether one variable causes the other. In fact, they may only be correlated because both are caused by another, unknown, factor. So these studies are only suggestive, but they have been important in creating etiologic hypotheses that can be tested using methods that can determine causality.

Case Control Studies

In these studies, cases of cancer are compared with similar people from the same population who do not have cancer (serving as the control group) for past exposures that may be related to the disease. These exposures are usually measured by respondent's answers to questionnaires or from historical records (such as health records).[25] If the cancer cases have had more exposures to the suspected carcinogen than the controls, then it can be inferred that the exposure increases one's odds or risk of having the cancer. The cancer registry is important in identifying the cases to be included in these studies, by providing access to all of the cases in a given population for sampling. The registry also facilitates case control studies by providing data that can be included in the analysis such as stage, treatment, and demographic characteristics.

It can be seen that case–control studies start with the cases and matching controls, and look backward in time at possible risk factors. This retrospective approach can be efficient and cost-effective.

Cohort Studies

This type of study begins with identification of a group, or cohort, with a known history of exposure. Exposures of interest are then measured and the study subjects are investigated or are followed over time to determine disease status. The exposures of those with and those without the disease are compared. If the disease of interest occurs disproportionately among the exposed group, it can be inferred that this exposure may be an important factor in the etiology of the disease.[251,252] In cohort studies in which the disease of interest is cancer, central cancer registries are often used to determine the disease outcome by linking the cohort members to all the cases in the registry. Here, too, the registry can provide additional data on the patients to be included in the analyses. If the registry includes follow-up as part of their operation, they can also add information on survival status and cause of death. This prospective following of originally healthy subpopulations may take place over years and be costly, but it allows analysis of all possible health outcomes not just the predefined disease as in case–control studies. Thus the famous Framingham, Massachusetts cohort study could uncover the unsuspected relationship of heart disease to smoking as well as lung cancer.

One type of cohort study is the retrospective cohort. In these studies the cohort is defined today to be some point in the past. For example we can decide now to study all employees who were employed at a particular nuclear facility on January 1, 1970. The registry is asked to link those early cohort members to today's registry files to determine who has developed the disease. Rates of the disease in the cohort are then often compared to an expected rate. The latter is determined from registry data for the entire population. Examples of these studies include linkages to rosters of occupational groups as identified from employment or union records, college students, and professional societies.

Genetic Studies

In recent years progress has been made in identifying genes that are related to different cancers. Consequently, there is interest in identifying high-risk families that can be studied and compared to the general population. Central registries are increasingly being asked to help identify these families.[253–256] After IRB approval, cancer cases of interest are identified, and then contacted to obtain a family history. Families of interest may then be asked to complete more detailed questionnaires, to give blood, and to allow access to pathologic material. Many central registries are in the best position to carry out these tasks, and the family registry becomes an extension of the cancer registry. Sometimes the registry can be linked to an existing database to facilitate genetic research (e.g., the Utah Cancer Registry's linkage to the Mormon genealogy database).

Basic Science Studies

Basic science research may look at the mechanisms by which cells become cancerous or metastatic, identify markers for early detection or progression, or identify new methods of screening, treatment, and palliative care. Population-based data have often been used to develop leads for basic science work. An example is the observation that cervical cancer occurred more frequently in some populations, and that it might be sexually transmitted. This eventually led basic scientists to look for the human papilloma virus.

Patterns of Care Surveillance (Clinical Studies)

Population data can also be used to look, in a general way, at the outcome of different treatments or screening procedures, although they cannot replace the randomized, controlled, clinical trial. The central registry can be used to measure treatment in different geographic areas, different types of hospitals (teaching hospitals, county hospitals, HMO hospitals), or different sub-populations. These general assessments can suggest areas where professional education may be appropriate. The NCDB and other CoC projects have performed patterns of care studies in large multihospital series for decades.[26,27,257–261] Hospital registrars use the aggregate data to evaluate their hospital against composite hospital data in terms of types of cancer seen, patient characteristics, cancer characteristics, treatment, survival and other factors. In addition, annual patterns of care studies are conducted through the SEER Program and periodically by the NPCR.

Survival Surveillance

Survival rates are considered a primary measure of the cancer burden.[22,23] In the same way that incidence surveillance can be maintained with regard to various demographic and other risk factors of the cases, the same comparative surveillance can be maintained for survival. For example, which anatomic stage of disease group survives best? Is there any difference between stages? Which ethnic/racial group survives best? Which treatment group survives best?

Cancer Control

Cancer control includes six areas: primary prevention; screening; early diagnosis; treatment; rehabilitation; and palliative care.[262-265] Cancer registries are integral to all of these areas. Without registries, how will we know which types of people (male, female; older, younger; black, white; which geographic areas; and so on) are at greatest risk for certain types of cancer, are diagnosed with late-stage disease, or have poor survival? If we do not know how often each type of cancer occurs in a specific population, how do we know where to focus our efforts and prioritize the use of our limited cancer control resources? How will we know that cancer control efforts had any effect, if we do not know how often the disease was diagnosed or treated, or what the survival was before and after the intervention efforts? How can we determine whether cases are found earlier if we do not know their stage at diagnosis before and after any intervention?

Thus, we see that central registries are an integral part of the cancer control process. Cancer registries not only provide data for prioritizing our limited cancer control resources to high-risk groups and geographic areas but also provide the mechanism to evaluate cancer control activities.

NAACCR Certification of Central Registries

NAACCR has instituted a program that annually reviews central cancer registries in the US and Canada for excellence based on pre-determined criteria. The certification process includes criteria for completeness, percentage passing edits, percentage of death certificate only information, timeliness, undetected duplicates, and missing data fields for sex, age, county, and race. NAACCR reports that in 2009, 6 Canadian and 52 U.S. registries were certified for their 2006 data. The percentage of the population that is reflected by certified registries for 2006 data is approximately 90%. The indicators and the levels required for central registry certification are listed in Table 36-13.

History of U.S. Central Cancer Registries

The initiation of registration of populations with cancer was a slow process, with many false starts.[266,267] In some instances, the early population-based efforts are closely intertwined with hospital registration, each one facilitating the other.

1920s

A first, but unsuccessful, cancer census took place in London in 1728. It was not until 1900, however, that many researchers and citizens demanded statistics about the

Table 36-13	Summary of Data Quality Criteria and Standards for NAACCR Call for Data

Level of Central Registry Certification		
Criterion	Silver	Gold
Completeness*	≥90%	>=95%
Passing EDITS	≥97%	≥100%
Death Certificate Only	≤5%	≤3%
Timeliness	within 23 months	within 23 months
Duplicate Reports in Data**	≤2/1,000	≤1/1,000
Missing, unknown		
Sex, Age, County	≤3%	≤2%
Race	≤5%	≤3%

*Calculated by using the NAACCR case completeness estimate method.
**Calculated by using the NAACCR duplicate protocol.

disease. Attempts were made to collect these statistics by physician questionnaires, but poor reporting led to many failures. The oldest known example of a modern successful registry is in Hamburg, Germany, where in 1929 a follow-up patient care service was instituted in the local health department.[267]

The activities of the ACoS in promoting cancer registries also goes back to the 1920s when the organization started a bone cancer registry by asking its members to submit information on living cases with that cancer.[82,273] This was followed by the CoC effort later in the 1920s by collections of cases of cancer of the cervix, breast, mouth and tongue, colon and thyroid.

The Massachusetts Cancer Registry began in 1926 in the State Health Department, centered in an abandoned state hospital, and was designed to establish cancer clinics throughout the state under the direction of Dr. Herbert Lombard.[269] Early in the data collection process, Lombard and his staff reported on the relationship of cancer to population density and a higher cancer rate in foreign born Americans and their children than in native born Americans with native grandparents. They also published one of the first studies linking oral cancer and the use of tobacco.

The registry did not report all cases of cancer in the state but did report and follow cases in the major hospitals. By 1953, 20 hospitals maintained state-aided cancer clinics. They offered multi-disciplinary diagnostic consultative services for referred cancer patients.

Following Dr. Lombard's retirement in 1959, the Massachusetts state cancer registry lost its funding. There was a brief resurgence of interest in the early 1960s when the NCI funded the program to assist in obtaining data for its End Result Program. Attempts were made to fund a cancer registry in Boston in the late 1960s but this initiative also failed through lack of state funding. The registry was reorganized in 1982 and now has complete coverage of cancer patients in the state.

1930s

In 1930, the CoC developed standards for hospital cancer clinics and by 1937 there were 240 accredited cancer clinics.

The first truly population-based registry in the United States was the Connecticut Tumor Registry, which was founded in 1941 but registered cases back to 1935.[270,271] This registry has been in continuous operation since then and is part of the SEER Program.

The Connecticut Cancer Registry was started when a group of New Haven physicians began compiling data, which showed a steady increase in the cancer rates in New Haven. They proceeded to form cancer clinics in their hospitals and maintain uniform records. From these beginnings, the State Medical Society formed a Tumor Study Committee to coordinate cancer control activity in the State, and this body was instrumental in getting state legislation passed which created a Division of Cancer and other Chronic Diseases in 1935. In 1941 the tumor registry began operating statewide with a team from the Division visiting each hospital and abstracting all cancer records for the period 1935-1940. Subsequently the tumor clinic registrar, trained by the state team, continued abstracting and sending abstracts of cancer cases to the central cancer registry. It is the oldest continuous state cancer registry in the United States and has served as a model for other state registries. The Connecticut Tumor Registry first published incidence data in 1947, and every year thereafter.

New York State's interest in cancer control goes back to the late 19th century, when Dr. Roswell Park received a grant from the State Legislature to set up a state pathology laboratory in Buffalo. The Roswell Park Memorial Hospital, a 300 bed state cancer research hospital developed from this beginning.[272]

A Division of Cancer Control was established in 1931 at the Institute. Cancer was made a reportable disease in 1939 in New York State, exclusive of New York City, and transferred operations to the State Health Department in Albany. Its function was expanded from public education to training, nursing and laboratory resources, and research. Cancer reporting started in 1940 with the endorsement of the Medical Society of the State of New York. The State Registry has been a source for a number of research projects. Under the direction of Dr. Peter Greenwald, studies on the clustering of Hodgkin's disease cases and a number of surveillance studies were instituted.

The earliest attempt in the United States to estimate cancer incidence for the entire country was in 1937. Since cancer was not a reportable disease nationally, the NCI performed a study of a sample of the cases in 1937 to determine the incidence of cancer. This was referred to as the Ten Cities Cancer Survey.[273] Under the direction of Harold F. Dorn, the survey was conducted over a period of three years, 1937-1939, in a convenience sample of ten areas, mostly urban, comprising about ten percent of the country's population.

Reports were obtained from every hospital and from all but 2% of the physicians. It is estimated that only 8.5% of the cases were reported by death certificates only. The data from the study was used for estimating the incidence of cancer for the US and for observing variations by site, age, race and region of the country. It served as a baseline for evaluating cancer trends in subsequent national cancer surveys. And it taught much about the techniques to use and pitfalls to avoid in achieving complete registration in cancer surveys.

1940s

In 1948-1949, the NCI conducted its 2nd National Cancer Incidence Survey in the same ten areas surveyed in 1937-1939.[274] This survey was expanded to include analysis not only of age, sex and race but also by marital status and income class and by stage of disease and histologic type of cancer. Another section of the survey showed trends by site since the first survey.

The American Cancer Society (ACS) realized the need for registering cancer cases in the late 1940s and started giving assistance to hospital, regional and state registries. Requests came from hospital administrators, county and state medical societies.

In California cancer registration in hospitals started in 1949 when the California Tumor Registry in the State Health Department was founded.[275] In that year abstracting of cases in hospitals began going back to 1942. Over the next 14 years many more hospitals were added so that by 1956, 53 hospitals had cancer registries.

1950s

A manual for hospital cancer programs was prepared by the CoC in 1954, including a section on methods for reporting end results. In 1956 the requirements were amended to specify that an accredited cancer program must have a cancer registry.

Personnel from the American Cancer Society helped establish cancer registries in Iowa and Puerto Rico in the early 1950s which remain viable today. They also started registries in Alabama, Kentucky, and Michigan (Calhoun County). Some of the registries failed through lack of continuing funding but were reinstituted at a later date.

The data from the Connecticut Cancer Registry was integrated with data from eleven other cancer centers to become part of the End Results Group of the NCI in 1956. The End Results Group issued four reports in the 1950s and 1960s.[217] These reports were attempts to present survival figures on newly diagnosed cases from a number of state cancer registries and large hospital cancer registries in different parts of the country. The reports showed survival rates by age, sex, race and stage by site of cancer for different time periods of diagnosis going back to the 1940s. While these data did not comprise a random sample of all cancer cases in the country, they were the major source for tracking national survival rates by site and time period.

The Utah Cancer Registry was founded in 1966 by Charles R. Smart, M.D., an early advocate of cancer registries and their computerization.[276] The Utah Registry was established by the incorporation of several hospital tumor registries into a central registry, and with the cooperation of the remaining hospitals in the state. The primary purposes of the Registry were to provide service to hospitals and physicians, to provide a mechanism to stimulate frequent physician examinations of patients for recurrent or secondary malignancies, and to serve as an educational resource for physicians treating cancer patients.

1960s

Another survey, the Third National Cancer Survey (TNCS), was conducted by the NCI in 1969-1971, with some different geographic areas added.[277] This was planned as a three year survey around a census year in seven metropolitan areas and two entire states. A three-year survey was planned to get adequate incidence data on rare sites and to expand the coverage on rural areas of the country. Seven of the ten cities included in the 1937 and 1947 surveys were also in the TNCS for trend analyses. The entire states of Iowa and Colorado were in the survey, and the Minneapolis-St. Paul Metropolitan area was added. The Commonwealth of Puerto Rico also participated in the survey. In addition to analyses by demographic variables, and by site, histologic diagnosis, and stage of disease, the survey included questions on a 10% sample of cases in regard to treatment, duration of hospitalization, cost of medical care, and the economic impact on the family. In addition to the all sites survey, a special survey on skin cancer was conducted in four of the ten areas.

The survey compiled over 180,000 new cases over the three-year period with 90.1% microscopically confirmed. In the earlier two surveys about 74% were microscopically confirmed. Only 2.1% of the diagnosed cases were by death certificate only.

The primary purpose of these surveys was to obtain morbidity, mortality, and prevalence data. Patients were not followed for outcome. Because patients could not be followed for survival from surveys conducted every ten years, and because of the cost of setting up registries every ten years, the Third National Cancer Survey in 1969-1971 was the last of its kind.

1970s

In the early years of the Connecticut Registry's operations, compliance by physicians and hospitals in the state to furnish basic data and follow-up data was voluntary. Cancer

became a reportable disease by law in 1971 in Connecticut and in 1973 the law was extended to apply to private pathology laboratories.[271] The NCRA was chartered in 1974.

By 1972 new CoC standards stated that accredited hospital cancer programs in hospitals with 300 or more cancer patients annually must have full facilities and personnel, an active cancer registry, and ongoing research in cancer. Activities by the CoC expanded in the late 1970s and 1980s to provide expert help in setting up cancer registries in hospitals, and to provide expert assistance in design of forms and coding and technical assistance with computer operations.

Regional population based registries were formed in Los Angeles County in 1972 and the San Francisco-Oakland Bay Area (SFO) in 1973. The primary purpose of, and funding for, the Los Angeles County registry was provided to facilitate population-based analytic epidemiologic studies. In 1973, the Utah Registry also began epidemiologic studies of the Utah population. The Utah Cancer Registry covers a low-risk population, with low levels of overall cancer incidence.

In 1973, the SEER Program was started by the NCI.[27] Originally the program was designed to give annual reports on cancer incidence, mortality and survival from areas comprising about 10% of the population of the United States.[278] The areas in the 1973 survey included the states of Connecticut, Iowa, New Mexico, Utah and Hawaii, and the metropolitan areas of Atlanta, Detroit, Seattle and San Francisco-Oakland. Data from Puerto Rico was also collected but published separately.

A fifth report from the End Results Group was published in 1976 and included data from two state cancer registries and two hospital registries.[23] Comparison of overall 5-year relative survival rates in whites showed an increase from 39% in cases diagnosed in 1950-1959 to 41% in 1967-1973. Among blacks the increase was from 29% to 32%. Survival rates, as published by the NCI, thereafter are obtained from data collected in the SEER Program.

Interest in central cancer registries grew with the start of the SEER Program in 1973, which gave continuing financial assistance to the existing cancer registries in its program. Nationally, by 1977, there were 20 state cancer registries, and by 1979, 797 hospital cancer programs had been accredited by the CoC.[72]

1980s

In 1980, the NCI published data on 5-year survival rates from the same four registries as their 1976 report for 1960-1963 and 1970-1973.[22] The report showed a statistically significant increase in 5-year survival rates in the latter period in 17 of 35 sites in males and 26 of 35 sites in females.

In the 1980s additional state governments decided to fund central cancer registries and seven additional registries began between 1980 and 1984 and ten additional started between 1985 and 1989.

In 1983 the NCRA started a credentialing process for cancer registrars (CTR).

In 1987, cancer surveillance and control leaders formed the American Association of Central Cancer Registries (AACCR). The founding sponsors of the organization include the NCI, the American Cancer Society, the National Cancer Registrar's Association, the ACoS, and the American Association of Cancer Institutes. In 1995, the name was changed to NAACCR to formalize the inclusion of Canada (first as AACCR then NAACCR).

By the 1980s statewide registries were operating in 37 states, DC, Puerto Rico and Virgin Islands.

1990s

An important event which led to further development of state registries was the passage of the U.S. Cancer Registries Amendment Act in 1992, which allocated money to fund and enhance registries in all states, under a program administered by the CDC, the NPCR.[7] In 1995, funds were allocated to forty-two states and territories and the District of Columbia, representing 93% of the U.S. population. By 1993 there were more than 1300 hospitals with CoC accredited cancer programs.[279]

In 1994 NAACCR developed and published a set of data standards and a standardized data transfer format for cancer registries, later in 1995, NAACCR published incidence data from forty-eight central registries in the United States and Canada. Additional registries were added each year as more of them become population-based and are able to identify at least 95% of the cases in their areas.[21] In 1997, NAACCR instituted a program to annually review and certify the completeness, accuracy and timeliness of central registry data from across North America. Silver or Gold recognition is awarded based on increasing levels of quality excellence.

2000s

In 2000, the NPCR program was providing funding for 45 states, 3 territories, and the District of Columbia. Forty-three of these grants were to enhance current statewide registries, and 2 were to plan new registries. As of 2010, the NPCR provided funding for central registries in 45 states, the District of Columbia, Puerto Rico, and the U.S. Pacific Island Jurisdictions. Funds for the remaining five states are provided by the SEER Program.

Much progress has been made in central cancer registries in the United States since the first attempt in Massachusetts in 1927. Major milestones in the history of U.S. central cancer registries are listed in Table 36-14.

All states now have central registries and legislation requiring cancer reporting. Central registries also share data on patients diagnosed in one area who reside in another. What has not changed, however, is the reliance central registries have on hospital registries. In fact, in this country

Table 36-14	Timeline of U.S. Central Cancer Registry History		
1926	Pilot Massachusetts Registry	1973	Connecticut law making cancer reportable by independent pathology laboratories
1935	Reference date for Connecticut Registry		
1937-39	Ten Cities Cancer Survey	1973	San Francisco-Oakland Registry started
1939	New York law making cancer reportable (excluding New York City)	1974	NCRA formed
		1977	20 state registries exist
1941	Connecticut registry started	1979	797 CoC Approved hospital cancer programs
1948-49	Second National Cancer Survey		
1949	California Tumor Registry started	1983	CTR credentialing began
1950s	Registries started in Alabama, Iowa, Kentucky, Puerto Rico, and Michigan (Calhoun County)	1987	NAACCR formed
		1989	37 state registries exist
		1994	Standardized data set established by NAACCR Uniform Data Standards Committee (UDS)
1954	CoC published manual for hospital cancer programs		
1956	End Results Group started	1996	Standardized edits established by NAACCR UDS
1960s	First survival publications by End Results Group	1998	First NAACCR Incidence Report
		1992	U.S. Cancer Registries Amendment Act passed
1966	Utah Registry started.		
1969-71	Third National Cancer Survey	1995	First SEER Incidence Report
1971	Connecticut law making cancer reportable by hospitals	1993	NPCR started
		1997	NAACCR registry certification program started
1972	Los Angeles County Registry started		
1973	SEER Program started		

central registries grew out of hospital registries, and most still rely on them to identify and report the bulk of the cancer cases. It continues to be essential for these two types of registries to work together to help each other accomplish their goals of reducing the incidence, morbidity, and mortality of cancer in the U.S.

Summary

The central registry, because of its comprehensive coverage, is an essential tool in community-based and other research. The central registry is essential for many types of research and should be utilized. As expressed by Greenwald et al., "We think that any registry-hospital, local, regional, or national—must devote at least as much resources, time, and talent to its use for research and control purposes as it does to data acquisition, computerization, and publication of annual reports. Otherwise, it is doubtful that the registry investment is being optimally utilized."[262]

Many thanks to the faculty members of the NAACCR Short Course.[197] The writings and teaching materials of the course were used extensively.

References

1. MacLennan, R., Muir, C., Steinitz, R., Winkler, A. *Cancer Registration and Its Techniques* (IARC Scientific Publications No. 21). Lyon, France: International Agency for Research on Cancer, 1978.
2. Jensen, O. M., Parkin, D. M., MacLennan, R., Muir, C. S., Skeet, R. G. *Cancer Registration Principles and Methods* (IARC Scientific Publication No. 95). Lyon, France: International Agency for Research on Cancer, 1991.
3. Menck, H. R., Smart, C. R., editors. *Central Cancer Registries: Design, Management and Use.* Langhorne, PA: Harwood Academic Publishers, 1994.
4. Menck, H. R., Deapen, D., Phillips, J. L., Tucker, T. C., editors. *Central Cancer Registries: Design, Management and Use.* Alexandria, VA: National Cancer Registrars Association, Inc., 2007.
5. Menck, H. R., West, D. "Central Cancer Registries." In *Cancer Registry Management Principles & Practice,* edited by C. L. Hutchinson, S. D. Roffers, A. G. Fritz. Dubuque, IA: Kendall Hunt Publishing Company, 1997.
6. McKeen, K. M., Davidson, A. N. M. *The Surveillance, Epidemiology and End Results Program: Cancer Registry Management Principles & Practice,* edited by C. L. Hutchinson, S. D. Roffers, A. G. Fritz. Dubuque, IA: Kendall Hunt Publishing Company, 1997.
7. Hutton, M. D., Simpson, L. D., Miller, D. S., Weir, H. K., McDavid, K., Hall, H. I. "Progress Toward Nationwide Cancer Surveillance: An Evaluation of the National Program of Cancer Registries, 1994-1999," *Journal of Registry Management,* 2001;28(3):113–120.
8. Howe, H. L. "Population-Based Cancer Registries in the United States" (pp. 1–10). In *Cancer Incidence in North America, 1988-1990, Vol. VI,* edited by H. L. Howe, et al. Springfield, IL: American Association of Central Cancer Registries, 1994.
9. *ELM National Oncology Data Base.* Rockville, MD: ELM Services Inc., 1988.
10. Liss, J. M. "The MRS National Data Set 1989. Part 1: Description and Overview" (pp. 1–5). *Medical Registry Reports 5.* Hackensack, NJ: Medical Registry Services, Inc., 1991.
11. Eberle, C., Fremgen, A., Wynn, G. The National Cancer Data Base. In *Cancer Registry Management Principles & Practice,* edited by C. L. Hutchinson, S. D. Roffers, A. G. Fritz. Dubuque, IA: Kendall Hunt Publishing Company, 1997.
12. Dorn, R: "Federal Registries." In *Cancer Registry Management Principles & Practice,* edited by C. L. Hutchinson, S. D. Roffers, A. G. Fritz. Dubuque, IA: Kendall Hunt Publishing Company, 1997.
13. ACTUR: Automated Central Tumor Registry (ACTUR), Defense Enrollment Eligibility Reporting System. Users Manual. UM1006EL R2. Washington, DC: The Assistant Secretary of Defense for Health Affairs and the Assistant Secretary of Defense for Force Management and Personnel, 1992.
14. Parkin, D. M., Sanghvi, L. D. "Cancer Registration in Developing Countries." In *Cancer Registration Principles and Methods* (IARC Scientific Publication No. 95), edited by O. M. Jensen, D. M. Parkin, R. MacLennan, C. S. Muir, R. G. Skeet. Lyon, France: International Agency for Research on Cancer, 1991.
15. IARC/IACR. *Cancer Incidence in Five Continents, Vol. 6* (IARC Publication No. 120). Lyon, France: International Agency for Research on Cancer, 1993.
16. Roffers, S. D. "Cancer Registries in Other Countries." In *Cancer Registry Management Principles & Practice,* edited by C. L. Hutchinson, S. D. Roffers, A. G. Fritz. Dubuque, IA: Kendall Hunt Publishing Company, 1997.
17. Health and Welfare Canada. "The Making of the Canadian Cancer Registry: Cancer Incidence in Canada and Its Regions 1969 to 1988." Bureau of Chronic Disease Epidemiology, Laboratory Centre for Disease Control, Health and Welfare Canada, Ottawa, Canada.
18. Skeet, R. G. "Manual and Computerized Cancer Registries." In *Cancer Registration Principles and Methods* (IARC Scientific Publication No. 95), edited by O. M. Jensen, D. M. Parkin, R. MacLennan, C. S. Muir, R. G. Skeet. Lyon, France: International Agency for Research on Cancer, 1991.
19. Young, J. L. "The Hospital-Based Cancer Registry." In *Cancer Registration Principles and Methods* (IARC Scientific Publication No. 95), edited by O. M. Jensen, D. M. Parkin, R. MacLennan, C. S. Muir, R. G. Skeet. Lyon, France: International Agency for Research on Cancer, 1991.
20. Austin, D. F. "Types of Registries: Goals and Objectives" (pp. 1–11). In *Central-Cancer Registries: Design, Management and Use,* edited by H. R. Menck, C. R. Smart. Langhorne, PA: Harwood Academic Publishers, 1994.
21. Clive, R. E., Miller, D. S. "Introduction to Cancer Registries." In *Cancer Registry Management Principles & Practice,* edited by C. L. Hutchinson, S. D. Roffers, A. G. Fritz. Dubuque, IA: Kendall Hunt Publishing Company, 1997.
22. Kosary, C. L., Ries, L. A. G., Miller, B. A., et al. "SEER Cancer Statistics Review, 1973-1992: Tables and Graphs

(NIH Publication No. 96-2789)." Bethesda, MD: National Cancer Institute, National Institutes of Health, 1995.

23. Myers, M. H., Ries, L. A. "Cancer Patient Survival Rates: SEER Program Results for 10 Years of Follow-up," *CA Cancer J Clin* 1989;39(1):21–32.

24. Parkin, D. M., Hakulinen, T. *Analysis of Survival, in Cancer Registration Principles and Methods* (IARC Scientific Publication No. 95), edited by O. M. Jensen, D. M. Parkin, R. MacLennan, C. S. Muir, R. G. Skeet. Lyon, France: International Agency for Research on Cancer, 1991.

25. Deapen, D., Berglund, L. C., Bernstein, L. C., Ross, R. K. "Cancer in Los Angeles County, A Bibliography 1972-2000." Los Angeles: Cancer Surveillance Program, University of Southern California School of Medicine, 2001.

26. Guinan, P., Stewart, A. K., Fremgen, A. M., Menck, H. R. "Patterns of Care for Metastatic Carcinoma of the Prostate Gland: Results of the American College of Surgeons' Patient Care Evaluation Study," *Prostate Cancer and Prostatic Diseases,* 1998;1:315–320.

27. Janes, R. H., Niederhuber, J. E., Chmiel, J. S., Winchester, D. P., Ocwieja, K. C., Karnell, L. H., Clive, R. E., Menck, H. R. "National Patterns of Care for Pancreatic Cancer: Results of a Survey by the Commission on Cancer," *Annals of Surgery,* 1996;223:261–272.

28. Steele, G. D., Osteen, R. T., Winchester, D. P., Murphy, G. P., Menck, H. R. "Clinical Highlights from the National Cancer Data Base: 1994," *CA Journal for Clinicians,* 1994;44:71–80.

29. *ACS Cancer Facts and Figures.* Atlanta, GA: American Cancer Society 2010. Found at: http://www.cancer.org/Research/CancerFactsFigures/index.

30. Hisserich, J. C., Martin, S. P., Henderson, B. E. "An Area-wide Cancer Reporting Network," *Public Health Reports,* 1975:90;15–17.

31. Parkin, D. M. "The Role of Cancer Registries in Cancer Control," *International Journal of Clinical Oncology,* 2008;13:102–111.

32. Armstrong, B. K. "The Role of the Cancer Registry in Cancer Control, *Cancer Causes Control,* 1992:3(6):569–579.

33. Deapen, D., Menck, H. R., Ervin, I. L., Leventhal, M., Niland, J. C. "Experience in Developing E-path Cancer Reporting for Rapid Case Ascertainment," *Journal of Registry Management,* 2002;29:2, 44–51.

34. National Cancer Data Base. Available at: http://www.facs.org/cancer/ncdb/index.html. Revised December 18, 2009.

35. Bilimoria, K. Y., Stewart, A. K., Winchester, D. P., Ko, C. Y. "The National Cancer Data Base: A Powerful Initiative to Improve Cancer Care in the United States," *Ann Surg Oncol* 2008;15(3):683–690.

36. Surveillance, Epidemiology, and End Results (SEER) Program Overview. Available at: http://www.seer.cancer.gov/about/. Accessed April 3, 2010.

37. National Program of Cancer Registries. Available at: http://www.cdc.gov/cancer/npcr/about.htm. Revised March 15, 2010.

38. Jensen, O. M., Whelan, S. "Planning a Cancer Registry." In *Cancer Registration Principles and Methods* (IARC Scientific Publication No. 95), edited by O. M. Jensen, D. M. Parkin, R. MacLennan, C. S. Muir, R. G. Skeet. Lyon, France: IARC, 1991.

39. Watkins, S., MacKinnon, J., Price, W. "Legislation, Affiliation and Governance." In *Central Cancer Registries: Design, Management and Use* (pp. 13–18), edited by H. R. Menck, C. R. Smart. Langhorne, PA: Harwood Academic Publishers, 1994.

40. Fisher, R., Haenlein, M. "Legislative Authorizations for Cancer Registries." In *State Cancer Legislative Database Update,* Bethesda, MD: National Cancer Institute, National Institutes of Health, 1991.

41. Centers for Disease Control and Prevention. "State Cancer Registries: Status of Authorization Legislation and Enabling Regulations—United States, October 1993," *MMWR Morbidity and Mortality Weekly Report,* 1994;43(4):71, 74–75.

42. Bates, P. M. "Proactive, Productive, and Progressive: New Legislation Helps Keep the "Pro" in Cancer Registries." *For the Record,* May 20, 2002.

43. Fritz, A., Roffers, S. "Marketing Cancer Information and Services." National Cancer Registrars Association. Available at: http://www.ncra-usa.org.

44. Desler, M. S. "Interfacing with Organizations." In *Cancer Registry Management Principles & Practice,* edited by C. L. Hutchinson, S. D. Roffers, A. G. Fritz. Dubuque, IA: Kendall Hunt Publishing Company, 1997.

45. Watkins, S., MacKinnon, J., Price, W. "Budgets and Staffing" (pp. 111–130). In *Central Cancer Registries: Design, Management and Use,* edited by H. R. Menck, C. R. Smart. Langhorne, PA: Harwood Academic Publishers, 1994.

46. Steban, D., Whelan, S., Laudico, A., Parkin, D. M. *Manual for Cancer Registry Personnel* (IARC Technical Report No. 10). Lyon, France: International Agency for Research on Cancer, 1995.

47. Ward, S., DeCoe, B. M. "Cancer Registry Personnel, Office Space, and Equipment." In *Cancer Registry Management Principles & Practice,* edited by C. L. Hutchinson, S. D. Roffers, A. G. Fritz. Dubuque, IA: Kendall Hunt Publishing Company, 1997.

48. National Cancer Registrars Association, Inc., American College of Surgeons Commission on Cancer. *Cancer Registry Staffing & Compensation Manual, Results of a Survey Conducted for the National Cancer Registrars Association.* Alexandria, VA: National Cancer Registrars Association, 2001.

49. Joneikis, V. K. "Cancer Registry Management." In *Cancer Registry Management Principles & Practice,* edited by C. L. Hutchinson, S. D. Roffers, A. G. Fritz. Dubuque, IA: Kendall Hunt Publishing Company, 1997.

50. Phillips, K. "How Much Time Would a Registrar Take If a Registrar Did Have Time." *Advance,* May 21, 2001.

51. Menck, H. R., Parkin, D. M., editors. *Directory of Computer Systems Used in Cancer Registries.* Lyon, France: WHO International Agency for Research on Cancer, 1985.

52. Watkins, S. "Cancer Registry Budget." In *Cancer Registry Management Principles & Practice,* edited by C. L. Hutchinson, S. D. Roffers, A. G. Fritz. Dubuque, IA: Kendall Hunt Publishing Company, 1997.

53. Weir, H. K., Berg, G. D., Mansley, E. C., Belloni, K. A. "The National Program of Cancer Registries: Explaining State Variations in Average Cost per Case Reported," Preventing Chronic Disease, 2005;2(3):A10.

54. Muir, C. S., Demeret, E. "Cancer Registration: Legal Aspects and Confidentiality." In *Cancer Registration Principles and Methods* (IARC Scientific Publication No. 95), edited by O. M. Jensen, D. M. Parkin, R. MacLennan, C. S. Muir,

R. G. Skeet. Lyon, France: International Agency for Research on Cancer, 1991.

55. Coleman, M. P., Muir, C. S., Menegoz, F. "Confidentiality in the Cancer Registry," *British Journal of Cancer,* 1992;66:1138–1149.

56. Stiller, C. A. "Cancer Registration: Its Uses in Research and Confidentiality in the European Community," *Journal of Epidemiology and Community Health,* 1993;47:342–344.

57. Chen, V. W. "The Right to Know vs. the Right to Privacy," *Journal of Registry Management,* 1997:125–127.

58. Hofferkamp, J., editor. *Standards for Cancer Registries, Vol. III: Standards for Completeness, Quality, Analysis, Management, Security and Confidentiality of Data.* Springfield, IL: North American Association of Central Cancer Registries, August 2008.

59. North American Association of Central Cancer Registries. *2002 NAACCR Workshop Report: Data Security and Confidentiality.* Springfield, IL: North American Association of Central Cancer Registries, May 2002. Available at: http://old. naaccr.org/filesystem/pdf/Data%20Confidentiality%20 Workshop%20Summary.pdf.

60. North American Association of Central Cancer Registries. "Policy Statement 99-01: Confidentiality." Available at: http://www.naaccr.org.

61. Office of Civil Rights Web site: http://www.hhs.gov/ocr/ privacy/hipaa/understanding/summary/index.html. Accessed April 2, 2010.

62. Berry, G. "HIPAA's Impact on the CTR Professional," *Advance,* February 18, 2002.

63. "The National Cancer Registrar Association Guide to the Interpretation of the Code of Ethics." In *Cancer Registry Management Principles & Practice,* edited by C. L. Hutchinson, S. D. Roffers, A. G. Fritz. Dubuque, IA: Kendall Hunt Publishing Company, 1997.

64. Coughlin, S. S., Clutter, G. C., Hutton, M. "Ethics in Cancer Registries," *Journal of Registry Management,* 1999;26:5–10.

65. Overton, P., McCracken, K. J. "Using the NCRA Code of Ethics: Responsible Reporting." *The Connection,* 1997;16.

66. Coughlin, S. S., Soskolne, C. L., Goodman, K. W. *Case Studies in Public Health Ethics.* Washington, DC: American Public Health Association, 1997.

67. Levine, R. J. The Institutional Review Board (pp. 257–273). In *Ethics and Epidemiology,* edited by S. S. Coughlin, T. L. Beauchamp. New York: Oxford University Press, 1996.

68. Johnson, C., Phillips, J. L. *Standards for Data and Data Management: Cancer Registry Management Principles & Practice,* edited by C. L. Hutchinson, S. D. Roffers, A. G. Fritz. Dubuque, IA: Kendall Hunt Publishing Company, 1997.

69. Gordon, B. "Data Set Planning." In *Central Cancer Registries: Design, Management and Use,* edited by H. Menck, C. Smart. Chur, Switzerland: Harwood Academic Publishers, 1994.

70. Howe, H. H. "Recommendations for Public Use Files of National Cancer Data. A Report of a Workshop Held at the Broadmoor, Colorado Springs, CO, August 25-27, 1997." North American Association of Central Cancer Registries, November 1997.

71. MacLennan, R. "Items of Patient Information Which May Be Collected By Registries." In *Cancer Registration Principles and Methods* (IARC Scientific Publication No. 95), edited by O. M. Jensen, D. M. Parkin, R. MacLennan, C. S. Muir, R. G. Skeet. Lyon, France: International Agency for Research on Cancer, 1991.

72. Thornton, M., O'Connor, L., editors. *Standards for Cancer Registries, Vol. II: Data Standards and Data Dictionary, Record Layout Version 12,* 14th ed. Springfield, IL: North American Association of Central Cancer Registries, February 2009, rev. August 2009.

73. Commission on Cancer. *Manual for Cancer Programs.* Chicago: American College of Surgeons, 1956.

74. SEER Program. *The Seer Program Code Manual,* rev. ed. Bethesda, MD: National Cancer Institute, 1992.

75. Shambaugh, E. "Comparability of Cancer Data," *Proceedings of Central Registry Workshop,* Chicago, American College of Surgeons, December 7–8, 1979.

76. *NAACCR Committee Manual and Guidelines.* Springfield, IL: NAACCR, March 2007. Available at: http://www.naaccr. org/LinkClick.aspx?fileticket=CuAfEe0Nw3A%3d&tabid =161&mid=523, accessed April 14, 2010.

77. "NAACCR New Data Item—Review Process Diagram." Springfield, IL: NAACCR, October 2007. Available at: http://www.naaccr.org/

78. Havener, L. editor. *Standards for Cancer Registries, Vol. I: Data Exchange Standards and Record Descriptions, Version 12.* Springfield, IL: North American Association of Central Cancer Registries, February 2009.

79. Commission on Cancer American College of Surgeons. *Facility Oncology Registry Data Standards Revised for 2010.* Chicago: American College of Surgeons, Supplement 2010.

80. Adamo, M. B., Johnson, C. H., editors. *SEER Program Coding and Staging Manual 2010* (NIH Publication number 10-5581). Bethesda, MD: National Cancer Institute, 2010.

81. Clive, R. "Major Standard Setters for Central Registries." Course materials for the NAACCR Short course: Central Cancer Registries: Design, Management and Use, provided annually at the NAACCR meeting.

82. Passaro, E., Organ, C. H. "Ernest A. Codman: The Improper Bostonian," *Bulletin of the American College of Surgeons,* 1999;84(1):16–22.

83. Brennan, M., Clive, R., Winchester, D. "The COC: Its Roots and Its Destiny," *Bulletin of the American College of Surgeons,* 1994;79(6):14.

84. Blankenship, C., Moore, M., Opaluch, G. M., Sylvester, J: *The American College of Surgeons Commission on Cancer and the Approvals Program: Cancer Registry Management Principles & Practice,* edited by C. L. Hutchinson, S. D. Roffers, A. G. Fritz. Dubuque, IA: Kendall Hunt Publishing Company, 1997.

85. Greene, F., Morrow, M., Sylvester, J. "New Initiatives Underway at the ACOS Commission on Cancer," *Oncology Issues,* 2000:22–23.

86. Morrow, M., Sylvester, J. "The Cancer Program of the American College of Surgeons," *Current Problems in Cancer,* 2001;25(2):98–112.

87. Menck, H. R., Blankenship, C., Fremgen, A. M. "The National Cancer Data Base and Physician Network," *Topics in Health Information Management,* 1997;17:45–59.

88. Sylvester, J., Blankenship, C., Carter, A., Douglas, L., Stewart, A. "Quality Control: The American College of Surgeons Commission on Cancer Standards, National Cancer Data Base, and Cancer Liaison Program," *Journal of Registry Management,* 2000;27(2):68–74.

89. McGinnis, L. "The Field Liaison Program: Why Bother?" *Bulletin of the American College of Surgeons,* 1983;68(9):22.

90. Jessup, J. M., Menck, H. R., Winchester, D. P., Hundahl, S. A., Murphy, G. P. "The National Cancer Data Base Report on Patterns of Hospital Reporting," *Cancer,* 1996;78:1829–1837.

91. Menck, H. R., Bland, K. I., Scott-Conner, C. E. H., Eyre, H., Murphy, G. P., Winchester, D. P. "Regional Diversity and Breadth of the National Cancer Data Base," *Cancer,* 1998;83:2649–2658.

92. Edge, S. B., Byrd, D. R., Compton, C. C., Fritz, A. G., Greene, F. L., Trotti, A., editors. *AJCC Cancer Staging Manual,* 7th ed. Chicago: American Joint Committee on Cancer, 2010.

93. Hutchinson, C. L., Roffers, S. D., Fritz, A. G. *Cancer Registry Management Principles & Practice.* Dubuque, IA: Kendall Hunt Publishing Company, 1997.

94. Seiffert, J., Young, J. L. *The North American Association of Central Cancer Registries. Cancer Registry Management Principles & Practice,* edited by C. L. Hutchinson, S. D. Roffers, A. G. Fritz. Dubuque, IA: Kendall Hunt Publishing Company, 1997.

95. Swan, J., Wingo, P., Clive, R., et al. "Cancer Surveillance in the US: Can We Have a National System?" *Cancer,* 1998;83(7):1282–1291.

96. World Health Organization. *International Classification of Disease for Oncology.* Geneva: World Health Organization, 1976.

97. World Health Organization. *International Classification of Diseases for Oncology,* 2nd edition. Geneva: World Health Organization, 1990.

98. World Health Organization. *International Classification of Diseases for Oncology,* 3rd edition, U.S. Interim Version 2000 (ICD-O-3). Geneva: World Health Organization, 2000.

99. Douglas, L. L. "Collaborative Stage: An Update," *Journal of Registry Management,* 2001;28(4):196–203.

100. "Collaborative Stage Data Collection System: About Us." Available at: http://www.cancerstaging.org/cstage/about.html. Revised January 2010.

101. Phillips, J. L., Gress, D. M. "Comparison of Registrar Collaborative Staging and Physician AJCC Staging Using Data Submitted to the National Cancer Data Base," *Journal of Registry Management,* 2008;35(1); 4–11.

102. Stewart, A. K. "The Rubber Meets the Road: Results of the CSv2 Field Study on the Collection of Site-Specific Factors," *Journal of Registry Management,* 2009;36(4):139–142.

103. Havener, L., editor. *Standards for Cancer Registries, Vol. V: Pathology Laboratory Electronic Reporting, Version 3.0.* Springfield, IL: North American Association of Central Cancer Registries, July 2009.

104. Tucker T, Howe H, Kohler B, Fulton JP. Adapting the HL-7 Standard for Cancer Registry Work, at: http://www.naaccr.org.

105. Health Level Seven (HL-7), at http://www.hl7.org.

106. Toal S, Lezin N. Working Toward Implementation of HL7 in NAACCR Information Technology Standards: Meeting Summary Report, at http://www.cdc.gov/cancer/npcr/npcrpdfs/ hl7mtg8.pdf

107. SEER Program. Book 2 Cancer Characteristics and Selection of Cases (1991). NIH Publication No. 92-993, at http://seer.canccr.gov/publications/onlinepubs/pubs.html.

108. Surawicz, Tanya; McCarthy, Bridget J.; Jukich, Patti J.; and Davis, Faith G. The accuracy and completeness of primary brain and central nervous system tumor data: Results from the Central Brain Tumor Registry of the United States. J of Registry Management 27(2):51-55, 2000.

109. Jean-Baptiste R, Gebhard IK (eds). Procedure Guidelines for Cancer Registries, Series IV. Cancer Case Ascertainment. NAACCR; February 2002.

110. Seiffert J., Hoyler SS, McKeen K, and Potts M, "Casefinding, Abstracting, and Death Clearance." In Menck, H. R., and C. R. Smart (eds.) Central Cancer Registries.- Design, Management and Use. Langhorne, PA: Harwood Academic Publishers, ISBN 3718605791, 1994, pp. 35-64.

111. SEER. Multiple Primary and Histology Coding Rules, January 01, 2007. Available at: http://seer.cancer.gov/tools/mphrules/2007_mphrules_manual_04302008.pdf.

112. Potts M, Hafterson J, Wacker FF, Serbent J: Case Ascertainment. In *Cancer Registry Management Principles & Practice* (eds CL Hutchinson, SD Roffers, AG Fritz), Dubuque, Iowa: Kendall Hunt Publishing Company; 1997.

113. Powell J: Data Sources and Reporting, in Cancer Registration Principles and Methods: (eds. OM Jensen, DM Parkin, R MacLennan, CS Muir, RG Skeet: Lyons: IARC; 1991. IARC Scientific Publication No. 95. ISBN 9283211952.

114. Menck HR. E-path Reporting: Electronic Casefinding. J Registry Management 2002;29:2, 37-38.

115. Dale D, Golabek JK, Chong N: The Impact of E-path Technology on the Ontario Cancer Registry Operations. JRM 2002;27(2):52-56.

116. Aldinger WL, Rydzewski S: Early Experiences with E-path Reporting in Pennsylvania: Non-Hospital Sources. JRM 2002;27(2):39-43.

117. Phillips JL, Menck HR: Computerization, in Central Cancer Registries: Design, Management and Use (eds. H Menck, C Smart), Chur, Switzerland, Harwood Academic Publishers; 1994.

118. Menck HR. Selecting Your Cancer Registry Software. Oncology Issues 2002;17:32-34.

119. NAACCR Procedure Guidelines for Cancer Registries, Series II. Calculating the DCO Rate, June 2000. Available at: http://old.naaccr.org/filesystem/pdf/SeriesIISection.pdf.

120. NAACCR, Death Clearance Procedures for Central Registrics, CD Training Module. Available at: http://www.naaccr.org.

121. Fulton JP, Wingo P, Jamison M, Roffers S, Howe HL, Chen VW. Exploring the Effects of Death Certificate Follow-Back on Cancer Registration, at http://www.naaccr.org.

122. NAACCR's Death Clearance Manual 2009. Available at: http://www.naaccr.org/LinkClick.aspx?fileticket=RD1FxWlmC24%3d&tabid=130&mid=470.

123. Johnson CH, Hutchinson CL: General Principles of Abstracting and Cancer Registry Files. In *Cancer Registry Management Principles & Practice* (eds CL Hutchinson, SD Roffers, AG Fritz), Dubuque, Iowa: Kendall Hunt Publishing Company; 1997.

124. LeTendre DC, Rosemary D, Riddle S and Creech CM. *Where did they really live? Resolving discrepancies in address at diagnosis.* J of Registry Management 27(2):57-58, 2000.

125. Dolecek TA, Lawhun G, Vann S, Snodgrass JL and Stewart SL: *Hispanic identification in the Illinois State Cancer Registry.* J of Registry Management 27(2):43-50, 2000.

126. Berry G: Collecting Race and Ethnicity Data in the Registry. Advance, December 17, 2001.

127. NAACCR Procedure Guidelines for Cancer Registries Series I: Interstate Data Exchange, January 2001. Available at: http://old.naaccr.org/filesystem/pdf/SeriesISection.pdf

128. Department of Defense Automated Central Tumor Registry (ACTUR), accessed April 13, 2010. Available at: http://www.afip.org/consultation/actur/.

129. NAACCR: Cancer Registry Management Reports (NAACCR Instructional Module for Cancer Registries), J. Seiffert, North American Association of Central Cancer Registries, 1998.

130. Coleman MP, Bieber CA: CANREG: Cancer Registration Software for Microcomputers, in Cancer Registration Principles and Methods: (eds. OM Jensen, DM Parkin, R MacLennan, CS Muir, RG Skeet: Lyons, France: IARC Scientific Publication No. 95. ISBN 9283211952, 1991.

131. Williamson TJ, McKelvey LW: Computer Principles. In Cancer Registry Management Principles & Practice (eds CL Hutchinson, SD Roffers, AG Fritz), Dubuque, Iowa: Kendall Hunt Publishing Company; 1997.

132. Rocky Mountain Cancer Data Systems - Research Park, 420 Chipeta Way, Suite 120, Salt Lake City, UT 84108. (801) 581-4307 http://rmcds6.med.utah.edu

133. Cancer Patient Data Management System, Kentucky Cancer Registry, 2365 Harrodsburg Road, Lexington, KY 40536-3381. (859) 219-0773 www.kcr.uky.edu

134. Registry Plus, a suite of publicly available software programs for collecting and processing cancer registry data. Atlanta (GA): U.S. Department of Health and Human Services, Centers for Disease Control and Prevention, National Center for Chronic Disease Prevention and Health Promotion; 2010. Available at: http://www.cdc.gov/cancer/npcr/.

135. Précis-Central Central Registry Data Management System IMPAC, Medical Systems Inc., 100 W. Evelyn Avenue, Mountain View, CA 94041. (650) 623-8800 www.impac.com

136. C/NET Solutions, 1936 University Ave., Suite 112, Berkeley, CA 94704-1024. (800) 366-2638 www.askcnet.org.

137. C/NExT – C/NET Solutions, 1936 University Ave., Suite 112, Berkeley, CA 94704-1024. (800) 366-2638 www.askcnet.org

138. Electronic Registry Services - 270 Northland Blvd, Suite 111, Cincinnati, OH 45246. (800) 824-9020 www.ers-can.com

139. METRIQ. Elekta IMPAC, Medical Systems Inc., 100 W. Evelyn Avenue, Mountain View, CA 94041. (650) 623-8800 www.impac.com

140. Oncolog, Inc. - 1665 Liberty Street SE, P.O. Box 2226, Salem, OR 97308. (800) 345-6626 www.oncolog.com

141. Van Holten V: Editing for Consistency of Data Items, in. Cancer Registration Principles and Methods: (eds. OM Jensen, DM Parkin, R MacLennan, CS Muir, RG Skeet: Lyons: IARC; 1991. IARC Scientific Publication No. 95. ISBN 9283211952.

142. NAACCR: Volume IV: Standard Data Edits, Standards for Cancer Registries, at: http://www.naaccr.org/StandardsandRegistryOperations/VolumeIV.aspx.

143. Commission on Cancer American College of Surgeons: Standards of the Commission on Cancer, Volume III: Data Edits, at http://www.facs.org/dept/cancer/index.html.

144. *NAACCR Call for Data Instructions*, at: http://www.naaccr.org/DataandPublications/CallforData.aspx.

145. NAACCR. Instructions for Using Metafiles and GenEDITS, at: http://www.naaccr.org/DataandPublications/CallforData.aspx

146. NAACCR Edits metafile, at http://www.naaccr.org/StandardsandRegistryOperations/VolumeIV.aspx

147. NAACCR Edits Changes, at http://www.naaccr.org/StandardsandRegistryOperations/VolumeIV.aspx

148. SEER Edit Documentation. Bethesda, MD: SEER Program, National Cancer Institute; 1993.

149. SEER Publications, at http://www.seer.cancer.gov, including ICD-O-2 to 3 and ICD-O-3 to 2, ICD-9 to ICD-10, ICD-10 to ICD-9, ICD-O-2 to ICD-9, ICD-O-2 to ICD-10, ICD-O-1 to ICD-O-2, ICD-0-2 to ICD-9-(CM), ICD-O-2 to ICD-10.

150. Clark PM, Gomez EG: Details on Demand: Consumers, Cancer Information, and the Internet. Clinical J of Oncology Nursing 5;1: 19-24, 2001.

151. Fritz, AG. Just trying to keep up: Journal scanning services. J of Registry Management 27(1):25-26, 2000.

152. Wiggins L. (ed.). Using Geographic Information Systems Technology in the Collection, Analyses and Presentation of Cancer Registry Data: A Handbook to Basic Practices. Springfield, IL: NAACCR, October 2002.

153. Thomas B. Generalized Record Linkage System at: http://www.naaccr.org.

154. Ulmer C, McFadden B, Nerenz DR (eds). Race, Ethnicity, And Language Data Standardization For Health Care Quality Improvement. Subcommittee on Standardized Collection of Race/Ethnicity Data for Healthcare Quality Improvement, Board on Health Care Services, Institute Of Medicine Of The National Academies, The National Academies Press, Washington, D.C., 2009.

155. Thoburn KK, Gu, D, Rawson. Fundamentals of Linking Public Health Datasets: Link Plus Probabilistic Record Linkage Software. Presented on the National Association of Health Data Organizations-CDC (Assessment Initiative) 2nd Probabilistic Record Linkage Conference Call, March 30, 2007.

156. Thoburn KK, Gu, D, Rawson, Rogers JD. Make the Most of Your Data with CDC's Link Plus: Free, Fast, and Efficient Probabilistic Record Linkage Program. Presented at the National Association of Health Data Organizations 22nd Annual Meeting, October 18, 2007.

157. Borges HT; Watkins J, Stafford R; and Biggar RJ. Linkage of selected AIDS and cancer registries in the United States. J of Registry Management 28(2):89-92, 2001

158. Cooksley C; Hwang L and Ford CC. HIV and cancer: Community-based analysis of trends and registry linkage. J of Registry Management 28(2):82-88, 2001.

159. Korzeniewski SJ, Grigorescu V, Copeland G, Gu G, Thoburn KK, Rogers JD, Young WI. Methodological Innovations in Data Gathering: Newborn Screening Linkage with Live Births Records, Michigan, 1/2007-3/2008. Matern Child Health J. 2009 Apr 8.

160. Johnson JC, Soliman AS, Tadgerson D, Copeland GE, Seefeld DA, Pingatore NL, Haverkate R, Banerjee M, Roubidoux MA. Tribal linkage and race data quality for American Indians in a state cancer registry. Am J Prev Med. 2009 Jun;36(6):549-54.

161. Weir HK, Jim MA, Marrett LD, Fairley T. Cancer in American Indian and Alaska Native young adults (ages 20-44 years): US, 1999-2004. Cancer 113(65):1153-1167, 2008.

162. Wilde ET. Do Response Times Matter? The Impact of EMS Response Times on Health Outcomes. Princeton University, 2007.

163. Balciau P. Comparison of two Probabilistic Record Linkage Software Programs: Link Plus and Automatch. Presented at the NAACCR Annual Meeting, 2004.

164. Campbell KM. Record linkage software in the public domain: a comparison of Link Plus, The Link King, and a 'basic' deterministic algorithm. Health Informatics Journal, Vol. 14, No. 1, 5-15 (2008).

165. SEER Stat and SEER Prep. Available at: http://seer.cancer.gov.

166. SEER Joinpoint Regression Program at http://seer.cancer.gov.

167. Kim HJ, Fay MP, Feuer EJ, Midthune DN. Permutation Tests for Joinpoint Regression with Applications to Cancer Rates. *Stat Med* 2000;19:335-351.

168. Skeet RG: Quality and Quality Control, in. Cancer Registration Principles and Methods: (eds. OM Jensen, DM Parkin, R MacLennan, CS Muir, RG Skeet: Lyons: IARC; 1991. IARC Scientific Publication No. 95. ISBN 9283211952.

169. Hilsenbeck SG: Quality Control, in Central Cancer Registries: Design, Management and Use (eds. H Menck, C Smart), Langhome, PA: Harwood Academic Publishers; 1994, ISBN 3718605791. pp. 131-78.

170. The NPCR Cyber Cancer Registry. Available at: https://apps.nccd.cdc.gov/dcpcccr/default/Login.aspx.

171. Parkin DM, Chen VW, Ferlay J, Galceran J, Storm HH, Whelan SL, eds. *Comparability and Quality Control in Cancer Registration*. Lyon: IARC; rev 1996. IACR Technical Report No. 19. ISBN 9283214331.

172. Ross F, Roffers SD: Quality Control of Cancer Registry Data. In Cancer Registry Management Principles & Practice (eds CL Hutchinson, SD Roffers, AG Fritz), Dubuque, Iowa: Kendall Hunt Publishing Company; 1997.

173. Roffers SD. Demystifying total quality management, The Abstract. 19:1, September 1992.

174. Gavin C. Improving Quality: Guide to Effective Programs. Meisenheimer, Aspen Publishers; 1992. ISBN 083402344

175. Fritz AG. The SEER Program's commitment to data quality. J of Registry Management 28(1):35-44, 2001

176. Berry G. Navigating the Gray Areas of Registry Data. Advance, November 19, 2001.

177. Hall HI, Gerlach KA, Miller DS. Methods of Quality Management. J Reg JRM. 2002:29;, pp 72-77.

178. Izquierdo, Jorge N; and Schoenbach, Victor J. The potential and limitations of data from population-based state cancer registries. J of Registry Management 27(4), 2000.

179. Malnar K, Phillips JL, Fritz AG, Fleming I, Landis SH, McKee R, White M; Stewart A; and Douglas, L. Quality of oncology data: Findings from the Commission on Cancer PCE Study. J of Registry Management 28(1):24-34, 2001.

180. Gross L. The Nuts and Bolts of Quality Control in the Cancer Registry. Advance, February 18, 2002.

181. Thoburn KK, German RR, Lewis M, Nichols PJ, Ahmed F, and Jackson-Thompson J. Case completeness and data accuracy in the Centers for Disease Control and Prevention's National Program of Cancer Registries. Cancer, Volume 109 (8); 1607-1616.

182. German RR, Wike JM, Wolf HJ, Schymura MJ, Roshala W, Shen T, Schmidt B, Stuckart E. Quality of cancer registry data: findings from CDC–NPCR's Breast, Colon, and Prostate Cancer Data Quality and Patterns of Care study. JRM 2008;35(2):67–74.

183. Roffers, S.D.; Case completeness and data quality assessments in central cancer registries and their relevance to cancer control. In: Howe HL, et al. eds. Cancer Incidence in North America, 1988-1990. Sacramento, CA: American Association of Central Cancer Registries; 1994:V1-7, at: http://www.naaccr.org.

184. NAACCR. at: http://www.naaccr.org/Standardsand RegistryOperations/VolumeIV.aspx

185. Fulton JP, Wingo P, Jamison M, Roffers SD, Howe HL, Chen VW. Exploring the effects of death certificate followback on cancer registration. In: Howe L, ed. Cancer Incidence in North America, 1988-1992; Section VI:1-8. Sacramento, CA: North American Association of Central Cancer Registries; April 1996, at: http://www.naaccr.org.

186. Fulton JP, Howe HL. Evaluating the incidence-mortality ratios in estimating completeness of cancer registration. In: Howe HL, et al. eds. *Cancer Incidence in North America, 1988-1991*. Sacramento, CA: North American Association of Central Cancer Registries; 1995:Sec VI:1-9, at: http://www.naaccr.org

187. Tucker TC and Howe HL. Measuring the quality of population-based cancer registries: the NAACCR perspective. JRM. 2001; 28(1):41-5.

188. NAACCR Standard to Assess the Completeness of Case Ascertainment. NAACCR Newsletter, Nov 1996, at: http://www.naaccr.org.

189. Dale, D, Chong N. Moving from Baseline to Certification, at: http://www.naaccr.org.

190. Howe H. Using the Feedback from Registry Certification, at http://www.naaccr.org.

191. Tucker TC. Registry Certification, at: http://www.naaccr.org.

192. Hotes J, Howe HL, Wu XC, Correa C. Hurdles in Achieving Registry Certification, 1995-1997, at http://www.naaccr.org.

193. SEER Program. Self Instructional Manuals for Tumor Registrars, Book 1 through 8. SEER Program, National Cancer Institute, Executive Plaza North, Room 343J, Bethesda, MD 20892

194. SEER Program. Principles of Oncology for Cancer Registry Professionals. National Cancer Institute, Rockville, MD 20852.

195. SEER PROGRAM. National Cancer Institute. Principles and Practice of Cancer Registration, Surveillance, and Control training program. National Cancer Institute, Rockville, MD 20852.

196. Cancer Registration and Surveillance Training Modules, at http://www.training.seer.cancer.gov.

197. NAACCR Short Course. Central Cancer Registries: Design, Management and Use - The short course given annually at the NAACCR meeting.

198. University of southern California Cancer Surveillance Program, Cancer Registrar Training Program, at http://www.ncra-org/training.html.

199. University of Pittsburgh in Pennsylvania, Health Information Systems Major, at http://www.him.upmc.edu.

200. Northeastern University, Boston, MA, at a.collins@nunet.neu.edu.

201. Santa Barbara City College, at http://online.sbcc.net.

202. Programs at Emory University, at http://cancer.sph.emory.edu.

203. Cancer Registry Training Program, Commission on Cancer, American College of Surgeons, at http://www.facs.org/dept/cancer.

204. CTR Corner, online at: http://www.facs.org/dept/cancer/index.html.

205. NAACCR Standards for Cancer Registries Query Database [on-line] at www.naaccr.org.

206. West DW, Flannery J and Dibble R, "Central Cancer Registries: Follow-up." In Menck, H. R., and C. R. Smart, (eds.), Central Cancer Registries: Design, Management and Use. Langhorne, PA: Harwood Academic Publishers, 1994, pp. 188-91.

207. Ashley P, Gress D, Towarnicj C: Monitoring Patient Outcome: Follow-Up. In Cancer Registry Management Principles & Practice (eds CL Hutchinson, SD Roffers, AG Fritz), Dubuque, Iowa: Kendall Hunt Publishing Company; 1997.

208. Dorn, HF, "Methods of Analysis for Follow-up Studies." Human Biology 22 (1950): 238-48.

209. NCRA, Follow-up Resources at http://www.ncra-usa.org/links.html#follow

210. Boyle P, Parkin DM: Statistical Methods for Registries, in Cancer Registration Principles and Methods: (eds. OM Jensen, DM Parkin, R MacLennan, CS Muir, RG Skeet: Lyons: IARC; 1991. IARC Scientific Publication No. 95. ISBN 9283211952.

211. Goodman MT, and Wilkens LR, "Calculation and Assessment of Incidence Rates." In Menck, H. R., and C. R. Smart, (eds.), Central Cancer Registries: Design, Management and Use. Langhorne, PA: Harwood Academic Publishers, 1994, pp. 195-231.

212. California Cancer Registry, Cancer Incidence and Mortality in California by Detailed Race/Ethnicity, 1988-1992. April 1995.27 (191)

213. Surawicz TA, Kupelian VA, and Davis FG. Changes in age-adjusted disease incidence using the Year 2000 standard population: An example using Central Brain Tumor Registry of the United States data. J of Registry Management 28(2):61-64, 2001.

214. Decoufle P, Thomas PL, and Pickle LW. Comparisons of the proportionate mortality ratio and standardized mortality risk measures. Am J Epidem 1980;111:263-268.

215. Wilkens LR, and Goodman MT, "Calculation and Assessment of Survival Rates." In Menck, H. R., and Smart, C. R. (cds.), Central Cancer Registries: Design, Management and Use. Langhorne, PA: Harwood Academic Publishers, 1994, pp. 233-57.

216. AJCC. Cancer Survival Analysis, in AJCC Cancer Staging Manual. 5th Ed. Philadelphia: Lippincott-Raven Publishers; 1997. ISBN 0397584148

217. AJCC. Reporting of Cancer Survival and End Results, in AJCC Staging of Cancer. 4th Ed. Philadelphia: Lippincott-Raven Publishers; 1992. ISBN 0-397-51264-3.

218. Shambaugh EM, Young JL, Zippin C, et al: Book 7: Statistics and Epidemiology for Cancer Registries. U.S. Department of Health and Human Resources, Public Health Service, National Institutes of Health, NIH Publication No. 94-3766, 1994.

219. Austin, DF, "Cancer Registries: A Tool in Epidemiology." In Lillienfeld, A. M. (ed.), Reviews in Cancer Epidemiology, vol. 2. New York: Elsevier North-Holland, 1983.

220. Aldrich, T., "Research Uses of Central Cancer Registries." In Menck, H. R., and C. R. Smart, (eds.), Central Cancer Registries: Design, Management and Use. Langhorne, PA: Harwood Academic Publishers, 1994, pp. 296-97.

221. Hoyler SS, Malnar K: Data utilization. In Cancer Registry Management Principles & Practice (eds CL Hutchinson, SD Roffers, AG Fritz), Dubuque, Iowa: Kendall Hunt Publishing Company; 1997.

222. Jensen OM, Storm HH: Reporting of Results, in Cancer Registration Principles and Methods: (eds. OM Jensen, DM Parkin, R MacLennan, CS Muir, RG Skeet: Lyons: IARC; 1991. IARC Scientific Publication No. 95. ISBN 9283211952.

223. Wingo PA, Parkin DM, Eyre HJ. Measuring the occurrence of cancer: impact and statistics. In Clinical Oncology, 3rd Edition, Lenhard R, Brady L, Osteen R, Gansler T (eds.). American Cancer Society, Atlanta, Georgia.

224. Hatzell T, Aldrich TE, Cates W, Shin E. Public Health Surveillance, in Public Health Administration: Principals for Population-based Management (eds. LF Novick, GP Mays),Aspen Publishers, Gaithersburg, MD, 2000.

225. Parkin DM, with Aslan A. A. Cancer Occurrence in Developing Countries. Lyons: IARC; 1986. IARC Scientific Publication No. 75. ISBN 9283211758.

226. Copeland G, Lake A, Firth R, Bayakly R,Wu XC, Stroup A, Russell C, Kimberley B, Niu X, Schymura M, Hofferkamp J, Kohler B (eds). Cancer in North America: 2003-2007. Volume One: Combined Cancer Incidence for the United States and Canada. Springfield, IL: North American Association of Central Cancer Registries, Inc. May 2010. Available at: http://www.naaccr.org/DataandPublications/CINAPubs.aspx.

227. Copeland G, Lake A, Firth R, Bayakly R,Wu XC, Stroup A, Russell C, Kimberley B, Niu X, Schymura M, Hofferkamp J, Kohler B (eds). Cancer in North America: 2003-2007. Volume Two: Registry-specific Cancer Incidence in the United States and Canada. Springfield, IL: North American Association of Central Cancer Registries, Inc. May 2010. Available at: http://www.naaccr.org/DataandPublications/CINAPubs.aspx.

228. Cancer Facts and Figures. 1998. Atlanta, GA: American Cancer Society National Headquarters. ISSN 00690147.

229. Harras A, ed. Cancer Rates and Risks, 4th ed. NIH Publication No. 96-691. May 1996.

230. Aldrich T: Statistics and Epidemiology: Cancer Registry Management Principles & Practice (eds CL Hutchinson, SD Roffers, AG Fritz), Dubuque, Iowa: Kendall/Hunt Publishing Company; 1997.

231. Howe HL, Wingo PA, Thun MJ, Ries LAG, Rosenberg HM, Feigel EG, Edwards BK. Annual report to the nation on the status of cancer (1973 through 1998), featuring cancers with increasing trends, JNCI 2001;93:824-842. Available at: http://seer.cancer.gov/report_to_nation/archive.html.

232. SEER Program. Racial/Ethnic Patterns of Cancer in the United States 1988-1992, SEER.

233. SEER Program. Cancer Incidence and Survival among Children and Adolescents: United States SEER Program 1975-1995

234. SEER Program. Prostate Cancer Trends 1973-1995, SEER

235. Histology of Cancer - Incidence and Prognosis (Cancer January 1, 1995 - Vol. 75, No. 1), SEER

236. Menck HR, Mills PK and Menck-Taylor JC. Time trends and metropolitan clustering of AIDS-related cancer: Cancer registry-based surveillance. J of Registry Management 28(2):70-76, 2001.

237. West M, Lynch CF and Wagner DM. Descriptive epidemiology of head and neck cancer in Iowa, 1973-1998. J of Registry Management 28(4), 2001.

238. Menck HR, Casagrande JC, Henderson BE, "Industrial Air Pollution. Possible Effect on Lung Cancer." *Science* 183 (1974): 210-12.

239. Perkins CI, Morris CR, Wright WE, and Young JL, Cancer Incidence and Mortality in *California by Detailed Race/Ethnicity, 1988*1992. Sacramento: State of California, Department of Health Services, 1995.

240. Fulton JP, et.al. Urbanization in cancer incidence, Unites States, 1988-1992. In Howe HL ed. *Cancer Incidence in North America, 1989-1993; Vol 1*. Sacramento, CA: North American Association of Central Cancer Registries; 1997:VI1-VI9.

241. Roche LM, Skinner R, Weinstein RB. Use of a geographic information system to identify and characterize areas with high proportions of distant stage breast cancer. J Public Health Manag Pract. 2002;8(2):26-32.

242. Thacker SB. "Time-Space Clusters: The Public Health Dilemma." Health and Environment Digest 3 (1989):4-5.

243. CDC. "CDC: Guidelines for Investigating Clusters of Health Events." Morbidity and Mortality *Weekly Report* 39(RR-1 1) (1990):1-23.

244. CDC. Guidelines for Investigating Disease Clusters. MMWR 39(RR-11)1-23, 1990.

245. Heath CW, Hasterlik RJ. Leukemia among children in a suburban community, 1963. CA Cancer J Clin 1990; 40:27-50.

246. Croner CM, Sperling J and Broome FR. Geographic Information Systems (GIS):New Perspectives in Understanding Human Health and EnvironmentalRelationships . Statistics in Medicine. 15:1961-88. 1996.

247. Clarke KC, McLafferty SL, and Tempalski BJ. On Epidemiology and Geographic Information Systems: A Review and Discussion of Future Directions. Emerging Infectious Diseases. 2(2):85-92.1996.

248. Aldrich TE, Andrews KW, Liboff AR. Brain Cancer Risk and EMF: Assessing the Geomagnetic Component. Archives of Environmental Health. Archives of Env.Health. 56(4):314-19.2001.

249. Aldrich TE, Griffin JR. Environmental Epidemiology and Risk Assessment. Van Norstrand Reinhold, New York, New York, 1993.

250. Houk VN., Thacker SB, "Registries: One Way to Assess Environmental Hazards." *Health and Environment Digest 1* (1 9 8 7):5-6

251. Horn-Ross PL, Hoggatt KJ, West DW, Krone M, Stewart SL. Anton-Culver H, Bernstein L, Deapen D, Pinder R, Peel D, Reynolds P, Ross RK, Wright W. Recent diet and breast cancer risk: the California Teachers Study Study. Cancer Causes Control 13:407-415, 2002.

252. Lew EA, Garfinkel L. Mortality at ages 75 and older in the Cancer Prevention Study (CPS I). CA Cancer J Clin 1990; 40(4):210-224.

253. Williams R. Clinical screening and genetic testing project of high-risk African-American breast cancer families. J of Registry Management 28(3):151-153, 2001.

254. Friedman DL. Multiple cancer familial syndromes. J of Registry Management 28(3):139-145, 2001.

255. Harrison B. Genetic testing and counseling for predisposition to cancer. J of Registry Management 28(3):146-150, 2001.

256. Ballinger L. Hereditary cancer susceptibility. J of Registry Management 28(3):134-138, 2001.

257. Steele, GD, Winchester DP, Menck HR, and Murphy GP, National Cancer Data Base *Annual Review of Cancer Patient Care 1992*. Atlanta, GA: American Cancer Society, 1992.

258. Spath P. Cancer Patient Care Evaluation Guide. Chicago: American College of Surgeons, 1987.

259. Wingo PA, Luke E, O'Brien K, Brogan DJ, Chen VW, Wu XC, Tucker T; Howe HW, Ross F; Vann S; Stewart A, Chmiel JS, Sylvester J, Bumpus R; and Shen T. Population-based patterns of care studies: Collaboration among state cancer registries, the American College of Surgeons, and the American Cancer Society. J of Registry Management 28(1):5-16, 2001.

260. Osteen RT, Steele GD, Menck HR, Winchester DP: Regional Differences in Surgical Management of Breast Cancer, CA 1992; 42: 39-43.

261. Steele GD, Winchester DP, Menck HR: The National Cancer Data Base: A Mechanism for Assessment of Patient Care, Cancer 1994; 73: 499-504.

262. Greenwald P, Sondik EJ, and Young JL, "Emerging Roles for Cancer Registries in Cancer Control." *Yale Journal of Biological Medicine 59* (1986):561-66.

263. Parkin DM, Wagner G, Muir CS. The Role of the Registry in Cancer Control. Summit, New Jersey: IARC; 1985, 1989. ISBN 9283211669

264. Friedell GH, and Tucker TC, "Central Cancer Registries: Prevention and Control." In Menck, H. R., and C. R. Smart (eds.), Central Cancer Registries: Design, Management *and Use*. Langhorne, PA: Harwood Academic Publishers, 1994, pp. 296-97.

265. Armstrong BK. "The Role of the Cancer Registry in Cancer Control." Cancer Causes *and Control* 3 (1992):569-79.

266. Garfinkel, L., "History of U.S. Central Cancer Registries." In Menck, H. R., and C. R. Smart, (eds.), Central Cancer Registries: Design, Management and Use. Langhorne, PA: Harwood Academic Publishers, 1994, pp. 303-309.

267. Wagner, G., "History of Cancer Registration." In Jensen, O. M., D. M. Parkin, R. MacLennan et al. (eds.), Cancer Registration Principles and *Methods*. IARC Scientific Publications No. 95. Lyon, France: WHO International Agency for Research on Cancer, 1991, pp. 3-6.

268. Stephenson GW: The Commission on Cancer. A Historical Review, Bull Amer Coll Surg Sept: 7-13, 1979.

269. US Dept of Health Education and Welfare: A history of Cancer Control in the United States 1946-71. Book 2, DHEW Publication No (NIH) 78-1518, Washington DC.

270. Flannery JT and Janerich DT: The Connecticut Tumor Registry: Yesterday, Today and Tomorrow, Conn Med 11: 709-712, 1985.

271. Griswold MH, Wilder CS, Cutler SJ and Pollack ES: Cancer in Connecticut 1935-51, Conn State Dept of Health, Hartford, Conn, 1955.

272. Ferber B, Handy VH, Gerhardt PR and Solomon M: Cancer in New York State, exclusive of New York City, 1941-1960. A Review of Incidence Mortality, Probability and Survivorship, N.Y. State Dept of Health, Albany NY, 1962.

273. Dorn HF: Illness from Cancer in the United States, U.S. Govt Printing Office, Washington DC, 1944.

274. Dorn HF, Cutler SJ: Morbidity from Cancer in the United States, Publ Health Monogr 56, U.S. Dept of Health Education and Welfare, Washington DC, 1959.

275. California Tumor Registry: Cancer Registration and Survival in California, Calif State Dept of Health, Berkeley, Calif, 1963.

276. Smart CR. Cooperative tumor registry. Rocky Mt Med J 1968;65(11):27.

277. Biometry Branch, National Cancer Institute: Third National Cancer Survey: Incidence Data, Monogr 41, DHEW Publ No. (NIH) 75-787, Bethesda, Maryland, 1975.

278. Surveillance Programs, Division of Cancer Prevention and Control: Cancer Statistics Review 1973-1986, NIH Publ No. 89-2789, National Cancer Institute, 1989.

279. Commission on Cancer, Data Acquisition *Manual.* Chicago: American College of Surgeons, 1988.

chapter 37

Geographic Information Systems

Frank P. Boscoe, PhD
David K. O'Brien, PhD, GISP
Colleen C. McLaughlin, PhD, CTR

Overview

Most people associate a geographic information system (GIS) with the production of maps. The real power of a GIS, however, goes beyond mapmaking to the acquisition, storage, linkage, manipulation, and analysis of geographic data. A GIS can range from simple to highly complex, from no cost to many thousands of dollars; in general, the higher the cost, the greater the functionality. Most North American central cancer registries are now using GIS for a variety of purposes. According to a survey of North American Association of Central Cancer Registries (NAACCR) conducted in 2005, more than 40 registries used GIS in the past year.

Object Topology

A GIS stores real-world entities that have geographic locations—whether people, hospitals, rivers, or counties—as spatial objects. Spatial objects can be points, lines, or areas. In GIS jargon, these are also referred to as *nodes, arcs,* and *polygons*. A collection of spatial objects stored together is variously known as a *table, layer,* or *theme*. The outstanding feature of a GIS, and what makes it different from ordinary database software, is that it stores information about how the spatial objects are connected to one another, a property known as *object topology*. A GIS can rapidly calculate which objects are adjacent, overlapping, or contained within each other. This makes it easy to calculate the number of cancer cases located within a particular distance of some location, or to calculate rates for geographic units not stored in a central cancer registry, such as school districts.

In addition to object topology, each table also contains attribute data about the objects. Typical attribute data for a county object might include county name, area, population, and poverty rate. Typical attribute data for a person object might include age, sex, address, and postal code (Figure 37-1). Most GISs store tables as multiple files, all of which must be in the same directory for the table to be accessed properly. GIS maps often contain data from multiple layers. For example, a state-level cancer mortality rate map can consist of one layer, with the state boundaries shaded by cancer rate and a second layer that indicates by symbols which states are part of the Surveillance, Epidemiology, and End Results (SEER) Program and which are funded through NPCR.

Obtaining Geographic Information System Layers

A table that stores geographic reference information, such as county boundaries or streets, is known as a *base table* or *base layer*. Learning how to produce a base layer by digitally tracing a paper map used to be a major part of an introductory GIS course. Today, though, nearly all of the base layers that a cancer registrar is likely to ever need are readily available via the Internet. Both the U.S. Bureau of the Census (www.census.gov/geo/www/cob/index.html) and Statistics Canada (http://geodepot.statcan.ca/Diss/Products/Products_e.cfm) offer GIS layers for all of the units for which population data are collected. Individual state GIS clearinghouses provide another rich source of state-specific GIS layers. (Links to the state clearinghouses are provided at: http://registry.fgdc.gov/serverstatus/.) An advantage to using data acquired via a GIS clearinghouse is that it also includes metadata, or data about the data, specifying when it was created, information about data accuracy and precision, and other useful information.

Spatial Queries

Information from different tables is combined through queries. These can be framed as conventional database queries, such as "join the cancer incidence table to the cancer mor-

Name	Opcert	Address	City	State	Zip
CORTLAND MEMORIAL HOSPITAL	1101000H	134 Homer Ave	Cortland	NY	13045
MARGARETVILLE MEMORIAL HOSPITAL	1226701C	Route 28	Margaretville	NY	12455
THE HOSPITAL	1227000H	43 Pearl St W	Sidney	NY	13838
DELAWARE VALLEY HOSPITAL	1229000H	1 Titus Pl	Walton	NY	13856
O'CONNOR HOSPITAL DELHI	1221000H	Andes Road Rte 28 Box 205A	Delhi	NY	13753
ST FRANCIS HOSPITAL-POUGHKEEPSIE	1302000H	35 North Rd	Poughkeepsie	NY	12601
VASSAR BROTHERS HOSPITAL	1302001H	45 Reade Place	Poughkeepsie	NY	12601
NORTHERN DUTCHESS HOSPITAL	1327000H	10 Springbrook Av	Rhinebeck	NY	12572
ST FRANCIS HOSPITAL-BEACON	1301000H	60 Delavan Ave	Beacon	NY	12508
BUFFALO GENERAL HOSPITAL	1401000H	100 High St	Buffalo	NY	14203
CHILDRENS HOSPITAL	1401002H	219 Bryant St	Buffalo	NY	14222
ERIE COUNTY MEDICAL CENTER	1401005H	462 Grider St	Buffalo	NY	14215
SHEEHAN MEMORIAL HOSPITAL	1401006H	425 Michigan Ave at Eagle St	Buffalo	NY	14203
MERCY HOSPITAL	1401008H	565 Abbott Rd	Buffalo	NY	14220

Figure 37-1. View of a Typical GIS Data Table (Point Locations of Hospitals in New York State)

tality table where the state names from the two tables are equal." This is how GIS tables are joined to spreadsheets, text files, SAS datasets, and other non-GIS files. Information from GIS tables can also be combined through spatial queries that make use of topology, for example, "join the cancer case table to the county table where the location of the cancer case point object falls within the county polygon object." Spatial queries typically use intuitive terms such as "adjacent," "within," "outside," and "intersect." One particularly useful spatial query is known as a *buffer*, defined as the set of all objects within a given distance of a reference object, such as the set of all property parcels located within one mile of a hospital.

Editing Geographic Information System Layers

Although most of the geographic layers of interest to a cancer registry are readily available, some cleaning or tweaking of the geographic data is often necessary. For example, a county base layer may include lakes or rivers as separate polygons, which can add unnecessary cluster to a cancer rate map. Islands are often stored as separate objects, which can complicate subsequent analyses; one available base layer of the United States has more than 300 separate objects for Alaska. The amount of resolution also needs to be appropriate for the mapping purpose. Some base layers render the Chesapeake Bay coastline in exquisite detail with many thousands of points, but on a national map fitted to a standard-size sheet of paper, all of that detail appears merely as a black smudge. A GIS contains commands for adding, editing, combining, deleting, aligning, and relocating spatial objects to deal with these various issues.

Coordinate Systems and Projections

A GIS stores points, lines, and polygons in terms of their exact location on the Earth's surface. Although many coordinate systems are in use, the most commonly used is latitude and longitude. The Earth is divided into 180 degrees of latitude (90 north and 90 south of the equator) and 360 degrees of longitude (180 west and 180 east of Greenwich, England). By convention, north latitude and east longitude are expressed as positive numbers, and south latitude and west longitude are expressed as negative numbers. Thus, all of Canada and the United States (with the exception of a few Alaskan islands, Guam, and a few other Pacific territories) fall in the negative longitude range. When GIS data mysteriously refuse to appear on a map, a common reason is that positive longitude values were mistakenly used, meaning that the data are actually on the opposite side of the globe.

The set of equations that define how the spherical surface of the Earth is represented on a two-dimensional printed page or computer screen is known as the *map projection.* Most GIS software can change map projections on the fly and can properly align multiple layers on the same map even if they were created using different projections. To envision how projections work, think of the Earth as a transparent globe with a light bulb in the center. Then imagine a piece of photographic paper as the projection surface. This surface can be made into various shapes and placed at various locations and orientations around the globe. Three common examples are as follows (Figure 37-2):

1. Cylindrical projections, based on the projection surface being wrapped around the globe like a cylinder
2. Conic projections, based on the projection surface being rolled into a cone and placed over the globe
3. Azimuthal projections, based on the projection surface being a flat plane placed against the globe so it is tangent at only one point

When a cylinder is placed over the globe vertically, intersecting it at the equator (see Figure 37-2a), the result is known as the *Mercator projection.* In this projection, traditionally used in classroom maps for many decades, the lines of latitude and longitude run parallel and perpendicular to each other. There is no distortion at the equator, but increasing distortion away from the equator, making Greenland and Antarctica look artificially large. A similar

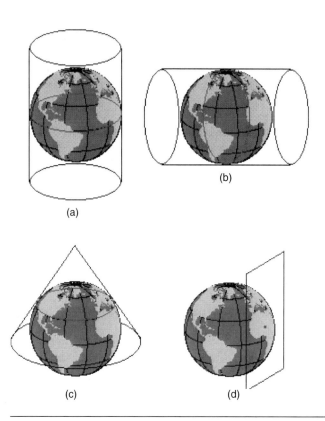

(a)

(b)

(c)

(d)

Figure 37-2. Examples of Surfaces Used to Develop Map Projections[1]: (a) Cylinder; (b) Cylinder (transverse); (c) Cone; and (d) Plane

projection system is the most widely used in GIS and is known as the *Universal Transverse Mercator,* or *UTM system.* In the UTM system, the cylinder is placed horizontally about the globe so it touches at the north and south poles (see Figure 37-2b). If the intersecting circle is made to follow the 0- and 180-degree longitude lines, then the result is a projection with no distortion along these lines and progressively increasing distortion away from these lines. By rotating the cylinder horizontally, a series of projections can be created with different distortion-free locations: one with no distortion at −6 and 174 degrees, another with no distortion at −12 and 168 degrees, and so on. The UTM system divides the Earth into 60 such zones of 6 degrees each. At the center of each zone, there is no distortion, and at the edge of a zone, the distortion is only about one part in 2,500. A map projected in one zone can span several zones with minimal visual distortion. For example, mainland Alaska spans zones 3 through 7, and a map of Alaska projected in zone 5 has the correct shape and orientation (Figure 37-3a). UTM coordinates are expressed in easting and northing values. The easting value describes the distance, in meters, east or west of the center of the UTM zone, where the center is defined as 500000 E. The northing value describes the distance, in meters, north of the equator, where the equator is defined as 0 N. Thus the location of the White House in Washington, DC, can be given as 323330 E, 4307410 N (zone 18).

When latitude and longitude values are treated as if they were simple x- and y-coordinates, the result is variously known as the *rectilinear, equirectangular,* or *geographic projection* (see Figure 37-3b). This is also referred to as *unprojected* because no mathematical transformation is involved. This projection distorts and compresses the landmasses as one travels farther from the equator, and the effect is noticeable within the United States. Many beginning GIS users inadvertently choose this projection. Figure 37-3c shows a conic projection better suited for the Continental United States than for Alaska.

In addition to a projection, every map has a datum. A datum is a coordinate reference system that takes into account the shape of the Earth. For most purposes, the Earth can be assumed to be a perfect sphere. The Earth is not a perfect sphere, however: its poles are somewhat flattened, its equator is somewhat bulged, and it has a slight pear shape, meaning that the Earth's shape is more accurately represented as a spheroid. As surveying techniques have improved, geodesists (people who study the shape of the Earth) have refined their spheroid models of the Earth's surface. In North America, the two primary datums in use are NAD-27 (North American Datum of 1927), based on the 1866 Clarke spheroid, and NAD-83 (North American Datum of 1983), based on the 1980 Geodetic Reference System spheroid. Most states in the United States have transformed their NAD-27 GIS data to the newer NAD-83 datum. A point with specific latitude/longitude coordinates in NAD-27 can be several hundred feet away from a point with the same coordinates in NAD-83.

Geographic Information System Use in Central Cancer Registries

Most central cancer registries now make use of GIS in some form. A number of states, including Kentucky and Florida, publish county-level rate maps in their annual reports (Figure 37-4). New York State published a round of zip-code–level incidence maps in 1999–2000 that indicated circular zones ("clusters") of statistically elevated rates (Figure 37-5). The use of GISs for the identification and/or mapping of clusters as part of ongoing surveillance activities has become widespread, with much recent attention focused on identifying clusters of late-stage disease or poor survival.[2] (More detail on clustering is given later in this chapter in the Spatial Analysis section.) Another popular application of GISs has been to measure and evaluate spatial variations in cancer treatment patterns. In particular, important differences have been found based on distance from a teaching hospital and between rural and urban areas.

The Dartmouth Atlas Project (www.dartmouthatlas.org) is a useful reference for learning more about geographic variation in medical practice.

The increasing number of GIS-themed presentations given at recent NAACCR annual meetings provides evidence that GISs have been gaining in importance and visibility. GISs have also been a featured topic in a variety of

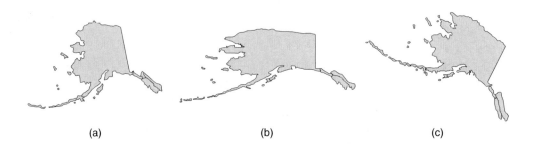

(a)   (b)   (c)

Figure 37-3. Three Different Projections of Alaska: (a) Universal Transverse Mercator (UTM) Zone 5; (b) Rectilinear or "Unprojected"; and (c) a Conic Projection Better Suited for the Continental United States

recent training courses offered by NAACCR and SEER. A NAACCR GIS committee has been very active in recent years. It has overseen publication of a handbook of basic practices in GIS and best practices in geocoding, both of which provide far more breadth and depth than what is in this chapter.[3,4] Both can be downloaded from the GIS Committee page of the NAACCR Web site (http://www .naaccr.org/committees/gis).

Cartography

Cartography, the science of mapmaking, has been described as "the meeting place of science and art." The primary purpose of a map is to convey information and to illustrate a geographical concept or relationship, but it is also desirable to produce attractive maps from an artistic perspective. Many excellent cartography textbooks describe how to create correct, clear, and attractive maps.[5]

Maps have a variety of roles. They are used as aids in thinking visually and spatially. Researchers use maps to generate questions and hypotheses. Maps are used to help confirm (or not confirm) hypotheses, communicate what analysts think they know, and synthesize and present findings. They are also used for persuasive and rhetorical purposes.[6]

Maps have limitations. Because a tremendous amount of information can be portrayed, map designers need to select, generalize, and simplify. If too much information is presented, it might hide the core theme of the map and obscure its understanding for the audience. Dividing the information over a series of maps is often a more effective tactic. If too little detail is included, it also can lose the audience.[7] A poorly designed map fails to communicate effectively and may, in fact, deliver the wrong message to the

All Sites, 1998–2002
Total Population 1998–2002
Age-Adjusted to the 2000 U.S. Standard Million Population

Rate per 100,000
☐ 326.25–462.43
◻ 463.06–496.38
▨ 497.41–522.22
■ 522.64–697.86

Figure 37-4. Age-Adjusted Invasive Cancer Incidence Rates by County in Kentucky

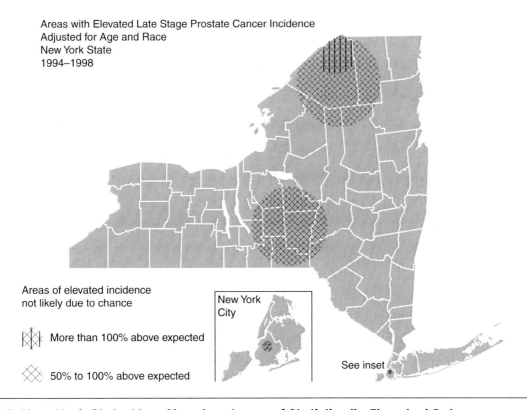

Areas with Elevated Late Stage Prostate Cancer Incidence
Adjusted for Age and Race
New York State
1994–1998

Areas of elevated incidence
not likely due to chance

More than 100% above expected

50% to 100% above expected

New York City

See inset

Figure 37-5. New York State Map Showing Areas of Statistically Elevated Rates

audience.[8] The underlying spatial analysis might be complex and effective, yet the audience might not be convinced if the final output fails to effectively portray the message of the results.

It is important to understand both the audience and the viewing environment of maps. The audience's age, educational level, map-reading experience, and familiarity with the map's subject matter must be considered. Color blindness and other accessibility issues must be considered as well. The viewing environment provides a context for map design. Will the map be in a newspaper, report for public information, scientific paper, or atlas? Will it be distributed on the Internet in either static or interactive formats? Will it be viewed on paper or in a room with a computer projection system? Will the reader spend a large amount of time studying the map or flip the page quickly?

Choropleth Maps

Maps fall into two broad categories. Maps depicting data are known as *thematic maps,* and maps depicting the positions of landscape features are known as *locational* or *reference maps.* While cancer registry staff use reference maps for various purposes, they tend to produce thematic maps almost exclusively. The most common type of thematic map is the choropleth map, in which each geographic area is shaded by a different color. Each shade corresponds to a range of values of some variable, such as a cancer incidence rate (Figure 37-6).[9] The geographic areas to map,

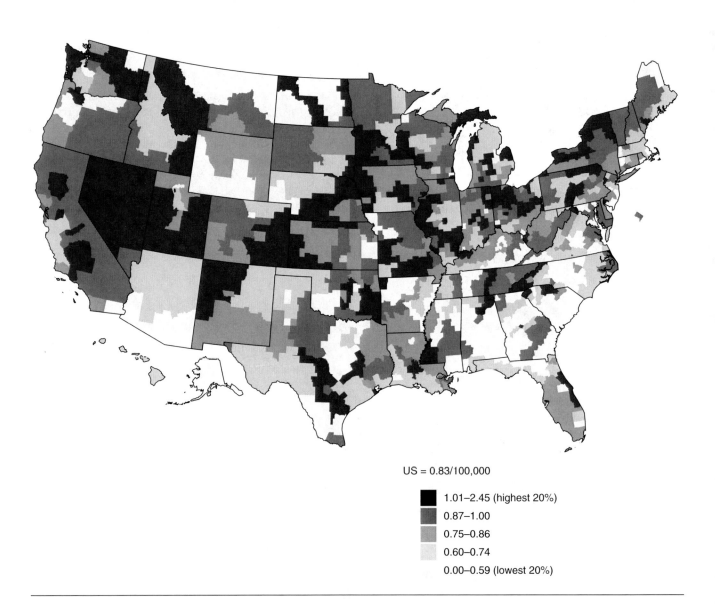

US = 0.83/100,000

■ 1.01–2.45 (highest 20%)
■ 0.87–1.00
■ 0.75–0.86
□ 0.60–0.74
□ 0.00–0.59 (lowest 20%)

Figure 37-6. Testicular Cancer Mortality, White Males, 1950–1969, by State Economic Area. An Example of a Choropleth Map with 5 Equal-count (Quantile) Ranges of about 102 State Economic Areas Each[9]

data ranges, and color scheme for a choropleth map must all be carefully chosen by the map designer.

Geographic Units

The choice of geographic units for a choropleth map depends on a number of factors. Showing more units adds more information, but showing fewer units results in more data within each unit and, thus, more reliable rates. Ideally, units should be of similar size and should contain similar numbers of people to limit interpretive problems (these are discussed in detail later in the Spatial Analysis section). Of course, these conditions conflict with one another because of the uneven distribution of human populations. Units that are equal in area (such as towns and townships in many states) have widely differing populations, whereas units roughly equal in population (such as census tracts, units of about 4,000 people) have widely differing areas. The final choice requires a compromise. Using a formal criteria evaluation approach, researchers have found that mapping counties represents the best overall compromise when working with national data for the United States, but each mapping project presents a unique situation.[10]

Other examples of geographic units that can be used for mapping include smaller census units (block groups in the United States, dissemination areas in Canada), postal codes, local health jurisdictions or local health department districts, and researcher-defined areas that are aggregations of counties, towns, and/or postal codes. The latter category includes entities such as health service areas, hospital service areas, and hospital referral regions.[11,12]

Because people in the United States tend to be more familiar with their own zip codes than with their census tracts, it is tempting to map at the zip-code level. However, zip codes were designed to aid in the delivery of the mail and not as a way to map health data. Therefore, they do not typically coincide with census tract or municipal boundaries. In addition, existing zip code boundaries frequently change—new zip codes are created, and old ones are retired. This makes mapping zip codes difficult, not to mention the problem of determining populations for zip-code areas.

Regardless of what geographic area the data analyst maps, care must be taken to limit situations where there are very small numbers of cases in the chosen geographic area. Even at the county level, there are states that have very large rural counties with small populations. Small counts will result in unstable rates—rates that may be very high for one diagnosis year and very low for another. In such situations, it is best to aggregate the cancer data being displayed by either aggregating the data over a longer period or aggregating the geographic areas.

Data Classification

A map designer needs to define both the number of data ranges and a scheme for classifying the data. The optimal number of data ranges depends on the purpose and scope of the map, but a rule of thumb is that between five and seven generally works well, providing a balance between informational content and map complexity. Common types of classification schemes are provided by most GIS software and include the following:

- *Equal count (quantiles):* Each range contains approximately the same number of records. The ranges are known as quantiles. Five ranges are known as quintiles, ten ranges as deciles, and so on.
- *Equal interval:* The difference between the top and bottom values in each range is the same. That is, each range covers an equal portion of the scale; for example, 0 to 100, 101 to 200, 201 to 300, and so on.
- *Natural breaks:* This is based on a mathematical procedure that examines the distribution of data points and puts similar data into each range. The range breaks are determined according to an algorithm such that within each range, the difference between the data values and the average of the data values is minimized.
- *Standard deviation:* A statistical method based on variability of the data. The middle range breaks at the mean of the data values, and the ranges above and below the middle range are within a fixed number of standard deviations above or below the mean. It is useful for identifying areas that differ significantly from an average value.
- *Equal area:* Ranges are computed such that an equal amount of land area falls into each range. This is one of the most complex ranging schemes to perform but is very effective visually because no range group dominates the map.
- *User defined:* Users supply their own classification scheme.

Although the quantile method has been shown to be a consistently reliable choice for typical large datasets,[13] a data analyst may have to experiment with several classification schemes to find the one best suited for the map. For example, if a dataset consists of 6 rates of [1, 2, 13, 14, 15, 100], the quantile method would put 15 and 100 into the same group, which is misleading. The equal interval method would be a better choice, or a user-defined grouping of 0 to 10, 11 to 20, and 21 to 100.

Color Schemes

The choice of color scheme is important when designing a choropleth map. People have expectations about color, and colors have connotations that can "make or break" a map. For example, people are accustomed to blue representing water and green representing vegetation, lowlands, and forests. When there is a strong expectation about colors, such as the historical use of reds for high rates and blues for low rates in cancer mortality maps, the reader will be confused if these conventions are violated, even when the legend is clear.[14]

Differences in hue (green vs. blue vs. red) are used on maps to signify qualitative differences, such as different health regions or land-use types. Differences in value (light blue vs. medium blue vs. dark blue) are used on maps to signify quantitative differences, with darker colors having higher values. Thus, a map with blues for the highest values and yellows for the lowest values will be confusing because it conflicts with the convention; it is not clear whether blue should be considered worth more or less than yellow.

There are two primary quantitative map color schemes: sequential and diverging. Sequential color schemes proceed from light to dark over a single hue, with the darker colors representing higher values. Sequential color schemes may also proceed from light to dark over a limited range of hues, such as dark red to medium red-orange to light orange. Diverging schemes use a neutral color such as gray to represent values near the mean, with values greater than the mean proceeding from light to dark in one hue and values less than the mean proceeding from light to dark in another hue. Diverging schemes are useful when one of the goals of the map is to show where rates are higher or lower than some middle value (e.g., the overall statewide rate).

Map designers must also consider whether their color maps will be largely circulated in grayscale. Maps posted on the Internet might be printed on black-and-white printers, or printed in color but subsequently reproduced on standard copy machines. Also, map users may be color-blind. In such cases, cartographers should consider using a color scheme in which there is enough contrast to distinguish among the various colors if they are produced in grayscale.

Other color considerations arise when the primary means of presentation is a flat plasma or liquid crystal display (LCD) screen, or a computerized projection machine. Some LCD screens, especially laptop computers, are difficult to view obliquely. Some computer projection devices, especially older ones, do not necessarily support all colors. Some colors on a computer screen look very different when viewed from a projector. Color schemes that utilize gradual change in hues may look like one solid color.

The ColorBrewer Web site (www.colorbrewer.org), based on research by Cynthia Brewer, contains recommended color schemes that address all of these concerns. The Web site provides numeric color specifications that can be entered into a GIS. Some GIS software already incorporates these color schemes directly.

In addition to considering color schemes, cartographers can use patterns to indicate high and low values. Many standard patterns are available in GIS packages, such as dots, lines, and cross-hatchings of varying densities, with denser patterns equating with higher values. Maps using patterns can be more difficult to interpret but have the advantage of being reproducible in black and white.

Other Types of Thematic Maps

Besides choropleth maps, several other styles of thematic maps can illustrate cancer data:

- *Dot density map:* Used to map the number of items in an area, where each dot corresponds to a fixed number of items. Note that the dots are typically distributed randomly throughout an area and do not represent actual locations.
- *Bar chart:* Symbolizes a quantity by the height or length of a bar placed over the corresponding geographic area. Can be useful for comparing two or more variables. For example, the difference in lung cancer incidence rates for male and female individuals by county can be illustrated by two bars of different colors placed at the center of each county.
- *Pie chart:* Similar to the bar chart, but the pie illustrates the relative proportion of the variables out of 100%.
- *Proportional symbol map:* Uses point symbols that vary in size. The size or area of a symbol is directly proportional to the data value it represents. For example, populations of multiple counties can be illustrated by proportional circles plotted at the center of each county.
- *Graduated symbol map:* Uses a discrete set of symbol sizes, with each size representing a range of data values. This design is similar to the choropleth map, in which each color represents a range of data values. This type of map is useful when there are many geographic areas illustrated because the user might have a difficult time distinguishing among similar-sized symbols.
- *Isopleth map:* Better known as a *contour map,* in which lines are drawn to represent equal values, such as elevation lines on a topographic map. The space between such lines can be shaded with specific colors, or colors can gradually change hue without a boundary line. Isopleth and choropleth maps are similar, but they differ in how the data are presented. Choropleth maps aggregate data within specific geographic areas, such as census tracts or counties. Isopleth maps imply data that are continuous and vary smoothly over space.

Some Uses of Rate Maps

Cancer rate maps serve a variety of functions. They can be used as a lookup table to identify rates in a specific geographic unit, and they can be used to assess broader patterns and trends across multiple geographic units. They can be used to help generate hypotheses about possible causes of cancer, or they can provide evidence in support of existing hypotheses (though maps by themselves cannot prove a cause-and-effect relationship). They can be used to communicate complex findings in a concise manner. They can also be used to argue in favor of particular actions or policies.

Some of these map functions are enhanced by combining cancer data with other data layers. For example, cancer rate maps can be overlaid with locations of specialty clinics in high-cancer-rate areas as a way to encourage the general public to pursue early detection, such as a map of bladder cancer rates combined with locations of urologists' offices. The relation between two variables, such as lung cancer mortality and smoking behavior in the population, can be explored by creating a cross map of areas that are high in both variables, high in either variable, or high in neither variable. But when many variables are of interest (as is usually the case), it is often more useful to combine them through some kind of statistical model rather than attempt to show them all on the same map. Using the lung cancer example, this would be essential if the additional influences of race, socioeconomic status, and air quality needed to be taken into account.

The ease of combining layers in a GIS leads many beginning map users to be seduced by the suggestion of cause-and-effect relationships between cancer and the environment. What needs to be remembered is that correlation does not imply causation. Lung cancer rates correlate to some degree with many variables—temperature, humidity, production of certain crops and animals for human consumption, and smoking behavior—but not all of these are causally related. The reverse can also be true. A specific pesticide may be related to a specific type of cancer, but an overlay map may not suggest any correlation if the cancer is also caused by unrelated factors or the quality of the pesticide data is low. When working with cancer data, it is important to remember that the time between exposure and onset of cancer symptoms can be several decades, and the population of many areas of the country is very mobile. Map analyses are best suited for illnesses that have a short time period between exposure and symptoms.

Maps on the Web

Rapid advances in technology have made it easy to perform many of the functions of GIS software via the Internet, without the need to purchase a commercial off-the-shelf product. For viewing cancer data, there are sophisticated mapping sites such as the Interactive Maps section of the National Cancer Institute/Centers for Disease Control and Prevention (NCI/CDC) State Cancer Profiles website (http://statecancerprofiles.cancer.gov). Users can map incidence or mortality data by site, race, sex, age, and time period, with some control over the map's visual appearance. The Kentucky Cancer Registry offers similar functionality on its Web site (www.kcr.uky.edu).

More recently, Google Earth (http://www.google.com/earth/index.html) and other similar "earth browsers" have revolutionized the GIS field by incorporating many of the features of commercial GIS software, but with a shallower learning curve, and at no or minimal cost. Geographic data can be easily created, viewed, manipulated,

and distributed using a program such as Google Earth, all over a high-resolution satellite view of the Earth's surface. A CDC researcher recently found that Google Earth was the simplest way to manage a polio outbreak along the Congo River—superior to any printed map or governmental source—from navigation to calculating fuel needs to determining jurisdictional boundaries.[15]

Google Earth and similar programs read and write KML, an open source language that mimics other Web-based languages. For projects that involve large numbers of geographic objects (as in the case of cancer rates by census tract in a state, or locations of all reporting sources in a province), it is possible to use traditional GIS software to convert data to KML or to write a program in a conventional programming language that outputs KML.

With ever-increasing computing power, the cost and difficulty of geographic analysis will undoubtedly continue to diminish. For the latest free software tools in this rapidly evolving field, visit the Free Geography Tools Web site (http://freegeographytools.com).

Geocoding

Geocoding is the process of assigning geographic information to a cancer patient's record based on the patient's usual place of residence. Usually, this means latitude and longitude coordinates, although the term is also used to describe the assignment of any more specific geographic information. Geocoding is accomplished by comparing address information in the cancer patient record with a reference file containing all possible addresses. This is a complicated process, and a variety of stand-alone software packages and private vendors have arisen to fulfill this need. Commercial GIS software packages include geocoding capabilities, but a GIS is not essential for geocoding.

Geocoding continues to get easier with each passing year. Address information on patient records supplied by hospitals has seen steady improvement, not least because there are more characters available in the address field, making for fewer creative abbreviations. The quality of address reference files and other reference materials also continues to improve, particularly those in the public domain. Numerous states are in the process of phasing out difficult-to-geocode rural route and post office box addresses to facilitate emergency response. Geocodes can now be automatically assigned to well more than 90% of incoming case reports in certain urban and suburban areas, and a modest amount of sleuthing is often all that is required for most of the remainder, though for large registries this still translates into a large amount of manual labor.[16,17]

Capturing the latitude and longitude coordinates of a cancer patient's residence is useful for several reasons. Sometimes in a cancer surveillance investigation, it is important to know the exact distance between a residence and a source of environmental exposure. For example, in one study, the risk for soft tissue sarcoma in a small Italian city was measured in 1-km increments from an industrial waste incinerator.[17] In addition, because latitude and longitude values never change, they easily can be used to aggregate upward to any past, present, or future geographic unit of analysis. A request for cancer counts by neighborhood, legislative district, zip code, or any other geographic unit can be easily met by spatially joining the cancer cases (points) to the geographic unit (polygons) in a GIS. (Calculating cancer rates for these areas might not be possible, though, if corresponding population counts are not available.)

The most important limitation of using latitude and longitude coordinates for analysis is that residential location tends to be a weak basis for assigning exposure. Populations in the United States and Canada are highly mobile. Given the long latency period of many types of cancers, it is often true that "exposed" cancer patients were actually living elsewhere during the relevant period of exposure. For some cancers, exposures throughout the life course, from in utero through childhood and early adulthood, appear to be relevant.[19] In such situations, the residence at diagnosis

may offer little explanatory value. Where the residence at diagnosis is simply used as an indicator of socioeconomic factors such as income levels or educational attainment, then population mobility is less of an issue because people tend to be similar to their neighbors in these respects no matter where they live.

Parsing and Standardizing Addresses

In the NAACCR record layout, a patient's address at diagnosis is stored in four fields (Figure 37-7).* A residential street address consists of up to 11 components in the United States and 9 components in Canada. Parsing refers to the process by which the address stored in the cancer registry

---

*A fifth field for supplemental address information, such as the name of a facility, nursing home, or apartment complex, is also available but not typically used for geocoding. In addition to address at diagnosis, there are also corresponding fields for current address.

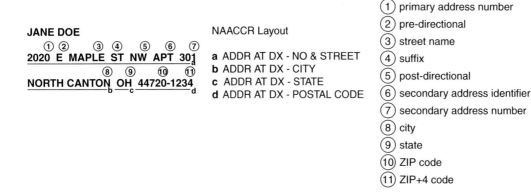

Figure 37-7a. Residential Address Components for U.S. Addresses

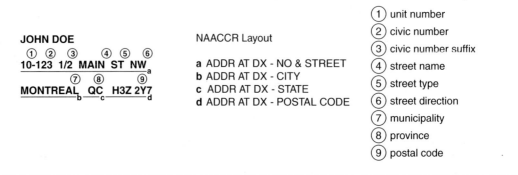

Figure 37-7b. Residential Address Components for Canadian Addresses

is broken into these more specific address elements. Once an address has been parsed, it is then standardized. Address standardization refers to the process of modifying an address so it conforms to conventions for format, abbreviation, and address components as defined by the U.S. Postal Service or Canada Post. In the United States, NORTH MAIN STREET is standardized as N MAIN ST, whereas the city N CANTON is standardized as NORTH CANTON. Registries may also develop useful custom standardizations, such as BKLYN for BROOKLYN and BDWY for BROADWAY in New York. Commercially available geocoding applications do these steps quite well (including, in some cases, automatic correction of minor spelling errors), though unusual addresses can sometimes produce unexpected results, so it is always useful to periodically review address records that fail to geocode to determine whether any systematic problems are present.

Address Matching

Once a cancer patient's address has been parsed and standardized, it is ready to be matched against a reference file. A reference file contains a complete set of addresses for a given geographic area. It might contain a separate record for each individual property or, more commonly, will store starting and ending house numbers, known as address ranges, for short street segments. Matching can be either deterministic or probabilistic. With the deterministic approach, a subset of the address components in the cancer patient address are compared with the same address components in the reference file, and they must agree exactly and uniquely for a match to be made. With probabilistic matching, multiple address components are compared, with each component having a different weight. The weights for the components that match are then summed to obtain an overall match score, which is sometimes represented as a standardized number ranging from 0 (no elements match) to 100 (all elements match). These methods form part of a broader set of statistical methods known as *record linkage* (see Chapter 36 for more information on record linkage).

A deterministic match typically consists of several passes, each with slightly more relaxed matching requirements (Table 37-1). There are many more possible passes that could be made in addition to those in Table 37-1 that could yield potential matches. As the matching criteria become more relaxed, however, the risk for making an incorrect match increases.

The probabilistic matching method involves assigning a weight to each field being compared. The weight is derived from two probabilities. The first is the probability that two fields agree given that they are truly a match, denoted as m. In general, this probability will be very high, close to 1. For example, if the true street name is "Maple," then we would expect the vast majority of all associated patient records to also have the name "Maple," but there may be a few with "Mapple" or some other minor spelling variation. The second probability is the probability that two fields agree at random, denoted as u. This probability is typically low. For example, there are about 1,600 zip codes in New York State, so the probability of two randomly selected records having the same zip code is about 1/1600 or 0.0006.* In a state or province with only four permissible values in the predirectional field (N, S, E, W), the u probability for predirectional would be 1/4.

Once m and u are known, the weight for each field can be calculated as:

$$\text{Weight} = \ln (m/u)$$

Thus, for zip code, assuming an m of 0.99 and a u of 0.001, the weight is 6.9. For predirectional, using an m of 0.99 and a u of 0.25, the weight is 1.4. Intuitively, it makes sense that the street name should have a much higher weight than the predirectional.

By way of example, suppose we wish to match on house number (assume a weight of 6.7), predirectional

Table 37-1	Illustration of Deterministic Matching of the Address 1060 W. Addison St., Chicago, IL 60613 (Wrigley Field)	
Pass	**Matching Variables**	**Addresses Yielding a Match**
1	Street number, Pre-directional, Street name, Suffix, ZIP code	1060 W ADDISON ST 60613
2	Street number, Pre-directional, Street name, ZIP code	1060 W ADDISON ST 60613
		1060 W ADDISON 60613
		1060 W ADDISON AVE 60613 etc.
3	Street number, Pre-directional, Street name, Suffix, City	1060 W ADDISON ST CHICAGO 60613
		1060 W ADDISON ST CHICAGO 60614
		1060 W ADDISON ST CHICAGO 99999 etc.

Table 37-2	Illustration of Probabilistic Matching of Two Different Addresses, One Correct and One Containing an Error	
Cancer Patient Address	**Candidate Matches (matching elements in bold)**	**Match Score**
1060 W ADDISON ST 60613	**1000–1098 W ADDISON ST 60613**	24.2
	900–998 **W ADDISON ST 60613**	17.5
	2000–2098 **W ADDISON ST** 60618	10.6
	1000–1098 W WAVELAND AVE **60613**	15.0
1060 W ADDISON ST 60618	**1000–1098 W ADDISON ST** 60613	17.3
	900–998 **W ADDISON ST** 60613	10.6
	2100–2198 **W ADDISON ST 60618**	17.5
	1000–1098 W WAVELAND AVE 60613	8.1

(1.4), street name (7.7), suffix (1.5), and zip code (6.9). Table 37-2 depicts several candidate matches for two different cancer patient address records; the first is complete and correct, and the second has the wrong zip code.

The first cancer patient address yields an exact match on every field, which is clearly the desired match. Note that match scores are calculated for all addresses, even ones that are obviously incorrect, such as the Waveland Avenue address. Because the Waveland Avenue address has a match score of 15, one can use this as a basis for categorically eliminating all candidate matches for all addresses with a score of 15 or less. For the second record, the highest match is for 2100–2198 West Addison, because the zip code has a higher weight than the street number. However, the zip code is off by only one digit (possibly because of a simple typo), whereas the street number is different in several digits. Based on this result, match scores in the 17.3 to 17.5 range may be considered questionable. Such possible matches are best reviewed manually (Table 37-3). One strategy to reduce the amount of clerical review is to conduct probabilistic matching using multiple passes with different combinations of variables. A pass that substituted city name for zip code in the second record in Table 37-1, for example, might yield a match with a score above the threshold. Note that the upper and lower thresholds will differ for each pass because different variables are being compared each time.

All geocoding software uses some version of the above methods. Users are generally able to exert control over the matching process by specifying the passes, minimum match scores, and other parameters. Simply using software directly out of the box with default settings is not likely to yield optimal results.

---

*Because zip codes are of unequal sizes, the actual u value is more like 1/1,000 or 0.001. Larger zip codes are more likely to be selected at random than small zip codes, which increases the overall probability of a random match.

Table 37-3	Interpretation of Probabilistic Match Scores
Match Score	**Action**
Above upper threshold	Automatically assign geocodes
Between upper and lower threshold	Clerical review
Below lower threshold	Reject as possible match

Assigning Geocodes

As mentioned earlier, geocoding reference files contain either a record for each individual address or, more commonly, one record for each street segment. House numbers and latitude and longitude coordinates for the beginning and ending of each street segment are stored in the reference file, and geocodes are assigned by interpolating between the beginning and ending house numbers and coordinates. For example, for a street segment ranging from 100 to 198 Maple Avenue, an address of 101 Maple Avenue would be placed near the beginning of the segment, whereas 196 Maple Avenue would be placed near the end. Geocoding software typically also allows users to specify the amount of setback between the house and the street.

Latitude and longitude values provided by geocoding software tend to be ridiculously precise. Reporting a value to six decimal places is common, which corresponds to a precision of about 1 cm. (It has been jokingly suggested that this allows us to geocode not only the patient's residence, but also the actual tumor!) Matching vendor practice, the NAACCR record layout allows for six decimal places in these fields. There is sometimes a temptation to become preoccupied with the details of geocoding—the level of precision, whether the geocode indicates the center of the house or the edge of the driveway, or whether interpolation along a street segment is sufficiently accurate. But given the broader limitations of geographic cancer studies (population mobility, disease latency, the fact that populations are counted only once every 10 years, and usually poor exposure assessment), the authors are unaware of any studies with results that have hinged on these kinds of details.

Other geographic identifiers that are often supplied by a geocoding reference file in the United States include the county subdivision (also known as *minor civil division;* these include cities, towns, townships, and boroughs), census tract (a statistical unit averaging about 4,000 people), census block group (a statistical unit averaging about 1,500 people), and census block (the smallest unit, consisting of an area bounded by roads, water, or other physical barriers). In Canada, a geocoding reference file may specify the census division (one or more municipalities or counties that typically share services such as police), census tract (similar to the United States, but defined for urban areas only), dissemination area (a statistical unit averaging about 500 people), and census block. While the latitude and longitude are sufficient to derive this information in a GIS, it is still convenient to have this information included in a geocoding reference file.

Central cancer registries may do their geocoding in-house or by submitting their cases to a commercial geocoding vendor or to a free Web-based geocoding service (for example, see https://webgis.usc.edu/Services/Geocode/). When choosing an outside vendor or service, it is advisable to send a small test dataset with known geocodes to gauge quality.

Handling Unmatched Records

Inevitably, even with the best possible reference databases and best matching algorithms, there will always remain some unmatched records. Cancer registries either leave the latitude and longitude fields for these records blank or fill in coordinates based on the smallest geographic area for which there is information, typically the zip code. Such records are disproportionately from rural areas, where rural route and post office box addresses are in more common use. Even in states such as New York that have replaced rural routes with standard addresses as part of an effort to improve the delivery of emergency services to rural areas, this remains true (Table 37-4).

When imprecise coordinates based on zip code or some other information are assigned, care must be taken to fill in the corresponding GIS Coordinate Quality field, new to Version 11 of the NAACCR record layout (Table 37-5). This data item is a two-digit code that indicates the basis of assignment of latitude and longitude coordinates from an address. Most records in most situations will be coded as 03 (for matched records), and 09 and 10 (for unmatched records), because nearly all cancer case records do contain a valid five-digit zip code.

Table 37-4	Percentage of Cases Geocoded in New York State Cancer Registry, Diagnosis Year 2001, as of December 2004

Geographic Area	% Geocoded
10 most populous counties	91.8
10 least populous counties	64.7
Statewide	88.1

Because one of the primary reasons for storing geocodes is to be able to flexibly aggregate cancer cases to any unit of choice (school district, 1-mile buffer around a hazardous waste site, etc.), records with GIS Coordinate Quality values of 9 or higher have limited analytic value. Values of 3 and lower are usable in all situations, whereas the inclusion of those between 4 and 8 could depend on the specific research or surveillance question.

Spatial Analysis

So far this chapter has covered how address data for cancer patients are collected, processed, and used to make maps of the geographic distribution of cancer. One may also want to use the geographically referenced cancer data to delve further into the patterns of cancer to answer more complicated questions, such as the following:

- What areas of the country have increased cancer rates?
- Are there clusters of cancer?
- Are cancer rates greater in rural farming areas?

To address these types of questions, spatial analysis is required. Spatial analysis is a form of data analysis that incorporates information about the geographic location of events. Like all data analysis, it can be used to uncover new patterns (generate hypotheses) or to investigate suspected relations or patterns (test hypotheses). One may also encounter the term *exploratory spatial data analysis,* which refers to using the geographically referenced data to explore and find new patterns. In this case, spatial analysis is used to develop new questions in addition to potentially answering research questions.

The Sparse Data Problem

Choropleth maps of cancer incidence or mortality are relatively easy to create and interpret. So why would we need more sophisticated spatial analysis to answer questions such as those listed earlier? The reason is that with maps, as with everything else, what you see is not always what

Table 37-5	Geographic Information Systems Coordinate Quality Codes[20]
00	Coordinates derived from local government-maintained address points, which are based on property parcel locations, not interpolation over a street segment's address range
01	Coordinates assigned by Global Positioning System (GPS)*
02	Coordinates are match of house number and street, and based on property parcel location
03	Coordinates are match of house number and street, interpolated over the matching street segment's address range
04	Coordinates are street intersections
05	Coordinates are at midpoint of street segment (missing or invalid building number)
06	Coordinates are address zip code + 4 centroid†
07	Coordinates are address zip code + 2 centroid
08	Coordinates were obtained manually by looking up a location on a paper or electronic map
09	Coordinates are address 5-digit zip code centroid
10	Coordinates are point zip code of post office box or rural route
11	Coordinates are centroid of address city (when address zip code is unknown or invalid, and there are multiple zip codes for the city)
12	Coordinates are centroid of county
98	Latitude and longitude are assigned, but coordinate quality is unknown
99	Latitude and longitude are not assigned, but geocoding was attempted; unable to assign coordinates based on available information
Blank	Geographic Information Systems (GIS) Coordinate Quality not coded

*A GPS is a device used to obtain highly accurate latitude and longitude coordinates in the field based on interactions with satellites.
†In a GIS, a centroid is usually defined as the point halfway between the northern and southern extents and halfway between the eastern and western extents of an area. This can vary depending on how the shape of the area is generalized, and whether uninhabited parts of the area such as water and parkland are included.

you get. Maps are subjective, and different viewers may interpret them differently. Research has shown that less-experienced viewers tend to overidentify clusters in rural areas, where random fluctuations might cause adjacent areas to all have high rates because of one or two excess cases. Conversely, more experienced researchers underidentify patterns in these same areas, attributing the patterns to random fluctuations, while missing an overall increased risk in the region. An example of a map that is difficult to interpret is a map of mortality rates from testicular cancer by State Economic Area for white male individuals for 1950 though 1969 (see Figure 37-6). On this map, almost all of Nevada and Utah are shown to have the greatest rates of testicular cancer mortality. But one might reason that because Nevada and Utah are mostly desert with few residents, it may be the high rates are driven by very small (and hence, unstable) numbers. Indeed, the two greatest rates in these two states accounted for only 36 deaths over the 20-year period. Spatial analysis can be used to offset the difficulties of map interpretation by using statistical methods to weed out the random fluctuation caused by sparse data.

Sparse data are one of the most pervasive problems in making maps and in spatial analysis. It boils down to the problem that, in areas with small populations, one or two additional cases of cancer may cause the rate of cancer in the area to become increased. Take Cheyenne County, Colorado, for example. Between 1999 and 2002, the prostate cancer mortality rate among men here was 11.3 per 100,000. This is not largely different from the rate for the nation as a whole, which was 10.9 per 100,000. And despite being slightly greater than the national average, Cheyenne County is actually in the 40th percentile for prostate cancer mortality, meaning that 60% of counties have greater rates. Only about 2,200 men were living in the county during this time period, though, with only one man dying of prostate cancer. One can easily imagine that an additional man could have died from prostate cancer. If that had happened, then the rate for the 4 years would have been double what was observed, or 22.6 deaths per 100,000 men. With just one additional death, Cheyenne County would have been close to the 90th percentile for prostate cancer mortality. On a typical red-to-blue choropleth map of prostate cancer mortality, Cheyenne County would have gone from a pale blue to a strong red. There are, indeed, several counties, including Treasure County, Montana, Keya Paha County, Nebraska, and King County, Texas, that had only one or two deaths from prostate cancer during the 4-year span but were among the counties with the greatest prostate cancer rates in the nation, with rates more than four times greater than the rate for the entire United States.

The reason sparse data is a particular problem when making maps is that large geographic areas with very small populations are easier to see on the map and they tend to be close to each other. Cheyenne County has less than 1/1,000 of the population of New York City but is about three times bigger in land area and, therefore, takes up more space on a map of the United States. One additional death caused by prostate cancer in Cheyenne doubles the rate, but one additional death caused by prostate cancer in New York City barely changes it (from 10.084 deaths per 100,000 to 10.087 deaths per 100,000 men). On a map, Cheyenne County is both easier to see than New York City and more likely to have unusually high or low rates. Cheyenne County is also surrounded by similar counties that are large in land area and small in population.

Types of Spatial Analysis

Spatial analysis takes many forms and is the subject of numerous textbooks and college courses. Covered here are just several of the more common types of spatial analysis that are widely used in central cancer registries.

Cluster Detection

Cluster detection is the process of identifying geographic areas that have unusually high or unusually low occurrences of cancer, whether in the entire population or among specific demographic groups. We can look for clusters of rare cancers, such as childhood brain tumors, or of fairly common cancers, such as female breast cancer. Cluster detection methods can be used at fine geographic scales, such as neighborhoods, or coarser scales, such as counties. Clusters of unusual stage distributions, treatment types, survival patterns, or any variable of interest can also be identified. Finally, cluster detection can include a temporal component in addition to the spatial component, allowing the identification of space-time clusters.

The search for cancer clusters has gained some attention in the media. In particular, there has been a lot of attention paid to clusters of childhood cancer in Woburn, Massachusetts (the basis for the book and movie *A Civil Action*), Toms River, New Jersey, and Fallon, Nevada.[21-23] Sometimes, the fact that there is an excess of cancer in an area is fairly obvious. For example, between 1997 and 2005, 17 leukemia cases were identified among children who had ever lived in Churchill County, Nevada (where Fallon is located). Given the size of the county, only one case would be expected among the children every 5 years. The probability of this pattern arising through chance is less than 1 in 100,000. Usually, though, the excess risk is more subtle, requiring statistical testing to confirm that the excess is not due to chance. In Dover Township, New Jersey (where Toms River is located), there were 87 newly diagnosed cases of cancer among children, whereas 67 would have been expected based on the size of the population. This 30% excess in the number of cases observed compared with expected

was deemed "statistically significant" because there was less than a 5% chance that this number of cases would be observed by chance alone. Specifically, this kind of finding would be expected by chance about 1 of every 100 times. Although these suspected clusters could have been identified through spatial analysis of cancer registry data, they were actually first identified by physicians or community members, which is how most cluster investigations have been triggered.

Sometimes the search for a cancer cluster is motivated by the possibility of exposure to specific carcinogens. A focused cluster detection method compares the cancer rates in the neighborhood of a potential exposure with the cancer rates in areas without the exposure to identify a difference in cancer risk. This approach has been used to assess the cancer risk around nuclear facilities. In one example, researchers at Columbia University evaluated the risk for cancer among people who lived within 10 miles of the Three Mile Island Nuclear Plant, which was the site of a reactor accident in 1979.[24] The results of this analysis showed that the accident at Three Mile Island was not correlated with an increase in cancer rates in the area. In the United Kingdom, much attention has been paid to the risk for childhood leukemia around nuclear facilities. Initially, it appeared as though the risk for cancer was increased among children living in the communities with nuclear facilities, but researchers pointed out that this did not mean that radiation release from the nuclear facilities into the environment caused the increased risk.[25] Alternative hypotheses include: (1) the fathers of the leukemia cases were more likely to work at the nuclear facilities, so maybe the increased risk was related to the father's radiation exposure; or (2) communities where nuclear facilities were built had rapid influxes of new residents, possibly introducing new viruses to the community. This example highlights the fact that spatial analysis of cancer is not different from other epidemiologic studies in that these studies cannot prove a causal relation between the cancer and the environment.

Global cluster detection methods involve scanning an entire geographic area for unusual patterns. An example of this type of cluster detection method is the spatial scan statistic (http://satscan.org), which has been used to analyze both cancer incidence and cancer mortality data. The scan statistic looks for clusters by grouping the data for neighboring geographic units together to find regions where there is a statistically significant excess of cases or deaths. The scan statistic is powerful for identifying relatively large geographic regions that have high cancer rates. This method averages the rates throughout the "cluster" area, meaning that individual geographic units within a cluster may actually have lower rates than average.

Using this method, Kulldorff and colleagues identified an excess of breast cancer mortality spanning the New York City and Philadelphia metropolitan areas (Figure 37-8).[26] Notably, this corridor has a significantly greater

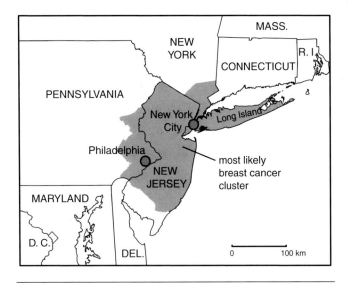

Figure 37-8. Breast Cancer Cluster in Northeast United States[29]

median income than the rest of the northeastern United States. Higher income is a risk factor for breast cancer because women with higher incomes and higher education levels may also be more likely to have better nutrition during childhood, later age for the birth of their first child, fewer children, moderate regular alcohol consumption, and other lifestyle factors associated with increased breast cancer risk. Thus, the presence of a cancer cluster does not automatically imply any environmental cause. In fact, it is best to try to account for known lifestyle risk factors statistically before entertaining environmental hypotheses.

Data Aggregation and Spatial Smoothing

Sometimes a choropleth map of cancer rates is difficult to interpret because there is a lot of noise in the map. Noise is a term used by researchers to say that the data jump around a lot. For example, the following string of numbers is generally increasing, but because there is noise in the data, each number may or may not be bigger than the one before it: 3, 5, 2, 7, 2, 8, 5, 9, 3, 5, 12, 7, 12, 6, 12, 15, 4, 8, 34, 9, 43. On a map, sparse data in large counties with small populations, such as Cheyenne County (discussed earlier), are a source of noise. Figure 37-9a[9] is an example of a map with a lot of noise. It is difficult to determine what areas of the Upper Midwest might have high kidney cancer mortality rates. Figure 37-9b shows the same data, but instead of being grouped by county, the counties are grouped together into state economic areas. This map is easier to interpret because there is less noise. Wisconsin is seen to have a much more uniformly above-average rate. Grouping the counties together this way is an example of data aggregation. Another way to aggregate the data would have been to use a longer time period, such as 50 years instead of 25 years.

Another way of removing noise on a map is to use the technique of spatial smoothing (Figure 37-10).[11] With this technique, an area's cancer rate is influenced by the rates of neighboring areas. One simple smoothing approach is to simply average each geographic area with its adjacent areas. Another approach is to use a spatial filter. In this method, cancer rates for geographic areas are assigned the rate of all of the surrounding areas falling within a filter of a certain

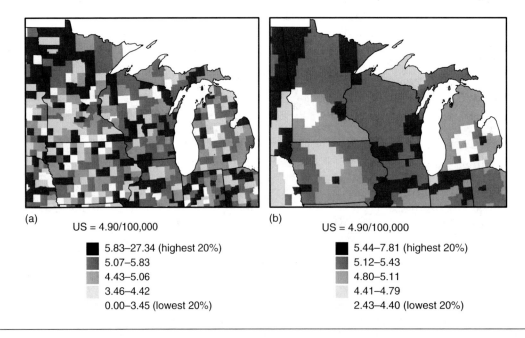

(a)   US = 4.90/100,000

- ■ 5.83–27.34 (highest 20%)
- ■ 5.07–5.83
- ▨ 4.43–5.06
- ▧ 3.46–4.42
- □ 0.00–3.45 (lowest 20%)

(b)   US = 4.90/100,000

- ■ 5.44–7.81 (highest 20%)
- ■ 5.12–5.43
- ▨ 4.80–5.11
- ▧ 4.41–4.79
- □ 2.43–4.40 (lowest 20%)

Figure 37-9. Examples of Noisy and Less-Noisy Maps: Cancer Mortality Rates for Kidney, Renal Pelvis, and Ureter; White Males, 1970-94; by County (left) and State Economic Area (right)[9]

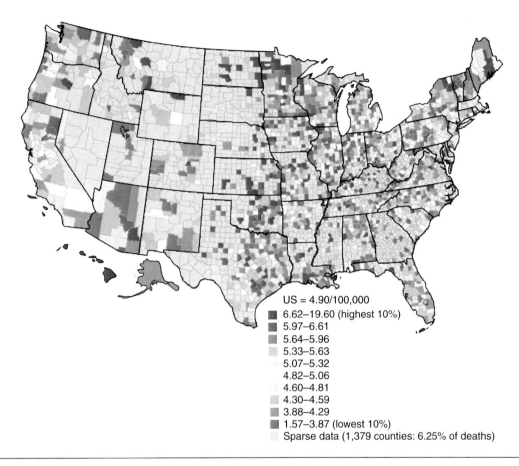

US = 4.90/100,000
- 6.62–19.60 (highest 10%)
- 5.97–6.61
- 5.64–5.96
- 5.33–5.63
- 5.07–5.32
- 4.82–5.06
- 4.60–4.81
- 4.30–4.59
- 3.88–4.29
- 1.57–3.87 (lowest 10%)
- Sparse data (1,379 counties: 6.25% of deaths)

Figure 37-10. Example of a Smoothed Map: Cancer Mortality Rates by County (Age-adjusted 1970 US Population) Kidney, Renal Pelvis, and Ureter: White Males, 1970–94. From the Centers for Disease Control and Prevention National Center for Health Statistics[11]

size.[27] For example, if the unit of analysis is the zip code, and the filter size is 25 km, then the cancer rate for a zip code will be equal to the overall cancer rate for every zip code within 25 km. There are many other smoothing methods, some involving complex mathematics. Regardless of the method chosen, smoothing tends to decrease high rates and increase low rates, thus providing a clearer overall picture.

Distance Studies

Distance studies are used to answer questions such as, "Does living far away from a major cancer center affect what treatment a patient receives?" Researchers using data from the New Mexico Tumor Registry found that women who lived farther away from a radiation treatment facility were less likely to have radiation therapy after undergoing breast-conserving surgery for breast cancer.[28] Only about half of the women who lived more than 75 miles from a radiation treatment center had radiation therapy, whereas more than 80% of women living less than 50 miles from the centers had the treatment. The researchers used the street address of the patients and the radiation treat-

ment center to calculate the distance. Researchers have also studied distance to care with respect to survival after cancer. They have found that patients who travel longer distances for cancer care have better survival rates, but this is probably because the patients with better prognoses are more likely to be referred for treatment. Patients with poorer prognoses tend to be treated closer to home to minimize their end-of-life burdens.

Summary

GISs have become an integral part of central cancer registry activities, from data presentation to surveillance to etiologic research. Ricketts' definition of GIS speaks to the needs and interests of the cancer registrar: "GIS is, at its heart, a simple extension of statistical analyses that join epidemiological, sociological, clinical, and economic data with references to space."[29]

The ability to produce a variety of map types is well supported in GIS, although care and experience are required to produce maps that are clear and informative. This

Table 37-6	Free Spatial Analysis Software of Interest to Cancer Registries	
Software	**Purpose**	**URL**
SaTScan	Cluster detection	satscan.org
Headbang	Spatial smoothing	srab.cancer.gov/headbang
GeoDa	Large variety of spatial analysis methods	geodacenter.asu.edu/software/downloads

chapter has attempted to cover some of the more important map design and cartography issues that a basic GIS user encounters. If any single point about map design is to be remembered, it should be that default settings within a GIS should be generally avoided.

GIS greatly facilitates geocoding, the assignment of spatial information to cancer cases. Within central cancer registries in the past decade, the emphasis of geocoding has been shifting from trying to correctly identify a patient's county of residence to assigning specific latitude and longitude coordinates. The ultimate advantage of this is that it allows for flexible aggregation, or the ability to combine cases into any geographic unit for analysis, whether county, zip code, school district, census tract, or even an arbitrary area such as a 1-km square that might be more relevant when considering air pollution exposure.

Spatial analysis encompasses various mathematical and statistical ways to find patterns and trends contained within spatial data that go beyond basic GIS output. Most types of spatial analysis cannot be performed within a GIS but require additional specialized software. There have long been calls for GIS software manufacturers to integrate more spatial analysis functionality into their products, but progress has been slow, probably in part because public health remains a small part of the overall GIS market. The good news is that many of the spatial analysis software tools of greatest utility in cancer surveillance are free of charge (Table 37-6).

References

1. Mackenzie, J. "FREC 480-GIS in Natural Resource Management, Projection Systems." University of Delaware. Available at: http://www.udel.edu/johnmack/frec480/480lec_projections.html. Last accessed July 26, 2010.
2. Abe, T., Martin, I. B., Roche, L. M. "Clusters of census tracts with high proportions of men with distant-stage prostate cancer incidence in New Jersey, 1995 to 1999." *American Journal of Preventive Medicine*, 2006;30(2 Suppl):S60–S66.
3. Wiggins, L., editor. *Using Geographic Information Systems Technology in the Collection, Analysis, and Presentation of Cancer Registry Data: A Handbook of Basic Practices.* Springfield, IL: North American Association of Central Cancer Registries, 2002.
4. Goldberg, D. W. *A Geocoding Best Practices Guide.* Springfield, IL: North American Association of Central Cancer Registries, 2008.
5. Robinson, A. H., Morrison, J. L., Muehrcke, P. C., Kimerling, A. J., Guptill, S. C. *Elements of Cartography.* New York: John Wiley & Sons, 1995.
6. DiBiase, D. "Visualization in the Earth Sciences." *Earth and Mineral Sciences, Bulletin of the College of Earth and Mineral Sciences (Penn State University),* 1990;59(2):13–18.
7. Buttenfield, B. P., McMaster, R. B., editors. *Map Generalization: Making Rules for Knowledge Representation* (pp. 172–186). London: Longman, 1991.
8. Monmonier, M. *Mapping It Out: Expository Cartography for the Humanities and Social Sciences.* Chicago, IL: The University of Chicago Press, 1993.
9. Devesa, S. S., Grauman, D. G., Blot, W. J., Pennello, G., Hoover, R. N., Fraumeni, J. F. Jr. *Atlas of Cancer Mortality in the United States, 1950-94.* Washington, DC: U.S. Gov't Printing Office, 1999.
10. Boscoe, F. P., Pickle, L. W. Choosing geographic units for choropleth rate maps, with an emphasis on public health applications. *Cartography and Geographic Information Science,* 2003;30(3):237–248.
11. Pickle, L.W., Mungiole, M., Jones, G. K., White, A. A. *Atlas of United States Mortality.* Hyattsville, MD: National Center for Health Statistics, 1996. Available at: http://www.cdc.gov/nchs/products/other/atlas/atlas.htm. Last accessed July 26, 2010.
12. Dartmouth Medical School Center for the Evaluative Clinical Sciences. *The Care of Patients with Severe Chronic Illness.* Hanover, NH: Dartmouth, 2006. Available at: http://www.dartmouthatlas.org/downloads/atlases/2006_Chronic_Care_Atlas.pdf. Last accessed July 26, 2010.
13. Brewer, C. A., Pickle, L. W. "Evaluation of methods for classifying epidemiological data on choropleth maps in series." *Annals of the Association of American Geographers,* 2002;82(4):662–681.
14. Carswell, C. M., Kinslow, H. S., Pickle, L. W., Herrmann D. "Using Color to Represent Magnitude in Statistical Maps: The Case for Double-Ended Scales." In Pickle, L. W., Herrmann, D., editors. *Cognitive Aspects of Statistical Mapping.* Working Paper Series No. 18. Hyattsville, MD: National Center for Health Statistics, 1995.
15. Kamadjeu, R. "Tracking the polio virus down the Congo River: A case study on the use of Google Earth in public health planning and mapping. *International Journal of Health Geographics,* 2009;8:4.
16. Boscoe, F. P., Kielb, C. L., Schymura, M. J., Bolani, T. M. "Assessing and improving census tract completeness." *Journal of Registry Management,* 2002;29(4):117–120.
17. McElroy, J. A., Remington, P. L., Trentham-Dietz, A., Robert, S. A., Newcomb, P. A. "Geocoding addresses from a large population-based study: Lessons learned." *Epidemiology,* 2003;14(4):399–407.

18. Comba, P., Ascoli, V., Belli, S., Benedetti, M., Gatti, L., Ricci, P., Tieghi, A. "Risk of soft tissue sarcomas and residence in the neighbourhood of an incinerator of industrial wastes." *Occupational and Environmental Medicine,* 2003;60(9):680–683.

19. Okasha, M., McCarron, P., Gunnell, D., Smith, G. D. "Exposures in childhood, adolescence and early adulthood and breast cancer risk: A systematic review of the literature." *Breast Cancer Research and Treatment,* 2003;78(2):223–276.

20. Thornton, M., O'Connor, L, editors. *Standards for Cancer Registries Volume II: Data Standards and Data Dictionary,* 14th ed., version 12. Springfield, IL: North American Association of Central Cancer Registries, February 2009.

21. Waller, L. A. "A civil action and statistical assessments of the spatial pattern of disease: Do we have a cluster?" *Regul Toxicol Pharmacol,* 2000;32(2):174–183.

22. Maslia, M. L., Reyes, J. J., Gillig, R. E., Sautner, J. B., Fagliano, J. A., Aral, M. M. "Public health partnerships addressing childhood cancer investigations: Case study of Toms River, Dover Township, New Jersey, USA." *International Journal Hygiene Environmental Health,* 2005;208 (1-2):45–54.

23. Steinmaus, C., Lu, M., Todd, R. L., Smith, A. H. "Probability estimates for the unique childhood leukemia cluster in Fallon, Nevada, and risks near other U.S. military aviation facilities." *Environ Health Perspect,* 2004;112(6):766–771.

24. Hatch, M. C., Wallenstein, S., Beyea, J., Nieves, J. W., Susser, M. "Cancer rates after the Three Mile Island nuclear accident and proximity of residence to the plant." *American Journal of Public Health,* 1991;81(6):719–724.

25. Laurier, D., Grosche, B., Hall, P. "Risk of childhood leukaemia in the vicinity of nuclear installations—findings and recent controversies." *Acta Oncol,* 2002;41(1):14–24.

26. Kulldorff, M., Feuer, E. J., Miller, B. A., Freedman, L. S. "Breast cancer clusters in the Northeast United States: A geographic analysis." *American Journal of Epidemiology,* 1997;146(2):161–170.

27. Talbot, T. O., Kulldorff, M., Forand, S., Haley, V. B. "Evaluation of spatial filters to create smoothed maps of health data." *Statistics in Medicine,* 2000;19(17-18):2399–2408.

28. Athas, W. F., Adams-Cameron, M., Hunt, W. C., Amir-Fazli, A., Key, C. R. "Travel distance to radiation therapy and receipt of radiotherapy following breast-conserving surgery." *Journal of the National Cancer Institute,* 2000;92(3): 269–271.

29. Ricketts TC. "Geographic Information Systems and public health." *Annual Review of Public Health,* 2003;24:1–6.

chapter 38

National Cancer Data Base

Andrew K. Stewart, MA

Purpose

The National Cancer Data Base (NCDB) was established to serve as a comprehensive clinical surveillance resource about cancer care in the United States. The NCDB was the first national database used to track and compare the treatment of most types of cancers. Working in conjunction with other activities of the Commission on Cancer (CoC), the purpose of the NCDB is to improve the quality of cancer care by providing cancer programs with the means to compare their management of cancer patients with the way in which similar patients are managed in other cancer care centers around the country. The NCDB resides in and is operated by the CoC of the American College of Surgeons (ACoS).

Overview

The forerunner to the CoC, the Cancer Campaign Committee, was founded in 1913 and was charged with "conducting a study of the efficacy of surgery and radiation therapy in the management of gynecologic cancers." By 1922, the CoC was formally established. Currently, the CoC is a group of 48 multidisciplinary professional organizations dedicated to the mission of reducing cancer morbidity and mortality through education, standard setting, and monitoring the quality of cancer care. The NCDB is central to the mission of the CoC as a means toward the active monitoring of cancer care in the United States.

The American Cancer Society (ACS) and the CoC of the ACoS have maintained a long-standing partnership in the fight against cancer. The ACS and the ACoS fund the activities of the NCDB. The NCDB was established in 1989 by these two organizations to provide important information to individuals and institutions interested in the care of cancer patients. The NCDB is a nationwide, institutionally based, oncology data set that currently captures 70% of all newly diagnosed malignant cancer cases in the United States annually and holds information on almost 25 million cases of reported cancer diagnoses for the period 1985 through 2007 and continues to grow. Data on all types of cancer are tracked and analyzed. Data collected include patient characteristics, tumor staging, histology characteristics, type of first-course treatment administered, disease recurrence, and survival information. These data elements are submitted to the NCDB from CoC-accredited cancer program registries using nationally standardized data transmission formats. Data confidentiality is of prime importance, and the NCDB has proactively worked to continually ensure and maintain compliance with the Health Insurance Portability and Accountability Act (HIPAA) of 1996 privacy regulations established by the Federal Government in 2003. Data residing in the NCDB can be linked to other reference data sources, such as U.S. census files to provide aggregate, zip-code estimates of various socioeconomic variables such as family income and educational achievement, or the American Hospital Association (AHA) files to obtain specific hospital characteristics. Data in the NCDB are analyzed and reported in a variety of ways, and allow for comparative analyses, which include hospital, state, region, or national reports to examine patterns of care and evaluate whether and how treatment patterns vary regionally or over time.

Organization

The CoC operates under the guidance of five standing committees: the Committee on Accreditation, the Committee on Cancer Liaison (Physicians), and the Quality Integration Committee (QIC). The QIC is the central advisory panel that guides and assists in the prioritization of the work conducted by the NCDB staff and prioritizes collaborative initiatives or projects with external agencies or investigators. The QIC is concerned with and represents the CoC in matters addressing the progress and direction of research and continuing education as it pertains to improving the care of patients with cancer. The committee members are selected from the CoC membership. Surgical specialties should represent the College Fellowship. Multidisciplinary balance, programmatic goals, potential member interests, and geography are considerations. Preferably, members are actively involved in cancer-related activities through clinical practice, accredited cancer programs, research activities, or by association with professional groups supporting cancer programs.

Data Cycle

The NCDB's data cycle consists of three parts: (1) an annual Call for Data, (2) data processing that includes edit checks and writing case records to the CoC's data warehouse, and (3) data analysis and evaluation. All documentation described in this section is maintained for the current and most recent Calls for Data on the NCDB page of the ACoS Web site (www.facs.org).

Call for Data

The annual Call for Data is sent electronically to all CoC-accredited cancer programs and is issued in the autumn of each year. Specific instructions are provided outlining case submission transmission file specifications and data format requirements. These guidelines are consistent with the North American Association of Central Cancer Registries (NAACCR) data transmission specifications established for the most current data year requested in the Call for Data. In addition, instructions are provided describing how registries can prepare, validate, and complete their data submission.

Data are requested for as many as 5 years at the time of each Call for Data, to facilitate obtaining the most recent data available, as well as follow-up recurrence and survival data for previously reported patients. For example, in the fall of 2009, the Call for Data requested that cases for the years 2008, 2003, 1998, 1992, and 1988 be submitted to the NCDB. The 2008 cases were the most recently abstracted and completed case records available that hospital registries could provide at that time. Case records from 2003 were used to update previously reported cases and included 5-year follow-up information. Cases from 1998 were used to update previously reported records and included 10-year follow-up information, and so forth, for 15- and 20-year follow-up from re-reported 1992 and 1988 cases.

Data are received from CoC-accredited cancer program registries via the secured CoC Datalinks Web application. On receipt of a data file, the corresponding registry is notified via e-mail confirming receipt of the transmission. As data files pass through the sequence of file validation, record-level data edit reviews and case writing to the CoC's data warehouse additional e-mail notifications are generated informing each respective registry of the status of the data submission. The NCDB staff monitors the participation of hospitals, tracks the accuracy and frequency with which data submissions are made, and checks for unexpected fluctuations in site-specific caseloads.

Data submission to the NCDB is a requirement of the CoC's accreditation program. Standard 3.6 of the CoC's *Cancer Programs Standards* specifies that complete data for all analytic cases are submitted to the NCDB in accordance with the annual Call for Data. Although this requirement had been in place since 1996, it was infrequently monitored until 2003, when a Web-based reporting application used by the NCDB started to simultaneously update each cancer program's Survey Application Record as data files are received, edited, and written to CoC databases, allowing compliance with Standard 3.6 to be easily reviewed and assessed.

Data Edits

In advance of transmitting data files to the NCDB, CoC-accredited cancer program registrars are advised to use the most current NCDB EDITS metafile to pre-edit their data transmission file to ensure that submitted records are of the highest possible quality. The NCDB EDITS metafile for each Call for Data is made available on the NCDB Web page 3 to 4 months in advance of the deadline for data submission. The NCDB EDITS metafile utilizes standardized and nationally accepted data edits using GenEdits software, freely available from the Centers for Disease Control and Prevention. Instructions for using the NCDB metafiles and EDITS software are available on the NCDB Web page.

Once data files are received, every case submitted undergoes three parallel editing processes. Each of these steps uses the same NCDB metafile made available to registries to pre-edit their data transmission file.

The first editing process evaluates the quality of the data reported for each case. With each Call for Data specified edits, both single items and interitem combinations are checked for validity. Cases that fail certain specified single

and interitem "rejection edits" will be automatically excluded from further processing and will not be written to the CoC's data warehouse. At minimum, these "rejection edits" include edit failures associated with codes reported in the data items: accession number, postal code at diagnosis, birth date, date of first contact, date of diagnosis, tumor morphology, primary site, sequence number, sex, and sex/primary site. Other additional "rejection edits" may also be included.

The second editing process is applied to all cases that did not fail any of the previously mentioned "rejection edits." Records are evaluated and scored depending on which and how many of the specified single and interitem edits a case fails. Cases that accumulate a data quality score equal to or greater than 200 points are subsequently rejected and are not written to the CoC's data warehouse. Cases with a data quality score of zero (0) are considered problem free, whereas those with a score between 1 and 199 are expected to be reviewed, corrected, and resubmitted in accordance with Standard 3.7 of the CoC's *Cancer Program Standards*. The data quality score assigned to each case is recorded as part of the case record in the CoC data warehouse. Documentation providing specific information describing edit names and the data quality score associated with each edit is posted on the NCDB Web page and is made available when the NCDB metafile is released.

Standard 3.7 of the *CoC Cancer Programs Standards* specifies that "cases submitted to the NCDB that were diagnosed in 2003 or more recently meet the established quality criteria included in the annual Call for Data."[1] This standard requires CoC-accredited cancer program registries to resolve errors that result in rejected records and to correct any other errors leading to the assignment of a data quality score of greater than zero (0) for all case records diagnosed in 2003 or later. For example, in the Call for Data requesting cases for the years 2008, 2003, 1998, 1993 and 1988, Standard 3.7 applies to cases for the years 2008 and 2003. Resolution of edit errors and data quality problems for cases from the remaining three years, though advised and strongly encouraged, is not required.

The third editing process includes the production of an edit report for each of the years included in every data transmission made by a CoC-accredited cancer program registry. These reports specify the exact nature of any identified edit errors or warnings and should be used by registries to review particular cases and data items in its registry database, thus providing both the cancer program and the CoC with better quality data. The hospital data edit reports are posted electronically and are made available to each respective program registry using the secured CoC Datalinks Web application. The electronic posting of each edit report includes information specifying the receipt date of the submission, the total number of records received in the submission file, the number of records rejected, and the number of records identified as having quality problems. In addition, a summary site/stage table showing the distribution of all quality accepted records by *International Classification of Diseases for Oncology* (ICD-O) topography code and American Joint Committee on Cancer (AJCC) Stage Group is generated to serve as a mechanism by which registries can confirm and validate the type and number of cases received and processed. Registries are notified via e-mail on completion of the editing process; summary information describing the status of the edits review of their data submission is provided in the notification.

Writing Cases to the Commission on Cancer Data Warehouse

The CoC data warehouse is maintained across a number of dedicated Oracle servers. Individually edited and data quality scored records are written to the CoC data warehouse as soon as the editing process is complete. Each case is assigned a contextual code that is used in the duplicate case elimination process. Cases are written to the CoC data warehouse after a primary key search is performed. This key is based on the specific code values made up of the CoC Facility Identification Number (FIN) of the submitting registry, the accession and sequence number of the case, and the year portion of the data item "Date of 1st Contact." If two case reports with the same key are identified, depending on the data quality score of the two cases, a case update is performed. If no match is found, the case is added to the database as a new case. Once a record is written to the database, a second key search is performed to identify clinical duplicates—that is, instances in which the same patient is reported by more than one registry. When clinical duplicate cases are identified, the contextual code is assigned to each case and used to flag one of the two or more cases for use in aggregate analyses. The remaining cases are preserved for use in generating registry-specific reports.

Data Quality

Data are reported to the NCDB from a variety of cancer programs, ranging from very large academic/research institutions to medium and small community providers. Cancer registry abstractors and coders, though trained in a variety of ways and representing a wide array of backgrounds, participate in the submission of data to the NCDB. Because of the importance of these data, both for local review and use of the data for broader aggregated cancer research and to promote the improvement of the quality of cancer care, data quality is essential. All reports, publication, and information disseminated using data entered into the NCDB are affected by the quality of the data reported from participating program registries. Therefore, it is mandatory that the data be assessed on a regular basis to ensure reliability. The primary method used by the staff of the NCDB is the establishment and regular monitoring of the data quality scores and edit errors generated as part of the data submission process.

In addition to data edit reports, further studies are performed to assess the impact of available data through quality evaluation and monitoring tools currently applied

to data reported to the NCDB. Various types of reabstracting studies have been done to satisfy this need. However, additional statistical approaches are being developed to monitor various parameters on an ongoing basis.

The data reporting and quality requirements set fourth in CoC's *Cancer Program Standards* represent an ongoing commitment by the CoC to maintain quality assurance efforts by the NCDB. In addition, the programmatic standard that case abstracting be performed or supervised by a CTR (Standard 3.1) is a continued demonstration of the CoC's recognition of the qualitative contribution certified cancer registry professionals bring to the task of accurate and consistent case abstracting and coding. Finally, the ongoing requirement that CoC-accredited cancer programs conduct studies evaluating quality and outcomes (Standard 8.1) provide opportunities for cancer programs to document carefully designed and thoroughly executed internal reviews of the quality of their registry data.

Data Confidentiality

The ACoS is committed to ensuring the strictest adherence to the CoC's policies on data confidentiality and has implemented all the appropriate policies, procedures, and information systems to comply with the rules and regulations concerning privacy of patient data under the HIPAA and is in compliance with the final regulations released in August 2002. The CoC has entered into a "business associate" (BA) agreement with each hospital with an accredited cancer program, and as such functions as an organization that performs activities such as quality assurance and improvement or accreditation functions for a covered entity (§160.103). In this function, the NCDB consists of a limited data set from CoC-accredited cancer program registries. A limited data set is defined as one that *does not include any* of the 14 following data elements: name, street address, phone/fax numbers, e-mail addresses, Social Security number, certificate or license numbers, vehicle identification numbers, URLs or IP addresses, full face photographs, medical record numbers, health beneficiary numbers, other account numbers, devise identifiers or serial numbers, and biometric identifiers.

Under these guidelines, the ACoS assures all covered entities that (1) any and all data that may lead to the identity of the any patient, research subject, physician, or other person are strictly privileged and confidential; (2) no patient, physician, or facility will be identified in published results; (3) data will be received, stored, analyzed, and reported in accordance with the confidentiality requirements as set down by HIPAA; and (4) secure data repositories will be used at all times.

Data Analysis and Evaluation

Case records reported to the NCDB are maintained in the CoC data warehouse in such a way as to maximize the analytic utility of the data, whether this is for aggregate analytic purposes or for generating hospital-based benchmark reports. All the data collected by the NCDB are frequently utilized in the analytic work and report generation conducted by the NCDB staff; however, much of the basic framework for this effort is informed by the following set of covariates.

More than 22 years of data are maintained by the NCDB. This longitudinal depth allows for the systematic evaluation of changing patterns of diagnosis, disease presentation, and first-course therapy by diagnosis year.

The NCDB organizes much of its analysis and reporting by disease site. There are 61 NCDB analytic disease sites, and every case reported to the NCDB is assigned to one of these categories. All cases reported with ICD-O morphology codes 9590 to 9948 are assigned to the appropriate hemic or lymphatic site. The remaining cases are assigned to the appropriate site group depending on the specified combinations of topography and morphology codes (Table 38-1). Tumor morphology, including tumor histology, behavior and grade, are coded for each case reported to the NCDB. Codes describing tumor histology are

Table 38-1	NCDB Analytic Site Groups		
Anatomic System	**Anatomic Site**	**ICD-O-2/3 Topography Code**	**ICD-O-2/3 Histology Code**
Head and Neck	Lip	C00.0-C00.9	8000-9582
	Tongue	C01.9-C02.9	8000-9582
	Salivary Glands	C07.9-C08.9	8000-9582
	Floor of Mouth	C04.0-C04.9	
	Gum and Other Mouth	C03.0-C03.9, C05.0-C05.9, C06.0-C06.9	8000-9582
	Nasopharynx	C11.0-C11.9	8000-9582
	Tonsil	C09.0-C09.9	8000-9582
	Oropharynx	C10.0-C10.9	8000-9582
	Hypopharynx	C12.9, C13.0-C13.9	8000-9582
	Other Oral Cavity and Pharynx	C14.0, C14.2-C14.8	8000-9582
Digestive System	Esophagus	C15.0-C15.9	8000-9582
	Stomach	C16.0-C16.9	8000-9582
	Small intestine	C17.0-C17.9	8000-9582
	Colon	C18.0-C18.9, C26.0	8000-9582
	Rectosigmoid Junction	C19.9	8000-9582
	Rectum	C20.9	8000-9582
	Anus	C21.0-C21.8	8000-9582
	Liver	C22.0	8000-9582
	Intrahepatic Bile Duct	C22.1	8000-9582
	Gallbladder	C23.9	8000-9582
	Other Biliary	C24.0-C24.9	8000-9582
	Pancreas	C25.0-C25.9	8000-9582
	Retroperitoneum	C48.0	8000-9582
	Peritoneum, Omentum, Mesentary	C48.1-C48.2	8000-9582
	Other Digestive	C26.8-C26.9, C48.8	8000-9582
Respiratory System	Nose, Nasal Cavity, Middle Ear	C30.0-C31.9	8000-9582
	Larynx	C32.0-C32.9	8000-9582
	Lung, Bronchus—Small Cell Carcinoma	C34.0-C34.9	8040-8045

(Continued)

Table 38-1   NCDB Analytic Site Groups (continued)

Anatomic System	Anatomic Site	ICD-O-2/3 Topography Code	ICD-O-2/3 Histology Code
Respiratory System (continued)	Lung, Bronchus—Non-Small Cell Carcinoma	C34.0-C34.9	8012-8035, 8046-8576
	Lung, Bronchus—Other Types	C34.0-C34.9	8000-8011, 8580-9582
	Pleura	C38.4	8000-9582
	Trachea, Mediastinum, Other Respiratory	C33.9, C38.1-C38.3, C38.8, C39.0-C39.9	8000-9582
Bones and Joints	Bones and Joints	C40.0-C41.9	8000-9582
Soft Tissue and Heart	Soft Tissue and Heart	C38.0, C47.0-C47.9, C49.0-C49.9	8000-9582
Skin (non-epithelial)	Melanoma—Skin	C44.0-C44.9	8720-8790
	Other Non-Epithelial Skin	C44.0-C44.9	8120-8713, 8800-9582
Breast	Breast	C50.0-C50.9	8000-9582
Female Genital System	Cervix	C53.0-C53.9	8000-9582
	Uterus	C54.0-C54.9, C55.9	8000-9582
	Ovary	C56.9	8000-9582
	Vagina	C52.9	8000-9582
	Vulva	C51.0-C51.9	8000-9582
	Other Female Genital	C57.0-C58.9	8000-9582
Male Genital System	Prostate	C61.9	8000-9582
	Testis	C62.0-C62.9	8000-9582
	Penis	C60.0-C60.9	8000-9582
	Other Male Genital	C63.0-C63.9	8000-9582
Urinary System	Bladder	C67.0-C67.9	8000-9582
	Kidney and Renal Pelvis	C64.9, C65.9	8000-9582
	Ureter	C66.9	8000-9582
	Other Urinary	C68.0-C68.9	8000-9582
Eye and Orbit	Eye and Orbit	C69.0-C69.9	8000-9582
Brain, Nervous System	Brain	C71.0-C71.9	8000-9523, 9540-9582
	Other CNS	C71.0-C71.9	9530-9539
		C70.0-C70.9, C72.0-C72.9	8000-9582
Thyroid/Endocrine	Thyroid	C73.9	8000-9582
	Endocrine	C37.9, C74.0-C74.9, C75.0-C75.9	8000-9582
Hemic and Lymphatic	Hodgkin Lymphoma	Any	9650-9667
	Non-Hodgkin Lymphoma	Any	9590-9596, 9670-9729
	Plasma Cell Tumors	Any	9731-9734
	Leukemia	Any	9800-9948
Other and Unspecified	Other and Unspecified	All other cases not otherwise specified above	

reported to the NCDB using either the *International Classification of Diseases for Oncology,* 2nd edition (1990; ICD-O-2), if diagnosed before 2001, or the 3rd edition (2000; ICD-O-3), if diagnosed 2001 or later. Cases diagnosed before 2001 that have not been converted forward to ICD-O-3 standards are converted as part of the process of writing cases to the CoC data warehouse. The reported ICD-O-2 morphology codes are retained.

Analyses utilizing patient characteristics typically involve consideration of age, sex, and race/ethnicity. Patient age is typically categorized into 10- or 5-year age ranges, depending on the analytic task. Adult cases are defined as those aged 19 or older at the time of diagnosis. Cases reported as men or women are retained for most analytic work; cases reported as hermaphrodites or transsexuals are infrequently encountered. Patient race/ethnicity is computed using a combination of the race codes and reported information describing Spanish/Hispanic heritage, and is frequently reported as White, African American, Hispanic, Native American, Asian/Pacific Islander (API), and Other/Unknown. Additional racial/ethnic information can be imputed using a combination of coded race and place of birth information depending on the analytic task. In addition, certain socioeconomic measures can be used such as insurance status and aggregate measures of family income and educational status. The latter two measures are derived from published U.S. census data and matched to NCDB case records based on the reported zip code of residence at the time of diagnosis for each case.

Cases reported to the NCDB are staged using the AJCC Staging System. In many analyses, pathologic stage group information is used whenever possible, supplemented by clinical stage group information when pathology is unknown. This method is used to minimize the number of cases under analysis without an AJCC stage designation. The stage grouping utilized in analyses is sensitive to the disease site under review and the *AJCC Cancer Staging Manual* in use at the time the case was diagnosed. The introduction of the Collaborative Staging System, starting with cases diagnosed in 2004, presents new opportunities to analytically evaluate and describe the extent of disease reported at the time of diagnosis and will complement the NCDB's past reliance on physician-based staging information.

The NCDB is particularly interested in treatment patterns. The first course of treatment represents the combination of treatment modalities used in the management of the disease. Surgery is among the principal recognized treatment modalities for cancer and includes the local excision or resection of the primary tumor. The type and description of surgical procedures are specific to the reported ICD-O primary site of disease, and have been clearly defined and described in CoC coding manuals, including the *Data Acquisition Manual (DAM), Registry Operations and Data Standards, Volume II (ROADS),* and *Facility Oncology Registry Data Standards (FORDS).* Radiation, which includes beam radiation, brachytherapy, or radioisotopes, and systemic therapy, separately reported as chemotherapy, hormone therapy, or immunotherapy (biological response modifiers), are also reported to the NCDB and are included in the analysis of treatment patterns. In some instances, no treatment is provided to certain cases. For many analyses, cases are categorized using one or a number of the following specified descriptions of first-course treatment: surgery alone; radiation alone; chemotherapy alone; hormone alone; surgery plus radiation; surgery plus chemotherapy; surgery plus hormone therapy; surgery plus BRM (immunotherapy); surgery, radiation plus chemotherapy; surgery, radiation plus hormone therapy; surgery, radiation, chemotherapy plus hormone therapy; radiation plus chemotherapy; radiation plus hormone therapy; other specified treatment modalities (which may include surgery, radiation, chemotherapy, hormone therapy, and/or immunotherapy); and no treatment. Treatment modalities are reported depending on the disease site and stage of disease under review; some treatment management strategies may be used in the treatment of one type of disease but not with another. Similarly, management of disease may depend on its stage at presentation, thus excluding certain treatment modalities from analytic review.

Data can be analyzed geographically. Frequently, U.S. census regions (Northeast, Atlantic, Southeast, Great Lakes, South, Midwest, West, Mountain, and Pacific) are used to provide a broad set of regional area analyses. Alternatively, reporting on a state or one of the 17 ACS divisions in which the reporting hospital is located can be used. Furthermore, facility characteristics, based on one or a combination of the scope of resources and services available and case volume can be used to review patterns of diagnosis, patient care, and outcomes. The cancer program category scheme used by the CoC accreditation standards are often used to combine programs.

Outcomes, or survival analyses, are performed by computing observed or relative survival rates, depending on the focus of the analytic task. Observed survival rates are computed using the actuarial method, compounding survival in 1-month intervals from the date of diagnosis, with death from any cause as the recognized end point. Relative survival rates are the ratio of the observed survival rate to the expected survival rate of persons of the same sex, age, and racial or ethnic background. Expected survival rates are computed in single-year increments using the most recent life-expectancy tables published by the National Center for Health Statistics. Using this methodology, the relative survival rates become risk-adjusted for the demographic variability in patient populations, and can be calculated in the absence of specific and reliable cause of death information for each patient. Outcomes analyses also include the application of multivariate survival techniques, particularly the use of Cox regression techniques, which model the relative risk of patient survivorship based on one or more covariates.

Reports and Publications

Benchmark Reports

A set of Web-based benchmark applications promotes access to NCDB data by the general public, researchers, and clinicians. The benchmark reports have been released in two formats. One release is explicitly designed to facilitate public use. The other is targeted for use by CoC-accredited cancer programs as a tool by which to evaluate and compare the cancer care delivered to patients diagnosed or treated, or both, at their facility. These reports are provided as a direct benefit of their CoC accreditation status.

The public benchmark reports are limited in scope to the 11 most commonly diagnosed and treated solid tumors in the United States. Users are provided access to data for a limited number of diagnosis years and can design queries using data from any one or a combination of three types of hospitals (small community, comprehensive community, and academic/teaching facilities), and specify a geographic region or state to narrow the scope of their analysis. As many as three covariates (including patient age, ethnicity, and sex; tumor histology and stage; first-course therapy and type of surgical resection) are available for users to define the type of information they wish to review. No facility identifiers are included as part of this reporting application, and queries that return aggregated data from fewer than six facilities are suppressed to ensure facility confidentiality. Since its release in early 2002, the public benchmark reports have been well received; on average, 80 queries per weekday are received. Breast cancer, followed by non-small cell lung cancer, colon cancer, and prostate cancer are the most frequently reviewed disease sites and account for approximately two thirds of all queries. These reports are updated annually as subsequent NCDB Call for Data cycles are completed.

The Hospital Comparison Benchmark Reports are similar in the design of the public reports but provide authorized users additional options and control to generate desired reports. Access to these reports is password protected and limited to designated persons affiliated with CoC-accredited cancer programs. These reports contain data starting with the diagnosis year 2000 and have expanded as subsequent NCDB Call for Data cycles are completed. In contrast with the public benchmark reports described earlier, these reports include data on each of the NCDB analytic disease sites, with the exception of cancers of other and unspecified sites that are not included. Users are allowed greater control over the type of cases selected and have a longer list of covariates from which to select, including patient insurance status, an aggregate measure of median family income and educational attainment, tumor behavior, and more detailed information on the type of radiation and/or systemic therapy administered as part of the first course of therapy. Although the public benchmark application only allows users to generate aggregate reports, the Hospital Comparison reports provide users with three options: (1) show data reported to the NCDB from their own program's cancer registry; (2) show aggregated data; or (3) display a comparative report that contains data reported from the user's registry alongside aggregated data. Aggregated data can be provided based on the user's selection of hospital characteristics. In addition, facilities that are part of cooperative or corporate systems (e.g., Veterans Administration hospitals, hospitals that are members of the Children's Oncology Group [COG], or other system hospitals) can compare their performance with that of other facilities in the same system. Specific geographical regions, either states or ACS Divisions, can also be used to further refine queries submitted to this application. Similar to the benchmark reports available to the public, breast, non-small cell lung, colon, and prostate cancers are the most frequently queried cancers. The reporting application handles approximately 22,000 queries from staff at CoC-accredited cancer programs annually.

This "point and click" application allows data to be displayed as tables, bar graphs, or pie charts. Programs can view their own data, and compare their patient mix, treatment patterns, and outcomes to peer groups (facilities similar to their own) or to different types of cancer programs. They can also review state, region, or national norms for treatment patterns and outcomes. These reports are intended to enable physicians and registrars at cancer programs to identify patterns of care within their own programs that may differ significantly from patterns in similar programs or differ from state, regional, or national norms. Such information can be useful for identifying issues for quality improvement studies, a requirement of the CoC's *Cancer Program Standards* (Standard 8.1). The information may also be useful for planning and marketing purposes.

The NCDB Survival Reports provide site-specific AJCC stage-stratified observed survival rates for all disease sites, and they are available to authorized persons affiliated with CoC-accredited cancer programs. Cancer program specific survival rates are provided as part of this application. However, in many instances, the number of cases reported from any one hospital may be quite small, thus limiting the generalizability of the computed rates for many types of cancer. The survival reports application handles approximately 11,000 queries from staff at CoC-accredited cancer programs annually.

In early 2005, the CoC released the first version of its Cancer Program Practice Profile Reports (CP³R). The first CP³R was designed to provide CoC-accredited cancer programs the opportunity to gauge processes of care for Stage III colon cancer. Using evidence from randomized clinical trials reported in the mid-1990s, and the development and wide dissemination of standards of care for colorectal cancers by organizations such as the National Comprehensive Cancer Network (NCCN), the initial release of the CP³R provided a comparative assessment of historical patterns of care using information routinely captured by hospital-based cancer registries and reported to the NCDB. Each CoC-accredited cancer program was provided with an estimate of its concordance rate for adjuvant chemotherapy for node-positive (Stage III) colon cancer, a commonly recognized standard of care. The CP³R was designed to enable cancer programs to identify specific cases and review the specific treatment information submitted to the NCDB by their cancer programs' registry. Each of the identified cases used in the development and generation of the tables and charts displayed in the CP³R can be reviewed, including specific information describing surgical therapy, chemotherapy, immunotherapy, hormone therapy, and radiation therapy administered to the patient and reported to the NCDB.

In the mid-2000s, a public/private partnership led by the National Quality Forum (NQF) brought together payers, consumers, researchers, and clinicians to promulgate performance measures for breast and colorectal cancers. The CoC was actively engaged in this process. Through a parallel process, the American Society for Clinical Oncology (ASCO) and the NCCN developed a similar set of measures for breast and colorectal cancer. These included:

- Radiation therapy is administered within 1 year (365 days) of diagnosis for women younger than 70 receiving breast-conserving surgery for breast cancer.
- Combination chemotherapy is considered or administered within 4 months (120 days) of diagnosis for women younger than 70 with AJCC T1cN0M0, or Stage II or III hormone receptor–negative breast cancer.
- Tamoxifen *or* third-generation aromatase inhibitor is considered or administered within 1 year (365 days) of diagnosis for women with AJCC T1cN0M0, or Stage II or III hormone receptor–positive breast cancer.
- At least 12 regional lymph nodes are removed and pathologically examined for resected colon cancer.
- Adjuvant chemotherapy is considered or administered within 4 months (120 days) of diagnosis for patients younger than 80 with AJCC Stage III (lymph node–positive) colon cancer.
- Radiation therapy is considered or administered within 6 months (180 days) of diagnosis for patients younger than 80 with clinical or pathologic AJCC T4N0M0 or Stage III receiving surgical resection for rectal cancer.

Facilitated by the NQF, the CoC, ASCO, and NCCN agreed to synchronize their developed measures to ensure that a unified set were put forth to the public. Of the six measures harmonized by these professional medical societies, four were endorsed by the NQF as *accountability measures,* meaning that these measures can be used for such purposes as public reporting, payment incentive programs, and the selection of providers by consumers, health plans, or purchasers. Additional measures relating to regional lymph node examination for resected colon cancers and radiation therapy for advanced stage rectal cancer are considered *quality improvement* measures and are intended to be used for internal monitoring of performance within an organization or group. These latter two *surveillance measures* can be used at the community, regional, and/or national level to monitor patterns and trends of care to guide practice change where appropriate, policy making, and resource allocation. None of these measures is designed to assess individual hospital or physician performance. Each of these six processes of care measures for breast and colorectal cancer were implemented through the CP³R Web-based application in the fall of 2008. This reporting tool, with its complement of measures, continues and expands the scope and detail of data feedback to CoC-accredited cancer programs to improve the quality of data across several disease sites, foster preemptive awareness to the importance of charting and coding accuracy, and improve clinical management and coordination of patient care in the multidisciplinary setting. Information describing non-surgical treatment can be modified, if necessary. The CP³R application handles more than 60,000 user sessions from staff at CoC-accredited cancer programs annually.

Publications

More than 300 peer-reviewed journal articles have been published using data submitted to the NCDB. Articles predominantly have focused on clinical surveillance of patterns of care and outcomes for almost all disease sites. The findings reported in these published articles and other projects initiated by investigators across the United States have prompted additional analytic questions and will undoubtedly spur the publication of further peer-reviewed articles. The dissemination of information maintained by the NCDB is limited only by the number of reporting tools, analyses, and publications that can be produced.

Interactions with Other National Organizations

Because of its function as a database of reported cancer diagnoses, the NCDB interacts with a number of other groups and organizations. Integral to many of the functions performed by the NCDB is the wide array of relationships maintained with other organizations interested in the surveillance and epidemiology of cancer and cancer care in the United States. These interactions include NCDB and CoC staff participation in coordinated activities involving the AJCC, ACS, the Canadian Association of Provincial Cancer Registries (CAPCR), the NAACCR, the National Cancer Registrars Association (NCRA), the National Program of Cancer Registries (NPCR) of the Centers for Disease Control and Prevention, and the Surveillance, Epidemiology, and End Results (SEER) program of the National Cancer Institute. Much, though by no means all, of the cancer surveillance interagency activity revolves around the setting of standards for data abstracting and recording, and optimal cancer registry management practices.

In addition, membership in the CoC includes 48 national professional organizations. Exhibits have been prepared for display at various medical conventions to help promote the profile and work of the NCDB. NCDB staff act as contact persons for a number of these organizations and are available at conventions to distribute NCDB materials and to answer questions from researchers and other potential users of the database. Among these national professional organizations are ASCO; College of American Pathologists (CAP), Society of Surgical Oncology (SSO), the American College of Radiology (ACR), the American Society for Therapeutic Radiation and Oncology (ASTRO), as well as a number of surgical specialty societies.

One of the missions of the NCDB is to help educate groups and individuals concerned with the development and maintenance of better cancer registry data, and the use and impact of that data. NCDB staff regularly schedule presentations to various organizations, including cancer registry data managers and other medical and oncology groups. These groups have the potential to use the information recorded in registry databases to manage and direct cancer care in facilities and cancer care centers.

Summary

Since its inception in 1989, the NCDB has collected diagnostic, staging, treatment, and outcomes information on almost 25 million cancer diagnoses. These data have been published, reported in several formats, and used by clinicians and hospitals throughout the United States. The uses of the data are many and include significant advances in the utilization of the database as a clinical and facility benchmarking tool. As the database continues to grow and becomes more widely recognized, it will be used to an even greater extent. Its potential is abundant. With millions of case records at its disposal, the NCDB is an enormous and valuable resource for patterns of care information on which quality improvement can be leveraged at the point of delivery of cancer care in the United States.

Further information is available through the NCDB Web page of the ACoS Web site (www.facs.org).

Reference

1. Commission on Cancer. Standard 3.7: Cancer Program Standards, 2009 Revised Edition. Chicago: American College of Surgeons, 2009, p. 46.

chapter 39

Federal Registries: Department of Defense and Department of Veterans Affairs

Elizabeth Butts, MPH, CTR, CPC

Raye-Ann Dorn, MPH, CTR

Sonja Jennings, CTR

Judy Tryon, CTR

The foundations of medicine may have been laid in Greece around 500 B.C., but no actual recording of diseases was published until the late sixteenth and seventeenth centuries.[1] The need for reliable cancer statistics became increasingly apparent during the early twentieth century when, in 1915, Frederick L. Hoffman, a statistician for the Prudential Insurance Company of America, published a compilation of cancer statistics from around the world.[2] Hoffman was instrumental in having the U.S. Census Bureau analyze cancer mortality in the United States for the 1914 data.

Ongoing interest and isolated studies into the disease process eventually led to a declaration of war on cancer by President Richard Nixon in 1971. Since then, billions of dollars have been spent on education, prevention, screening, treatment, and research. Fundamental to any research was the need to develop databases for long-term acquisition and validation of knowledge about the different disease processes in human patients.[3] The federal government has become the leader in the data collection arena, maintaining registries in all branches of the military establishment, the Department of Veterans Affairs (VA), the National Institutes of Health, the Indian Health Service, and the Centers for Disease Control and Prevention.

Registries

The VA and the Department of Defense (DoD) administer, through the respective branches of the armed forces, registries for the tracking of cancer incidence and mortality at all medical centers. A summary of cancer programs within these departments of the federal government is presented in Table 39-1.

Table 39-1	Cancer Registry Programs Administered by the Department of Veterans Affairs and the Department of Defense		
Cancer Registry Programs		Total Programs	CoC* Accredited
Administered by the Department of Veterans Affairs			
Veterans Affairs		140	60
Administered by the Department of Defense			
U.S. Air Force		34	4
U.S. Army		28	10
U.S. Navy		21	3
Total		83	17

*Commission on Cancer of the American College of Surgeons

Programs at federal institutions are similar to their nongovernmental counterparts. The guidelines established by the American College of Surgeons' Commission on Cancer (ACoS CoC) Accreditation Program are followed. External peer review of the programs and accreditation by the ACoS CoC is desirable and highly encouraged.

Although the data collection methods and the external approval standards are the same as for the private sector, a major difference between federal cancer registries and nongovernmental registries is in the way the programs are organized. Directives from subject matter experts at the national level provide registry oversight, general direction, and guidance. However, the actual implementation and establishment of these directives are left to the individual facilities, thereby preserving local program autonomy and flexibility.[4-6] Another difference between federal registries and the private sector is that both the VA and the DoD have centralized repositories of data. VA data are collected and maintained locally in the software program (OncoTraX). The DoD cancer data repository is called ACTUR (Automated Central Tumor Registry). ACTUR is a component of the Defense Enrollment Eligibility Reporting System (DEERS) program and is administered for the three DoD military services (Army, Navy, and Air Force) by the Armed Forces Institute of Pathology (AFIP).

Department of Veterans Affairs

To care for him who has borne the battle, his wife and his orphan.
—Abraham Lincoln

The VA was established on March 15, 1989, succeeding the Veterans Administration, and is responsible for providing federal benefits to veterans and their families. Headed by the Secretary of Veterans Affairs, it is the second largest of the 15 Cabinet departments and operates nationwide programs for health care, financial assistance, and burial benefits.

Of the 23.4 million veterans currently alive, nearly three-quarters served during a war or an official period of conflict. About a quarter of the nation's population is potentially eligible for VA benefits and services because they are veterans or family members or survivors of veterans.

Continuum of Care

Perhaps the most visible of all VA benefits and services is health care. From 54 hospitals in 1930, VA's healthcare system now includes 153 medical centers, with at least one in each state, Puerto Rico, and the District of Columbia. VA operates more than 1,400 sites of care, including 909 ambulatory care and community-based outpatient clinics,

135 nursing homes, 47 residential rehabilitation treatment programs, 232 Veterans Centers, and 1,008 comprehensive home care programs. VA healthcare facilities provide a broad spectrum of medical, surgical, and rehabilitative care. The Veterans Health Administration (VHA) healthcare and research budget ($37.2 billion in obligations) constituted 43% of the VA's total obligations in fiscal year 2008.[7]

The VA manages the largest medical education and health professions training program in the United States. VA facilities are affiliated with 107 medical schools, 55 dental schools, and more than 1,200 other schools across the country. Each year, more than 90,000 health professionals are trained in VA medical centers. More than half of the physicians practicing in the United States had some of their professional education in the VA healthcare system.

There are about 23.4 million living veterans, 7.5% of whom are women. There are about 37 million dependents (spouses and dependent children) of living veterans and survivors of deceased veterans. Together, they represent 24% of the U.S. population. In 2008, VHA provided healthcare services to approximately 5.58 million unique patients out of the projected U.S. veteran population. Vietnam Era veterans, about 7.9 million, comprise the largest segment of the veteran population.

In 2008, the median age of all living veterans was 60 years old, 61 for men and 47 for women. Median ages by period of service were 37 years old for Gulf War, 60 for Vietnam War, 76 for Korean War, and 84 for World War II.

Sixty percent (60%) of the nation's veterans live in urban areas. States with the largest Veteran populations are California, Florida, Texas, Pennsylvania, New York, and Ohio, respectively. These six states account for about 36% of the total veteran population.

Veteran population by race breakouts are: white, 79.7%; black, 11.1%, Asian/Pacific Islander, 1.4%; Hispanic, 5.7%; American Indian/Alaska Natives, 0.8%; and others, 1.3%. The percentage of the veteran population 65 years or older is 39.4%.[8]

Registries

Like the DoD after the National Cancer Act of 1971, the VA joined the war on cancer and in 1986 initiated the development of the Decentralized Hospital Computer Program (DHCP) Oncology Program, a hospital-based cancer registry software program fully integrated into the medical centers' main computer system for capturing cancer incidence in a uniform and consistent way. Initially, the program was implemented at only 50 of the department's largest medical teaching centers, but in 1992, after the release of *Criteria and Standards for VA Oncology Programs,*[9] cancer registration was expanded from tertiary care centers to include secondary care facilities, increasing the number of hospitals with cancer registration to 65. With the establishment of a permanent centralized presence at VA Central Office in the Office of the National Coordinator for Cancer Programs in 1995, the final push for establishing cancer registration at

all VA medical centers diagnosing and/or treating veterans with the disease was realized, bringing the total of active cancer registration centers to 140.

Cancer programs in the VA are similar in composition and nature to their nongovernmental counterparts in that the fundamental program elements of the guidelines established by the ACoS CoC for cancer programs are followed. The essential functions of casefinding, abstracting, follow-up, statistical reporting, and research facilitating are the same.

A significant difference is that all of the VA's cancer registries utilize a standardized centrally maintained software program (OncoTraX) assuring uniformity and consistency in data collection. Although the data elements collected adhere strictly to the standards established by the national standards setter organizations, the VA collects numerous additional data elements of interest to the organization for researching patterns of care and outcomes. OncoTraX is a fully integrated program decentralized in its completeness to each VA medical centers' main computer system permitting the fully automated functioning of a paperless registry. The VA patients are highly mobile and because the program is fully integrated into the hospital's main computer systems, the data collected are readily available to local staff, as well as regionally and nationally. The completed abstracts have been part of the electronic health record since 1992. Providing continuity of service and care, abstracts can be accessed at any VA medical center.

VA Central Cancer Registry

VA Central Cancer Registry (VACCR) was established in 1995 as an adjunct project by the Office of the National Coordinator for Cancer Programs to ascertain compliance in data collection at the VA's medical centers, and as a method for testing and resolving issues with data extraction tools for the releasing of data to the state central cancer registries.

The scope and mission of VACCR was updated in 1997 to become a multi-hospital central registry collecting, merging, and consolidating the 50,000 yearly cancer cases being collected by the VA's medical centers for the veteran population presenting for care. Although not strictly defined as a population-based registry, the primary purposes are to combine incidence reporting with expanded patient care, reporting outcomes, and supporting of research and cancer control activities. The ultimate goal of VACCR is the use of its collected data for analysis by physicians, health officials, and researchers within the VA community making decisions about healthcare policy and implementation, physician and staff recruitment, equipment and space needs, patient referral patterns, treatment outcomes, and unmet patient needs.

VACCR, in conjunction with the Office of the Chief Patient Care Services Officer, established formalized processes for data request and access in 2007 via peer protocol reviews and data transfer/use agreements. In addition, a searchable 600,000 case intranet public use file of deidentified data is also available to all VA employees.

Additional roles of the VACCR include the training/mentoring/support of all cancer programs in the VA and the maintenance of the OncoTraX program to assure continued adherence to nationally released standards.

Department of Defense

The Military Health System mission is to provide optimal health services in support of our nation's military mission—anytime, anywhere.[10]

Continuum of Care

The U.S. Military Health System consists of the Office of the Assistant Secretary of Defense for Health Affairs; the medical departments of the Army, Navy, Marine Corps, Air Force, Coast Guard, and Joint Chiefs of Staff; the Combatant Command surgeons; and TRICARE providers (including private sector healthcare providers, hospitals, and pharmacies). TRICARE is the major component of the Military Health System providing access to high-quality healthcare services, whereas maintaining the capacity to support military operations. There are more than 9,500,000 TRICARE beneficiaries, approximately 3% of the U.S. population. Beneficiaries include active duty service members, retirees of the seven uniform services (U.S. Army, U.S. Air Force, U.S. Navy, U.S. Marine Corps, U.S. Coast Guard, Commissioned Corps of the Public Health Service, and the Commissioned Corps of the National Oceanic and Atmospheric Association), their family members, survivors, and others who are registered in the DEERS. TRICARE is also available to members of the National Guard and Reserves and their families.

TRICARE beneficiaries can be found worldwide from Africa to the Philippines. Ninety-three percent are stationed or reside in the United States. More than a half million of the beneficiary pool are stationed or reside abroad. Of the total beneficiary pool, about 15% are active duty, 21% are dependents of active duty, and 21% are retirees.[11]

DoD cancer registries focus primarily on active duty service members, families of service members, and retirees presenting to the DoD military treatment facilities for health care.

Mirroring trends in the civilian population, the aging beneficiary population, age 65 or older, is projected to comprise 47.8% of the beneficiary pool in 2015.[12] Care is provided through military facilities worldwide, which include 59 military hospitals and 413 medical clinics, as well as a network of civilian providers.

Risk amelioration programs such as alcohol education, smoking cessation, and weight loss are part of TRICARE health promotions.

Registries

The Automated Central Tumor Registry was established in 1986 by the Assistant Secretary of Defense for Health Affairs to satisfy ACoS CoC requirements for a comprehensive cancer data reporting system. ACTUR is the central repository of more than 300,000 reported incidence cases.

Although ACTUR is similar to its civilian counterparts in terms of adherence to data collection guidelines established by ACoS, CoC, Surveillance, Epidemiology, and End Results (SEER) Program, North American Association of Central Cancer Registries (NAACCR), and National Program of Cancer Registries (NPCR), ACTUR differs from private sector data collection programs in several ways. The DoD requires that ACTUR data sets are military specific and include documentation of the sponsor's (military participant) Social Security number, sponsor's branch of service, and active duty status. DoD registrars collect sponsor participation in military campaigns such as Desert Storm (Persian Gulf), Enduring Freedom (Afghanistan), and Iraqi Freedom (Persian Gulf II), as well as exposure to toxic agents such as Agent Orange. These data are collected for historical and epidemiologic purposes.

Another practice particular to DoD registries is the maintenance of a patient convenience chart. Pertinent pathologic, diagnostic, and operation reports are kept within the patient files maintained in the registries. Patient data are preserved because outpatient and inpatient files are transferred to the DoD repository in St. Louis, Missouri, if there has been no outpatient activity for 2 years, or 5 years for inpatient charts. With the expansion of the DoD's electronic medical record to include all inpatient and outpatient episodes of care, future maintenance of a paper registry chart may become redundant.

The DoD discourages changes in inception dates to provide relief to follow-up incidence in compliance with ACoS CoC Standards 4.4 and 4.5. Because of this, some DoD registries have follow-up statistics that date as far back as 1953. Also, unlike civilian registries, the patient is the first point of contact for DoD registries. The emphasis on the patient as the primary source for follow-up information is due to communication challenges precipitated by rotation and transfer of DoD physicians. Patient status, however, can be changed only by clinical documentation.

Each of the triservices has a consultant to provide guidance to the registries under their purview. Overall program direction is established by the DoD ACTUR Coordination Committee composed of the three triservice consultants, representatives from the AFIP, DoD Central Registry staff, database experts, and service physician consultants.

The size and makeup of the service registries differ somewhat. For instance, the Navy has recently adopted a regionalized approach to cancer data collection. Each of the three Navy Medicine Regions will have a Navy Regional Tumor Registry Supervisor (NRTRS) who, together with the Navy Tumor Registry Consultant (NTRC), will coordinate data collection in each respective region. These regions include overseas sites and shipboard medical facilities (SBMF) as well. Each regional supervisor will be housed in one of the three Navy medical centers located in Portsmouth, Virginia

(Navy Medicine East), San Diego, California (Navy Medicine West), and Bethesda, Maryland (Navy Medicine Capital Region). The consultant and the regional supervisor are responsible for ensuring the timely and accurate cancer data submission into the ACTUR database and to serve as subject matter experts to the registrars within the specific regions.

Central Registry

The DoD Central Cancer Registry is part of the AFIP located on the campus of Walter Reed Army Medical Center. With an inception date of 1998, the central registry is a repository of more than 85,000 cases, including data on 71,000 patients. Breakdown by service is as follows: Army, 47%; Air Force, 30%; and Navy, 23%. These data are available for internal review board sanctioned research projects.

Abstracts in ACTUR are run through National Program of Cancer Registries' Prep Plus™, an editing module available in Registry Plus™. After computer-generated edit review, all cases undergo visual review, editing, and consolidation. Central Registry certified tumor registrars assist DoD registrars on a one-to-one basis and participate in the training of DoD registrars at the annual ACTUR conferences.

References

1. Shimkin, M. B. "Contrary to Nature" (National Institutes of Health Report 76-720). Washington, DC: U.S. Government Printing Office, 1977.

2. Hoffman, F. L. *The Mortality from Cancer Throughout the World.* Newark, NJ: Prudential Press, 1915.

3. DeVita, V. T., et al. *Cancer: Principles & Practice of Oncology* (p. 219), 6th ed. Philadelphia: J. B. Lippincott, 2001.

4. "MEDCOM Reg (Medical Command Regulation) 40-1." Ft. Sam Houston, San Antonio, TX: U.S. Army, 1996.

5. "Air Force Instruction 44-110." Washington, DC: US Air Force, 1996.

6. "BUMEDINST 6320.92." Navy Cancer and Tumor Registry Program. Bureau of Medicine and Surgery. Washington, DC: U.S. Navy, 2009.

7. "Performance and Accountability Report, 2008". Department of Veterans Affairs, Office of Budget, Produced by the National Center for Veterans Affairs Analysis and Statistics (008A-3).

8. *Criteria and Standards for VA Oncology Programs* (VA Regulation M9, Chapter 9, Appendix 9D, Change 12). Washington, DC: Department of Veterans Affairs, 1992.

9. "VHA Directive 2003-034." *National Cancer Strategy.* Washington, DC: Department of Veterans Affairs, 2003.

10. U.S. Department of Defense Military Health System. "What Is the MHS?" Available at: www.health.mil/About_MHS/index.aspx. Accessed July 9, 2010.

11. TRICARE Operations Center. "Eligible Population 2009." Available at: http://www.tricare.mil. Accessed July 27, 2009.

12. TRICARE Management Activity, Health Program Analysis and Evaluation Directorate (TMA/HPA&E) in the Office of the Assistant Secretary of Defense (Health Affairs) (OASD/HA). *Beneficiary Trends and Demographics. Evaluation of the TRICARE Program, Fiscal Year 2009 Report to Congress* (p. 21). Falls Church, VA: Office of the Assistant Secretary of Defense Health Affairs, 2009.

Clinical Trials

Therese Richardson, RHIA, CTR

Clinical trials are medical research studies designed to answer questions about new drugs or devices. They are the final step in the research process of moving scientific research from the laboratory to treatments for people. The terms *clinical study, clinical trial,* and *protocol* are often used interchangeably; however, each has a different meaning.[1]

History

In 1937, President Franklin D. Roosevelt signed the National Cancer Institute Act, which established the National Cancer Institute (NCI) as a division of the National Institutes of Health (NIH). The National Cancer Institute Act mandates funding to support cancer research and training.[2]

Cooperative Oncology Groups

In the mid-1950s, the NCI began to fund cooperative oncology groups in an effort to expand enrollment in clinical trials. Cooperative oncology groups are composed of groups of physicians at various institutions who collaboratively design and implement clinical trials. Examples of these include the Eastern Cooperative Oncology Group (ECOG), Southwest Oncology Group (SWOG), Cancer and Leukemia Group B (CALGB), National Surgical Adjuvant Breast and Bowel Project (NSABP), Radiation Therapy Oncology Group (RTOG), and Pediatric Oncology Group (POG). Cooperative oncology groups are overseen by NCI's Cancer Therapy Evaluation Program (CTEP), a branch of the NCI's Division of Cancer Treatment.[3]

The National Cancer Act of 1971 resulted in a large increase in NCI funding as approved by Congress. The NCI was charged with the responsibility of conducting basic scientific research in oncology and applying the results to clinical practice.[4]

By 1973, most clinical trials were conducted at NCI-approved Comprehensive Cancer Centers that received core grants from NCI to fund operations. However, only about 20% of patients with cancer were treated at these facilities and enrolled in clinical trials. Most cancer patients were still being treated by community oncologists.[3]

In 1976, the NCI's Division of Cancer Treatment established the Cooperative Group Outreach Program (CGOP). CGOP enabled community physicians to affiliate with a cooperative group to offer their patients access to cooperative group trials. The Community Clinical Oncology Program (CCOP) was instituted in 1983. CCOP differs from the CGOP program in its funding source, research focus, accrual requirements, and affiliation policies. CGOPs are funded by the NCI's Division of Cancer Prevention and Control (DCPC). In addition to cancer treatment, DCPC-sponsored clinical trials focus on prevention and early detection of cancer.[4]

Sometimes two or more clinical trial groups join forces to form an "intergroup" so that a large number of patients from a wider geographical area can participate in their studies. In this manner, specific diseases of a rare nature can be carefully studied in an expeditious manner, because patients are accrued more rapidly than if only one group conducted the study. Each cooperative group is held accountable to the NIH for the performance of its members.

Where Do Clinical Trials Take Place?

Clinical trials take place in doctors' offices, cancer centers, community hospitals and clinics, as well as military hospitals and veterans' hospitals throughout the United States and in other countries.

Growth of Regulation

Research on vulnerable populations such as prison inmates, the mentally handicapped, the poor, and minority groups was conducted in this country from the mid-1800s to the mid-1900s without informed consent.[5] It was not until the exposure of medical atrocities performed on prisoners during World War II that a code of ethics for human experimentation was developed. The Nuremberg Code of 1947 serves as the foundation for ethical principles governing clinical research today.[6]

In 1974, the National Commission for the Protection of Human Subjects of Biomedical and Behavioral Research developed written policies to protect human subjects from such atrocities. These policies were made operational by the Food and Drug Administration (FDA), a division of the Department of Health and Human Services (DHHS). *The Belmont Report,* published in 1978, mandated the establishment of institutional review boards (IRBs), outlined protocol design criteria, and required that written informed consent be provided to all research subjects.[3]

Federal Requirements

To be approved to perform research, each institution must comply with the regulations set forth by the DHHS. A written general assurance must be sent to the secretary of DHHS covering the requirements listed in Table 40-1.[7] There are certain minimal standards in the composition of IRB membership that must be met by each institution. Some of these are listed in Table 40-2.[7] In addition, each IRB member must have certain specific qualities as listed in Table 40-3.[7]

Institutional Review Board

An IRB is a committee whose membership, composition, purpose, and functions are specified by federal law. Before any clinical trial can be initiated in a hospital or clinical setting, federal law required that it be approved by an IRB.

Table 40-1	Responsibilities of Institutions Participating in Clinical Trials

1. Principles governing the institution must be defined.
2. Institutional responsibilities toward protecting the rights and welfare of human subjects must be defined.
3. An institutional review board must be established.
4. Adequate meeting space must be available for the institutional review board.
5. Provisions must be made for sufficient staff to support institutional review board review and record-keeping duties.
6. Written procedures for the institutional review board to follow when conducting research reviews must be defined.
7. A current list of members including name, profession, earned degrees, and other pertinent information must be maintained.
8. Records with reviews of research being conducted must be kept.
9. Unforeseen risks to subjects or others from research must be reported to the Department of Health and Human Services

Table 40-2	Partial List of Institutional Review Board Membership Composition Requirements by the Office for Protectin from Research Risk

1. Minimum of five members
2. Male and female members
3. More than one profession represented
4. Minimum of one nonscientific member (e.g., law, clergy)
5. Minimum of one member not affiliated with the institution and not part of any employer's immediate family

The Office for Protection from Research Risks (OPRR), a division of NIH, issues OPRR *Reports,* which present discussions of IRB functions, as well as updated IRB rules and regulations.

Three purposes were given for establishing these IRBs:

Protection of the rights and welfare of individuals involved in clinical research studies
Guarantee of the appropriateness of the methods used to secure informed consent from research subjects
Articulation of the risks and benefits potentially involved in the experiments[6]

Table 40-3	Required Qualities of Institutional Review Board Membership

1. Expertise in matters relating to each member's particular field
2. General knowledge of clinical medicine and clinical research, with the exception of members in nonscientific professions
3. Knowledge of the institution's commitments and regulations, the laws applicable to it, and its expected standards of professional conduct
4. Concern for the welfare of vulnerable subjects
5. Sensitivity to, and knowledge of, community attitudes
6. Ad hoc consultants (nonvoting) with special skills and competencies

Clinical Trial Protocol

Clinical trials follow strict scientific guidelines. These guidelines clearly state the purpose of the study and who will be able to participate. The principal investigator (PI) is the person in charge, usually a physician. The PI prepares a plan for the study, called a *protocol,* which acts like a "recipe" for conducting a clinical trial.

The protocol explains the purpose of the trial, how the study will be carried out, and why each part of the study is necessary. It includes the following information:

The reason for doing the study
The number of people who will be enrolled in the study
Who is eligible to participate in the study (requirements might involve type of cancer, general health, age)
Any agents that the participants will take, the dosage, and how often they will be administered
What medical tests participants will have and how often
What information will be gathered about the participants
The end points of the study

An end point is what the researchers will measure to evaluate the results of a new treatment being tested in a clinical trial. Research teams establish the end points of a trial before it begins. It is important to note that end points differ, depending on the type and phase of the clinical trial. Examples of end points are toxicity, tumor response, survival, and quality of life.[5]

Phases of a Clinical Trial

There are four phases of clinical trials. Each phase is designed to answer different research questions (Table 40-4).[6]

Who participates in Phase I treatment trials? People with cancer who are eligible for Phase I clinical trials have

Table 40-4	Phases of a Clinical Trial			
	Phase I	**Phase II**	**Phase III**	**Phase IV**
Number of Participants	15–30 people	Less than 100 people	Generally, from 100 to thousands of people	Several hundred to several thousand people
Purpose	• To find a safe dosage • To decide how the agent should be given • To observe how the agent affects the human body	• To determine whether the agent or intervention has an effect on a particular cancer • To see how the agent or intervention affects the human body	• To compare the new agent or intervention (or new use of a treatment) with the current standard	• To further evaluate the long-term safety and effectiveness of a new treatment

no known effective treatment options, or they have already tried other treatment options.

Phase I: Looking at Safety

In Phase I cancer trials, small groups of people with cancer are treated with a certain dose of a new agent that has already been extensively studied in the laboratory. During the trial, the dose is usually increased group by group to find the highest dose that does not cause unacceptable harmful side effects, called *toxicity*. This process determines a safe and appropriate dose to use in a Phase II trial.

Phase II: How Well the New Treatment Works

Phase II trials continue to test the safety of the new agent and to begin to evaluate how well it works against a specific type of cancer. In these trials, the new agent is given to groups of people with one type of cancer or related cancers, using the dosage found to be safe in Phase I trials.

Who participates in Phase II trials? People with cancer who have been treated with chemotherapy, surgery, or radiation, but the treatment was not effective. Participation in these trials is often restricted based on the previous treatment received.

Phase III: Comparing a New Treatment to the Standard Treatment

Phase III trials focus on learning how a new treatment compares with standard, or the most widely accepted, treatment. Researchers want to learn whether the new treatment is better than, the same as, or worse than the standard treatment.

In Phase III trials, participants have an equal chance to be assigned to one of two or more groups (called *arms*). In a study with two groups:

One group gets the standard treatment. This group is called the *control group*.
The other group gets the new treatment being tested. This group is referred to as the *investigational group*.

Placebos are almost never used in cancer treatment trial. In rare cases in which there is no standard treatment for a cancer, a new treatment may be compared with a placebo.

Who participates in Phase III trials? Participants in Phase III studies range from people newly diagnosed with cancer to people with extensive disease. Phase III studies are designed to answer research questions across the disease continuum.

Phase IV: Continuing Evaluation

Phase IV trials are used to further evaluate the long-term safety and effectiveness of a treatment. Less common than Phase I, II, and III trials, Phase IV trials take place after the new treatment has been approved for standard use.

Randomization

How Participants Are Assigned in Randomized Trials

The process of assigning participants to groups is called *randomization*. Phase III studies are randomized, clinical trials. Some Phase II trials may also be randomized.

Randomization is a method used to prevent bias in research. It ensures that unknown factors do not influence the trial results. Participants are assigned to either the investigational group or the control group by chance, via a computer program, or with a table of random numbers.

Anyone who is considering participating in a randomized, clinical trial needs to understand that the doctor does not choose the group for the participant. She or he has an equal chance to be assigned to one of the groups.

Randomization is important because it eliminates bias and ensures that the study results are caused by the treatments rather than by chance or other factors.

Informed Consent

The NCI defines informed consent as "the communication process that allows individuals to make an informed choice about participation in a clinical trial." The informed consent document contains specific, required information about the clinical trial and is a legal document. It is the patient's formal authorization to participate in the trial, and it must be reviewed and approved by each center's IRB.[8]

There are two acceptable ways to obtain written informed consent from a patient participating in a clinical trial. A consent form that contains all of the required elements may be read to the patient or the patient's legally authorized representative. The investigator is responsible for ensuring that the patient or legally authorized representative receives a written copy and has adequate time to read it and ask questions before signing it.[9] The consent form should be written in language that the patient understands. Non-English-speaking patients must be presented with a consent form written in the patient's native language. In such cases, the IRB must approve both the English version and the foreign language version.

The second way to provide informed consent is in the form of an oral presentation of consent. A short, written form clearly stating that the required elements of the informed consent have been presented orally to the patient or legal representative is signed by one of the aforementioned individuals. A witness must be present during the oral presentation, and the IRB must preapprove a written summary of what is presented. The person giving the oral presentation must sign the summary, and the patient receives copies of both the short form and the summary.[9]

The patient has the right to withdraw from a clinical trial at any time.

Aspects of the Clinical Trial (No Change)

Patient Eligibility

Patient populations are defined in detail in the study protocol. Records of prospective subjects must be reviewed to determine which are eligible for the study. If a patient meets the study eligibility criteria, the attending physician usually discusses the study with the patient or family members. Most studies specify a time frame for a patient's diagnosis date and specific diagnostic tests that must be completed before the patient is eligible for registration. Clinical criteria are defined and may include stage of disease, performance status, and specific values for many required diagnostic tests.

The consent form is presented to the patient after the study has been explained. The form must be written in language that a layperson can understand. It is read to or by the patient or guardian. All questions must be adequately answered. If the patient agrees to participate in the study, the consent form is signed by the patient or guardian, the PI, and other witnesses.

Patient Registration

Patients must be registered for the study by the clinical trials group. This is usually done by telephone or facsimile. The various treatment arms or branches of the study are defined within the protocol, which should also include a schema of the treatment arms. The schema defines the treatment modalities and dosages for each arm.

In studies with more than one treatment arm, the patient is placed on a study arm by randomization, or chance, to eliminate statistical bias and ensure valid results. This is done by personnel at the trial group operations office, who key specific patient information into a computer programmed to choose an arm at random. To make certain that each arm of the study will accrue subjects with varying prognoses or expected outcomes, some studies further separate, or stratify, certain factors (such as histology, stage of disease, age, and similar variables). The study arm chosen by the computer is then revealed and a case number assigned at the operations office. In a blind study, the study arm is not known to the patient and or the doctor (double-blind).

Data Collection

After patient registration has been completed, the treatment plan is arranged by the physician following the chosen study arm. Each study has a set of forms designed by the clinical trial group. Two basic types of initial data are required by the trial group: clinical data and films, and treatment plan information. These data must be collected in a timely fashion and submitted on approved forms.

The clinical trial groups rate the timeliness and accuracy of data submissions. These ratings and the number or percentage of patients accrued are part of the overall score that institutions receive from trial groups. Some trial groups allocate grant monies based on this scoring system.

Drug Accountability

It is a federal requirement that all drugs used in clinical trials be stored securely at all times when they are not being dispensed or inventoried. Drug inventory and accountability are evaluated by the clinical trial group during site visits. This is another factor in determining the institutional score previously mentioned.

Follow-up Data

After a patient completes the initial treatment, a follow-up examination schedule is arranged according to the requirements of the study. Follow-up is typically conducted on a progressive scale (e.g., starting at once a month, then going to once every 3 months, then every 6 months). After 5 years of survival, annual follow-up visits are usually recommended for the duration of the patient's disease-free interval. The protocol specifies required follow-up intervals and tests to be performed. As with other aspects of the patient's care, the follow-up data are recorded on forms and submitted to the trial group according to the assigned schedule.

Summary

A clinical trial group consists of several institutions with investigators who design and administer research studies. Clinical trials are medical research studies designed to answer questions about new drugs or devices. They are the final step in the research process of moving scientific research from the laboratory into treatments for people.

Clinical trials are categorized in three phases. Phase I trials are preliminary trials that test toxicity of the investigational techniques and establish basic safe dosage levels of investigational drugs. Phase II trials determine safety and efficacy of investigational drugs or techniques. Phase III trials are the final testing phase for clinical trial groups. Phase IV trials are used only by drug or device manufacturers to gain additional information about the product being tested.

Each clinical trial has a PI who is responsible to the clinical trials group for conducting research. Most national oncology clinical trial groups are funded through the NCI of the NIH. An IRB must review and approve a clinical trial and its informed consent form before patient accrual can begin.

The IRB is governed by strict federal guidelines. It must review all new and ongoing research studies within its institution. The composition of the IRB committee is regulated by specific federal requirements. The committee must have both scientific and nonscientific members with various stated qualifications and backgrounds. The IRB's main function is to protect the rights of human subjects participating in research.

The informed consent form is an important document that contains information for the subjects who participate in research studies. The subject must understand the information before signing the informed consent form.

Advances in medicine are the ultimate result of clinical trial studies. It is important for clinical trial investigators to report their findings to the medical and research communities to advance longer survival periods and enhance quality patient care.

References

1. Spilker, B. *Guide to Clinical Trials* (pp. xxi–xxiii). New York: Raven Press; 1991.
2. Jenkins, J. F., & Lake, P. C. "Celebration of an Era of Public Service at the National Institutes of Health and the National Cancer Institute." *Cancer Nursing,* 1988;11:58–64; White-Hershey, D., & Nevidjon, B. "Fundamentals for Oncology Nurse/Data Managers: Preparing for a New Role." *Oncology Nursing Forum,* 1990;17:371–377.
3. Cheson, B. D. "Clinical Trials Programs." *Seminars in Oncology Nursing,* 1991;7:235–242.
4. Jenkins, J., & Hubbard, S. "History of Clinical Trials." *Seminars in Oncology Nursing,* 1991;7:228–234.
5. McCarthy, C. R. "Historical Background of Clinical Trials Involving Women and Minorities." *Academic Medicine,* 1994;69:695–698.
6. Merkatz, R. B., & Junod, S. W. "Historical Background of Changes in FDA Policy on the Study and Evaluation of Drugs in Women." *Academic Medicine,* 1994;69:703–707.
7. U.S. Department of Health and Human Services. *OPRR Reports: Code of Federal Regulations Title 45-Public Welfare, Part 46-Protection of Human Subjects* (National Institutes of Health Publication No. 02-5050 [2001]). Bethesda, MD: Public Health Service Act, 1991:6-9,137.
8. National Cancer Institute. *Informed Consent* [online]. Available at: http://cancertrials.nci.nhi.gov/NCI_CANCER_TRIALS/zones/TrialInfo/DecidingInformedConsent/templt.html#top. Accessed October 30, 1998.
9. U.S. Food and Drug Administration. *Code of Federal Regulations* (Title 21, Vol. 1, Part 50.27). Washington, DC: U.S. Government Printing Office, 1998.

chapter 41

Cancer Registries in Other Countries

Brenda K. Edwards, PhD
Lynn Ries, MS
Judith Swan, MHS

Cancer registration in other countries has grown substantially over the last few decades. Scientists and policy makers worldwide are relying on cancer registries to provide important data for research and for developing evidence-based cancer care and cancer-control plans. There is also a growing number of collaborative efforts among countries in the area of cancer registration and reporting.

Many of the collaborative activities are conducted through international organizations such as the World Health Organization (WHO) and its International Agency for Research on Cancer (IARC), which is described in detail later in this chapter, together with the International Association of Cancer Registries (IACR), a professional society dedicated to fostering cancer registries worldwide. For Volume IX (2007) of the IARC/IACR publication *Cancer Incidence in Five Continents* (CI5), 313 registries in 80 countries submitted data.[1] Another prominent international group is the International Union Against Cancer (UICC), which connects public health scientists and practitioners, epidemiologists, public health educators, behavioral scientists, and investigators to move the cancer-control agenda forward in communities worldwide.

Using international data for comparison of cancer rates is important to the understanding of the disease and its control.[2] For example, scientists have been able to link differing patterns of stomach cancer to risk factors such as diet or infection. Migrant studies have provided additional information on the cause of cancer, for example, when populations move from countries of high risk to low risk and succeeding generations acculturate to the adopted area. Also evident from international comparisons of cancer incidence and survival, where available, are differences in application of early detection and treatment.

History of Cancer Registration

There were early attempts to collect data on cancer, such as the 1728 cancer census, but these were eventually abandoned as unreliable until the start of the twentieth century.[3] In 1900, the German government sent questionnaires to all physicians to determine the number of cancer patients in the country. Although the survey was considered a failure because only half of the physicians responded, the same process was initiated over the following decade by Holland, Spain, Portugal, Hungary, and Denmark. A 1927 pilot in the United States of cancer registration in Massachusetts brought in only one third of the cancer cases, and it was suggested that registration be made compulsory to collect more accurate counts.

The first cancer registry began in Hamburg in the late 1920s, but continuous reporting of patients with cancer did not begin until 1937 in Mecklenburg, Germany. In the United States, the Connecticut Tumor Registry began operations in 1941, covering cases back to 1935. Denmark became the first to collect national data in 1942.

In 1946, a dozen cancer-control experts met in Copenhagen and recommended to the WHO that worldwide cancer registries be established with comparable data recording, and that an international body correlate the reported statistics.[4] The meeting was called by Dr. Clemmesen, Director of the Danish Cancer Registry, and it provided the initial stimulus to develop population-based cancer registries where none had previously existed. Among the group's findings were the following:

1. Great benefit would follow the collection of cancer data from as many countries as possible.
2. A plan should be instituted for such data to be recorded in a comparable way.
3. Each country should have a central registry to arrange for the recording and collection of the data.
4. There should be an international body whose duty it is to correlate the data and statistics obtained in each country.[3]

As a result of this conference, WHO's "Subcommittee on the Registration of Cases of Cancer as Well as their Statistical Presentation" met in Paris in 1950. This group continued to make recommendations for developing cancer registries for epidemiologic study over the years. Another important meeting was the UICC's International Symposium on Geographical Pathology and Demography of Cancer in 1950, which called for the enumeration of all new cases of cancer in defined areas. In 1965, the IARC was established as a specialized cancer research center of the WHO. The IACR was initiated in 1966 in Tokyo as a membership organization for cancer registries "concerned with the collection and analysis of data on cancer incidence and with the end results of cancer treatment in defined population groups."[5] The association collaborates closely with the IARC. By 1975, more than 100 cancer registries were established around the world.

In 1956, the Commission on Cancer (CoC) of the American College of Surgeons (ACoS) formally adopted a policy to encourage establishment of hospital-based cancer registries through their Approvals Program. The purpose was to periodically review results of cancer treatment regimens, examining patterns of care and disease. Early hospital registries were based on paper and card files of data.

The introduction of microcomputers to hospital record-keeping in the 1970s and 1980s enabled the expansion of hospital and central registries. Standardization of data collection made it possible to pool data from multiple U.S. hospital registries in the CoC's National Cancer Data Base (NCDB) and population-based registry systems such as the National Cancer Institute's (NCI's) Surveillance, Epidemiology, and End Results (SEER) Program and the Centers for Disease Control and Prevention's (CDC's) National Program of Cancer Registries (NPCR) in the United States and population-based registries in Europe through the European Network of Cancer Registries (ENCR).

International Association of Cancer Registries and International Agency for Research on Cancer

The establishment of the IACR was proposed in 1966 during an informal meeting of approximately 60 scientists during the 9th UICC International Congress in Tokyo, Japan. Bylaws and a constitution were drafted, and the IACR was formally announced in 1967.[6] In January 1979 at the World Health Assembly, IACR became a nongovernmental organization in official relations with WHO.[7] The aims of the IACR are to improve cancer incidence and survival information; to standardize definitions, coding, and reporting; and to foster the exchange of scientific research between countries. IACR is composed of member organizations, mostly population-based cancer registries from around the world. The IACR has annual meetings held in different parts of the world to foster the exchange of scientific research including epidemiologic studies based on registry data, cancer registry operations, and the development of statistical methods to analyze data.

The IARC began in May 1965 based on a resolution of the 18th World Health Assembly and is a WHO agency. IARC's current (2010) membership is 21 countries and is based in Lyon, France.[8] Its mission is cancer research for cancer prevention. IARC coordinates research across countries and organizations. IARC has also been instrumental in describing the global burden of cancer in publications and databases. IARC has had a pivotal role in establishing population-based cancer registries in developing countries. IARC provides administrative support for IACR in Lyon, France.

IARC and IACR have worked together for many years in the area of cancer control to facilitate the exchange of cancer information among countries and the compilation of cancer incidence and survival information to better describe the burden of cancer around the world. Joint publications such as *Cancer Incidence in Five Continents* allow cancer researchers to evaluate differences and similarities among countries in cancer incidence and to monitor cancer trends around the world. Free software called CanReg (currently version 5) was developed to provide the basis of an operational cancer registry from data entry to analyses of cancer incidence information. CanReg4 was used in more than 150 registries in at least 75 countries, and its manual is published jointly by IARC and IACR.[9] Jointly, IACR and IARC have published several technical reports such as computer edits called *Check and Conversion Program for Cancer Registries* (http://www.iacr.com.fr/TechRep42-MPrules. pdf), *Guidelines on Confidentiality for Population-Based Cancer Registration* (http://www.iacr.com.fr/confidentiality2004. pdf), and *International Rules for Multiple Primary Cancers* (http://www.iacr.com.fr/MPrules_july2004.pdf). These technical reports have aided in standardization of codes, coding rules, and recodes for data analyses. Standardization for the coding of primary site and histology is made possible through the WHO publication *International Classification of Diseases for Oncology* (ICD-O).[10]

North America

The North American Association of Central Cancer Registries, Inc. (NAACCR) was established in 1987 as a collaborative umbrella organization to develop and promote uniform data standards for cancer registration in the United States and Canada. As part of this goal, NAACCR provides education and training for registry staff and certifies population-based registries. It annually aggregates and publishes data from central cancer registries in the United States and Canada that meet its quality standards as *Cancer in North America* (CINA). Data from the United States are from population-based cancer registries that participate in NCI's SEER Program or CDC's NPCR Program, or both.

Canada is the second largest country in landmass in the world, and Statistics Canada has collected data on cancer incidence since 1969. In recent decades, the incidence and survival data have been compiled by the Canadian Cancer Registry. Data reporting is coordinated by the Canadian Council of Cancer Registries, which has representatives from 10 provinces and 2 territories. SEER has been working with the Council, the Canadian Partnership Against Cancer (CPAC), and NAACCR to develop a framework for a data quality program in Canadian cancer registries.

Europe

The ENCR was established in 1989 to improve the quality, comparability, and availability of cancer incidence data and develop a basis for monitoring cancer rates in the European Union. It also promotes the use of cancer registries in healthcare planning, cancer research, and cancer control. ENCR is affiliated with IACR. Because of the marked differences in registry practices, ENCR is working to establish cancer registration standards across its membership.

Middle East

The Middle East Cancer Consortium (MECC) was established through an official agreement of the Ministries of Health of Cyprus, Egypt, Israel, Jordan, and the Palestinian Authority. The agreement, orchestrated largely through the efforts of NCI, was signed in Geneva in May 1996. Turkey officially joined the Consortium in June 2004. The objective of the MECC is to reduce the incidence and impact of cancer in the Middle East through the solicitation and support of collaborative research. MECC's first regional activity was the Cancer Registry Project (CRP). The CRP, which started in January 1998, supports cancer registration in all MECC jurisdictions. Population-based registration can be used to inform public health planning and cancer-control programs and research. A monograph was published in 1996 comparing cancer registry data from Cyprus, Israel, Egypt, Jordan, and the NCI's SEER Program.[11] The publication includes age-adjusted and age-specific incidence rates by sex and country, age distribution of cases, histology and subsite, and basis of diagnosis. In a region where few countries maintain cancer registries, and where cancer statistics are scarce, MECC's main areas of focus include cancer surveillance, information, and education. In 2007, MECC published a report on palliative care in the Middle East.

Asia

To facilitate regional data sharing and epidemiologic studies, Asian countries began formation of the Asian Cancer Registry Network (ACRN) in 2010. The new network plans eventually to include cancer registries from the Philippines to Turkey, an area covering approximately two thirds of the world population, and to standardize data for use in research and cancer control planning.[12] The network could benefit less-developed countries through improvements to diagnostic and coding systems that will enable cross-regional comparisons. An organizational meeting was held at the Fall 2010 IARC meeting in Yokohama, Japan.

International Uses of Cancer Registry Data

EUROCARE

EUROCARE is the EUROpean CAncer REgistry-based study on survival and CARE of cancer patients, a cancer epidemiology research project on survival of cancer patients in Europe. The study resulted from a collaboration established in 1989 between the Istituto Nazionale Tumori (Milan, Italy), the Istituto Superiore di Sanità (Rome, Italy), and population-based cancer registries from 12 European countries with incidence and survival data available. The project has had four editions, analyzing survival data on patients diagnosed from 1978 to 1984 (EUROCARE-1), from 1978 to 1989 (EUROCARE-2), from 1983 to 1994 (EUROCARE-3), and from 1988 to 2002 (EUROCARE-4). The fourth edition of EUROCARE includes data on more than 13 million cancer diagnoses provided by 93 population-based cancer registries in 23 European countries. EUROCARE-5 is being planned. The collective studies thus far are the source

for more than 90 publications (http://www.eurocare.it/Publications/tabid/61/Default.aspx).

CONCORD

The CONCORD study compares population-based relative survival from cancer using data from cancer registries in 31 countries representing 5 continents.[13] Designed as a follow-on to the EUROCARE study, CONCORD included North America, Australia, Japan, Algeria, Cuba, and Brazil, as well as all regions of Europe. Begun in 1999, it reported survival for 1.9 million adults diagnosed with a primary cancer of the breast, colon, rectum, or prostate during 1990–1994 and followed up until 1999. The data came from 101 population-based registries, and the results showed greater survival in countries with higher income. The analysis was identical for all data sets, and quality control was standardized. Adjustment was made for differences in background mortality in the general population and age structure of the patient population, and 2800 life tables were constructed for the many participating countries.[14]

The CONCORD study demonstrates the value of population-based cancer registries for the comparison of cancer outcomes and evaluation of how countries fare in cancer control. In particular, it suggests a wide variation in access to prevention, diagnosis, and treatment services. As economic development proceeds, a country's healthcare expenditures can be tracked and compared with changing cancer survival rates.

GLOBOCAN

The GLOBOCAN database was first built using the huge amount of data available to IARC for 2002.[15] In its most recent release, GLOBOCAN provides access to the 2008 estimates of the incidence of, and mortality from 27 major cancers worldwide.. It is an Internet application with graphing and mapping capabilities, and is available using the online GLOBOCAN software. Incidence data available from cancer registries cover entire national populations or samples of such populations from selected regions. Mortality data by cause are available for many countries through the registration of vital events, although the degree of detail and quality of the data vary considerably across countries. The validity of the estimates is dependent on the extent and accuracy of locally available data.

Cancer Incidence in Five Continents

Cancer Incidence in Five Continents (CI5) is a series of international data compilations begun in the mid-1960s and repeated about every 5 years since. It presents incidence data that meet acceptable quality criteria from population-based cancer registries around the world.[16] Originally a publication of the UICC, from the third volume it has been a collaborative project for IARC and IACR.[17] Including data from 32 registries in 29 countries in its first volume, CI5 Volume IX contains data from 225 registries in 60 countries, covering 11% of the world population.[18] The continental coverage is Africa 1%, Asia 4%, South and Central America 4%, Europe 33%, Oceania 73%, and North America 80%. The data and software for extended analyses of the content of each volume are available electronically, and a subset of registries with annual data of at least 15 years' duration has been compiled into an additional analytic database, the Annual Detailed Database.[19]

Summary

Despite global politics, cancer registration is making inroads in many countries. Much collaborative work in compiling global statistics and international comparisons is done under the auspices of IARC and IACR. Large international studies and databases are providing more information than ever previously available on the cancer burden around the world. Future follow-on study results from CONCORD and EUROCARE will add to our global knowledge of cancer and cancer care, and the reach of cancer registration will continue to expand.

References

1. Curado, M. P., Edwards, B., Shin, H. R., et al. *Cancer Incidence in Five Continents, Volume IX* (IARC Scientific Publications No. 160). Lyon, France: International Agency for Research on Cancer, 2007

2. Menck, H. R. "Cancer Registries in Other Countries." In *Cancer Registry Management: Principles and Practices, 2nd ed.* Hutchison C et al, eds. National Cancer Registrars Association. Dubuque, IA: Kendall Hunt Publishing Co., 2004.

3. Wagner, G. "History of Cancer Registration." In O. M. Jensen, D. M. Parkin, R. Maclennan, et al., editors. *Cancer Registration Principles and Methods* (IARC Scientific Publications No. 95, pp. 3–6). Lyon, France: WHO International Agency for Research on Cancer, 1991.

4. Roffers, S. D. "Cancer Registries in Other Countries." In C. L. Hutchinson, S. D. Roffers, A. G. Fritz, editors. *Cancer Registry Management: Principles and Practices*. Dubuque, IA: Kendall Hunt Publishing Co., 1997.

5. Clemmesen, J. *Symposium on the Geographical Pathology and Demography of Cancer*. Paris: Council for the Coordination of International Congresses of Medical Sciences, 1951.

6. International Association of Cancer Registries Web site: http://www.iacr.com.fr/. Accessed May 2010.

7. Whelan, Sharon L. *The International Association of Cancer Registries: A History, draft version 2009.*

8. International Agency for Research on Cancer Web site: http://www.iarc.fr/en/about/. Accessed May 2010.

9. International Agency for Research on Cancer/International Association of Cancer Registries. *CanReg4 Manual.* Available at: http://www.iacr.com.fr/canreg4%20manual%20_June2008.pdf. Accessed May 2010.

10. Fritz, A., Percy, C., Jack, A., Shanmugaratnam, K., Sobin, L., Parkin, D. M., Whelan, S., editors. *International Classification of Diseases for Oncology,* 3rd ed. Geneva: World Health Organization, 2000.

11. Freedman, L. S., Edwards, B. K., Ries, L. A. G., Young, J. L., editors. *Cancer Incidence in Four Member Countries (Cyprus, Egypt, Israel, and Jordan) of the Middle East Cancer Consortium (MECC) Compared with US SEER* (NIH Publication No. 06-5873). Bethesda, MD: National Cancer Institute, 2006.

12. Moore MA, Shin HR, Curado MP, Sobue T. Establishment of an Asian Cancer Registry Network: Problems and Perspectives. Asian Pacific J Cancer Prev; 9: 815-832..

13. Coleman, M. P., Quaresma, M., Berrino, F., et al. "Cancer Survival in Five Continents: A Worldwide Population-Based Study (CONCORD)," *Lancet/Oncology,* 2008;9:730–756.

14. Baili, P., Micheli, A., De Angelis, R., et al. "Life tables for world-wide comparison of relative survival for cancer (CONCORD study)," *Tumori,* 2008;94:658–668.

15. Ferlay, J., Bray, F., Pisani, P., Parkin, D. M. "GLOBOCAN 2002: Cancer Incidence, Mortality and Prevalence Worldwide" (IARC CancerBase No. 5. version 2.0). Lyon: IARC Press, 2004.

16. Doll, R., Payne, P., Waterhouse, J., editors. *Cancer Incidence in Five Continents: A Technical Report.* Berlin: Springer-Verlag (for UICC), 1966.

17. Waterhouse, J., Muir, C., Correa, P., Powell, J., editors. *Cancer Incidence in Five Continents, Volume III* (IARC Scientific Publication No. 15). Lyon, France: International Agency for Research on Cancer, 1976.

18. Curado, M. P., Edwards, B., Shin, H. R., Storm, H., Ferlay, J., Heanue, M., Boyle, P. *Cancer Incidence in Five Continents, Volume IX* (IARC Scientific Publication No. 160). Lyon, France: International Agency for Research on Cancer, 2007.

19. Parkin, D. M., Ferlay, J., Curado, M. P., Bray, F., Edwards, B., Shin, H. R., Forman, D. *Fifty Years of Cancer Incidence: CI5 I-IX.* (In press).

Other Registries

Elaine Collins, RHIA, CTR

A registry is a structured system for the collection, storage, distribution, and analysis of a defined segment of health data on individuals. All registries rest on the premise that the focused collection and interpretation of data are integral to the maintenance of health, and the understanding and treatment of disease. The traditional registry database accumulates information on the experience of many individuals with a specific health condition or procedure, facilitating the generalization of individual experience to broader populations. Traditionally, registries have been secondary sources of data, abstracted from the primary source of individual health information records created by treating medical practitioners. However, this distinction is blurring at the treating facility level, as disease-specific registry modules integrated into the electronic health record are used to directly monitor and document individual patient care, especially for chronic conditions. Cancer registries are well established nationally and internationally, with a long history that has evolved from paper-based data collection to electronic methodologies. Electronic technology, in promoting the standardization of data definitions, collection of information in standardized formats, interchange of data among systems, and transmission of data between databases, has fostered an information environment in which registries of many types are proliferating and flourishing. Analytic software functions and programs applied to large databases convert the wealth of accumulated data into meaningful information supporting each registry's mission.

Disease-specific registries support investigations into the causes of disease by identifying for researchers many individuals with the same condition, with the potential for gathering information on suspected risk factors, genetic disorders, and prior exposures. Disease registries support quality improvements in treatment facilities through monitoring of therapies and outcomes. Where a disease or condition is a rare event, registries gathering data from multiple facilities allow meaningful conclusions to be drawn from the pooled information. Disease registries support public health surveillance by providing disease-specific incidence information and survival data, and by revealing trends in severity, treatment, and delivery of services over time and geographic areas. Procedure, device, and drug registries support assessment of the efficacy of new techniques, technologies, and pharmaceuticals by tracking complications and outcomes for patient recipients. Registries support the delivery of certain routine health services, such as vaccinations, by maintaining and updating records on individuals who have received these services. Trauma and disaster registries track care rendered to and effects on persons subjected to harmful external events. Registries are used to gather data in anticipation of future need, for example, donor registries, state special needs and advance directives, and the DNA registry for military personnel. And registries provide an avenue for ongoing communication with the individuals whose data are stored, in some instances recruiting them into special studies, in others informing them of implant device problems, available services, new therapies, and periodic routine provider contacts.

Registry Standards

Registry activities exist across a wide spectrum of interest in health care, from a custom registry monitoring a particular aspect of care rendered by the staff at a single facility, to an international pooling of information from multiple national registries describing the global experience of a disease such as cancer. Every registry has a stated purpose or mission, which determines the cases to be entered into the registry database and the data to be collected.

Case definition, or identification of the individuals about which data will be collected, may be expressed as both inclusion and exclusion criteria. Essential elements of a case definition are listed in Table 42-1.

A set of defined items that will be collected for each individual entered into the database, and a coding structure for each data item, assure completeness and uniformity in collection and interpretation of data. The registry identifies standard health information coding systems that may be used in data collection or creates new data definitions and codes that will support the collection of pertinent information. Table 42-2 lists types of data items that may be included in a registry database.

Policies and procedures govern all aspects of registry operations. Major categories of policies and procedures are presented in Table 42-3.

Table 42-1	Elements of a Case Definition

Description of the condition, procedure, or other subject of interest

Date at which data collection starts, for the entire registry and for each case in the registry

Date at which data collection ends, generally for each case in the registry, but potentially for the entire registry

Population covered, including mandatory versus voluntary inclusion of eligible participants

Identification of persons within the registry: personal identifiers retained versus anonymous data

Time orientation: prospective, retrospective, or concurrent

Table 42-2	Registry Data Elements

Case Identification
- Accession number
- Medical record number
- Study number
- Facility

Demographic Variables
- Patient name
- Date of birth
- Social Security number
- Address
- Sex
- Race/ethnicity
- Occupation

Diagnosis Parameters
- Disease/condition
- Anatomic site
- Pathology
- Procedure
- Comorbidities
- Injury/Event

Diagnostic Workup
- Clinical examination
- Radiology procedures
- Laboratory tests
- Cardiac tests
- Genetic profile
- Surgical procedures

Therapy/Treatment
- Surgery
- Chemotherapy
- Radiation
- Medications
- Respiratory therapy
- Physical/occupational therapy
- Providers
- Complications

Services
- Genetic counseling
- Social services
- Psychiatric services
- Rehabilitation services
- Nutritional services

Management Schedules/Monitoring
- Recurring clinical examinations
- Recurring laboratory tests
- Recurring radiology examinations

Follow-up/Outcomes
- Quality of life
- Status
- Disease free
- Recovered with/without disability
- Chronic controlled/uncontrolled
- Vital status

Table 42-3	Registry Policies and Procedures

Identification of all eligible cases from multiple sources

Collection of quality data, with quality-control activities to assure collection of consistent, timely, and accurate data

Preservation of integrity and security of information

Controls on computer procedures for data entry and update, storage, and access

Maintenance of patient confidentiality

Reporting and dissemination of information

Registry Time Orientation

A prospective registry collects information on the health status of a defined population over a long period. The Framingham Heart Study is an example of a prospective registry, investigating the causes, prevention, and treatment of heart disease; this study began in 1948 with 5,209 subjects from Framingham, Massachusetts, and is now in its third generation of participants. The Agricultural Health Study, beginning in 1994, gathers information about the health of pesticide applicators and their families in Iowa and North Carolina. The Nun Study is a study of aging and Alzheimer's disease, started in 1986 as a pilot study on aging and disability using data collected from the older School Sisters of Notre Dame living in Mankato, Minnesota, and expanded in 1990 to include older Notre Dame sisters living in the midwestern, eastern, and southern regions of the United States.

Retrospective registries collect data on individuals with a definitive diagnosis, related to their diagnostic workup, treatment, and progression of disease. Cancer and birth defect registries are familiar examples of such registries, which are managed to collect data both to assess treatment outcomes at the facility level and to conduct public health surveillance for the allocation and assessment of public resource use.

Concurrent registries support ongoing clinical research and evaluation of specific events, procedures, or treatments. Included in this category would be a family genetic registry, a drug effects registry, or a trauma registry.

Registries by Funding and Management

Registries are funded and managed by both public agencies and private organizations, with many collaborations between public funding and nonprofit organizational management.

Federal Government

In the United States, at the federal level, specific registries have been mandated by law, where Congress has identified a compelling national interest in data collection. Agencies within the National Institutes of Health (NIH) support numerous registries through grants to health research contracting entities, in furtherance of the NIH's general mission of research into the causes and treatment of disease. Organ transplant registries, although not directly funded or managed by the federal government, are subject to federal statutory requirements, setting the framework for a system of organ allocation throughout the country and providing for federal reimbursement of transplant service costs.

The Agency for Toxic Substances and Disease Registries, within the Centers for Disease Control and Prevention (CDC), established in 1980 to implement health-related sections of laws that protect the public from hazardous wastes and environmental spills of hazardous substances, supports registries as data resources and also uses them to monitor long-term consequences for affected persons.

The National Exposure Registry, maintained from 1986 to 1999 and now archived, listed persons with low-level exposures to certain hazardous substances, and included subregistries focusing on trichloroethylene, trichloroethane, dioxin, and benzene. Data included demographic, residential, and health information including tobacco use.

The Tremolite Asbestos Registry follows the health of residents of Libby, Montana, who were exposed to this very toxic form of asbestos.

The World Trade Center Health Registry, a partnership with the New York City Health Department, was established in 2002 to monitor over a 20-year period the physical and mental health of people most directly exposed to the events of September 11, 2001.

The National Institute of Arthritis and Musculoskeltal and Skin Diseases supports a number of patient research registries: Alopecia Areata, Ankylosing Spondylitis, Juvenile Rheumatoid Arthritis, Lupus, Muscular Dystrophy, Neonatal Lupus, Rheumatoid Arthritis, and Scleroderma. Many of these registries focus on family history, may enroll families as well as individuals, and collect DNA samples for investigation of genetic causes for these diseases. The registries are housed in university and other specialized hospital facilities.

The Armed Forces Institute of Pathology (AFIP) houses a DNA Registry for all military personnel, to assist in identification of remains. The International Tissue and Tumor Repository for Chronic Arseniasis and Chronic Arsenic Effects Registry are also maintained by AFIP, to share and transfer information on diagnosis, training, and development of research programs on environmental pathology, toxicology, and use of chemical measurements in arsenic health effects studies.

The National Marrow Donor Registry began operation in 1986, established by the U.S. Navy as directed by Congress after the passage of the National Organ Transplant Act in 1984. The National Marrow Donor Program (NMDP) became a not-for profit organization in 1990, taking over the administration of the federal contract from the American Red Cross, with its functions further defined and expanded by the Transplant Amendments Act of 1990. Renamed "Be the Match" Marrow Registry in 2009, the NMDP is the hub of a worldwide network of more than 500 medical facilities in marrow and blood cell transplantation. The NMDP facilitates an average of 200 marrow or blood cell transplants each month. The program uses an electronic infrastructure, the Search, Tracking and Registry System (STAR), to collect donor and cord blood unit information needed for donor search, manage and facilitate all donor searches, and track patient and donor status after transplant.

The United Network for Organ Sharing Registry, under contract with the U.S. Department of Health and Human Services (HHS), administers the Organ Procurement and Transplantation Network (OPTN), established by the Congress in the National Organ Transplant Act of 1984. HHS implemented a Final Rule in 2000 establishing a regulatory framework for the structure and operations of the OPTN. Policies intended to be binding on OPTN members are developed through the OPTN committees and Board of Directors, and then submitted to the Secretary of HHS for final approval. Sections of the rule cover listing requirements, organ procurement, identification of organ recipients, allocation of organs, designated transplant program requirements, reviews, evaluation, enforcement, record maintenance and reporting requirements, and an advisory committee on organ transplantation.

State Government

State governments support many types of registries. The registries are created by state legislation, funded with state money that may be supplemented through federal programs, and collect information covering all state residents. Reporting of cases to the registries may be set up as voluntary or required by statute. Registries maintained by many states include:

- Birth defects registry: to track the incidence of birth defects, to support investigations into their causes, and to inform families of available services
- Trauma registry: to gather data from and provide infrastructure support for designated trauma center facilities within the states

- Central registry for child abuse and neglect: to aid social services agencies in the investigation, treatment, and prevention of child abuse cases and to maintain statistical information for staffing and funding purposes; the registry records may also be used to screen persons who will be entrusted with the care of children
- Immunization registry: to promote and maintain records for pediatric immunizations
- Organ and tissue donor registry: to record willingness to donate organs/tissues on death
- Advance directive registry: repository of advance directives or living wills, accessible to healthcare providers with patient consent
- Paul Coverdell Stroke Registries: CDC-supported program to implement state-based stroke registries, eight prototype registry projects funded in 2001 and 2002, including evaluation of emergency transportation, emergency department services, and in-hospital services

See Table 42-4 for selected state registries.

Tribal Governments

The Alaska Native Tribal Health Consortium through the Alaska Native Epidemiology Center maintains, or collaborates with other organizations in the support of, special registries to monitor and measure Alaska Native Health: Tumor Registry, Cardiovascular Disease Registry, Stroke Registry, Trauma Registry, and Alaska Area Diabetes Program.

Health Research Centers

Universities, specialty hospitals, and health research centers participate in the collection of registry information, and in many cases, DNA and tissue specimens, at facility, national, and international levels of organization, which may be dictated by the size of the population required to gather sufficient data for valid statistical analyses. Thus, a university may manage a registry to monitor cardiac care for its patient population, may contribute data to a pediatric cardiomyopathy registry that has recruited a group of hospitals to be data centers, and may send data on pancreatic transplants to an international registry housed in another academic center.

The Early Rheumatoid Arthritis Treatment Evaluation Registry, at Vanderbilt University in Nashville, Tennessee, enrolled a cohort of 452 patients, diagnosed with disease for 3 years or less, between 2001 and 2004, to study the long-term outcomes of biological therapies. The subjects were drawn from hospital clinics, a rheumatoid practice, and from other contributors. The program was also adopted at facilities in New York and Massachusetts, which enrolled about 100 patients each.

The Johns Hopkins Center for Hereditary Eye Diseases, founded in 1972, maintains a DNA registry of blood samples that are made available to interested investigators within the Johns Hopkins Medical Institutions, across the United States, and throughout the world.

The University of North Carolina at Chapel Hill, in collaboration with the National Institute of Environmental Health Sciences, established an Environmental Polymorphism Registry in 2004. This is a DNA repository maintaining personal identifiers to recruit individuals with genetic polymorphisms or variants in environmentally sensitive genes into studies to define environmental risk factors.

The National Congenital Cytomegalovirus Disease Registry, at Baylor College of Medicine, gathers information on infants born with cytomegalovirus (CMV) symptoms, tracks trends, identifies risk groups, and provides basic data needed for evaluation of future intervention programs. The registry also provides an outreach educational program for families and healthcare providers, and a support network for parents.

The University of Minnesota houses a Temporomandibular Joint Implant Registry and Repository, sponsored by the National Institute of Dental and Craniofacial Research. This registry collects patient information, temporomandibular joint (TMJ) tissue specimens, and also retrieved TMJ implants, to improve understanding and treatment of TMJ disorders.

Table 42-4	Selected State Registries
California	Parkinson's Disease Registry, 2007
Colorado	Stroke Registry, 2006
Georgia	Special Needs Registry
Illinois	Occupational Disease Registry
Kentucky	Women's Health Registry, 2006
Missouri	Autism Project Registry, 2004
Nebraska	Parkinson's Disease Registry, 1996
Nevada	Sentinel Events Registry, 2002
New Hampshire	Registry for Autism Spectrum Disorders, 2008
New Jersey	Cardiac Catheterization Data Registry
New York	Occupational Lung Disease Registry
Rhode Island	Special Needs Emergency Registry, 2009
South Carolina	Alzheimer's Disease Registry, 1988
Utah	Registry of Autism and Developmental Disabilities, 2003
Vermont	Blueprint for Health, Chronic Care Information System, 2006
West Virginia	Autism Spectrum Disorders Registry, 2004
	Alzheimer's Disease Registry, 2008

The Jesse E. Edwards Registry of Cardiovascular Disease, founded in the early 1960s and currently located at the John Nasseff Heart Hospital in St. Paul, Minnesota, is a cataloged collection of more than 20,000 human hearts and 85,000 photographic slides. The specimens and slides are obtained from hospitals, medical examiners, medical device companies, and organ procurement facilities nationally and internationally, and are used in cardiovascular research, education, and training.

The University of Rochester, New York, was the primary grantee in 1995 of an award from the National Heart, Lung, and Blood Institute to establish The North American Pediatric Cardiomyopathy Registry; collaborators on the award included Boston Children's Hospital; Texas Children's Hospital, Houston; New England Research Institutes, Watertown, Massachusetts; and Albany Medical College, New York. The registry was established to describe epidemiologic features and the clinical course of selected cardiomyopathies in patients 18 years or younger and to promote etiology-specific treatments, recruiting patients from clinical centers in New England and the Central Southwest.

The International Pancreas Transplant Registry, located at the University of Minnesota and supported by the National Institute of Diabetes and Digestive and Kidney Diseases and the United Network for Organ Sharing and Eurotransplant, maintains a database of all reported pancreas transplants worldwide. In cooperation with more than 200 centers, the pretransplant and posttransplant courses of nearly 24,000 patients who have received pancreas transplants are followed. Biostatistical analyses are performed regularly and the results are published or presented at international and national scientific meetings. It is believed that almost all transplants performed since 1966 are represented in the database. The collection of information on pancreatic transplants was initiated in 1977 by the American College of Surgeons (ACoS). The International Pancreas and Islet Transplant Registry was created in 1980 and organized in the Department of Surgery at the University of Minnesota. The islet cell transplant data moved to the International Islet Transplant Registry located at the University of Giessen, Germany, in 1987.

The Intestinal Transplant Registry was established in 1994 to review the worldwide experience for the IV International Symposium on Small Bowel Transplantation. A report is prepared every 2 years based on data collection for the biannual international symposium. International centers performing intestinal transplantation, from 21 countries, participate in the database, which has been funded by educational grants from pharmaceutical companies.

Nonprofit Groups

Private, not-for-profit organizations collect registry data to support the populations they serve, in most cases, either patients with a specific disease diagnosis or providers offering a specific treatment methodology or care for a particular disease.

The National Trauma Data Bank and the National Cancer Database of the ACoS are examples of registries created by an organization of providers, designed to gather information from treating facilities that agree to contribute standardized data items and comply with program requirements and review by the organization. The ACoS also manages an approval process for Bariatric Surgery Center Networks, gathering outcome information from the surgery centers through an online data entry process. The surgery centers also submit data to the International Bariatric Surgery Registry, first established in 1979 as a national data analysis center and then expanded in 1996 to international data collection. The registry is housed at the University of Iowa Hospitals and Clinics in Iowa City.

The United States Eye Injury Registry, a federation of individual state eye injury registries, documents serious eye injuries (injuries judged by the reporting ophthalmologist to have a likelihood of resulting in permanent structural or functional damage to the eye or orbit, or both). The registry is a volunteer, bylaws-driven organization governed by officers regularly elected by the directors of participating state registries. All ophthalmologists are invited to participate, and the registry database includes cases from hospitals, trauma centers, and individual ophthalmologists. Formed in 1988, and located in Birmingham, Alabama, in the offices of the founders, the registry receives financial support from the Helen Keller Eye Research Foundation.

The Prospective Registry Evaluating Myocardial Infarction: Events and Recovery (PREMIER) is a project of Cardiovascular Outcomes, Inc. (CV Outcomes), a nonprofit, 501(c)(3) corporation dedicated to the advancement of outcomes research and quality assessment/improvement in cardiovascular disease, founded in 1992. CV Outcomes serves as the administrative coordinator for the Cardiovascular Outcomes Research Consortium. The registry was designed to gather information on the longitudinal care and outcomes of patients after myocardial infarction (MI), to further improve the quality of MI care. Patients with MI were prospectively screened and enrolled from 19 U.S. centers between January 1, 2003, and June 28, 2004. Consenting patients had detailed chart abstractions of their medical history and processes of inpatient care, supplemented with a detailed, patient-centered interview, with centralized follow-up at 1, 6, and 12 months to quantify patients' postdischarge care and outcomes, with a focus on their health status (symptoms, function, and quality of life).

Patient-oriented organizations supporting registries include the Cystic Fibrosis (CF) Foundation and the Chronic Obstructive Pulmonary Disease (COPD) Foundation. The CF Foundation was created in 1955 and established its patient registry in 1966, to gather data from patients treated at CF Foundation-accredited care centers. The registry focuses on the delivery of care for patients; data are also used in the design of clinical trials to test new therapies. The CF Foundation depends on donations from individuals, corporations, and other foundations and fund-raising events to support its activities.

The COPD Foundation Registry was established in 2007 to facilitate research initiatives and to promote the development of improved treatments and a cure for COPD. The registry operates under the direction of the COPD Foundation's Board of Directors and is guided by an oversight committee composed of leaders in the medical, ethical, scientific, and COPD communities. The National Jewish Health in Denver, Colorado, serves as the data coordinating center for the registry. The primary function of this database is to recruit individuals to participate in clinical trials of new therapeutic approaches and other research opportunities. All individuals older than 18 with COPD are eligible for self-enrollment into the database. In contrast, the Bronchiectasis Research Consortium Registry, a collaboration of the COPD Foundation, the University of North Carolina at Chapel Hill, and 10 academic and medical centers from across the United States, contains patient data used to support collaborative research and assist in the development of multicenter clinical trials for the treatment of non-CF bronchiectasis.

The National Breast Implant Registry (NaBIR) was founded by the Plastic Surgery Educational Foundation (PSEF) in July 2000 to concurrently collect data on the patterns of use and reasons for re-operations associated with breast implants. The scope of the registry was expanded in May 2002 when the International Breast Implant Registry was formed. In 2003, the European Parliament mandated tracking and registries for breast implants. Data collected by NaBIR include the type of implant, position of implant, incision site, manufacturer, and indications for operations. Information on tumor detection and staging was added at the request of the Food and Drug Administration (FDA). The registry is voluntary and data submitted are anonymous, protecting the patient's and surgeon's confidentiality. PSEF controls access to the data, which are stored at Data Harbor, Inc.

Commercial Sponsorship

Commercial enterprises may establish registries to collect information on the use of drugs in treatment of specific conditions, drug exposures, the performance of implant devices, or the adoption of particular procedural technologies. The commercial entities may be the sole managers of registry data or may collaborate with other organizations in the collection of data in which they have some commercial interest.

GlaxoSmithKline establishes pregnancy registries in consultation with the CDC to collect information on the effects of exposure to specified drugs on pregnancy outcomes. Information collected at the time of registration includes timing, dose, and duration of the drug exposure; estimated date of delivery; and sufficient contact information to allow for follow-up of the subsequent pregnancy outcome. Open registries in 2009 included Antiretroviral Pregnancy Registry, Lamotrigine Pregnancy Registry, LYMErix® Pregnancy Registry, Twinrix® Pregnancy Registry, Boostrix® Pregnancy Registry, and Sumatriptan/ Naratriptan/Treximet Pregnancy Registry.

The Gastrointestinal Stromal Tumors (GIST) Registry is sponsored by MD Anderson Cancer and Novartis Pharmaceuticals Corporation, the producer of Gleevec (imatinib mesylate) used in the treatment of Kit+ GIST (Kit is a protein on the surface of normal cells signaling cell division and growth). The registry is an observational database designed to describe variations in management of patients with GIST, overall and by patient and provider characteristics. The registry provides participating physicians with information regarding management of their patients with GIST compared with the aggregate experience of all physicians participating in the registry.

The Lifeline Registry for Endovascular Aneurysm Repair represents a collaboration among clinicians and industry to evaluate and report on long-term survival of endovascular graft patients with varying risk profiles. The registry is funded by manufacturers of endovascular grafts, Boston Scientific, Cook Inc., Edwards Lifesciences LLC, Endologix INC, W.I. Gore and Associates, Guidant Corporation, Medtronic Vascular, and Trivascular. The registry was organized in 1998 by the Lifeline Foundation, now the American Vascular Association, the nonprofit foundation of the Society for Vascular Surgery.

Facilities

Facilities maintain registry databases to monitor treatment outcomes for their own patients. As with cancer databases, the registry information may be reported to other entities including accrediting organizations and state governments. However, the primary purpose for the investment of facility resources is to improve the quality and effectiveness of services provided to the local patient population through the collection and analysis of data reflecting local diagnosis, treatment, and outcomes.

The Pittsburgh Regional Healthcare Initiative (PRHI) provides an example of a cardiac registry organized by physicians at a regional level to describe and improve the quality of care for patients in their facilities. The PRHI provided the structure for cardiac surgeons from 12 regional hospitals to gather and establish a regional registry in 2001 to monitor the quality of cardiac care and improve coronary artery bypass outcomes, initially focusing on four indicators of care: use of internal mammary artery instead of vessel from leg, use of preoperative aspirin, use of beta-blockers to depress pulse rate at start of surgery, and avoidance of anemia caused by blood dilution while on the bypass pump. The multihospital pooling of data provided the weight of evidence for evaluation of the effectiveness of modified procedures.

The Breast Health Registry database established by the Providence St. Vincent Medical Center in Portland, Oregon, exemplifies a facility registry initiative, designed to gather all pieces of information about women's breast care into one comprehensive database. When a woman is diagnosed with breast cancer, she may see 10 care providers during her course of care, including a surgeon, a medical oncologist, a radiation oncologist, a physical therapist, an integrative medicine provider, a visit to a social support center, and meetings with a counselor. The registry was designed to improve the patient's experience and quality of care, allowing care providers to more easily follow the entire course of medical care experienced by each patient.

Diabetes registries provide the model for facility databases structured to support long-term care of a chronic disease process. The University of Washington Physicians Network (UWPN) is a nonprofit primary care delivery system in Seattle with nine clinics linked by a computerized, networked clinical information system. In 1998, UWPN initiated a diabetes management program in collaboration with the Institute for Healthcare Improvement. The program is based on a conceptual model of chronic care, which assigns complementary responsibilities to patients and their caregivers for disease management. On the provider side, healthcare systems must assure delivery of interventions proved to be effective, empower patients to take responsibility for their care, and provide information, support, and resources to assist patients in self-management tasks. The model defines available resources as community services and policies, decision support, delivery system design, and clinical information systems. The organization of clinical data from patient medical records through a registry system is perceived as crucial in the management of the chronic illness population. The electronic registry automates monitoring of individual patient disease, including clinical visits, laboratory values, alerts, and patient notifications. The registry also allows analyses of aggregate data drawn from multiple patient records and assessment of costs, treatment methodologies, complications, disparities, and genetic components in the development of disease.

Registry Infrastructure

The continuum of registry infrastructure ranges from the worldwide elaboration of cancer data definition, collection, and reporting to a spreadsheet maintained by a physician in his or her office to track some element of interest across his or her patient population. The infrastructure tends to reflect the magnitude of the problem at the societal level and the resources that society has agreed to expend, the complexity of the problem and the amount of data required for understanding and resolution, and the points at which information and practice intersect to affect outcomes for individuals. Registry infrastructure is composed of organizations supporting and funding registries, defining and monitoring data standards, collecting, report-

ing, and transmitting data; individuals gathering and entering data into the registry databases, and organizations providing education and monitoring their performance; and the designers and providers of the electronic programs and networks through which registry data are collected and transmitted.

Registry reporting relationships depend on funding sources, levels of collaboration, and commitments to data sources. Government-sponsored and -funded programs are required to submit data to their sponsoring agencies. Registries that serve the requirements of standardized accrediting programs must periodically submit data for review, both to ascertain data quality and to provide the data for analysis and interpretation.

Registry data collection may be conducted by medical personnel, assistants, or professional registry staff. Cancer registrars, trauma registrars, and data managers for clinical trial organizations are recognized professionals in the collection of health registry data, with their own professional associations supporting basic and continuing education and certification in the field. Data management tasks may range from database design and data definition through case identification and data abstraction to data reporting and analysis, depending on the scope, volume, and complexity of data gathered into the registry database.

The quality and usefulness of registry data depend on the quality of database design and data item definition, the fit of the data to the intended purpose of the registry, and the policies and procedures that ensure that data are collected in a uniform, consistent, and timely manner. Validation may be built into the data entry process in electronic registry systems, edit routines may assure consistency among related data items, and logical review of overall data patterns can confirm their reasonableness and relevancy.

Registry Software

Registry software built on database technologies facilitates the collection, management, reporting, and analysis of large volumes of data. Many registry-specific systems have been designed and made available, both as commercial products and as custom systems built by users on a standardized database system. Current registry informatics activities focus on the following tasks:

Interoperability: developing connectivity among systems. Data collected in one system become transmissible among all systems, or accessible from all systems. Affected are communication between registries and broader facility electronic record systems, communication within networks of related registries, and communication between registry systems and the universe of all electronic health data systems.

Functional modularity: developing programs that perform defined registry functions required across the spectrum of registries of a specific type, which can be interfaced with multiple database systems. Edits programs and stage, severity, or prognostic calculators are examples.

Development of generic registry programs: either as standalone systems or modules attached to larger electronic health record systems, which can be tailored to specific disease types. Registries for the management of chronic disease, especially diabetes, are targeted markets for these programs. Also targeted are clinical practices that see a need for a type of registry-focused data collection but do not have the resources to purchase an existing customized registry program. Generic registry programs are also adapted to special uses where custom programs do not exist in the commercial or open software market. Literature is available to assist clinical practices in the evaluation and selection of such software products.

Transformation of existing registry systems into disease or case management modules: as with the generic registry programs, these modules may be linked with the facility-wide electronic health record. They guide the healthcare provider through diagnostic workup, treatment, and follow-up care of patients with the (usually chronic) condition, whereas also collecting in the process a standardized set of data items that meet registry requirements.

Summary

Registries serve facilities, research institutions, state governments, and federal governments, and through them the people about whom data are collected and interpreted, in understanding and managing disease and other health-related concerns. Registries have focused on toxic environmental exposures, prescription drugs, implant devices, chronic conditions, cardiac events, and myopathies. Registries have collected health-related data that might be of critical importance at some future point in a person's life; they have also collected data on the health effects of a person's involvement in some past event. Registries embody the concept that information is key to understanding and managing health and well-being, that defined data in designed systems can provide that information, and that definition and design are evolving processes informed by and built on the analysis of accumulated data. The conformation of registries within an integrated system of electronic health information is evolving. An integrated system of electronic health information, encompassing both clinical and research data, offers immense possibilities for focusing knowledge and resources on the resolution and management of health issues that form the core of the registry mission.

With grateful acknowledgment to the health information technology students at Anoka Technical College, Minnesota, who have investigated and reported on many types of registries.

References

Health data registries, as well as commercial software organizations providing registry software, are readily identifiable on the Internet.

The following are information sources for general chronic disease registries:

"The Chronic Care Model," Improving Chronic Illness Care, supported by the Robert Wood Johnson Foundation: http://www.improvingchroniccare.org/

"Using Computerized Registries in Chronic Disease Care," California HealthCare Foundation, prepared by First Consulting Group, February 2004: http://www.chcf.org/topics/view.cfm?itemID=21718

glossary of registry terms

Herman R. Menck, BS, MBA, CPhil, FACE

The following terms appear in one or more chapters of this textbook. In many cases, the term is well defined in the text and can be located through the index. In other cases, a definition has been obtained from another source. Most terms are listed under the noun form; a few are listed under the first word in the phrase or descriptive term. Phrases that include the same term are usually grouped together. Primary terms and cross references to other terms are shown in *bold italics.* A term used a second time in the same definition is abbreviated. *Italics* are used for equivalent terms or subcategories of a term that are not listed independently. The names of publications are shown in **bold**.

abscissa   see *axis.*

abstract   a summary, abridgment, or abbreviated record that identifies pertinent cancer information about the patient, the disease, the cancer-directed treatment, and the disease process from the time of diagnosis until the patient's death. The *a.* is the basis for all of the registry's functions.

abstracting   the process of collecting and recording pertinent cancer data from a health record. *Concurrent a.* starts when the patient is in the hospital and is usually completed by the time the first course of therapy has begun and the health record is sent for filing.

abstractor   an individual who collects and codes cancer registry data.

acceptance sampling   the inspection and subsequent approval (acceptance) or rejection of a product; for example, computerized *edit checks* for registry data.

accession register   an annual, sequential listing of all reportable cancers and reportable-by-agreement cases included in the registry.

accession   to enter a case into a registry and assign it a number.

accession number   a unique number assigned to the patient by the registrar, indicating the year in which the patient was first seen at the reporting institution and the sequential order in which the patient was identified by the registry or abstracted into the database. The *a. n.* is used for all additional primaries the patient may develop, regardless of the year in which subsequent reportable tumors occur.

accreditation   in registry terms of a *hospital a., h.a.* means meeting specific standards for the quality of a *cancer program* and passing a survey by the Commission on Cancer of the *American College of Surgeons. Categories of a.* are based on the facility's *caseload,* staff qualifications, available services, and other factors. Categories include National Cancer Institute–designated, teaching, community, comprehensive community, special, freestanding, integrated, managed care, and affiliate. Term previously used was *approval.*

accrue   to enter into a research study.

accuracy   correctness; in registry terms, a true representation on the *abstract* of the facts in the *source document.* See also *consistency, reliability, validity, reproducibility,* and *concordance.*

Acquired immunodeficiency syndrome (AIDS)   a usually fatal viral (human immunodeficiency virus [HIV]) disease spread by sexual contact or contact with blood from an infected person that gradually destroys a person's immune system.

active reporting   see *casefinding.*

Active Server Pages (ASP)   generates HTML pages from a server using ActiveX scripts and displays the pages with an .asp extension.

actuarial method   see *survival calculation.*

address standardization   process of modifying an address so it conforms to conventions for format, abbreviation, and address components as defined by the U.S. Postal Service (USPS) or CanadaPost.

adjuvant therapy   a treatment modality given in conjunction with another treatment modality, such as chemotherapy given after surgery or radiation for localized disease, with the intent to destroy *micrometastases.*

administration   the part of a healthcare facility that deals with day-to-day operations of the facility rather than direct patient care. *A.* usually includes the chief executive officer of the facility, medical staff office, accounting, housekeeping, human resources, and other departments.

advisory board   group that provides direction for cancer surveillance programs or central cancer registries. It includes representatives from the major stakeholders in the registry catchment area, helps to reinforce program goals, and solicits support.

age-adjusted incidence rate (AAIR)   summary incidence rate where the age effect is adjusted. It is used in comparisons with other rates adjusted in the same manner. Common adjustment methods include direct standardization, indirect standardization, and the cumulative rate methods.

Agenda for Change   a program of the *Joint Commission* that emphasized *continuous quality improvement* of all facets of healthcare services. The *A. f. C.* shifted the focus from examining an institution's capabilities to deliver quality care to monitoring their performance in healthcare delivery and evaluating the actual improvements achieved in their results.

age-specific incidence rate (ASIR)   incidence rate calculated within age groupings.

aggregate data   information about a group of patients, combined without personal identifiers; the opposite of *confidential data. a. d.* is considered nonconfidential because it does not name specific people or facilities.

aggregation (in statistics)   grouping of data in time or space to increase statistical strength

AJCC staging   see *TNM staging* and *American Joint Committee on Cancer.*

algorithm   set of rules that solve a problem in a finite number of steps.

alkylating agent   a chemotherapeutic drug that causes crosslinking of DNA strands, abnormal base pairing, or DNA strand breaks, thus interfering with DNA replication.

allele   one of two or more alternative forms of a gene in the same position on a chromosome.

allied health worker   person who works in a health sciences field, excluding physicians.

allocation of resources   decisions made regarding how equipment, personnel, and other components of an operation or service (in other words, resources) are to be used; management of resource consumption.

allowable code check   a type of *edit check* in which the computer reviews a single data element to see that it contains a correct code. For example, allowable codes for the data item "sex" might be 1, 2, and 9; the case would not pass the edit check if this field contained an "F." See also *range checks.*

alpha error   see *hypothesis.*

alpha-fetoprotein (AFP)   a protein made by fetal liver cells (hepatocytes) that serves as a biological marker for hepatoblastoma.

alternative hypothesis   statement that is true when the null hypothesis is false.

ambiguous terminology   a list of commonly used descriptive terms that may or may not indicate tumor involvement; for example, a "probable" metastasis is to be interpreted as tumor involvement, but a "possible" metastasis is not.

ambulatory   walking or moving; in other words, not confined to a hospital bed; sometimes referred to as *outpatient.*

American Association of Cancer Institutes (AACI)   an organization composed of member representatives from U.S. academic cancer treatment institutions; one of the sponsoring organizations of NAACCR.

American Association of Central Cancer Registries (AACCR)   see *North American Association of Central Cancer Registries (NAACCR).*

American College of Radiology   a professional organization of medical specialists in radiology (diagnostic imaging); among its responsibilities is setting standards for mammography facilities in the United States.

American College of Surgeons (ACoS)   a professional organization of surgeons and physicians founded in 1913. In addition to surgical issues, the ACoS has supported cancer and trauma registries and standards for hospitals.

American Cancer Society (ACS)   a national organization founded in 1913 that is devoted to fund-raising for cancer research and disseminating information about cancer treatment to the public; formerly the American Society for the Control of Cancer.

American Health Information Community (AHIC)   federally chartered advisory committee that provides input and recommendations to the *Department of Health and Human Services (HHS)* on how to make health records digital and interoperable, and assure that the privacy and security of those records are protected.

American Joint Committee on Cancer (AJCC)   the parent organization guiding the development of the *TNM staging* system in the United States; formerly the American Joint Committee for Cancer Staging and End Results Reporting.

American National Standards Institute (ANSI)   body that coordinates the development and use of voluntary consensus standards in the United States and represents the needs and views of U.S. stakeholders in standardization forums around the globe.

American Standard Code for Information Interchange (ASCII)   Common denominator of all modern computer character sets that was published in 1968 as ANSI X3.4.

analytic   a category of *class of case* that indicates that the cancer was initially diagnosed and/or treated at a specific healthcare facility and is eligible for inclusion in that registry's statistical reports of treatment efficacy and survival; the opposite of *nonanalytic.*

ancillary drugs   agents that enhance the effects of cancer-directed treatment but that do not directly affect the cancer; for example; colony-stimulating factors improve the speed of repopulating the bone marrow after a cycle of chemotherapy.

Ann Arbor staging   a specialized staging system for malignant *lymphoma* (Hodgkin's disease and non-Hodgkin's lymphoma).

annual incidence rate   incidence rate that is calculated for a per year period.

annual report   a publication produced on a yearly basis that describes the activities of an organization. A cancer program's *a. r.* also includes statistics on the types of cancers diagnosed and treated at a healthcare facility.

Annual Review of Patient Care   a yearly publication of the National Cancer Data Base that describes patterns of treatment and provides a benchmark for participating institutions to compare facility data with national aggregate data.

anomaly   a marked deviation from normal standard. In anatomic terms, an incorrectly formed or placed organ. A *congenital a.* is one that is present at birth, such as an improperly developed heart valve. A *horseshoe kidney* is a type of *a.* in which both kidneys are united at their lower poles.

ANOVA   analysis of variance; a *statistical technique* comparing the means from multiple samples simultaneously; also called *F-test.*

antimetabolite   a chemotherapeutic agent that replaces natural substances as building blocks in DNA molecules, thereby altering the function of enzymes required for cell metabolism and protein synthesis.

antitumor antibiotics   chemotherapy agent *natural products* that prevent nucleic acid synthesis and block DNA translation and ribonucleic acid (RNA) transcription.

artificial intelligence   branch of computer science and engineering that deals with intelligent behavior, learning, and adaptation in machines.

ascertainment   see *casefinding.*

Association of Community Cancer Centers (ACCC)   an organization of member cancer treatment centers, mostly in healthcare facilities, whose purpose is to promote quality cancer care in all aspects (including research, prevention, screening, diagnosis, and treatment) for patients with cancer and the community.

astrocytoma   a type of *glioma* (brain tumor) noted for its star-like extensions into the surrounding tissue.

at risk   a statistical and epidemiologic term meaning that a person has the chance or opportunity to experience development of a disease. A person exposed to asbestos is said to be *a. r.* for development of *mesothelioma.*

AUA staging   a specialized staging system for prostate cancer developed by the American Urological Association; sometimes called *Whitmore staging.*

audit   a formalized, retrospective review of patient records to determine quality of care, case completeness, or data quality.

autopsy   the pathologic examination of a dead person; a postmortem examination of a body; also called *necropsy.* An *a. report* is the detailed information about organs and structures in the body. Occasionally, the only diagnosis of a cancer is noted at the time of autopsy; *a. reports* are used in casefinding.

autopsy staging   in the *TNM staging* system, a *staging basis* designating that the information used to assign the *T, N,* and *M* categories was obtained from the postmortem examination of the patient.

average annual incidence rate   incidence rate calculated for 2 or more years by dividing the sum of the annual numerators by the sum of the annual denominators.

axis   the vertical or horizontal scale on a graph. The horizontal scale is the *x-axis,* or *abscissa,* which is labeled for categories being graphed. The vertical scale is the *y-axis,* or *ordinate,* which is labeled with the actual count or value.

backlog   the number of cases yet to be identified and/or abstracted within a specified time; for example, if a registry is expected to abstract 600 cases in 6 months and has completed only 400, that registry has a *b.* of 200 cases.

backup   system used to archive and retrieve computer files.

bar chart   a graphic presentation of information that displays the magnitude of one *variable* at various points in time or compares the magnitude of several variables. Types of *b. c.* include *stacked columns* or *component columns,* where the length of the column is the sum of the totals in the segments, and *paired bar charts,* where the zero point is in the center of the graph and distributions of two variables can be shown at the same time.

base layer   *GIS* layer containing basic reference information such as county boundaries or street locations. These are typically not modified by cancer registries.

basement membrane   a microscopic anatomic structure in most organs that forms the deep boundary of the mucosal surface. Tumor invasion or penetration through the *b. m.* indicates that the tumor is no longer *in situ* and has become invasive or *localized.*

batch   a group of similar items produced, processed, or gathered together and treated as a single unit. Also, an adjective used to describe when in production: batch production and batch processing.

Bayesian statistical methods   methodology typically assuming prior (historical) probabilities.

behavior   how a tumor acts; for example, benign, malignant (noninvasive or invasive), or metastatic.

bell-shaped curve   see *kurtosis.*

benchmark   a term borrowed from physics, where marks were actually made on the bench surface to gauge or measure something, to compare a facility's performance or outcomes with another source. *Internal b.* measure the facility's results against itself, usually from a previous period. *External b.* compare the facility's outcomes with another facility's or with aggregate data (a *reference database*) from a standard-setting organization.

benign   not malignant; not invasive; usually harmless; favorable for recovery.

beta error   see *hypothesis*.

bias   systematic errors in the analysis of data. The principal sources of bias are *misclassification* (when subjects are assigned to the wrong groups), *selection* (when all of the subjects in a population do not have the same opportunity to be included in a study), and *confounding*.

biological response modifier (BRM) therapy   see *immunotherapy.*

biopsy   to remove part of a tumor to determine a microscopic diagnosis. An *aspiration b.* uses a needle to suction into a syringe some fluid, cells, or tissue, which are then reviewed under a microscope. An *excisional b.* usually removes the entire, or most of, the tumor. An *incisional b.* removes only a portion of the tumor with the intent of diagnosis.

biostatistics   see *statistics.*

blank space   see *white space.*

blanket permission   in registry terms, a general approval by a facility's medical staff for the registry to contact patients directly (by letter or phone) to obtain current *follow-up* information.

blood–brain barrier   a mechanism of the vascular system of the brain that filters out or inhibits the flow-through of certain molecules, such as chemotherapy drugs.

Board of Regents   the governing body of the *American College of Surgeons.*

bone marrow transplant (BMT)   a type of immunotherapy in which a patient is given myeloablative doses of chemotherapy to destroy all tumor cells, after which bone marrow is returned to the body to restore marrow and immune system function. The types of *b. m. t.* are *autologous* (the bone marrow being restored is that of the patient), *allogenic* (the bone marrow is from another person and has been matched to the patient), or *syngeneic* (from an identical twin). Nowadays, often *stem cell transplants.*

borderline   a disease process that cannot be determined to be completely benign, yet that does not meet all criteria for malignancy; also described as *uncertain whether benign or malignant. B.* cases are not usually *accessioned* into a cancer registry.

brachytherapy   a type of *radiation therapy* where the radiation source is placed in direct contact with the tumor, for example, cesium capsules inserted into the uterus for treatment of endometrial cancer.

Breslow's microstaging   for malignant melanoma, a quantitative measurement in millimeters of the depth of invasion from the basal lamina of the skin to the greatest depth of tumor penetration.

budget   a document listing anticipated costs and income for a particular department or organization. The *capital b.* is used to plan and purchase major equipment with a life expectancy of 2 or more years. The *expense b.* includes the allocation of expenditures for personnel, supplies, office equipment, postage, maintenance, and other planned outlays of funds. The *operating b.* includes revenues and expenses. A *program planning b.* is built around identifiable projects that must be accomplished. A *production b.* is a list of expenses anticipated when a document is published, such as size and type of paper, number of copies, binding, and so forth. The *revenue b.* forecasts income from various sources to offset anticipated expenses. A *traditional b.* is based on previous experience and uses forecasting to account for inflation and other variables. A *zero-based b.* is a resource allocation method that requires budget makers to examine every expenditure during each budget period and to justify that expenditure in light of current budget needs.

budgetary control   the use of a budget to regulate and guide activities requiring and using resources for the development of new services, expanding or contracting services, increasing revenues, or decreasing operating expenses.

budgeting   the process of planning future activities and expressing those plans in a formal manner in terms of cost.

buffer (in a GIS)   set of all spatial objects within a given distance of a reference object; often used in environmental studies (e.g., a 1-mile buffer around a hazardous waste site)

Bureau of Labor Statistics (BLS)   principal fact-finding agency for the federal government for labor economics and statistics.

bypass surgery   an operation that creates a passage around a tumor or other lesion, usually performed to relieve symptoms in cancer patients.

calendar year   a 12-month period starting January 1 and ending December 31; see also *fiscal year.*

Call for Data   a request for submission of cancer cases to the *National Cancer Data Base* or other aggregate databases.

Canada Health Act   legislation that established national standards related to insured healthcare services.

Canadian Association of Provincial Cancer Agencies (CAPCA)   interprovincial organization of cancer agencies and programs that facilitates communication, advocacy, and collaboration for cancer control.

Canadian Cancer Registry   the organized data collection system of full population-based cancer data that began January 1, 1992. The registry is housed at Statistics Canada.

Canadian Cancer Society (CCS)   national group supported by a network of community-based volunteers dedicated to reducing the burden of cancer and improving the quality of life for those living with cancer.

Canadian Council of Cancer Registries   oversight body for cancer registry activities in Canada and for the operation of the Canadian Cancer Registry; created in the early 1990s.

Canadian Strategy for Cancer Control   funded health initiative allowing stakeholders to create and implement the comprehensive cancer plan to reduce cancer cases, enhance quality of life for cancer patients, and lessen cancer mortality.

cancer   a cellular tumor exhibiting the characteristics of *invasion* and *metastasis;* a *malignant* tumor. The term *c.* does not by itself indicate where the malignancy arose.

Cancer and Leukemia Group B (CALGB)   a *clinical trial group,* formerly the Acute Leukemia Group B, which has developed *protocols* for both adult and childhood cancers. The pediatric section separated from *CALGB* in 1980 to form the *Pediatric Oncology Group.*

cancer burden   estimate of the financial, emotional, or social impact that cancer creates within the population.

cancer cluster   the observation that an unusual number of a specific type of cancer case appears during a certain period or in residents of a small, well-defined area, such as a street, school district, or in the path of exhaust from a polluting smokestack. These clusters are usually the subject of epidemiologic investigation by a state cancer registry.

cancer committee   in hospitals, an organized group of healthcare professionals (physicians and nonphysicians) that directs the long-range planning and general activities of the cancer services in a healthcare facility.

cancer conference   a meeting of medical professionals to discuss the diagnosis and treatment of patients; sometimes called *tumor board.*

cancer control   actions taken to reduce the frequency and impact of cancer; any effort to provide information and procedures to help reduce the financial and medical burden of cancer in a population. *c. c.* programs are specific efforts to reduce the amount or severity of a particular type of cancer; for example, screening activities for prostate, colon, or breast cancer. *c. c.* type registries are operated primarily to support the targeting and evaluation of control programs. Also, use of proven prevention, early detection, diagnosis, treatment, and continuing care intervention strategies to reduce cancer incidence, morbidity, and mortality in defined populations.

cancer-directed treatment   procedures that destroy, modify, control, or remove primary, regional, or metastatic cancer tissue.

cancer identification   the section of an *abstract* that contains data items that describe the disease, such as the primary site, histology, date of initial diagnosis, diagnostic confirmation, stage at diagnosis, and so forth.

Cancer Incidence in Five Continents   summary published every 5 years by the International Agency for Research on Cancer; this book reports cancer incidence and mortality figures of member cancer registries of the International Association of Cancer Registries.

Cancer Incidence in North America   an annual publication of the North American Association of Central Cancer Registries (NAACCR) that reports age-specific and age-adjusted incidence rates and data quality indicators for registries that meet its standards for completeness and timeliness, and submit aggregate data to NAACCR.

Cancer Information Management   college-level curriculum covering the fundamentals of data management, computer principles, cancer as a disease, staging, coding, abstracting, follow-up, quality assurance, statistics, and other aspects of collecting and managing cancer data.

Cancer Liaison Physician Program (CLP)   a grassroots network of physicians designated by the *Commission on Cancer* to assist healthcare facilities in developing their cancer programs.

CancerLit   a database of cancer literature available from the *National Library of Medicine (NLM).*

Cancer Management Course   a physician-oriented program of the *Commission on Cancer* that presents extensive site-specific information on state-of-the-art cancer diagnosis and treatment.

cancer mortality atlas   a map or series of maps that show mortality rates caused by various types of cancers. In most cases, the maps are drawn to the level of county detail.

cancer notification form   see *confidential morbidity report.*

cancer prevention   efforts to develop methods to stop cancer before it develops; stop-smoking programs are efforts at preventing lung cancer. See also *cancer control.*

Cancer Program Manual   the Commission on Cancer document used between 1981 and 1995 that defined the guidelines for quality cancer programs; replaced by **Standards of the Commission on Cancer, Volume I: Cancer Program Standards.**

Cancer Program Standards   a publication of the *Commission on Cancer* used between 1996 and 2003 that lists the specific guidelines for evaluating the full spectrum of cancer care in a facility in 10 areas; replaced by *Commission on Cancer, Cancer Program Standards, 2004.*

cancer program   all of the departments and services in a healthcare facility involved in diagnosing, treating, and rehabilitating cancer patients. The activities of the *c. p.* are overseen by the *cancer committee.* An *accredited c. p.* is a facility that has been surveyed and has met the standards of the Commission on Cancer. The *c. p. manager* is the person responsible for maintaining *c. p. accreditation* by the Commission on Cancer.

cancer registrars   cancer data management professionals who collect, abstract, and report cancer statistics for or to various healthcare agencies.

Cancer Registries Amendment Act   *Public Law 102-515,* enacted in 1992, which provided funding for establishing or enhancing central cancer registry operations in all states.

cancer registry   a data collection system that assesses the occurrence and characteristics of reportable neoplasms; a data system designed for the collection, management, and analysis of data on persons with the diagnosis of a malignant or neoplastic disease (cancer). Two main types of *c. r.* are *hospital based* and *population based.* A *central c. r.* is a registry that collects cancer information from more than one facility and consolidates multiple reports on a single patient into one record. A *multihospital c. r.* is a *c. c. r.* consisting of cases from a group of hospitals and is generally not *population based.* A *national c. r.* is a central registry that collects information on all residents within a nation and can produce incidence and mortality rates based on a known population. A *regional c. r.* is a central registry that collects information on all residents within a defined geographic area, such as a city, county or counties, a valley, or multiple states. A *special purpose c. r.* is one that collects data on only one type or aspect of cancer, such as ovarian tumors, pediatric malignancies, or leukemia. A *state c. r.* is a central registry that collects information on all residents of a state, regardless of whether they were treated within the state.

cancer surveillance   process of monitoring various aspects of cancer, usually on a well-defined population; process of monitoring the *incidence* and *mortality* of cancer.

CAP cancer protocols   structured cancer case summaries produced by the *College of American Pathologists (CAP)* as a resource to pathologists in effectively delivering the information necessary to provide quality patient care. The protocols consist of checklists accompanied by background documentation including detailed outlines, explanatory notes, and references.

carcinogen   something that has been shown to cause or is linked with the development of cancer. *c.* include the tar in cigarettes, asbestos, and ionizing radiation.

carcinogenesis   the start of a cancer; a two-step process (*initiation* and *promotion*) in which a neoplasm becomes a cancer.

carcinoma   a *malignant* tumor of *epithelial* origin, in contrast with malignancy of supporting structures (*sarcoma*) or *hematopoietic* structures (*lymphoma* and *leukemia*).

carcinomatosis   invasion of many organs of the body at the same time by *metastases.*

card sorting   method for organizing a Web site. A group of users is presented with a set of cards, each of which describes a function of the Web site or a part of the content. The users make logical groupings of the cards, which can give the Web designer an insight into how to categorize the information content of the Web site.

cartography   science and art of making maps.

case   an occurrence of a primary cancer. A patient with two *primary* cancers represents two *c.s. c. consolidation* combines data from multiple sources pertaining to the same person or case into a single record containing the most complete information from all sources; also called *record linkage;* commonly a function of a central registry. *c.* definition is the process of establishing the criteria for inclusion and exclusion for *case ascertainment.* See *casefinding.*

case–control study   a type of epidemiologic research in which cases of cancer are compared with otherwise similar people from the same population who do not have cancer (the control group).

casefinding   the systematic process of identifying all cases of a disease eligible to be included in the registry database for a defined population, such as patients of a hospital or residents of a state. Also called *case ascertainment. Active c.* is performed by registry personnel who screen the *source documents* themselves. A *c.* completeness log is a list by year and month in which the number of cases identified each month can be compared. *Combination c.* is the use of active review by the registrar for critical casefinding sources and passive review of other sources as provided by reliable participants in other departments. *Passive c.* is performed by other healthcare professionals whom the registry relies on to notify the registrar of potentially reportable cases; also called *self-reporting.* See also *rapid case ascertainment.*

caseload   the number of records handled by a registry in a period of time, usually the number of new cancer cases annually entered into the registry.

case-sharing agreement   a contract between agencies or facilities wherein the parties agree to provide confidential information under carefully controlled circumstances for the purposes of research or patient follow-up.

catchment area   specific geographic area for which the cancer registry collects all cancer reports and maintains population-based information; see *service area.*

category   see *tabular list.*

cause-specific survival   net survival where the end point is the cause of death for which survival is being estimated, such as a specific cancer site. Deaths from other causes are considered censored.

CCH Pediatric Grouping System   a specialized way of categorizing childhood cancers and benign conditions by morphology and topography codes to simplify gathering or reporting cases, developed by the Columbus (OH) Children's Hospital (CCH).

censor   to exclude or remove an observation from a ***survival calculation*** because the subject was eligible at the beginning of the interval but did not complete the interval.

censoring   withdrawal of patients from survival analysis because their survival times are unknown, such as when they are lost to follow-up or still alive at the end of the interval of observation.

census block   Subdivision of a census tract averaging about 1,500 people; the smallest unit for which population data are typically tallied. It consists of an area bounded by streets or other well-defined natural or man-made features. It is used in both the United States and Canada.

census division (Canada)   one or more municipalities or counties that typically share services such as police.

census tract   statistical unit averaging about 4,000 people containing a relatively homogeneous population. In the United States, the entire country is described by census tracts. In Canada, only urban areas are so described.

Centers for Disease Control and Prevention (CDC)   a federal agency of the Department of Health and Human Services. Federal government agency based in Atlanta, Georgia, that tracks and investigates public health trends and epidemics. It publishes reports on all deaths through its National Center for Health Statistics and on all reportable diseases in the United States. It houses the National Program of Cancer Registries (NPCR) in its Cancer Surveillance Branch. In particular, one of the centers of the CDC, the National Center for Chronic Disease Prevention and Health Promotion (NCCDPHP), is responsible for the administration and conduct of the ***National Program of Cancer Registries (NPCR)*** and other cancer-related programs in the United States.

central cancer registry   a regional or statewide organized system for the collection, management, analysis, and dissemination of data on persons with the diagnosis of cancer, in a defined population. See ***cancer registry.***

central registry software systems   One or more computer applications that typically provide data import and data entry, record consolidation, record linkage, quality assurance, reporting and analysis, data exchange and export, security, and task and record management.

certification   the process of testing a person to assure that he or she meets established standards of knowledge to perform a specific job. *c.* is often accomplished by means of a standardized test. ***CTR c. examination*** is the test itself, administered twice per year by the ***National Board for the Certification of Registrars.***

certification (for central cancer registries)   act of recognition as having met special cancer data critical elements and qualifications set forth by the NAACCR for data completeness, timeliness, and quality. Annually, two levels of certification, gold and silver, are awarded to registries contingent on achieving that level of excellence.

certification-training programs   instruction that, once completed, validates ability to perform certain tasks and demonstrates expertise to employers, clients, and peers.

Certified Clinical Research Associate (CCRA)   the credential awarded to data managers who pass a certification examination testing clinical trials and general oncology knowledge.

Certified Tumor Registrar (CTR)   credential earned by persons successfully completing the National Cancer Registrars Association (NCRA) certification examination.

CGI (Common Gateway Interface)   standard interconnection for programs that are executed when called by Web pages.

Charter of Rights and Freedoms   enacted in 1982, part of the Canadian Constitution that promulgates basic rights and freedoms for Canadian citizens.

charts   visual displays of information, such as line graphs, pie graphs, and bar graphs; see also ***graphics.*** Also, healthcare jargon for the patient medical record.

chemotherapy   the use of cancer-killing drugs to treat cancer; types of *c.* include ***alkylating agents, antimetabolites, antitumor antibiotics,*** and ***natural products.***

CHI (Consolidate Health Informatics)   initiative of the Office of Management and Budget (OMB) that is a collaborative effort to adopt health information interoperability standards, particularly health vocabulary and messaging standards, for implementation in federal government systems.

Children's Cancer Group (CCG)   an international ***clinical trial group*** devoted to the treatment of children's cancer that has developed a series of staging systems for various children's malignancies. Its former name was the Children's Cancer Study Group.

choropleth   map in which geographic areas are shaded based on the values of some classified variable, such as cancer rates; the most common map type in cancer registration.

CIHI (Canadian Institute of Health Information)   independent, nonprofit, national organization aimed at improving the health of Canadians by providing high-quality, reliable health information.

Clark's level of invasion   for malignant melanoma, a descriptive measurement of tumor involvement of specific layers of the skin.

class of case   a registry term describing whether a case can be included in the statistical analysis of the database and based on where the initial diagnosis and treatment of the patient occurs. The main categories of *c. of c.* are *analytic* and *nonanalytic.*

classification an organized system of names; a way of grouping concepts or cases based on specific criteria that shows relationships among the groups but does not necessarily imply ***prognosis.***

classification (in GIS) grouping of data values into classes for mapping purposes.

classification of subjects the capability of a study to distinguish participants or cases in the study on the basis of various factors (such as exposure and end point). For example, if the study asks "Do persons with a certain exposure experience a different pattern of disease than do persons without that exposure?" or "Do people with a specific disease have more of a history of a certain exposure than persons without the disease?" the same four groups are described for the study.

clearinghouse (in GIS) source of freely obtainable GIS base layers maintained by a government agency.

clinical indicator a quantitative measure of an aspect of patient status that can be used as a guide to monitor and evaluate the quality and appropriateness of healthcare delivery.

clinical practice guidelines carefully consensus developed standards of medical practice outlining strategies for patient management that describe a range of acceptable ways to diagnose, manage, or prevent specific diseases and conditions; sometimes referred to as *clinical guidelines.* Often, *c. p. g.* are developed by hospitals or by managed care organizations to provide optimal care to their patients.

clinical protocol studies see ***clinical trials.***

clinical staging in the ***TNM staging*** system, a ***staging basis*** designation that the information used to assign the *T, N,* and *M* categories was obtained before any definitive treatment for the tumor was begun.

clinical study a scientific approach used to evaluate disease prevention, diagnostic techniques, and treatments; see also ***clinical trials.***

clinical trials carefully planned scientific studies used to compare one treatment with another. In-house *c. t.* are studies designed by physicians or other staff at an institution and sometimes shared with affiliate members at other institutions. A *c. t.* is a subset of a ***clinical study*** that evaluates investigational (nonstandard) medications, treatments, and diagnostic or preventive techniques or devices, or a combination of these elements; also called ***clinical protocol.*** See also ***phase.*** A *c. t. group* is an organization of researchers that formulates and conducts scientific studies involving specific medical conditions, diseases, or target populations to improve treatment and outcomes; also called *cooperative group. Generally patients are randomly assigned to treatment arm.*

cluster Geographic area, often circular in shape, with a statistically unusual pattern of cancer rate, stage distribution, treatment, or some other variable.

CoC see ***Commission on Cancer.***

code of ethics a document, or list of guidelines, describing appropriate professional behavior.

code a symbol or value assigned to a concept; a set of symbols arranged systematically for easy reference. The verb form ***to c.*** is the process of assigning a symbol or value. *c. categories* are the names or concepts represented by symbols or values, such as race codes or morphology codes; for example, the *c. c.* is "adenocarcinoma" and the code itself is 8140/3. Often used to facilitate analysis. Also, the sentences in a computer program.

coding the process used to transpose text into codes; the assignment of a case to a category using standardized rules.

cohort method study method using a defined group of subjects (e.g., the population of Framingham, Massachusetts, on January 1, 1960). For example, a method for calculating multiyear survival based on an initial group of patients diagnosed in a single year; preferred method of calculating multiyear survival for examining trends over time.

cohort study a type of epidemiologic research in which a group of individuals who are disease-free but who have a known risk or exposure are followed for a period to see who will experience development of the disease under study. This is a ***prospective*** type of research. A ***retrospective*** *c. s.* is one in which the cohort has been previously identified and the registry is asked to link cohort members to the registry to determine who has experienced development of the disease, for example, case–controls.

ColdFusion macromedia product that uses a language similar to HTML called *ColdFusion Markup Language.*

collaborative staging system cancer staging system designed to derive the extent of disease at the time of diagnosis based on a complex computer algorithm based on tumor size, extension of the primary tumor, lymph node involvement, and metastases. It assigns both the ***American Joint Committee on Cancer (AJCC) TNM stage*** and the ***Surveillance, Epidemiology, and End Results Program (SEER)*** Summary Stage 1977 and 2000. It was developed jointly by the national standards-setting organizations.

College of American Pathologists (CAP) professional organization for pathologists in the United States.

combination reporting see ***casefinding.***

Commission on Cancer (CoC) multidisciplinary organization that sets standards for cancer care in hospitals, established in 1922 by the ***American College of Surgeons (ACoS).***

Commission on Cancer (CoC) a division of the *American College of Surgeons (ACoS)* that consists of more than 100 representatives from professional organizations involved in cancer control; originally called the *Cancer Campaign Committee*. The standing committees of the *CoC* are Accreditation, Quality Integration, Cancer Liaison, Education, and Executive.

Commission on Cancer, Cancer Program Standards, 2004 a publication of the *Commission on Cancer (CoC)*, which lists specific standards and guidelines in eight areas for *cancer program accreditation.*

Committee on Accreditation the segment of the *Commission on Cancer (CoC)* that administers the activities of the Accreditation Program.

comorbidity the presence of another disease or diseases that affect the management of the disease currently under treatment; for example, diabetes is a *c.* that affects how quickly a patient can heal after surgery.

comparative data see *reference database.*

comparison groups persons representing the general population or background situation used in lieu of a true control group (having no exposure other than that of the study) to be compared with the study group.

complete method (in survival) method for calculating multiyear survival using the cohort of all patients diagnosed in the most recent years with available data; used in estimating current survival.

completeness the comprehensiveness of the data set collected, the specification of code values (as opposed to blank and unknown code values), and the avoidance of omissions; assurance that all cases in a specific population have been included in the disease registry.

complication an adverse effect or unfavorable result of a procedure or process; for example, infection is a potential *c.* of a surgical procedure.

component columns see *bar chart.*

computer hardware laptops (notebooks), desktops, servers, and peripheral devices such as printers

computerized axial tomography (CT) a radiographic method of examining the body by creating an image from cross-sectional computerized "slices" of tissue; also called *CAT scanning*. The computer calculates the degree of multiple X-ray beams that are not absorbed by all the tissue in its path and creates a computer image showing the geography and characteristics of tissue structures within solid organs.

concordance agreement between abstractors and coders given the same information and coding guidelines; see also *reproducibility.*

confidence interval statistical measure, typically presented as a range of values containing the true value of a statistic with a particular level of certainty (e.g., 95%).

confidential morbidity report (CMR) a standardized data collection form required by many central cancer registries to notify the registry of a new case of cancer; also called *cancer notification form.*

confidential private or secret. *c. data* is information that identifies a specific patient, physician, or facility, and includes the patient's name, address, phone number, or social security number.

confidentiality the concept of maintaining the privacy of personal information obtained in the process of work. A *c. agreement* is a written statement describing a facility's confidentiality policies, which is signed by an employee, contractor, or data requestor, who agrees to abide by the policies and protect private information from becoming public. A *c. pledge* is a brief statement in which an employee or contractor agrees to keep patient information private.

conformance testing extent that an implementation or message conforms to one or more standards

confounder factor that is known to be associated with the occurrence of a health event that can influence a related measurement. For example, most health events are associated with age, race, sex, etc. If such a known risk factor is not taken into account, the study results may be confounded (incorrect), so an effect caused by the study factor may be indistinguishable from the already known factor. In the study's analysis, the influence of a confounder can be separated from the effects of the study factor by stratifying the results based on the confounding factor or otherwise adjusting for it. The two factors can be analyzed together for combined effects.

Connection, The the official quarterly newsletter of the *National Cancer Registrars Association (NCRA).*

connective tissue body structures that connect, support, and surround other tissues and organs including muscle, tendon, fat, nerves, fibrous tissue, blood vessels, and lymph vessels. *Sarcomas* arise in *c. t.*

consent form see *informed consent.*

consistency in registry terms, application of abstracting and coding rules or guidelines in the same way for every case.

consultant in registry terms, a technical-level representative of the *Commission on Cancer (CoC)* who provides assistance with cancer program problems and registry questions.

contact in registry terms, a person or office that is likely to know the whereabouts and status of a patient for follow-up purposes.

contiguous directly adjacent; continuously adjoining; without lapse or intervening space; used in reference to *regionalized* cancers and extent of disease.

continuing education ongoing learning process required by most medical and allied health professional organizations to maintain credentials or licensure (e.g., Certified Tumor Registrars [CTRs] are required to complete 20 hours of continuing education in a 2-year period to maintain their credential).

continuity (in coding)   ability of a data item to be used productively over time, despite changes in coding or the underlying medical technology.

continuous quality improvement (CQI)   the uninterrupted process of evaluating *outcomes* and the processes to achieve the goals of *total quality management.*

contract personnel   staff working under a business arrangement for a defined set of services at a fixed price.

control list   a printout or other document that identifies all patients due for *follow-up* at a given point in time, such as a specific month and year. The *c. l.* is compared with the hospital admission and outpatient records to identify and update cases that have been seen at the facility since the *date of last contact.*

cooperative group   see *clinical trial group.*

correlation   the statistical analysis of the variation between two variables that is related to their dependence on one another. The value of the *c.* is the *rho statistic.* The two principal types of *c.* are *Pearson's* and *Spearman's.*

correlational study   a type of epidemiologic research in which rates of cancer or mortality are analyzed against some other factor measured in the population, such as dietary fat or amount of sunlight; also called *ecologic study.*

costs   the expenses incurred in running a business. *Direct c.* are those that originate in and are directly charged against a department's budget, such as personnel expenses. *Fixed c.* are those that tend to remain unchanged over a period of time even when the volume of activity changes, such as equipment leasing. *Indirect c.* are those that are general in nature and benefit several departments or services, such as electricity, building maintenance, and Human Resource services. *Semivariable c.* are those that increase or decrease with changes in activity but are directly proportional to changes in operative volume. *Variable c.* are those that change in response to changes in the volume of activity, such as staffing and supplies.

Council of State and Territorial Epidemiologists (CSTE)   professional organization that promotes the effective use of epidemiologic data to guide public health practice and improve health through training, capacity development, peer consultation, developing standards for practice, and advocating for resources and scientifically based policy.

Council of State Governments   multibranch organization forecasting policy trends for the community of states, commonwealths, and territories on a national and regional level.

Council on Certification   National Cancer Registrars Association (NCRA) group responsible for promoting stan-

dardization in the collection and use of cancer data through examination and certification of cancer registrars and other cancer data specialists.

cover sheet   the registration form or patient information portion of a health record; includes the patient's name and address, contact information, insurance information, and other data items useful for matching and following the case.

Cox regression model   semiparametric modeling technique used in survival analysis that allows for partitioning risk between risk factors, and that requires few assumptions about the underlying distribution.

CPU (central processing unit)   hardware component that performs the processing in a computer.

critical pathway   a description of key elements in the process of care that should be accomplished to achieve maximum quality at minimum cost. The *c. p.* defines the optimal sequence and timing of functions performed by physicians, nurses, and other staff for a particular diagnosis.

cross-classifying   a process, usually computerized, in which records are sorted in a variety of ways to identify any anomalies in the data; for example, comparing age with site to identify any cancers that would be unusual for a particular age group.

crude incidence rate   incidence rate calculated for an entire population without regard to age.

CSS (Cascading Style Sheets)   Web-designing method that applies style changes throughout a Web site by making a change to a single file.

cumulative hazard (in survival)   sum of the instantaneous hazard through time *t,* which is more easily estimated than the hazard function.

cumulative incidence   method for creating an age-adjusted rate by summing the age-specific incidence rates, weighted by the lengths of the age intervals, to adjust for the different age distributions in the study populations; for rare diseases, this provides an estimate of the cumulative risk of the disease over the age groups being summarized

curative   with the intent to remove all cancer so that it will not return.

Current Procedural Terminology (CPT)   a coding book for operations, tests, and other healthcare services.

customer   a *marketing* term meaning any person who makes use of a product or service. In registry terms, a *c.* is anyone who requests data from the registry.

cycle   in chemotherapy terminology, the administration of one phase of a planned sequence of chemotherapy. Several *c.* may be part of a planned *regimen.*

cytogenetic   pertaining to chromosomes, the cellular constituents of heredity.

cytology   the microscopic review of cells in body fluids obtained from aspirations, washings, scrapings, and smears; usually a function of the pathology department. The *c. report* is the documentation of the microscopic examination of cells in body fluids and their diagnosis.

DAD (Discharge Abstract Database)   system for reporting of all in-patient discharges of the hospital maintained by the CIHI.

Data Acquisition Manual (DAM)   the standardized registry data definitions and collection instructions published by the Commission on Cancer (CoC) used in approved cancer programs between 1986 and 1995.

data dictionary   list of terms that comprehensively defines the data items in a registry data set, including coding instructions, code definitions, and allowable codes; it may also include a history of data item changes, applicable edits, and guidelines or examples for item usage.

data edit report a listing of the failed or reviewable *edit checks* for a database.

data element   a fact, category of information, or specific item of information; also called a *field.* See also *data set.* Sex, race, name, and primary site are examples of *d. e.*

data item or element   each single value in a computer record; also referred to as *field.*

data manager   a specialist in collecting cancer information for *clinical trials* and maintaining the paperwork required by federal guidelines; also called *clinical research associate.*

data security   measures taken to protect confidential information about patients in any form (electronic, paper, or film) from unauthorized viewing, including locked cabinets and rooms, encrypted files, and passwords.

data set   a list of *data elements* that must be collected to meet the minimal needs of a group's goals, often with an additional list of elements that are recommended for the most effective operation. An *optional d.s.* is the nonrequired items that enhance registry reporting and analysis; also called *supplemental data set.* A *required d.s.* is the minimum set of information mandated by an organization.

data submittals   process of extracting an appropriate data set from the central registry database system to be submitted to another entity. Data are typically submitted to the funding source(s) and NAACCR but can be submitted for other purposes.

Data Use and Publication Committee (Canada)   committee that establishes process and procedure related to the Canadian Cancer Registry.

data utilization   the process of analyzing collected cancer data and converting it into information about treatment, survival, and other factors that affect cancer patients.

data   a fact, statement, or specific piece of information. In statistical terms, there are four types of *d.: qualitative* (classifying into related groups), which is subcategorized as *nominal* (naming, such as race or sex) and *ordinal* (ranked or placed into an order, such as stage of disease); and *quantitative* (actual values or measures),

which is subcategorized as *interval* (measures or amounts based on an arbitrary starting point, such as body temperature) and *ratio* (measures or amounts based on a scale on which zero means there is none, such as tumor size or age).

database design   information management system usually set up to store various data elements in logical groupings known as records or tables (e.g., storing all patient demographics together in one record and case-specific information in another record). The patient records must be linked to their case records using a key variable that is common to both types of records and unique to the patient record (e.g., the NAACCR patient ID number).

database engine   specialized software application that manages the storage and retrieval of data.

database system   series of software programs and files responsible for organizing and storing data so it may be manipulated and retrieved efficiently; usually includes a database engine and tools that support the database.

date of first recurrence   the point (month, day, and year) a cancer reappears after a *disease-free* interval.

date of initial diagnosis the first time (month, day, and year) that a recognized medical practitioner says there is cancer (either clinically or pathologically).

date of last contact   the most recent point in time (month, day, and year) that a patient's health status is known.

datum (in GIS)   network of highly accurate known point locations that are used as the basis for determining the locations of all other points on the Earth's surface. In North America, the datum in widest use is the North American Datum of 1983 (NAD83).

death certificate only (DCO)   a case that has been reported to a central registry through the state's vital statistics office based on a cancer diagnosis on the death certificate. The ratio of *d. c. o.* cases to incident cases in a period can be used as a measure of casefinding completeness in the central registry. *d. c. o.* cases are those that remain after *follow-back* procedures have been completed.

death clearance   the process of linking death certificates from a state's vital statistics office with registry records to obtain death data for previously registered cancer cases. See also *follow-back.*

death (mortality) rate   number of deaths that occur from cancer in the population at risk during a specific period.

debulking   the surgical removal of as much tumor as possible, with or without total removal of the primary tumor, so that adjuvant therapy will be more effective; also called *cytoreductive surgery.*

dedicated   intended for a specific purpose. A *d.* oncology nursing unit treats only cancer patients.

definitive treatment   see *cancer-directed.*

degrees of freedom   a statistical term that describes the number of individual values that are free to vary once the sum and the number of observations are specified; used for calculating *variance.*

deidentified data (individual)   information that represents individual persons without personal identifiers.

delinquent   a *follow-up* status indicating that there has been no contact with the patient for more than 15 months since the *date of last contact.*

demographic data items   data items that describe the patient (e.g., name, sex, age).

demography, demographics   the statistical and quantitative study of characteristics of human populations. *Demographics* are those data elements that describe the patient, physical environment, and geographic location.

Department of Health and Human Services (HHS)   the part of the executive branch of the federal government that is the principal agency for protecting the health of all Americans and providing essential human services. The *National Cancer Institute,* the *Centers for Disease Control and Prevention,* and the Food and Drug Administration are all parts of *HHS.*

designed studies   optimizing a system by investigating the current level of quality through a formalized plan and analysis; for example, a reabstracting study to evaluate the accuracy and completeness of the original abstracting and coding.

deterministic record linkage   process of matching cases that uses a static or predefined set of rules to compare data. These rules are defined before the linkage begins.

DHTML (Dynamic Hypertext Markup Language)   variety of Web technologies that allow Web pages to change depending on circumstances and the visitors' interaction with the site.

diagnosis   the identification of the nature and extent of a tumor or other condition. The *admitting d.* is a tentative or working diagnosis that distinguishes whether the cancer diagnosis was made before admission or whether the diagnosis was unknown at the time of admission. The *d. index* is a listing, usually computerized, of patients discharged from the hospital, organized by disease or diagnosis code (usually *ICD-9-CM*), usually prepared by the Health Information Department.

Diagnosis-Related Grouping (DRG)   a method of grouping illnesses to categorize the cost of treatment and the reimbursement rate paid by Medicare or Medicaid. Originally the approach involved coding with ICD-9-CM and grouping by homogeneous costs, using major diagnosis, length of stay, secondary diagnosis, surgical procedure, age, and type of services required. *DRGs,* in short, put the burden of responsibility on hospitals to closely monitor a patient's length of stay and the services provided.

differentiation   how much or how little a tumor resembles the normal tissue from which it arose; also called *grade. d.* is often categorized as well differentiated (closely resembling normal cells), moderately differentiated, poorly differentiated, or undifferentiated (having no resemblance to normal cells; anaplastic).

direct extension   a term used in *staging* to indicate *contiguous* growth of tumor from the primary into an adjacent organ or surrounding tissue.

direct standardization   method for creating an age-adjusted rate where the age distribution of a standard population is used to weight the age-specific rates of the study populations to adjust for the different age distributions in the study populations.

Disaster Recovery Plan   plan designed to prevent the loss of registry data in the event of a hardware failure or natural disaster.

disclosure   divulging information about a patient under appropriate circumstances, such as by written authorization of the patient; see also *release of information.*

discontinuous   tumors that are not connected; tumors in more than one area with normal tissue between them; often a sign of metastatic disease.

disease index   see master patient index file.

disease-free   having no clinical evidence of active cancer.

disseminated   in registry terms, a tumor that has spread throughout the body. Some tumors, such as leukemias, are *d.* at diagnosis; others become *d.* as the result of *metastasis.*

dissemination area (in Canada)   statistical geographic unit averaging about 500 people; all of Canada is described by dissemination areas.

distance study   type of spatial analysis in which the distance to medical care is analyzed as a possible explanation for observed geographic variations in outcomes.

distant   a category of the *summary staging* system in which there is a tumor at sites in the body remote from the organ of origin; tumor cells may have arrived at the *d.* site by traveling in the lymphatic system or the vascular system (*hematogenous*), by floating to the surface of another organ in the fluid of a body cavity (*implantation*), or by direct growth through an organ adjacent to the primary.

distribution   the dispersal or variation of a series of values for a variable; see *frequency distribution. Normal d.*: see *kurtosis.*

diverging color scheme (in GIS)   map classification scheme that represents values above the mean with colors proceeding from light to dark in one hue, values below the mean with colors proceeding from light to dark in another hue, and values near the mean using a neutral color such as gray.

DMZ (demilitarized zone)   part of a computer network controlled by a firewall that allows computers (such as Web servers) to be accessible from the Internet but isolated from the internal network.

DNA   deoxyribonucleic acid, the carrier of genetic information for all living organisms.

Dominion Bureau of Statistics (Canada)   federal government department responsible for collecting statistics (home of the first Canadian Cancer Registry); now called *Statistics Canada.*

double-blind study   a clinical research experiment in which the agent being tested or its action is not known to the patient or the investigator.

Dukes' staging   a specialized staging system for cancers of the rectum and colon, initially described in 1929 by Dr. C.E. Dukes. Several modifications of *D. s.* have been published by different researchers, and these are frequently referred to as *D. s.*

duplicate detection (deduplication or unduplication)   type of record linkage within the registry database system that matches each record against all others to find undetected duplicate patients and tumors.

dynamic map   multiple map images in an animated sequence.

early stage   a cancer diagnosed when it is minimally invasive and more easily treated than if it were found at an advanced stage. Early-stage cancers are potentially more curable than *late-stage* tumors.

earth browser   computer software for viewing, manipulating, and sharing geographic information and imagery, but lacking the analysis capabilities of a GIS.

ecologic study   see *correlational study.*

ectoderm   the outermost of the three cell layers in a developing embryo; the origin of epidermal tissues such as the skin, nails, hair, nervous system, and external sense organs.

edit check   computerized comparison of data fields for logic and accuracy in any of several ways: *allowable code checks, range checks, interitem checks, interrecord checks,* and *interdatabase checks.*

edit set   a group of edits used to edit a data file; edits may be grouped for a specific purpose, such as *National Cancer Data Base (NCDB)* or *North American Association of Central Cancer Registries (NAACCR) Call for Data* edits.

editing   reviewing the information on a case for logic, consistency, and possible errors.

edits   individual edits containing the logic for editing data fields.

EDITS   free software program developed by the CDC that provides tools for creating and running intrarecord and interrecord cross checks for cancer registry data; components include EditWriter, GenEDITS, and the EDITS API (EDITS Engine).

EDITS API (Application Program Interface)   sometimes called the *EDITS Engine.* It can be incorporated into programs of many descriptions, including programs for interactive data entry, after-the-fact verification of data, and more. Any language product for Windows should be able to use the EDITS API.

EDITS Metafile (NPCR-EDITS Metafile)   file containing everything needed to edit a data file except the data. Metafiles provide portability of edits so that the same edits may be used for different purposes. They are created and modified using EditWriter.

EditWriter   component of EDITS that is used to define data items; create record layouts; specify algorithms, logic, and documentation; and maintain reference tables.

educational standards   a list of criteria describing the minimum knowledge required to perform a specific job. *National Cancer Registrars Association (NCRA)* has published *e. s.* for cancer registrars.

efficacy   the power to produce a desired effect; effectiveness.

electronic health record (EHR)   the totality of electronic or digitally stored information about a patient throughout the healthcare system; including the *electronic medical record (EMR)* PHR (Personal Health Record), and *Health Information Exchange (HIE)/Regional Health Information Organization (RHIO).*

electronic medical record (EMR)   subset of the *electronic health record (EHR)* referring to the medical information contained within a healthcare facility, such as a hospital, clinic, or physician's office.

electronic pathology (e-path) reporting   electronic transmissions of pathology reports from a laboratory information system to a hospital or central registry, or both.

electronic reporting   electronic transmission of healthcare system data into cancer registry database systems.

eligibility   determination of qualification to participate or be chosen.

eligible case   a record meeting the criteria for inclusion in a registry; also described as *reportable.*

Employer Identification Number (EIN)   number used to identify a business entity; generally, businesses must have an EIN. It is also known as the Federal Tax Identification Number.

encrypted   electronic data modified in a secret way, or encoded, so as to make it unintelligible to unauthorized parties.

encryption   process of encoding electronic data, making it unintelligible to unauthorized parties; typically involves use of a "key" to encode data in such a way that a unique key is required to decode the data. Keys must be securely communicated between the sender and the recipient.

End Results Program   a federal program between 1956 and 1972 consisting of hospitals affiliated with medical schools across the country that monitored the survival of hospitalized cancer patients; predecessor of the *Surveillance, Epidemiology, and End Results (SEER) Program.*

end results   the evaluation of cancer therapy through the analysis of patient survival after treatment.

endocrine therapy   see *hormone therapy.*

endoscopy   the use of a fiberoptic instrument to visually examine passages (such as the colon) or the inside of hollow organs (such as the bladder) or viscera (such as the contents of the abdomen). Procedures are usually described by the organ they inspect, such as bronchoscopy (bronchus of lung) or gastroscopy (stomach).

end point   the health consequence of some *exposure,* usually an undesirable health event such as the occurrence of disease or death but occasionally a beneficial event such as recovery from an illness or healing of a wound. To view the exposure/end point relationship as being a cause-and-effect sequence is unrealistic in epidemiology. Exposure/end point associations imply a risk relationship, not certain causation.

enzyme   one of many complex proteins that are produced by living cells and catalyze specific biochemical reactions in the human body. *Topoisomerase* is a DNA repair *e.*

EOD   the 10-digit anatomic coding system developed by the *Surveillance, Epidemiology, and End Results (SEER) Program* to describe *extent of disease,* incorporating three digits for tumor size, two digits for extension of tumor, one digit for lymph node involvement, and two digits each for the number of regional lymph nodes pathologically examined and involved by tumor.

epidemiologic reasoning   a three-step sequence used in the study of disease: (1) determination of an association between an *exposure* and an *end point*; (2) formulation of a biologic inference (in other words, a *hypothesis*) about that relationship; and (3) testing of the hypothesis.

epidemiology   literally, the study of epidemics; a branch of medical science concerned with studying the patterns of incidence, distribution, and control of disease in human populations; the basic science of public health. The basic attributes of *e.* study are evaluating person, place, and time in relation to the disease. Also, the study of the distribution and determinants of disease in human populations.

epithelial   pertaining to the covering (epithelium) of internal or external surfaces of the body. *e.* cells include *squamous, columnar,* and *transitional* types.

error   see *hypothesis.*

error of omission   incorrect information as a result of the unavailability of correct information; for example, a tumor size marked as unknown because the correct tumor size was in a pathology report that was misfiled.

estimate (in statistics)   statistic, such as the survival probability, calculated from a sample to approximate the true value of the statistic for the entire population (survival probability).

estimated annual percent change (EAPC)   estimate of the average annual change in risk over a specified period. The calculation involves fitting a straight line to the natural logarithm of the data when it is displayed by calendar year.

ethics   moral philosophy pertaining to acceptable professional behavior in circumstances where actions may be interpreted as questionable. *Biomedical e.* deals with moral decisions in medicine. *e. issues* concern human experimentation (see *clinical trials*) and issues of life and death.

etiology   the cause of an event, usually a disease. *e.* is also the general name for the study of causes of disease.

experimental therapy   treatment that has not been approved by the Food and Drug Administration of the federal government, usually involving clinical research trials of prospective new chemotherapy drugs. See also *investigational.*

exploratory spatial data analysis (ESDA)   *set of informal techniques for identifying patterns and relationships in spatial data,* useful in generating hypotheses that can then be tested using more formal methods.

exposure (in epidemiology)   risk (precedent) factor associated with a likelihood of one experiencing some health event or end point. Exposures can range from an ambient environmental factor (air pollution), to the individual's environment (smoking or diet), to personal characteristics (age, race, and sex).

exposure   an ambient environmental factor (such as air pollution), a factor in the individual's environment (such as smoking or diet), or a personal characteristic (such as age, race, or sex) considered to be a precedent factor associated with a likelihood of one's experiencing some health event or end point. A person with such an *e.* is said to be *at risk.* Also, factor associated with a likelihood of one experiencing some health event or end point. Exposures can range from an ambient environmental factor (air pollution), to the individual's environment (smoking or diet), to personal characteristics (age, race, and sex).

extent of disease   the detailed description of how far a cancer has spread from the primary site at the time of diagnosis; a type of classification based on human anatomy that pertains to cancer spread in an individual case.

extramural research   federally funded research conducted by investigators at nonfederal institutions such as universities and teaching hospitals; the opposite of *intramural research.*

FAB (French-American-British) classification   a specialized morphological categorization of acute lymphocytic and acute myelogenous leukemias.

Facility Oncology Registry Data Standards (FORDS)   a 2002 publication of the Commission on Cancer (CoC) that details the CoC-required data set and codes, data collection rules, and other information necessary to accurately abstract and manage cancer cases.

Federal Health Architecture (FHA)   part of the Office of the National Coordinator for Health Information Technology (ONC) that is responsible for creating a federal framework derived from a national health information technology (IT) infrastructure; supporting federal activities in the development and adoption of health IT standards; and ensuring that federal agencies can seamlessly exchange health data between and among themselves, with state, local, and tribal governments, and with private sector healthcare organizations.

fiduciary   of or being a trustee or trusteeship.

field   each single value in a computer record; also referred to as *data item.*

field (in entry field)   defined screen area where text is entered (e.g., the subject field in an e-mail message where the subject is entered by the sender).

FIGO   the French acronym for the International Federation of Gynecology and Obstetrics; the major international proponent of staging systems for gynecologic cancers.

file blocking (in record linkage)   process used to reduce the number of pairs of records that need to be compared; useful when large files and several data items are to be compared. Two files each containing 10,000 records would require 100 million comparisons. Blocking partitions the two files into smaller comparison groups.

file preparation/standardization (as in record linkage)   process of preparing both data files for record linkage and adopting common conventions and formats, thus standardizing identical data items (e.g., Dr. and Drive).

final diagnosis   See *pathology report.*

firewall   computer or dedicated hardware device that restricts access between a protected network and the Internet, or between other sets of networks

first course of therapy, first course of treatment   medical care that is planned or given at the time of initial diagnosis when it has the greatest chance of eliminating the cancer; also called *initial treatment.*

fiscal year   a financial term indicating a 12-month period that does not necessarily coincide with a calendar year. For example, a *f. y.* may run from July 1 of a given year to June 30 of the following year.

Fisher's exact test   see *nonparametric statistics.*

flag   in registry and computer terms, a data field that indicates a special status; for example, an incomplete case or a data field requiring an *override.*

flow cytometry   a series of clinical tests to measure and describe the cellular and DNA activity of a tumor.

follow   in registry terms, to maintain annual contact with a patient or his or her physician to monitor the patient's health after a diagnosis of cancer. See *follow-up.*

follow-back   reviewing a patient's medical history to ascertain whether a case reported first by a death certificate ever had that cancer diagnosed at any other source while the patient was alive. Also, process of requesting more information from physicians, hospitals, or other healthcare providers for cancer death nonmatches from the death clearance process.

follow-up   an organized system of long-term surveillance of patients; the activities involved in monitoring patients after discharge; the process of obtaining annually updated information regarding a patient's health status to ensure continued medical surveillance. *Active f.* refers to someone, usually a physician or cancer registrar, initiating direct contact with patients to encourage them to see their physician. *F. data* in an *abstract* include those fields useful for tracking the patient after he or she has left the hospital, including the name, address, telephone number, and relationship of a relative, friend, or neighbor who is most likely to know how to locate the patient. *F. letters* are written requests for information on a patient's health status, which can be addressed to a physician, the patient, or a *contact.* The *f. rate* is a calculation of the percentage of patients who have current information (within 15 months) on their health status; the target rate is 90% successful *f. f. staff* are the individual(s) in a registry who conduct all patient tracking activities. *Passive f.* refers to methods that do not require contact with hospitals, physicians, or patients, to determine the patient's vital status, such as linkage with voter registration records or driver's license lists.

formal education   planned, structured course of study usually resulting in a certificate or degree from a recognized educational institution or accrediting body.

Framework for Improving Performance   a part of the Joint Commission's *Agenda for Change;* describes specific objectives for ascertaining quality of care.

freestanding   a diagnosing or treatment facility (which may or may not be affiliated with or owned by a hospital) that maintains its own patient records. Usually *f.* facilities are in a separate building, such as a surgery or radiation oncology center, and have their own management structure.

frequency   how many observations of a variable have a certain value. The *absolute f.* is the raw number of observations having a certain value. The *cumulative f.* is the percentage of observations having a specific value or less than that value. The *relative f.* is the proportion or percentage of observations that have a specific value.

frequency distribution   a visual depiction of the pattern of occurrence over the range of values for a variable. Common *f. d.* are the **histogram** and **frequency polygon.** See also **kurtosis** and **skew.**

frequency polygon   a type of **histogram** in which a line connects the top midpoint of each bar; sometimes called an *area chart.*

friable   prone to crumbling or breaking. A *f.* tumor can fall apart when grasped by an instrument.

frozen section   a pathologic examination technique where part of a biopsy specimen is quickly frozen, sliced thinly, and microscopically examined to determine the presence or absence of cancer cells.

F-test   see **ANOVA.**

full-time employee (FTE)   a person who works 40 hours per week or the equivalent; for example, two people each working 20 hours per week would be the equivalent of one FTE.

function   computer programming subprogram logic that is used repeatedly. The EDITS software provides date, string, table, and miscellaneous other functions; also used when writing individual edits using EditWriter.

GenEDITS (Generic EDITS Batch Driver)   batch application for editing any data file with any EDITS Metafile.

genetic study   a type of epidemiologic research in which patients and their families are evaluated for the presence of genes that may cause or contribute to the development of cancer.

geocode   *v.* to perform the act of geocoding; *n.* geographic information assigned to a cancer patient record.

geocoding   process of assigning geographic information, such as latitude/longitude, census geography, or minor civil division, to a cancer patient record.

germ cell tumor   a neoplasm that arises from cells that develop into sperm or eggs or cells that resemble those that create sperm or eggs.

gigabyte (GB)   unit of storage in a computer equivalent to 1024 megabytes (MB); 1 MB is equivalent to 1024 kilobytes (KB); 1 KB is equivalent to 1024 bytes; 1 byte is equivalent to 8 bits of binary information and is necessary to store a single ASCII character.

GIS (geographic information system)   computer software for the acquisition, storage, linkage, manipulation, analysis, and mapping of geographic data.

glioma   a type of tumor arising from the supporting or glial cells of the brain, including **astrocytoma,** oligodendroglioma, and ganglioglioma.

global pricing agreement   a written contract that provides a single reimbursement fee for a service, regardless of how costly the treatment is for an individual patient.

Governor General   Canada's link to the British monarchy, a position appointed by the prime minister of Canada

grade   how much or how little a tumor resembles the normal tissue from which it arose; the aggressiveness of a

tumor; also called *differentiation.* *g.* is also the description or name of the sixth digit of the **ICD-O** morphology code.

graduated symbol (in GIS)   type of map symbolization in which data are represented by point symbols that vary in size, with the size of a symbol directly proportional to the data value it represents; also known as *proportional symbol.*

grand rounds   an educational meeting of medical professionals.

Grants Administration   see **Office of Sponsored Research.**

graphics   the various ways to present data in pictures or visual detail, including such methods as a **table, bar chart,** or **line graph;** also called *charts.*

Greenwood's formula   mathematical formula used in the calculation of the standard error of the survival estimate as calculated by either the Kaplan–Meier or life-table method.

gross description   see **pathology report.**

growth fraction   the number of cells undergoing division at any one time. See also **S-phase.**

gynecologic   pertaining to women's health and female reproductive organs.

hardware   see **computer hardware.**

hazard function   instantaneous failure rate at time *t,* or number of deaths per unit of time.

hazard rate   instantaneous failure or death rate; the measure on which regression models for survival analysis are based.

HCN   Health Care Number.

Health Canada   Department within the Canadian federal government, now called the *Public Health Agency of Canada.*

healthcare reform   the process of reviewing and adjusting patient management patterns and services to reduce costs.

health information management (HIM)   professionals responsible for the development and administration of healthcare data collection and reporting systems (patient health records). Formerly referred to as *medical records management.*

health information management department   the part of a healthcare facility that gathers, analyzes, and stores the medical documents for each patient, ensuring completeness and coding, and indexing the records for future reference; also called *health record department.*

health record   the detailed medical information maintained on a patient; also called *chart.*

hematogenous   blood-borne; referring to tumor cells that have been carried through the bloodstream to a distant site where they were filtered out and began to grow.

hematopoietic   pertaining to the tissues that generate blood components, such as the blood marrow and stem cells.

heterozygosity   having different *alleles* at a given locus in a chromosome.

high risk (in quality control)   quality improvement term indicating a topic prone to error that can be improved through training or change in procedures.

high volume (in quality control)   quality improvement term indicating a topic where a large number of cases will be impacted if quality improves through training or a change in procedures. Also referred to as a *quantity* issue.

HIPAA (Health Insurance Portability and Accountability Act)   U.S. medical law tightening confidentiality and privacy requirements, materially affecting cancer registration, among other matters.

histogram   a graphic presentation of information that displays the magnitude of a continuous variable.

histologically confirmed   a diagnosis made on the basis of a microscopic examination of tissue.

histology   the study of the microscopic structure of tissue.

history   the portion of the health record that provides the background of the current illness, including type and duration of symptoms, exposures, and other information that might affect the diagnosis.

history file   a list of nonreportable cases that have been identified by the registry but not included in the registry database. Usually the reason for not accessioning the case is that it was diagnosed before the registry's *reference date.*

HITSP (Healthcare Information Technology Standards Panel) cooperative partnership between the public and private sectors under the umbrella of the American Health Information Community (AHIC). Its purpose is to achieve a widely accepted and useful set of standards specifically to enable and support widespread interoperability among healthcare software applications, as they will interact in a local, regional, and national health information network for the United States.

HL7 (Health Level Seven)   both a not-for-profit volunteer organization and a formatting standard for structuring, storing, and messaging clinical data.

HL7 parser   software application that interprets an HL7 data stream or file, separating it into the individual HL7 data elements that may then be translated, stored in a database, and/or further processed.

hormone   a natural substance produced by the body that controls reproduction, growth, or metabolism in organs distant from where the hormones are produced. *H. therapy* can be the use of surgery, radiation therapy, or drugs to interfere with hormone production, thereby preventing or delaying recurrence of the cancer; also called *hormone manipulation* or *endocrine therapy.* *H. replacement therapy* is the administration of a drug or hormone to restore normal levels of a needed hormone after removal of a gland that produces hormones.

horseshoe kidney   see *anomaly.*

hospice   an inpatient or outpatient program of nursing and supportive care for terminal patients.

hospital-based registry   a registry that collects information on all patients who use the services of a hospital or healthcare facility.

host performance scale   a classification system describing a patient's *quality of life.* The *Karnofsky scale* and the *Eastern Cooperative Oncology Group (ECOG) scale* are two types of *h. p. s.* that record the physical status of the patient.

HTML (Hypertext Markup Language)   common language of the World Wide Web; using a series of commands enclosed in less-than and greater-than signs that specify the appearance of the page.

human subjects committee   formal group within research organizations (e.g., universities) set up to review and approve the conduct of scientific research with human beings as participants in accordance with the ethical principles of respect for persons, beneficence, and justice, as well as applicable rules and law. Used interchangeably with *institutional review board (IRB).*

hypothesis   in statistics, a scientific observation or statement that is to be proved or disproved by research and testing. The *alternative h.* is a statement that there is a real difference between two groups, for example, as a result of a different type of treatment. The *null h.* is a statement that there is no difference between the two measurements being compared. Two types of errors can occur when a *h.* is tested: *type I* or *alpha error* occurs when the *n. h.* is true when the statistical test finds that it is false; and *type II* or *beta error* occurs when the *n. h.* is false, but it is accepted as true.

ICD (International Classification of Diseases) see *International Statistical Classification.* Various editions of this disease coding system include *ICD, 1965 revision* (*ICD-8*); ICD, adapted for use in the United States 1967 (*ICDA-8*); the *Hospital Adaption of ICD* (*HICDA*); *ICD, ninth revision* (*ICD-9*), *ICD, ninth revision—Clinical Modification* (*ICD-9-CM*), and *ICD, tenth revision* (*ICD-10*).

ICD-10-CA   Canadian version of the World Health Organization's *International Classification of Diseases, tenth revision* (*ICD-10*).

ICD-O   see *International Classification of Diseases for Oncology.*

ill-defined site   in registry terms, a cancer that originated in an area of the body that cannot be precisely described or coded to a single organ, such as the arm (a general term) or the abdomen (composed of many organs).

immunotherapy   treatment that boosts, directs, or restores the body's normal immune system and enhances the body's own ability to fight the cancer; also called *biological response modifier therapy.*

implantation   a tumor that has begun to grow on the surface of an organ because tumor cells floated from a primary site in the fluid (ascites) of a body cavity and settled on the surface of another organ.

implementation of changes   process of planning for a change in rules or reference materials before the change actually occurs, including training individuals on the changes and making any necessary changes in software.

in situ   Latin for "in place"; a tumor confined to the organ of origin without invasion; a tumor that fulfills all microscopic criteria for malignancy except invasion of the organ's *basement membrane;* malignant tumor that has not begun to invade; also described as *intraepithelial, noninvasive,* or *noninfiltrating.*

incidence   how many times something occurs; for example, the number of times new cancer is diagnosed in a defined population during a defined period such as a year. A new occurrence of a cancer is called an *incident case.* See also *rate.*

incidence data   information on each new occurrence of cancer.

incidence rate   number of new cancers of a specific site/type that occur in a defined population during a year divided by the number of individuals who were at risk for the given cancer in the population, generally expressed as the number of cancers per 100,000 persons.

incidence ratio   see *relative risk.*

in-depth report   part of an *annual report* in which information on one or more types of cancer is presented in detail; one of the required content items for approval of the annual report by the Commission on Cancer (CoC).

indirect standardization   approximate mathematical method for creating an age-adjusted rate where the age-specific incidence rates from a reference or standard population are applied to the age distribution of the study population; used when the age-specific rates for the study population are unavailable or unstable because the number of cases is small.

informed consent   the description of a scientific study and its procedures, written in nontechnical language, which is explained to and must be understood and voluntarily signed by the patient, parent, or guardian before he or she is accepted into a *clinical trial.* Also, legal and ethical obligation to ensure that the prospective subject has sufficient knowledge and understanding to make an informed, educated, and enlightened decision on whether to participate.

infratentorial   see *tentorium cerebelli.*

infusion   the administration of chemotherapy over an extended period by mixing the drug with a diluting solution and letting it flow into a blood vessel or body cavity. *He-patic artery i.* is the insertion of a catheter into the hepatic artery to deliver a concentrated dose of chemotherapy to the liver. The *i. center* is the part of a healthcare facility that administers chemotherapy to inpatients or outpatients.

initial treatment   see *first course of therapy.*

initiation   the transformation of a normal cell to one that has the potential for malignant growth; one of the two steps of *carcinogenesis.*

inpatient   a person spending at least one night in a healthcare facility to be diagnosed or treated.

institutional review board (IRB)   a committee in a healthcare facility whose membership, composition, purpose, and functions are specified by federal law and whose purpose is to provide a complete and adequate review of human research activities commonly conducted by the institution and to protect the rights (confidentiality and ethical issues) of all human subjects participating in scientific research.

interactive   use of a computer where the computer interacts with the user, after each step; contrasts with batch operations.

interactive map   computer-based map for which a user can influence the map content and appearance

interdatabase check   a type of *edit check* in which the computer checks two or more databases for consistency. For example, if the cancer registry shows that a patient has lung cancer, the hospital billing record should also show a diagnosis of lung cancer.

interdisciplinary   coordinated activity between various health specialists. Cancer treatment frequently involves *i.* communication, interaction, and planning among nurses, surgeons, and radiation or medical oncologists.

interfield edits   edits that compare the codes of one data item with the codes of other related data items within the same record.

intergroup   cooperative studies conducted by more than one *clinical trial group* to *accrue* larger numbers of patients from a wider geographical area into a study. For example, the *Children's Cancer Group (CCG)* and *Pediatric Oncology Group (POG)* combine efforts to study diseases such as the *I.* Rhabdomyosarcoma Study Group.

interitem check   a type of *edit check* in which the computer compares two or more data elements for logic. For example, an *i.* edit might check the fields "Primary Site" and "Sex"; this edit would fail if the primary site was prostate and sex was female.

International Agency for Research on Cancer (IARC)   an independently financed organization within the framework of the World Health Organization, based in Lyon, France, dedicated to worldwide research on the epidemiology of cancer and the study of potential carcinogens in the human environment; affiliated with the *International Association of Cancer Registries.*

International Association of Cancer Registries (IACR)   an organization based in Lyon, France, created in 1965, and consisting of member population-based registries throughout the world. The purposes of IACR include improving the quality of data on cancer incidence and mortality, and comparability between registries by standardizing methods of registration, definitions, and coding, and to disseminate information on the multiple uses of cancer registry data in epidemiologic research and the planning and evaluation of cancer prevention and therapy; affiliated with the *International Agency for Research on Cancer.*

International Classification of Diseases for Oncology (ICD-O)   the worldwide standard coding system for cancer diagnoses, now in its third edition *(ICD-O-3)* used worldwide for assigning morbidity and mortality codes to health records and death certificates. For names of predecessors, see *ICD.*

International Union Against Cancer   the name in English of the French-named Union Internationale Contre le Cancer (UICC), the international organization that promotes the use of the *TNM staging* system worldwide; also referred to in English as the UICC.

interrecord check   a type of *edit check* in which the computer checks multiple records for consistency. For example, the same patient cannot be coded as alive on one primary and coded as dead on another primary.

interval   see *data.*

intervention   an action is taken in an attempt to effect a change. For example, publicity about the availability of mammography in a non–English-speaking community is an *i.* that can be studied or evaluated to determine its success in reducing the number of late-stage cancers diagnosed in that community.

intramural research   federally funded research conducted at the *National Institutes of Health* Clinical Center in Bethesda, Maryland; the opposite of *extramural research.*

intramuscular   injection of a drug or chemotherapy agent into a muscle.

Intranet   network that belongs to an organization and is designed to be accessible only by the organization's members, employees, or others with authorization. An intranet's Web site looks and acts just like other Web sites but has a firewall surrounding it to fend off unauthorized users.

intraperitoneal   injection of a drug or chemotherapy agent into the peritoneal cavity.

intrathecal   injection of a drug or chemotherapy agent into the cerebrospinal fluid surrounding the brain and spinal cord to reach tumor cells in the brain or spine with an agent that cannot cross the *blood–brain barrier.*

intravenous   administration of a drug or chemotherapy agent by injecting it directly into the bloodstream through a vein.

intussusception   the telescoping of the large bowel or small intestine on itself, sometimes caused by a tumor mass in the bowel wall.

invasive cancer   cancer that has spread beyond the basement membrane.

investigational   a technique, drug, or treatment that is being evaluated by means of a scientific or research study. *i.* drugs have not yet been approved by the Food and Drug Administration for general use but can be used in a *clinical trial.*

involved   in registry terms, considered to contain or be affected by cancer.

IT (information technology)   technology involving the development, maintenance, and use of computer systems, software, and networks for the processing and distribution of data; formerly called *information systems.*

JavaScript and VBScript   programming (scripting) languages that add dynamic and interactive features to Web sites such as navigation tools, forms, animation, and other multimedia displays.

job description   see *position description.*

joinpoint   a knot or point, identified using the joinpoint modeling technique, at which the slope of a regression line changes.

joinpoint model   statistical technique that characterizes cancer trends using statistical criteria to determine how many times and when the trends in incidence or mortality rates have changed. The results of joinpoint analysis are given as calendar year ranges and the annual percent change (APC) in the rates over each period.

Joint Commission (JC)   the agency that establishes and oversees quality standards for hospitals and psychiatric, long-term care, and certain other health facilities in the United States. Formerly the joint Commission on Accreditation of Hospitals and also the *Joint Commission on Accreditation of Healthcare Organizations (JCAHO)*

Journal of Registry Management (JRM)   the official quarterly journal of the *National Cancer Registrars Association (NCRA)* that publishes scientific articles on registry science.

Kaplan–Meier calculation   see *survival calculation.*

Kaplan–Meier survival   statistical method where the survival probability is estimated at each time point when a death occurs, and censored observations are taken to occur at the end of the time interval; suitable for small (<30) and large cohorts of patients.

Kruskal–Wallis test   see *nonparametric statistics.*

kurtosis   the statistical description of the spread or dispersal of values along a range of data. Types of **k.** include *platykurtosis* (flatter and wider than a normal distribution), *leptokurtosis* (higher and narrower than a normal distribution), and *mesokurtosis* (the normal distribution or bell-shaped curve).

LAN (local area network)   network that operates only within a local area such as an office; often used for sharing resources such as a printer and file storage devices.

Langerhans cell histiocytosis (LCH)   a condition consisting of a proliferation of histiocytes, eosinophils, and lymphocytes.

late stage   a cancer that has spread beyond anatomic boundaries and that can no longer be treated with localized surgery or radiation therapy.

latency   the interval from the start of a disease until it is clinically detected. The **l.** period for most cancers is believed to be 10 to 20 years.

latitude   distance north or south of the equator, measured in degrees. The equator is defined as 0 degrees; the north pole, positive 90 degrees; and the south pole, negative 90 degrees. One degree is approximately 111.1 kilometers.

layer (in GIS)   collection of spatial objects stored together in a GIS; also referred to as a *table* or *theme*.

Lead Educator   National Program of Cancer Registries (NPCR) term for person in charge of educational efforts for a central registry. Also called *Training Coordinator.*

legal   pertaining to the law. In registry terms, usually pertaining to the **release of information** about a patient. **L. aspects** of policies imply circumstances pertaining to regulations of administrative agencies, common law, and statutory law.

legislative mandate   in registry terms, a law, regulation, or other governmental ruling empowering a central registry to establish and maintain a mechanism for cancer data collection and related surveillance activities. A **l. m.** can include funding, confidentiality policies, and penalties for not reporting eligible cases to the central registry. Legal requirements (via statutes and regulations) and political support for cancer reporting.

leptokurtosis   see **kurtosis.**

leukemia   the presence in the blood of malignant cells that developed in the bone marrow.

leukocoria   a white spot on the eye indicative of possible **retinoblastoma.**

life-table method   statistical method where the survival probability is estimated at set time intervals (e.g., weeks, months), and censored observations are taken to occur evenly throughout the time interval; not suitable for small (< 30) cohorts of patients. See also **survival rate.**

lifetime risk   probability of developing cancer in the course of one's life span. Lifetime risk may also be discussed in terms of the probability of developing or dying of cancer.

line graph   a graphic presentation of information showing a trend over time by displaying an increment of time on the *x*-axis, and the amount, frequency, or percentage on the *y*-axis.

LIS (Laboratory Information System)   data system for (anatomic) pathology laboratories into which most cancer diagnoses in the form of pathology reports are entered.

list   a graphic display of information about a single variable in text format.

localized   a category of the **summary staging** system in which the tumor is confined to the organ of origin without extension beyond the primary organ.

log-rank test   statistical test, using logarithms, for comparing the survival times for two or more groups.

LOINC (Logical Observation Identifiers Names and Codes)   standard coding system or a set of universal names with associated codes for identifying laboratory and clinical observations.

longevity   the length of time a registry has been established, based on the **reference date.**

longitude   distance east or west of the prime meridian, the north-south line passing through Greenwich, England, measured in degrees. The prime meridian is defined as 0 degrees. East of the meridian, longitudes are given using positive numbers to a maximum of 180 degrees exactly halfway around the globe from the prime meridian. West of the meridian, longitudes are given using negative numbers to a minimum of −180 degrees, corresponding to the same location as +180 degrees. The distance in a degree of longitude varies by latitude, being approximately 111.1 kilometers times the cosine of the latitude.

lost to follow-up   a case for which all **contacts** for **follow-up** have been exhausted without successfully obtaining current information on the patient's health status at a point in time more than 15 months after the **date of last contact;** see also **delinquent.**

lymphadenopathy   enlargement of lymph nodes, but not necessarily indicating tumor involvement.

lymphoma   malignancy of lymphoid tissues, in other words, those tissues and organs that produce and store cells that fight infection and disease; subdivided into **Hodgkin's disease** and **non-Hodgkin's lymphoma.** Burkitt **l.** is a rapidly growing tumor first described by Dr. Dennis Burkitt in Africa; African Burkitt is characterized by massive cervical node and jaw involvement; American Burkitt has a more disseminated presentation with an abdominal mass and malignant peritoneal and pleural effusions.

M   in the *TNM staging* system, the element that describes the presence or absence of distant metastases.

magnetic resonance imaging (MRI)   a diagnostic imaging technique that uses strong magnetic fields that take advantage of cellular properties to define internal structures.

malignancy   an invasive, uncontrolled growth of cells capable of invading surrounding structures and producing a *metastasis.*

managed care   the process of monitoring patient treatment to maximize quality and minimize cost. *m. c. organizations* are groups of healthcare providers whose purpose is to deliver quality medical services in the most cost-effective means possible in an attempt to reduce healthcare costs.

management   in registry terms, how the patient is diagnosed, treated, and followed; sometimes called *case management.*

manager   the individual in a registry who handles administrative and staffing issues and supervises others in the registry.

Manchester (UK) Children's Tumour Registry classification   a specialized scheme for the classification of cancer in children, divided into 12 main diagnostic groups containing several subclassifications.

Mann–Whitney U test   see *nonparametric statistics.*

Manual for Tumor Nomenclature and Coding (MOTNAC)   the earliest publication providing topography and morphology codes for cancer diagnosis, first published by the American Cancer Society in 1951.

manual   by hand; in registry terms, not involving a computer program. A *tickler file* is a *m.* follow-up system.

margin   in medical terms, the edge of a surgical resection or the rim of normal tissue surrounding a tumor; usually referred to as normal, clear, or uninvolved if there is no evidence of tumor at the edge. In business terms, *m.* is the profit and loss incurred as a result of an activity. A registry can perform this type of margin study on a cancer service (such as mammography screening) if it has access to a patient's financial records.

marketing   the process of informing others of the usefulness of a service or product. *M.* is a combination of publicity and customer education about the service or product. For example, a cancer registry markets its data (a product) to make its *customers* aware of the services it offers.

market-share studies   analysis of *referral patterns* and *treatment patterns* together with other information to determine a facility's or organization's market share (proportion of "available" business activity). For example, *m. s.* could determine that a hospital was treating a smaller proportion of all of the breast cancer cases in a city because of competition from a newly opened facility.

master file   main, or primary, file of patient data in the registry.

master file organization   method by which the data items and records are stored and indexed within the master file.

master patient index (MPI) file   the alphabetized, computerized list or card file that includes every patient, alive and dead, who has been accessioned into the registry since the *reference date;* also called *patient index.*

matching (in epidemiology)   design strategy used in epidemiology to make the study groups as comparable as possible. For example, if the study groups are made to be comparable with respect to age, any difference between them cannot be because of the influence of age. Matching can be for the whole study group or for individuals. One, or more than one, comparison person (control) can be selected for each study subject.

matching   a design strategy used in epidemiology to make the study groups as comparable as possible. For example, if the study groups are made to be comparable with respect to age, any difference between them cannot be caused by the influence of age. *M.* can be for the whole study group or for individuals. Individual *m.* may be one-to-one or many-to-one, which means that more than one comparison person is selected for each study subject.

matting   in registry terms, the lumping together of lymph nodes into a single mass, usually the result of tumor growth between the nodes.

mean   the average of a series of numbers.

measures of central tendency   statistical calculations that describe how alike the values in a range of numbers are; a collective term for *mean, median,* and *mode.*

median   the midpoint or middle value in a series of numbers.

MEDLINE   a database of indexed medical literature available through the National Library of Medicine.

medulloblastoma   a radiosensitive tumor of undifferentiated neuroepithelial cells arising in the cerebellum.

mesenchymal   pertaining to the mesenchyma; the diffuse network of cells forming the embryonic mesoderm and creating the blood and blood vessels, the lymphatic system, and cells of the reticuloendothelial system.

mesokurtosis   see *kurtosis.*

metadata   description of the quality, accuracy, precision, provenance, and other useful characteristics of a data set. Applies to all data sets but frequently encountered in GIS.

metafile   computer file containing everything needed to edit a data file except the data. They are created and modified using EditWriter.

metastasis, metastases (plural form)   any tumor spread to a part of the body away from the primary. See also *distant spread. Drop m.* is a specific type of tumor spread into the spinal cord and cauda equina from the brain.

microinvasion   tumor extension through the *basement membrane* (a histologic landmark in an organ), visible only through the microscope; an indication that the tumor is invasive and no longer in situ.

micrometastases   secondary tumors that are not visible to the unaided eye. *m.* can grow and develop into distant recurrences if they are not treated and destroyed by systemic therapy.

microscopic confirmation   diagnoses that include hematology, cytology, and tissue examinations.

microscopic description   the part of the *pathology report* that describes what the pathologist diagnoses with the aid of a microscope.

minor civil division   term used to refer to any subcounty governmental unit, such as town, township, borough, and city. Not all locations within the United States fall within a minor civil division.

mitosis   that part of the cell cycle in which the cell is actively dividing.

mode   one of the measures of central tendency that describes the most frequently occurring value in a series of numbers. *Bimodal* means that a range of numbers has two most common values.

morbidity   a *complication* or other effect of disease, such as impaired organ function as a result of a surgical procedure.

morphology   the science of structure and form without regard to function; the name of the *ICD-O* code describing the specific type of tumor.

morphology groupings   ranges or categories of *ICD-O* histology codes; usually used for aggregate reporting or data analysis of related types of cancer.

mortality   death.

mortality rate   number of deaths from a disease for a specified period, divided by the total number of population-at-risk.

multicentric, multifocal   in registry terms, the presence of more than one area of tumor in an organ or tissue.

multidisciplinary   consisting of representatives from many health specialties; for example, surgery, pathology, radiology, medical oncology, and radiation oncology. The *Commission on Cancer (CoC)* requires that the *cancer committee* be *m. multihospital registry.* See *central cancer registry.*

multiple primaries   the situation in which a patient has more than one cancer. See also *primary.*

myeloablative   lethal to bone marrow cells, usually referring to a drug or radiation administered before a *bone marrow transplant.*

myelodysplastic syndrome   a unique preleukemic state in which the bone marrow shows progressive deterioration in red blood cell production, platelet formation, and white blood cell maturation.

MySQL   popular free-of-charge database system for Web applications; often coupled with PHP scripts to create dynamic Web sites.

N   in the *TNM staging* system, the element that describes the presence or absence of tumor in regional lymph nodes.

NACRS (National Ambulatory Clinic Reporting System)   Canadian system for the reporting of all outpatient and clinic activities of the hospital that is maintained by the CIHI.

National Board for Certification of Registrars (NBCR)   an independent organization responsible for developing and administering the *certification examination* for cancer registrars.

National Cancer Act of 1971   a federal law that mandated the collection, analysis, and dissemination of data for use in the prevention, diagnosis, and treatment of cancer; the legal authorization for the establishment of the *Surveillance, Epidemiology, and End Results Program (SEER) Program* of the *National Cancer Institute.*

National Cancer Data Base (NCDB)   a clinically oriented electronic database of cancer cases submitted to the Commission on Cancer by approved cancer programs in the United States, which can be used as a *reference database* to compare the management of cancer patients in one facility or region with similar patients in other regions or nationally. Also, nationwide oncology outcomes database from more than 1,500 hospitals in 50 states, founded as a joint project of the American College of Surgeons Commission on Cancer (ACoS CoC) and the American Cancer Society. Each year, the NCDB issues a Call for Data to its participating hospitals and publishes numerous scientific articles. Also, a clinically oriented electronic database of cancer cases submitted to the CoC by approved cancer programs in the United States, which can be used as a *reference database* to compare the management of cancer patients in one facility or region with similar patients in other regions or nationally.

National Cancer Data Committee   the committee that oversees the *National Cancer Data Base (NCDB)* and patient care evaluations; see *Commission on Cancer.*

National Cancer Incidence Reporting System   first Canadian national cancer registry system; an event-based database.

National Cancer Institute (NCI)   one of the 24 institutes of the *National Institutes of Health (NIH),* established under the earlier "National Cancer Act" (of 1937) as the federal government's principal agency for cancer research and training. The National Cancer Act of 1971 broadened the scope and responsibilities of the NCI, and legislative amendments have maintained the NCI's authorities and responsibilities, and added new information dissemination mandates, as well as a requirement to assess the incorporation of state-of-the-art cancer treatments into clinical practice. NCI is the governmental agency that houses the *Surveillance, Epidemiology, and End Results Program (SEER) Program.* Also, federal government agency within the NIH that fights cancer by supporting and conducting groundbreaking research in cancer biology, causation, prevention, detection, treatment, and survivorship.

National Cancer Institute of Canada (NCIC) sister organization to *National Cancer Institute (NCI)* that assists in channeling funds raised by CCS into peer-reviewed research including clinical trials and targeted areas within basic science and sociobehavioral realms.

National Cancer Registrars Association (NCRA) a professional organization composed of cancer data specialists, whose purpose is to promote the education and professional development of cancer registrars and cancer registries; formerly the *National Tumor Registrars Association (NTRA).*

National Center for Health Statistics a federal center of the *Centers for Disease Control and Prevention* that provides population and mortality data that are used by the *Surveillance, Epidemiology, and End Results Program (SEER)* Program and others to derive cancer incidence, mortality, and survival rates.

National Committee on Vital and Health Statistics (NCVHS) group that serves as the statutory public advisory body to the secretary of *Department of Health and Human Services (HHS)* in the area of health data, statistics, and national health information policy.

National Institutes of Health (NIH) originally established in 1887 and now composed of 24 separate institutes, centers, and divisions, the *NIH* is one of eight health agencies of the Public Health Service, which, in turn, is part of the *U.S. Department of Health and Human Services (HHS).* *NIH* is federally mandated and funded to support and conduct biomedical research.

National Program of Cancer Registries (NPCR) *Centers for Disease Control and Prevention (CDC)* program that provides funding to state health departments to support and enhance state cancer registries. This program supports efforts by states and territories to do the following: improve existing cancer registries; plan and implement registries where they do not exist; meet standards for data completeness, timeliness, and quality; develop model legislation and regulations to enhance the viability of registry operations; train registry personnel; and establish a computerized reporting and data processing system. NPCR was funded by the *Cancer Registries Amendment Act.*

National Wilms' Tumor Study Group an *intergroup study* of the treatment of patients with Wilms' tumor with a goal of developing more effective treatments for children with Wilms' tumor, as well as looking for the causes of this cancer.

natural breaks data classification scheme in which classes are made to be as internally similar as possible (i.e., within-class variation is minimized, whereas between-class variation is maximized).

natural language processing process by which digital text from online documents stored in the organization's information system is read directly by software and automatically parsed, coded, or both.

natural product a chemotherapeutic agent that is derived from a plant or other organism rather than a chemical compound; *n. p.* include *antitumor antibiotics, plant alkaloids,* and *enzymes*.

necropsy see *autopsy.*

NEDSS (National Electronic Disease Surveillance System) Centers for Disease Control and Prevention (CDC) initiative that promotes the use of data and information system standards to advance the development of efficient, integrated, and interoperable surveillance systems at federal, state, and local levels. A primary goal of NEDSS is the ongoing, automatic capture and analysis of data that are already available electronically.

Nelson–Aalen statistic preferred statistical estimate of the cumulative hazard function.

neoplasm a new growth; the term *n.* itself does not carry any association of being *benign* or *malignant.*

nephroblastoma see *Wilms' tumor.*

nested design procedure that combines two study designs, one within another, to optimize choices; more data, quicker, and at lower costs.

net survival estimation of the survival probability adjusting for competing causes of death.

neuroblastoma a tumor of childhood arising from immature nerve cells in the neural crest ectoderm.

neuropeptides chains of protein building blocks that act on nerve cells.

NHII (National Health Information Infrastructure) initiative set forth to improve the effectiveness, efficiency, and overall quality of health and healthcare in the United States. It is a comprehensive, knowledge-based network of interoperable systems of clinical, public health, and personal health information that would improve decision making by making health information available when and where it is needed.

NHIN (National Health Information Network) one of several affiliates of the National Health Systems with the mission of providing the foundation for interoperable, secure, and standards-based health information exchange nationally.

noise variability in data that can obscure the ability to detect an underlying pattern or trend.

nomenclature   a system of names; an organized way of naming things.

nominal   see *data.*

nonanalytic   a category of *class of case* that indicates that the case was referred to the reporting facility for recurrence or subsequent therapy after the cancer was initially diagnosed and treated at another facility; the opposite of *analytic.* A *n.* case is generally not included in statistical reports of treatment and survival but may be included in administrative reports.

non–cancer-directed   procedures that do not attempt to modify, control, remove, or destroy cancer tissue; for example, bypass surgery, radiation to a single tender area of bone metastases, or removal of a painful primary or metastasis tumor mass.

noncontiguous   see *discontinuous.*

noninfiltrating, noninvasive   see *in situ.*

nonparametric statistics   various statistical techniques that can be used for small numbers of subjects or severely skewed distributions, including the *Kruskal–Wallis test, Mann–Whitney U test, Fisher's exact test,* and the *Wilcoxon signed rank test.* Also, methods that make no strong assumptions about the distributions of the variables being assessed.

nonreportable   not meeting the criteria for inclusion into a registry; see *reportable.* For example, a malignant diagnosis identified in the disease index may not be supported by the medical record itself (in other words, miscoded), rendering the case *n.*

North American Association of Central Cancer Registries (NAACCR)   an organization of member cancer registries established in 1987, whose purpose is to promote standardized data collection, quality, and consistency of central cancer registry operations, and exchange of information among population-based central cancer registries in North America. This organization was formerly known as the *American Association of Central Cancer Registries (AACCR).*

NPCR-CSS (National Program of Cancer Registries Cancer Surveillance System)   Centers for Disease Control and Prevention (CDC) database system resulting from annual data submissions from NPCR-funded state registries. State data meeting existing NPCR requirements are included in the aggregate NPCR-CSS database and proceed to be included in the United States Cancer Statistics (USCS) publication.

NPI (National Provider Identifiers)   unique identification number for healthcare providers scheduled for implementation by the Centers for Medicare & Medicaid Services (CMS) as part of *HIPAA (Health Insurance Portability and Accountability Act).*

nuclear medicine   a medical specialty or department of a healthcare facility that uses *radioactive isotopes* to diagnose and treat patients.

null hypothesis   statement that is either accepted or rejected based on the results of a statistical test and generally proposes that there is no difference in rates between groups

object topology   information about the relation between spatial objects in a GIS, such as whether they are adjacent or overlapping.

objective(s)   the measurable ends to which a person or organization strives; for example, one *o.* for a cancer registry is to maintain a 90% successful follow-up rate.

objects   metafile objects are the components of the metafile. They consist of Agency, Data Dictionary, Record Layout, Edits, Edit Sets, Error Messages, and User Tables.

observed survival   estimation of the actual observed survival probability.

Occupational Outlook Handbook   publication compiled by the U.S. Bureau of Labor Statistics that includes a description of the work, training, and education for various occupations.

Office of Sponsored Research   a federally required office in any institution involved in research that serves as a liaison or clearinghouse for communications between the facility and the *clinical trial group, Department of Health and Human Services (HHS),* or other organizations that grant funds for research, as well as controlling and coordinating the funding of research activities; also called *Grants Administration.*

Office of the National Coordinator for Health Information Technology (ONC)   the office that serves as the secretary of *Department of Health and Human Services' (HHS)* principal advisor on the development, application, and use of health information technology. To the extent permitted by law, it develops, maintains, and directs the implementation of a strategic plan to guide the nationwide implementation of interoperable health information technology in both the public and private healthcare sectors.

oncology   the study of cancer as a disease process; the study of tumors.

oncology indicators   specific *outcomes measures* designed to assess the quality of cancer care in an institution; see also *clinical indicator.* An example of an *o. i.* for lung cancer is "the number of unresectable tumors determined at thoracotomy."

online coursework   curriculum or training using a computer and the Internet.

open source software   applications and development tools that are freely distributed and licensed. Distributions include source code and are supported by a community of users and developers.

operating system   special master computer program that controls the resources and operations performed by a computer.

operations manual   in a registry, the specific instructions for initiating and terminating the computerized cancer registry program, including instructions for completing routine tasks, backup and data loss prevention procedures, and descriptions of edit checks and potential problems and their resolution, and a disaster recovery plan.

operative report   a summary of pertinent observations noted during the course of a surgical procedure dictated by the surgeon; also called a *surgery report.* The *o. r.* is useful to the registry because it contains detailed information about the location of the tumor and any extension, nodal involvement, or metastasis spread that did not undergo biopsy or was resected.

optional data   see *data set. o. d.* includes financial data (insurance payer information, as well as charges and reimbursements), laboratory studies, service utilization, and other items of specific interest to the facility collecting them.

oral   administration of drugs or chemotherapeutic agents by mouth (swallowing them) so that the drug can be absorbed through the gastrointestinal tract into the bloodstream.

ordinal   see *data.*

ordinate   see *axis.*

other cancer-directed therapy   a category of treatment that includes cancer treatments whose action or efficacy has not been clearly defined, such as *experimental therapy, unproven therapy,* and *double-blind studies.*

outcome   the result of an interaction between a patient and the healthcare system, usually the results of a study. Examples of measurable *o.* include *survival, patient satisfaction,* and time to recurrence. *o. measurement* is the process of analyzing whether a plan executes what it is capable of doing and, when it does, what the results are. *o. measures* are statistical statements that describe the expected results; for example, one *o. m.* for breast cancer is "the proportion of all breast cancers of known stage diagnosed at an in situ stage."

outpatient   a person treated without having to occupy a bed overnight at a healthcare facility. An *o. clinic* is a facility, usually affiliated with a hospital, where patients are examined and treated, but they do not stay overnight. Also called *ambulatory clinic.*

outsource   to procure (as some goods or services needed by a business or organization) under contract with a vendor.

override   to indicate that a data edit advising a possible inconsistency has been reviewed and the information is correct.

override flags (in editing)   checks that are set by a user to indicate that the data in the record(s) have been reviewed and, although unlikely, are correct.

paired bar chart   see *bar chart.*

palliative   intended to relieve symptoms or make the patient more comfortable; action taken to maximize the well-being of patients who cannot be cured. *p. treatment* is considered *non–cancer-directed* treatment.

Pap smear   a type of cytology examination used for the detection of abnormal cervical cells; named for its developer, Dr. George Papanicolaou.

parameter   a specific datum or characteristic; an aspect or criterion being studied; for example, an analysis of survival in white female patients with breast cancer includes three *p.*—race, sex, and primary site.

parametric statistical methods   methods that assume that the distributions of the variables being assessed belong to known parameterized families of probability distributions.

parse   to divide, and possibly understand, a text string (e.g., address) into smaller component parts.

passive reporting   see *casefinding.*

pathologic staging   in the *TNM staging* system, a *staging basis* designating that the information used to assign the T, N, and M categories included the resection of the primary tumor and, for most primary sites, the removal and examination of regional lymph nodes, in addition to the clinical examinations and diagnostic tests.

pathologist   a physician specializing in the microscopic diagnosis of disease.

pathology   the scientific study of the nature of disease, its causes, processes, development, and consequences, especially through the microscopic examination of tissues and cells. The *p. department* is the section of a healthcare facility responsible for microscopic analysis of tissues and body fluids.

pathology report   the written description of the microscopic examination of a tissue. The *gross description* reports the physical characteristics of the tissue: size, color, and abnormalities visible with the unaided eye. The *microscopic description* reports the cellular characteristics aided by the use of a *microscope:* what cells are involved, the behavior, and the aggressiveness or grade of any abnormality. The *final diagnosis* is a summary of the findings and indicates the pathologist's impression of what was found in concise terms.

patient   individual person with one or more primary cancers/reportable conditions; the complete demographic record for a person with cancer/reportable condition

patient brochure   a publication describing the services of the cancer registry, designed for patient education.

patient identification a part of the *abstract* containing data items that identify a specific person, such as a patient's name, address, social security number, health record number, sex, date of birth, race, and so forth.

patient index see *master patient index file.*

patient linkage process of using defined criteria to determine whether source records refer to the same patient based on the degree of agreement between demographic and other data fields. This can be automated, manual, or a combination of the two. Automated patient linkage can be performed using either deterministic or probabilistic methods. Also known as "record linkage or matching."

patient log a listing of the patients treated in a specific department such as radiation or medical oncology; useful for *casefinding.*

patient privacy the right of a patient to have his/her medical and other information protected from dissemination to unauthorized persons or agencies.

patient satisfaction a way of measuring the success of a healthcare encounter by analyzing the answers to questions asked of the person who received services or treatment.

PDF (Portable Document Format) widely used, standardized document format created by Adobe that preserves the original layout of documents when printed or viewed online. The Acrobat Reader, which is available as a free download, is needed to view or print PDF documents.

PDQ (Physician Data Query) a database of current cancer treatment and protocol information available through the *National Cancer Institute (NCI).*

Pearson's correlation see *correlation.*

Pediatric Oncology Group (POG) a pediatric *clinical trial group,* composed of the former pediatric sections of *Southwest Oncology Group (SWOG)* and *Cancer and Leukemia Group B (CALGB),* that has developed a series of staging systems for various children's malignancies.

peer review monitoring of the activities of medical professionals by other professionals with the same level of knowledge; usually the monitoring of physicians by other physicians.

percent change in rates estimate of the percent change in rates from the beginning to the end of a specified period, typically calculated as the difference between the average rate of the first interval and the average rate of the last interval, divided by the average rate of the first interval.

performance evaluation a review of the accomplishments and effectiveness of an individual in handling a job. *p. e.* are conducted by a supervisor to help an employee improve job skills.

performance improvement plan documentation of a healthcare facility's strategy to make its services more effective; part of a *Joint Commission on Accreditation of Healthcare Organizations (JCAHO)* survey.

performance measurement system an interrelated set of outcomes measures, process measures, or both, that supports internal comparisons of an organization's performance over time and external comparisons of performance among organizations at comparable times.

period prevalence measure of prevalence where the numerator includes the number of cases in a population during a specified period.

period survival method for calculating multiyear survival based on the last yearly conditional survival probabilities for each of the most recent years of survival data; used in estimating current survival.

person-year a statistical calculation in which the number of cases in the population is multiplied by the years *at risk;* used to express a *rate* over a period of time. For study designs where subjects are followed through time, each person contributes a *p.* for each year of participation; for example, a group of 100 persons studied from January 1, 1990, to December 31, 1999 (10 years) contributes 1,000 *p.* to the study (10 years × 100 persons). Also, 1 year that a person is at risk, as counted in the denominator of an average annual incidence rate; individuals may be counted multiple times if they are at risk for more than 1 year. For study designs where subjects are followed through time, each person contributes a "person-year" for each year of participation (e.g., a group of 100 persons, studied from January 1, 1995, to December 31, 2004 [10 years] contribute 1,000 person-years to the study).

phase one of the series of steps necessary to complete a *clinical trial. P. I* (Phase I) clinical trials test the initial safety of new drugs, devices, treatment modalities, or combinations of these elements. *P. II* (Phase II) clinical trials focus on dose responses, frequency of drug dosage, and other areas of safety, as well as drug efficacy; also called *pivotal trials. P. III* (Phase III) clinical trials compare the research drug, method, or device with current standard treatment. *P. IV* (Phase IV) clinical trials provide additional details regarding a drug's safety and efficacy.

PHIN (Public Health Information Network) *Centers for Disease Control and Prevention (CDC)* national initiative to implement a multiorganizational business and technical architecture for public health information systems. The five key components are detection and monitoring, data analysis, knowledge management, alerting, and response.

PHP (Hypertext Preprocessor) a scripting language that augments the HTML code on a Web page. It is often used to interact with online databases, especially MySQL.

physical examination the careful inspection of the body, looking for signs of disease. For cancer patients, the *p. e.*

can yield information on the size and location of the tumor, involved lymph nodes, organ enlargement, or other abnormalities resulting from the disease process.

pictorial chart a graphic presentation of information that uses symbols to display volume or magnitude. Maps and anatomic drawings are also considered *p. c.*

pie chart a graphic presentation of information that displays the relation of parts to a whole in circular format.

piggy-backing a research term where one test or procedure is used for two purposes to reduce costs for a scientific study; for example, using a blood test that diagnosed a leukemia as the required blood test for a study.

pivotal trial see *phase.*

plant alkaloids a chemotherapy agent of *natural products* derived from specific types of growing plants, which interfere with cell division by inhibiting *mitosis.*

Platform/Architecture hardware-related elements of the computerization used. It reflects baseline configuration, including whether the system will be Web based or local, whether a file server or client server architecture will be used, what operating system will be used, and whether data sources are hard copy or electronic.

platykurtosis see *kurtosis.*

ploidy the number of sets of chromosomes in a cell.

PNET (primitive neuroectodermal tumor) a tumor of the embryonal neural cells arising in the central nervous system or soft tissues.

point prevalence measure of prevalence where the numerator includes the number of cases in a population at a particular point in time or date.

Poisson regression statistical method used to model disease incidence where the outcome variable is a rate; assumes that the event occurrences are independent and occur constantly over time.

population in statistical terms, the individuals who make up a certain category defined for scientific study. In demographic terms, the residents of a specified area.

population-at-risk the specific set of individuals within a defined population who are susceptible to development of a specific disease. (For example, women are the population-at-risk who are susceptible to development of ovarian cancer. Thus, the denominator [population-at-risk] used to calculate incidence rates should be only women living in the population.)

population-based registries cancer registries that collect and maintain information on all newly diagnosed cancer patients within a defined geographic area (i.e., a state, a province, or a city). Also, a *registry* that collects information on all residents of a defined geographic area with a known census. *p.* registries are the only type of registry that allows the calculation of incidence and mortality

rates. The two types of *p.* registries are *incidence-only* and *multipurpose,* which combine incidence reporting with patient care, end results, and various other research and cancer-control activities.

position description a document delineating all of the responsibilities and other requirements of a named work activity, such as cancer registry abstractor; also called *job description.*

positive predictive value in *screening,* the percentage of all persons tested for a disease who are actually found to have the disease.

postal code (in Canada) six-digit alphanumeric code that describes a postal delivery location. Canadian postal codes are very specific. In urban areas, each side of a city block typically has its own code.

power in statistical terms, the effectiveness of a sample to represent the population of which it is a subset.

practice parameters carefully developed guidelines for treating a patient with a specific diagnosis, usually describing the minimum or maximum circumstances for administering that treatment.

prevalence how many cases of a particular disease there are in a population at a given point in time. *p.* is a combination of *incident cases* and cases that have been diagnosed and treated in previous years.

primary the organ of origin of a cancer; see also *site.* A *new p.* is one that has been diagnosed as separate and not related to a previous cancer. A *subsequent p.* is any distinct cancer diagnosed after the first one and not related to it. These concepts are synonymous; a cancer is usually called a *n. p.* during the diagnosis and treatment phase and a *s. p.* when referred to retrospectively. A patient with more than one *p.* is said to have *multiple primaries.* An *unknown p.* is a cancer that was first diagnosed from a metastasis site and whose point of origin cannot be determined.

primary prevention a type of *cancer control* effort intended to reduce the exposure to agents causing cancer or to reduce genetic predisposition to a cancer; preventing the occurrence of disease through occupational, environmental, and regulatory controls, and lifestyle and behavior modification. See also *secondary prevention.*

primary site table graphic presentation (usually a table of rows and columns) describing the number and characteristics of cases of various types of cancers in the cancer program *annual report;* a way to display a registry's *site distribution* information.

primary tumor a tumor that is at the original site where it first arose.

principal investigator (PI) in a healthcare facility, the leader of research activities who is responsible for conducting the studies designed by the *clinical trial group.*

probabilistic linkage   algorithms using a fluid or dynamic relation between data items that takes into account various attributes of the data that are important for increasing the probability of match situations. The rules that govern the process are developed as the project evolves. Two key attributes are error rates within any specific element and frequency analysis of the values of any specific element. The error rate associated with an element can be thought of as how often that particular element does not agree within a truly matched pair. Frequency analysis takes into account the commonness of any given value for a data item and uses this knowledge as a component in the matching process.

procedure manual   a document that describes in detail how each function or component of an activity is conducted; for example, a *p. m.* should describe each step in the case ascertainment process, whom to contact, and what to do with the information that is gathered.

process controls   statistical methods to measure the state of a procedure or function and trigger a review when the result exceeds established limits; for example, monitoring timeliness of reporting in a registry.

product line   in hospitals, a group of diagnoses or services that are managed (administratively and financially) as a unit. For example, obstetrical, orthopedic, and oncology services can be considered separate product lines because their patients are usually mutually exclusive. Radiation therapy and chemotherapy might be considered separate *p. l.* or included under a more general umbrella of oncology services. The *oncology p. l.* may also include nursing units, the *infusion center,* rehabilitation, and other services directly related to the treatment of cancer.

product moment calculation   see *survival calculation.*

productivity standards   quantifiable guidelines for performing a specific task; for example, stating that, on average, an experienced employee in a facility can complete eight abstracts per day uninterrupted by other tasks. *p. s.* are used to measure employee achievement at the time of *performance evaluation* or salary review.

product-limit method   see *Kaplan–Meier survival.*

prognosis, prognostic   the anticipated outcome of a procedure or status in terms of *survival* or *quality of life;* for example, early stage cancers usually have a good prognosis, meaning that a patient will live a reasonable length of time. *Prognostic* pertains to the factors that help to assess that outcome; for example, the number of involved axillary lymph nodes is a prognostic factor for breast cancer.

progress notes   the part of the health information record that summarizes diagnostic findings on a daily basis, usually handwritten by the health professionals taking care of the patient.

progression of disease   the advancement of the cancer to other organs despite treatment. Unlike *recurrence,* there is not a *disease-free* interval before *p. o. d.* begins.

projection (in GIS)   set of equations that define how the spherical surface of Earth is represented in two dimensions. This necessarily results in some distortion of area, shape, and/or distance.

promotion   causing a cell to grow rapidly and to metastasize as a result of uncontrolled growth; one of the two steps in *carcinogenesis.*

prophylaxis, prophylactic   the use of a specific action to prevent disease; for example, radiation to the central nervous system to prevent brain metastases from lung cancer.

proportion   a mathematical representation showing the relation of a part to the whole; the elements that make up the numerator (upper part of a fraction) are a subset of the elements that make up the denominator (lower part of a fraction).

proportion   ratio in which the numerator is part of the denominator.

proportional hazards assumption   assumption that the effect of independent variables is constant over time. Required by the Cox regression model.

proportional symbol   see *graduated symbol.*

prospective study   looking forward from the exposure to the later occurrence of disease or injury. A *p. s.* begins collection of cases at the present time for a specific period, such as a year; also called *cohort study.*

protocol   a detailed description of the study question, the plan for conducting the study, and assurances about the process of conducting a *clinical trial* or other research study.

Provincial Cancer Agency   organization responsible for the delivery of cancer services in the province or territory.

psychometric   of, or relating to, the psychological theory or technique of mental measurement.

PTCR (Provincial and Territorial Cancer Registries)   population-based central registries for provinces or territories.

Public Law 102-515   the Cancer Registries Amendment Act, law number 515 of the 102nd Congress of the United States, which established the *National Program of Cancer Registries (NPCR).*

public use file   line listing of individual person records, after removing variables that would permit identification of individuals; unlike aggregate data in which frequencies from multiple patients are combined, and no personal identification is possible.

p value   statistic expressing the probability, given the null hypothesis is true, of observing data as extreme as that observed; large **p** *values* provide evidence supporting the null hypothesis, and smaller **p** *values* provide evidence against the null hypothesis; the result of a statistical test indicating the probability that this statistic is the result of a random observation.

qualitative see *data.*

quality fitness for use; excellence. In registry terms, assurance that the information collected is accurate, complete, and usable for analysis. *Q. assurance* is the ongoing objective assessment of important aspects of patient care and the correction of identified problems. *Q. control,* in general terms, is a carefully planned set of activities by which database managers monitor current quality and take appropriate remedial action to positively affect future quality, maximizing correct reporting and characterizing the reporting process in measurable terms. Specifically, *q. control* is the process of checking data for accuracy and timeliness.

quality control/quality assurance/quality management program to assure the quality of the data collected. The rigor and comprehensiveness of a registry's quality management program is another important and defining characteristic. A variety of methodologic alternatives can be selected including staffing decisions, sampling methods, hospital feedback, reabstracting studies, recoding audits, benchmarks used, computer edits, visual edits, *death certificate only (DCO)* methods, correction procedures, and documentation of *q. c.* procedures. *q. improvement* is the process of reviewing various facets of a job or project to determine what factors about it can be made better.

quality of life those factors reflecting a patient's general status, not just cancer-related disabilities; an important concern in treating a patient and returning him or her to a fully functional life. Also called *quality of survival.*

quantile data classification scheme in which each class contains the same number of records. Five such classes are known as quintiles, 10 such classes are known as deciles, and so on.

quantitative see *data.*

race/ethnicity/nationality (as used in cancer registration) Related terms used to characterize cancer patients (e.g., race equals African American, ethnicity equals Hispanic, nationality equals Mexican). There is not scientific agreement on racial definitions. Default classifications used in decennial censuses are sometimes assumed.

radiation oncology department that section of a healthcare facility that treats patients using beam radiation (*teletherapy*) or *brachytherapy;* also called the *radiation therapy* department.

radiation therapy cancer-directed treatment by radioactivity that kills cells by damaging *DNA,* thereby affecting the ability of the cell to divide. *r. t.* is treatment using invisible, high-energy rays emitted by radiation sources that can be at a distance from the tumor (*teletherapy*) or close to it (*brachytherapy*).

radioactive isotopes natural substances (elements) that emit radiation (invisible rays) that can be used for cancer diagnosis and treatment. *r. i.* can be attached to small molecules and given intravenously. The *r. i.* is attracted to a particular type of tissue, such as thyroid, and concentrates there, providing lethal doses of radiation to cancer cells.

radiocurable the ability to administer a sufficient dosage of radiation therapy to completely kill the tumor and cure the patient without excessively damaging the normal tissue surrounding the tumor.

radiographic study see *X-ray.*

radiosensitive responding to *radiation therapy.*

RAID (Redundant Array of Independent Disks) disk storage computer disk configuration that allows one or more disk drives to fail whereas maintaining the integrity of the data they are storing. Failed components may be replaced before they lead to a loss of data.

RAM (Random Access Memory) hardware component in a computer where data and programs are temporarily stored during processing.

random sample a method of statistical selection in which every individual in the *population* has an equal and independent chance of being chosen for study.

randomization the assignment to a *treatment arm* of a *clinical trial* by chance, to eliminate statistical bias and assure valid results to the study.

range checks computerized *edit checks* that test that a code is within the scope of acceptable codes; for example, a code 7 would fail a *r. c.* if the code structure included only the values 1 through 5. See also *allowable code check.*

rapid case ascertainment (RCA) special *casefinding* procedures that allow early or preliminary reporting of certain types of cases to get notification of eligible study subjects to researchers. Also, rapid notification of reportable cases to the cancer registry quickly after diagnosis. This method of case identification can take extra resources for technicians to perform independent and early path report screening at a wide range of organizations, or it can be accomplished through electronic reporting of path report information to the registry. Some registries are *RCA* for research purposes (e.g., early or preliminary reporting of certain types of cases to get notification of eligible study subjects to researchers).

rate the measurement of change in a variable over a period of time. An *age-specific r.* is calculated for cases within a range of age at diagnosis, for example, younger than 50 years. The cancer *mortality r.* is the measurement of how many persons in the general population die of cancer during the time period of interest. A *crude r.* is calculated for an entire population. The *incidence r.* measures the frequency at which people at risk experience development of a disease over a specified period. An *age-adjusted i. r.* minimizes the effects of differences in age distributions across time or in different study groups by using standardized population tables to allow comparison of rates in populations that have different age distributions. The *annual i. r.* is the incidence rate calculated for a 1-year period. A *site-specific r.* is calculated for a particular cancer primary, such as lung or breast. A *specific r.* is one calculated for a subgroup of the population. See also *survival rate.*

ratio   a fraction formed of two independent measures, where the numerator is not a subset of the denominator. See also *data.*

reabstracting study   a formal procedure conducted to check the accuracy of data in the cancer registry against the *source document(s).*

real-time reporting   automatic identification of case information through electronic transmission to the central registry as it is entered/digitized in the originating facility.

recoding study   a quality-control mechanism in which source documents are reviewed and assigned codes by a second abstractor to evaluate the accuracy of the data in the registry.

record   building block of data sets. Data items, or fields, are combined into records, which are then combined into files, which comprise a data set.

record consolidation   the process of combining data from two or more linked records for the same patient and tumor to produce a single "best" value for each patient and tumor variable. This can be automated, manual, or a combination. Also known as *data item consolidation, resolution, merging, summarization,* or *record cleanup.*

record layout   the named grouping and organization of data items, typically defined in a data dictionary.

record linkage   combining information from several sources on the same patient, usually by means of computerized matching programs. Also, method for assembling the information contained in two or more electronic records or data sources typically by means of computerized matching programs. Record linkage is used in case ascertainment, duplicate detection, coding, follow-up, and collaboration with external research projects.

recruitment   process of adding new individuals to staff.

recurrence   the return of a cancer that was not previously clinically apparent symptomatic, usually at a site distant from the primary (*metastasis*). *Local r.* is a return of the primary tumor itself. *Regional r.* is return of the tumor in an area beyond the limits of the original organ. *Distant r.*

is *disseminated,* or in an area remote from the original tumor.

recurrent staging   in the *TNM staging* system, a *staging basis* designating that the patient had been previously treated for this cancer but was *disease-free* for a period before experiencing a *recurrence,* and that the information used to assign the *T, N,* and *M* categories was based on the recurrence, not the original cancer.

reference database   a compilation of information that can be used as a comparison, or *benchmark;* also called *comparative data.*

reference date   the starting date established for a registry, usually January 1 of a given year, after which all cases diagnosed or treated at the facility, regardless of *date of initial diagnosis,* must be entered into the registry.

referral patterns   information on why physicians treat their patients at specific facilities or why patients choose to use the services of a specific facility.

regimen   a combination of chemotherapy drugs administered in a planned sequence to act at different points in the cell cycle. A *r.* may consist of several *cycles* of chemotherapy.

regional lymph nodes   those lymph nodes that are the first level of lymphatic drainage from an organ; *r. l. n.* can usually be removed as part of the *cancer-directed treatment.*

regionalized   a category of the *summary staging* system in which the tumor involves more than the organ of origin by means of *direct extension* or spread to regional lymph nodes.

Registered Health Information Administrator (RHIA)   the credentials given to health information management professionals who pass a test that establishes management-level knowledge of health information management department operations.

Registered Health Information Technician (RHIT)   the credentials awarded to health information management professionals who pass a test that establishes baseline knowledge about health information management department operations.

registry   see also *cancer registry;* a comprehensive health information system designed for the collection, analysis, and dissemination of a specific set of health data; a database that identifies and enumerates every instance of a reportable disease in a defined population. A *concurrent r.* collects data on cases that meet specified criteria on an ongoing basis. A *prospective r.* collects data on a specific population with no clinical evidence of the disease at the time of entry into the database, and based on defined study criteria, monitors the disease's incidence or natural history for a specified length of time. A *retrospective r.* collects data on a previously identified specific population meeting a specified criterion such as an established diagnosis of a particular disease. A *special purpose r.* collects data on cases with a specified criterion, disease process, population, or device.

registry certification   see *certification.*

registry director   person entrusted with the overall direction of cancer surveillance activities in a registry.

registry manager   person charged with managing the daily registry operations.

Registry Operations and Data Standards (ROADS)   a publication, volume II of *Cancer Program Standards* of the Commission on Cancer (COC), used between 1996 and 2002, which details the CoC-required data set and codes.

rehabilitation   the process of returning a patient to normal or near-normal function after treatment.

relapse   the return of a cancer after a clinically disease-free interval. The term *r.* is usually used to describe the return of a leukemia, lymphoma, or other hematopoietic malignancy, rather than the return of a carcinoma; see also *recurrence.*

relational database design   database organization usually designed to store various data elements together in logical groupings known as *records* or *tables.*

relative risk   a measure of disease frequency in which a comparison is made between a measure that is *expected* (a point of reference such as the general population) and a measure that is *observed* (found to have the disease or condition being studied); also called the *incidence ratio.*

relative survival   measure of net survival where other causes of death are adjusted for by dividing the observed survival for a cohort of patients by the expected survival from published life tables in a population with similar characteristics (e.g., age, sex, race, and period of observation) to those of the study population; contrasts with *observed survival.*

release of information   the sharing of facts about a patient; also called *disclosure. r. o. i.* can be authorized (intentional) or unauthorized (deliberate or unintentional).

reliability   the agreement of different coders using the same information and coding guidelines; see also *reproducibility.*

remission   complete or partial disappearance of the signs and symptoms of disease in response to treatment; the period in which a disease is under control.

reportable   meeting the criteria for inclusion in a registry. The *r. list* identifies all diagnoses and types of cases to be included in the cancer registry database and should also specify which diagnoses are *nonreportable. r.-by-agreement* cases are those *benign* or *borderline* disease processes that a facility's cancer committee has decided should be collected because they are of local interest.

reporter   individual responsible for submitting cancer abstract to central registry from a facility that does not have a full registry; also called *data collector.*

reporting delay   amount of time between the cancer diagnosis and when that diagnosis is reported to the registry. For example, there is currently a standard delay of 22 months between the end of the diagnosis year and the time *Surveillance, Epidemiology, and End Results Program (SEER)* cancer registries first report cancers to the *National Cancer Institute (NCI).* Cancers are reported on November 1 for all years including 2 years previous to the current year. However, SEER cancer registries continue to update registry data indefinitely, so statistics will change as cases are added for periods previously reported.

reporting error   inaccuracy in the data reported.

reproducibility   in registry terms, the ability of another person to replicate the same codes given the same information and coding guidelines; also referred to as *reliability.*

required data   see *data set.*

research protocol   see *protocol.*

resection   the removal of tissue from the body, usually an organ and its regional lymph nodes. A *surgical r.* removes a tumor with margins of normal tissue with the intent to remove the entire tumor. A *total r.* removes the primary tumor, surrounding tissue, and regional nodes.

residual tumor   the amount of primary cancer remaining after the most definitive *resection.*

resource consumption   see *allocation of resources.*

retention   the maintenance of presently employed cancer registry staff (e.g., low turnover).

retinoblastoma   a tumor that is the most common primary eye malignancy in children.

retrospective study   looking back to the exposure history after the disease or injury has occurred; for example, cases already in a registry database that meet specific criteria for analysis. In many instances, the cancer registry identifies cases to be included from its files and the researcher then collects any information not available in the database.

rhabdomyosarcoma   a common soft-tissue malignancy of muscle origin.

RHIO (Regional Health Information Organization)/HIE (Health Information Exchange)   group of healthcare entities in a particular region with a business stake in improving the quality, safety, and efficiency of healthcare. The terms *RHIO* and *HIE* are often used interchangeably. RHIOs are the building blocks of the proposed National Health Information Network (NHIN) initiative proposed by the Office of the National Coordinator for Health Information Technology (ONCHIT).

rho statistic   see *correlation.*

risk   the relation between the health experience observed for a study group and what would have been expected on the basis of the ***comparison group's*** health experience. When this value is expressed as a ratio (risk = observed/expected), it is a measure of the strength of association that exists between an ***exposure*** and an ***end point.*** It may be shown as a decimal fraction (e.g., 1.5) or multiplied by 100 to give a percentage (150%). ***r.*** may imply either an adverse (>1.0) or a beneficial (<1.0) relation; no risk is shown by a value of 1.0.

RSS (Really Simple Syndication)   system using XML that allows users to subscribe to "feeds." Feeds are web documents that can be subscribed to by using software called *aggregators.* Aggregators collect updated feeds and display them for the user. The feed displays like a regular Web page and usually has links back to the originating Web site.

salvage therapy   treatment given after the failure of *first course of therapy* to prolong survival or to improve quality of life; a second attempt to cure the patient; see also ***subsequent treatment.***

sample   in statistical terms, a subset of a ***population.***

sampling   the process of selecting data to represent the population being studied. Types of ***s.*** include *simple, random, convenience,* and *stratified.*

sarcoma   tumor arising in the supporting structures of the body (bone, muscle, connective tissue). A ***s.*** does not have a basement membrane and cannot be described or staged as ***in situ. Ewing's s.*** is a particular type of childhood tumor that can arise either in bone (osseous) or in soft tissue (extraosseous). ***Soft-tissue s.*** is a term for any tumor of ***mesenchymal*** origin arising in nonskeletal ***connective tissue,*** such as muscles, tendons, and blood vessels.

scan   a visual report or image of a body part created by computerized tomography, magnetic resonance imaging, or tracing the absorption of a radioactive isotope.

screening   a search for occult, undetected, or early-stage disease in a population to determine the prevalence of a disease.

screening effect   increases in cancer incidence rates in a population that are a direct result of new or increased screening activities in the population.

SDO (Standards Developing Organizations)   groups responsible for developing and sometimes implementing standards for cancer reporting for central registries (e.g., NAACCR develops many standards for central registries).

second course of treatment   see ***subsequent treatment.***

secondary prevention   efforts to deter a disease from incapacitating or threatening the life of a patient after the disease has occurred; the type of disease prevention practiced by conventional medicine. Also, activities that cannot prevent the disease from occurring but are directed at limiting the consequences of disease once it is detected.

secretary/clerk   Person who handles routine correspondence, files, accounts, and procurement for an office.

section   see ***tabular list.***

security   methodology for protecting confidential patient data against loss caused by breech, computer failure, or natural disaster.

SEER Program   see ***Surveillance, Epidemiology, and End Results Program.***

self-reporting   see ***casefinding.***

semiparametric statistical methods   statistical methods that make parametric assumptions about some components of the variables being assessed and no strong assumptions about other components.

sensitivity   in ***screening,*** the search for people with a particular disease. Also, proportion of true positives, or the proportion of cases correctly identified by the test as meeting a certain condition (e.g., in mammography testing, the proportion of patients with breast cancer who are correctly identified by mammography). See also ***specificity.***

sequence number   a unique identifier for each separate primary for a patient that describes the chronology of diagnoses, allowing the registry to identify patients who have ***multiple primaries.*** The ***s. n.*** indicates the number of primary cancers the patient has had in his or her lifetime, not just the number of primary cancers included in the reporting registry. The ***s. n.*** is numeric for cancers, and alphabetic for benign or borderline tumors.

sequential color scheme (in GIS)   a map color scheme proceeding from light to dark over a single hue, with darker values signifying higher quantities.

server   computer that provides access to a shared file system and/or increased computing capacity.

service area   the geographic region from which patients come to a healthcare facility; the region from which a hospital chooses to attract patients; also called *catchment area.*

single-field edits   edits that examine only one field at a time (e.g., sex).

site   in registry terms, where a cancer is growing in the body. The ***primary site*** is the organ of origin; where the cancer started in the body; also called the *topographic site.* A ***metastatic s.*** is where the cancer has spread to; also called a *metastasis. s. distribution*— see ***primary site table.***

site-specific   pertaining to a particular primary cancer; for example, ***s.*** surgery codes are individualized to each type of cancer (breast, colon, lung, etc.).

site visit   formal inspection by members of a ***clinical trial group*** of a facility that participates in clinical trials to assure that the facility meets all standards for research and documentation.

skew   the shape of a frequency distribution that is not symmetrical. When the longer tail of a curve trails to the left, it is called *left-skewed* or *negatively skewed.* When the longer tail of the curve trails to the right, it is called *right-skewed* or *positively skewed.*

smoothing   method for reducing variability in data by borrowing information from nearby areas or times.

SNOMED   see *Systemized Nomenclature of Medicine.*

Society of Clinical Research Associates (SoCRA)   a professional organization of *data managers* and other healthcare professionals involved in clinical trials.

source code   the programming language code that is used to write a computer program or application.

source documents   the medical records, disease indices, patient lists, pathology reports, or other original records from which *reportable* cases can be identified and cancer information can be abstracted.

source record   input data record for the central registry (i.e., an individual report on a tumor sent from a reporting facility to the central registry and stored in electronic format). This record may be from a hospital, pathology laboratory, clinic, other central registry, death certificate, etc.

Southwest Oncology Group (SWOG)   formerly the Southwest Cancer Study Group, a *clinical trial group* established in 1956. Now strictly for adult tumors, the pediatric section separated in 1980 to form the *Pediatric Oncology Group.*

sparse data   data with small numbers of counts; can present many difficulties in analysis and interpretation.

spatial analysis   a set of techniques that make use of the geographic location of events.

spatial object (in GIS)   a real-world entity with a geographic location represented as a point, line, or area.

spatial scan statistic   a method for identifying cancer clusters that is in wide use by cancer registries and for which free software exists.

Spearman's correlation   see *correlation.*

specificity   in *screening,* the search for persons who do not have the disease under study. See also *sensitivity.*

S-phase   the point in the cell cycle when cells are actively synthesizing *DNA;* in *flow cytometry,* it is the percentage of cells in active DNA synthesis.

stacked columns   see *bar chart.*

stage, stage of disease   categories that describe how far a cancer has spread, usually at the time of diagnosis. The *s. o. d.* is that part of the *abstract* that contains the data items that identify cancer spread, and confirm and support the assigned *s.* See also *staging.*

stage grouping   in the *TNM staging* system, the process of assigning a general category (I, II, III, and so forth) conveying disease progression and *prognosis* information for a specific case, based on specific criteria.

staging   a common language developed by medical professionals to communicate information about a disease to others. *s.* usually conveys anatomic *extent of disease* or *prognostic* information about an individual case; a shorthand method of describing disease. Also, the grouping of cases into broad categories based on *extent of disease. s.* usually refers to groups of cases with the same characteristics.

staging basis   in the *TNM staging* system, the point of evaluation; the time at which information on the tumor is collected. See also *clinical staging, pathologic staging, autopsy staging,* and *recurrent staging.*

staging laparotomy   a careful operative exploration of the abdomen to rule out occult abdominal disease and accurately determine the stage of disease; used to stage Hodgkin's disease.

standard(s)   guidelines that indicate the optimum achievement level for a particular function or activity; for example, the *s.* for case abstracting is to have the abstract completed within 6 months of the patient's first discharge from the healthcare facility. *Data s.* are guidelines that provide uniformity of definitions and code structures for data elements and consistent use of codes. *s. of care* are carefully developed guidelines for the treatment of patients with a specific condition, such as *critical pathways* and *practice parameters.*

standard deviation   the measure of variation about the mean, or average, in a series of numbers.

standardization   in registry terms, the use of uniform guidelines that describe data elements and their codes and how those codes are applied, assuring that cases from registries adhering to those standards are coded by the same rules and edited and updated according to the same guidelines.

Standards of the Commission on Cancer   a publication of the *Commission on Cancer (CoC)* issued since 1996 that provides specific guidelines for *cancer program accreditation.* See **Cancer Program Standards** and **Registry Operations and Data Standards.**

statistical techniques   using information gained from a sample, which is a subset of a larger group, to make statements about the *population* of interest; mathematical methods used to help distinguish between a true association and one that results from chance. Statistical techniques include *hypothesis testing,* the *z test* (which measures the difference between an observation and the sample mean), *t test* (which compares one distribution with another to determine whether they represent two different distributions or populations), the **chi-square test** (which assesses variability about an expected value), **ANOVA** (analysis of variance or the **F-test**), **multivariable regression, correlation,** and **nonparametric statistics**.

statistics   a branch of mathematics dealing with the collection, analysis, interpretation, and presentation of masses of numerical data. **Biostatistics** are mathematical analyses having to do with living organisms, such as survival analyses for cancer patients.

stem cell transplant   a type of **bone marrow transplant** in which stem cells (the immature cells from which all blood cells develop) are obtained from the bloodstream and then used to restore the bone marrow.

stereotactic   approached from more than one direction, usually two. **s. radiosurgery** involves focusing radiation beams on a small area and delivering very high doses of **radiation therapy.**

steroid   a type of **hormone therapy** that is specifically toxic to lymphoid malignancies. **s.** are also used to alter immune system response and the reaction of cancer cells to chemotherapy, thereby improving treatment response.

subcategory   see **tabular list.**

subclassification   see **tabular list.**

subcutaneous   injection of a drug or chemotherapy agent under the skin.

subsequent primary   see **primary.**

subsequent treatment   any additional therapy administered after the failure of the first course of therapy, because of either progression of disease or the lack of response to initial treatment.

summary staging   a system of describing the anatomic spread of cancer in broad or general terms: **localized, regionalized,** and **distant;** sometimes called *general staging*. **s. s.** was originally developed in California, was later adopted by the **Surveillance, Epidemiology, and End Results Program (SEER) Program**, and was last updated in 2001.

supervisor   any individual directly responsible for overseeing daily operations of a program, department, or its staff.

Supplement on the Tumor Registry   the **Commission on Cancer (CoC)** document used between 1981 and 1986 that provided standardized guidelines and coding mechanisms for cancer data; replaced by the **Data Acquisition Manual (DAM)** (1986–1996) and later by **Standards of the Commission on Cancer, volume II: Registry Operations and Data Standards (ROADS) (1996–2002).** The **Facility Oncology Registry Data Standards (FORDS)** is the current CoC-required data set and coding manual used to collect accurate data and manage cancer cases.

supplemental data   see **data set.**

supportive care   treatment that enhances the patient's quality of life but does not directly affect the cancer, such as administering drugs to improve appetite or reduce brain swelling.

supratentorial   see **tentorium cerebelli.**

surgery   most often includes the removal of tissue from the body; see also **resection. Cytoreductive s.** removes as much gross disease as possible to improve the efficacy of adjuvant treatment; also called *debulking*. **Diagnostic s.** identifies the histologic type of cancer and estimates the stage of disease but leaves gross tumor in the body; see also **biopsy. Function-preserving s.** is treatment to remove as much tumor as possible without affecting mobility or activity level; for example, a wide excision of a rhabdomyosarcoma of the arm is a more **f. s.** than amputation. **Palliative s.** attempts to reduce pain or correct functional abnormalities to improve quality of life, but it does not modify, control, remove, or destroy cancer tissue. **Preventive s.** is intended to avoid the development of cancer by removing a diseased organ before it becomes malignant. **Reconstructive s.** restores the function or appearance of organs or tissues that were either removed or changed by cancer-directed treatment. **Tissue-sparing s.** is an attempt to remove all tumor from an organ whereas maintaining the organ's form and structure. An example of **t. s.** is lumpectomy for breast cancer.

surgery report   see **operative report.**

surveillance data   information that is used to monitor changes in cancer in a population. Included are measures of cancer incidence, morbidity, survival, prevalence, and mortality. Also included are the assessment of genetic predisposition, environmental and behavioral risk factors, screening practices, and the quality of care from prevention through palliation.

Surveillance, Epidemiology, and End Results (SEER) Program   program of the **National Cancer Institute (NCI)** a federally funded consortium of population-based cancer registries representing approximately 14% of the U.S. population, established by the **National Cancer Act of 1971** to collect and publish information on cancer incidence, mortality, survival, and trends over time from selected geographic areas in the United States. **SEER Program** participants were selected primarily for their ability to operate and maintain a population-based cancer reporting system and for their epidemiologically significant population subgroups.

survey   in registry terms, a detailed review of a cancer program comparing it with established standards for availability of services, patient management, and dissemination of cancer information.

Survey Application Record (SAR)   a **Commission on Cancer (CoC)** Web-enabled cancer program that is a primary source of cancer program information and provides a summary of facility demographic information, resources, services, and description of annual cancer program activity of the cancer program. Information recorded in the SAR is used by both the CoC surveyor(s) and CoC staff to evaluate and rate the program's compliance with the CoC standards at the time of cancer program survey.

survival   how long a patient has lived since diagnosis or some other beginning point. See also *survival calculation.* In general terms, the probability of living a given length of time (such as 5-year survival) based on the characteristics of a group of patients. The *s. curve* is the graphed series of *s.* calculations at intervals. The *s. rate* is a calculated number or percentage reflecting the proportion of persons in a defined population who remain alive during a specified time interval. *Adjusted s.* calculations take into account whether the patient died of cancer. *Cumulative s.* is the dependency of the later time periods on the earlier survival rates, for example, third interval survival is a proportion of the patients living through the second interval, which is a proportion of patients who lived through the first interval. *Observed s.* calculations include all patients regardless of their cause of death. *Relative s.* calculations factor in the survival rate of a similar population without the characteristic (such as cancer) in question.

survival calculation   a mathematical formula for determining the survival rate at a set of intervals. The *direct method* requires that all subjects be available for survival throughout the complete interval of interest; in other words, all patients would have to be diagnosed at least 5 years ago to calculate a 5-year survival by this method. The *life-table method* creates a series of calculations based on the number of patients who die and who are withdrawn alive during an interval (usually a year or month); also called the *actuarial* or *cohort method* of calculating survival. The life-table method takes the data for the time that a subject has survived and uses them for analysis as long as possible. The *Kaplan–Meier* or *product moment* calculation is a variation of the life-table method in which the *s. c.* is made each time a patient dies, rather than at the end of an interval.

survival probability   likelihood of remaining alive for a certain time after diagnosis among a cohort of patients.

survivor's day   a public event, usually sponsored by a healthcare facility, which honors patients who have successfully fought and survived cancer.

survivorship function   the shape of a survival curve, based on individual survival rates at various points in time; also called the *survival function.*

suspense   in registry terms, awaiting further action. The *s. file* or *s. list* is an inventory or document identifying potentially reportable cases that have not been abstracted; a list

of cases that have been ascertained but not yet completed. A *s. case* is a reportable disease awaiting completion and entry into the registry database.

syndrome   a group of symptoms or characteristics that appear together and identify a specific disease. For example, *superior vena cava s.* consists of venous engorgement, hepatic enlargement, and edema resulting from lymphatic or metastatic disease obstruction of the superior vena cava.

synthesis   the part of the cell cycle in which DNA is replicated as the cell prepares to divide.

system administrator   person who is responsible for maintaining the server and communications infrastructure, such as the network devices, wireless, and cabling systems (disaster recovery planning, virus scanning and security, software updates, database management system, basic system development).

Systematized Nomenclature of Pathology (SNOP)   a 1965 publication of the *College of American Pathologists (CAP)* that provided codes for most tissue diagnoses, including cancer morphology; replaced by SNOMED.

systemic   throughout the body; pertaining to or reaching all organs. Chemotherapy is *s.* treatment because it circulates throughout the body in the bloodstream and reaches all organs.

Systemized Nomenclature of Human and Veterinary Medicine   a comprehensive coding system for all medical and veterinary diagnoses, procedures, causative factors, and other descriptors of disease, originally published by the *College of American Pathologists (CAP).*

Systemized Nomenclature of Medicine—Clinical Terms, SNOMED Clinical Terms® (SNOMED CT®)   comprehensive and precise clinical reference terminology that healthcare providers, healthcare information technology suppliers, providers, payers, purchasers, and institutional researchers can use to improve the comparability of data. CT allows for consistent capture of detailed clinical information and provides a common language that enables a consistent way of capturing, sharing, and aggregating health data across specialties and sites of care.

T   in the *TNM staging* system, the element that designates the size and invasiveness of the primary tumor.

table   a graphic display or arrangement of information into rows and columns comparing more than one variable to summarize and present detail that would be cumbersome in narrative form.

tabular list   a listing or table of items in numerical order; in registry terms, the sequential list of topography and morphology codes in ICD-O or the numeric list of diagnoses in ICD-9. The divisions of the tabular list in ICD-9-CM are *chapter* (major disease concept), *section* (usually site-specific disease groupings within a range of three-digit codes), *category* (a specific three-digit code number), **sub-category** (further definition of the category at the decimal or fourth-digit level), and **subclassification** (the fifth-digit detail of the code).

target population   specific subset of individuals within a defined population that are at greatest risk for developing or dying of a specific type of cancer. These are the groups to which cancer-control interventions should be directed. For example, cancer-control interventions to increase cervical cancer screening are often directed at African Americans within a defined population because they are at greater risk for developing or dying of cervical cancer.

targeting education   selection of educational topics based on assessment of areas of weakness in the data, so as to improve the overall quality of the data through further training.

telemedicine   the practice of medicine, usually the process of diagnosing and recommending treatment, at a distance from the patient. Videoconferencing, television linkage, and computer imaging allow a patient in a rural area to be reviewed by physicians at a major referral facility without either the patient or the physician having to travel a great distance.

teleprocessing   the linkage of computers via telephone lines to transfer data or access the files of a central computer from a second, remote computer.

teletherapy   a type of **radiation therapy** where the radiation source is at a distance from the tumor, which is treated by a focused beam of radiation; also called *beam radiation* or *external beam radiation.*

tentorium cerebelli   a flap of meninges that separates the posterior fossa from the cerebral hemisphere. *Infratentorial* tumors are those that arise in the cerebellum or brainstem; *supratentorial* tumors are those that arise in the forebrain or cerebrum.

teratogen   an agent (chemical or other factor) causing physical defects in a developing embryo.

thematic map   map that depicts data, as opposed to one that depicts locations of features on the Earth's surface.

therapy   see **treatment.** *Induction t.* attempts to induce or achieve remission or reduction in bone marrow blasts after a diagnosis of leukemia. **Consolidation t.** is a more intensified treatment intended to cure the patient. **Maintenance t.** is the continuation of therapy as part of the initial treatment after evidence that the cancer is in remission; also called *continuation treatment.* **Prophylactic t.** is given to certain cancer patients in an effort to prevent central nervous system disease.

Third National Cancer Survey   a federally funded program between 1969 and 1971 that monitored the incidence and prevalence of cancer in the United States by surveying

certain population areas covering about 10% of the population; a predecessor of the **SEER Program.**

threshold (in record linkage)   level at which decisions are made regarding linking patient records. The preferred approach is to set the threshold quite high during the automated process and rely on manual review for the more complex situations where conflicts in the data elements exist.

tickler   in registry terms, a reminder. A *t. card,* also called a *follow-up card,* contains patient identifiers, contact information, and the date of last contact. It is used to remind the registrar to obtain follow-up on the patient at a 12-month interval after the last contact date. A **dual t. file** is a card file containing two sets of monthly guides. The card for a case that has been successfully followed is moved from the current year to the appropriate month for the following year. The *t. file* is the **manual** equivalent of the **control list.**

time-and-motion study   an analysis of work activity that involves measuring how long a task takes to accomplish and how much physical activity is involved (e.g., sorting, moving, organizing, and filing patient records).

timeliness   the degree to which various stages of the registration process occur on schedule; assurance that all cases have been included in a disease registry within a specified period, for example, within 6 or 12 months after diagnosis.

TNM staging   a method of describing how far a cancer has spread from its point of origin in terms of the tumor (T), involved regional lymph nodes (N), and distant metastases (M), plus a **stage grouping** and a **staging basis;** also called *AJCC staging.*

topography   in registry terms, the name of an anatomic site and its related code.

toxicity   the negative effect of a cancer treatment on normal tissue. Adriamycin is an anticancer drug that has an adverse effect of cardiac *t.*

TQM   total quality management; the process of quality; quality from start to finish. A corporation-wide belief that everyone in the organization is responsible for assuring that every step or activity of the organization is subjected to improvement in the level of excellence; also called *TQI* or *total quality improvement.* See also **continuous quality improvement.**

training   formal comprehensive instruction provided to cancer registry staff in the area of cancer reporting and cancer surveillance topics.

treatment   the attempt to cure a cancer or relieve symptoms of a cancer by various methods such as surgery, radiation therapy, chemotherapy, hormone therapy, or immunotherapy. Also called *therapy.* **Cancer-directed t.** is an attempt to modify, control, remove, or destroy the cancer; also called *definitive treatment.* **Non–cancer-directed t.** is that which diagnoses the cancer or relieves symptoms but does not attempt to cure the cancer. A *t. arm* is one of the therapy options being studied in a *clinical trial*. *T. patterns* are the therapy options for curing cancer; some types of cancer can be treated in a variety of ways and it is important to know which method results in the best survival and other outcomes. A *t. plan* is the therapy decision(s) determined by a physician for an individual patient based on a number of disease-specific and patient-specific factors.

trend   an increase or decrease in a *variable* over time.

Triad Clinical Cancer Control Program   a cooperative arrangement among Cancer Liaison Physicians, American Cancer Society divisions and units, and members of the *National Cancer Registrars Association (NCRA)* to identify issues, develop strategies, implement programs, and evaluate the effects of these activities on cancer control at state and local levels.

triad of disease   an epidemiologic concept that disease can be prevented by eliminating any one of the three elements (triad) necessary for a disease to occur: the *agent* (the actual biologic cause of the disease process), *host* (a person who is at risk for or susceptible to contracting the disease), or *environment* (the place where the agent and the host encounter each other).

truncated incidence rate   summary rate calculated for only the specific ages where disease occurrence is likely.

tumor   a swelling or mass; a new growth of tissue or cells.

tumor board   a meeting of medical professionals where the diagnosis and treatment of patients is discussed; see also *cancer conference.*

tumor linkage   process of using defined criteria to determine whether source records for the same patient refer to the same tumor or cancer, based on the degree of agreement between data fields with disease-related information. The process can be automated, manual, or a combination.

tumor marker   a substance in the blood or other human tissue that can assist in determining the presence or absence of cancer. *alpha-Fetoprotein* is a type of *t. m.*

tumor record   complete set of information on a single primary cancer or a reportable neoplasm, compiled from one or more source records from one or more facilities. Tumors are the entities that are counted in incidence surveillance.

type I error, type II error   see *hypothesis.*

UICC   see *International Union Against Cancer.*

UML (Unified Modeling Language)   general-purpose notational language for modeling (specifying, visualizing, constructing, and documenting) all the parts of a real-world system.

uncertain malignancy   see *borderline.*

Uniform Data Standards (UDS) Committee   a standing committee of *North American Association of Central Cancer Registries (NAACCR)* charged with compiling and resolving issues in coding, editing, and data exchange standards among NAACCR member organizations. Also, NAACCR group that provides the forum to discuss data issues and reach consensus on data standards. It includes members from all of the major standard-setting organizations, as well as several central registries and registry software providers. By June of each year, new and revised standards are released for implementation in January of the subsequent year as the **Standards for Cancer Registries, Volume II: Data Standards and Data Dictionary.**

Universal Serial Bus (USB) port   a connector, often on the side of a computer, that follows a widely used interface specification and allows peripheral devices to be connected to the computer.

Universal Transverse Mercator (UTM)   widely used geographic projection system that divides the globe into 60 longitudinal zones of 6 degrees each. Area, shape, and distance distortion is minimal within a zone.

unproven therapy   treatment of cancer by means of drugs or other methods that have not been shown to be effective according to the American Cancer Society.

unstable rate   incidence rate that is calculated for a population that has a very small number of cases. When a population has fewer the 16 incident cases, the rate calculated using these cases is considered to be unstable.

UPS (uninterruptible power supply)   redundant backup power source used to protect computers in the event of a power surge or temporary power outage.

usability   measure of the quality of the Web visitor's experience.

utilization review   the assessment of all hospital admissions for their appropriateness and medical necessity, as well as for *allocation of resources.*

validation   to declare or make legally valid.

validity   in registry terms, assessment of whether a specific piece of information in the registry is true or correct when compared with the *source document* from which it was taken.

variable   a category of information; for example, race and sex are two demographic *v.*

variance   the dispersal of observations about a *measure of central tendency.*

viscera   plural of viscus; internal organs.

visual editing   the manually checking of all aspects of the abstract, comparing codes with supporting text, and using judgment. This method contrasts with computer editing.

visual review   the process of editing an abstract by visually comparing data fields; a supplementary quality-control procedure to computerized edit checking.

vital status   whether a patient is alive or dead.

War on Cancer　President Richard Nixon's phrase describing increased efforts to reduce the morbidity and mortality of cancer, established by the ***National Cancer Act of 1971.***

Web conferencing　increasingly popular training medium in which two-way communication is established via the Internet for presentations and question/answer sessions between trainers and students. Also called *webinars* or *webcasts.*

Web server　software application that allows data and information to be accessed from the Web. Web servers do not necessarily require specialized hardware.

Web-based education　planned course of study (long or short), primarily using the Internet as the medium to convey knowledge. Also known as distance learning or on-line training. During Web-based education, the student communicates with the instructor via the Internet.

white space　the unprinted margin around a table or text; part of the graphic design of a report; also called *blank space.*

wide area network (WAN)　network of computers (as the Internet) in a large area (as a country or the globe) for sharing resources or exchanging data. Contrasts with ***LAN.***

Wilcoxon signed rank test　see ***nonparametric statistics.***

Wilms' tumor　an embryonal malignancy (***nephroblastoma***) that almost always arises in the kidney.

withdrawn alive　a term used in ***survival calculation*** that means that a patient has been excluded (***censored***) from the life-table calculation without dying. For example, a disease-free patient diagnosed 2 years ago would be ***w. a.*** at 24 months in a life table, even though the survival was calculated to 5 years.

World Health Organization (WHO)　an international agency of the United Nations responsible for health matters in many countries; for registries, the sponsor and publisher of the **International Statistical Classification of Diseases and Related Health Problems** and the **International Classification of Diseases for Oncology.**

written authorization　a paper signed by the patient that permits a facility to release information about him/her to another person or facility for the purpose of research, continuation of care, or administrative planning.

x-axis　see ***axis.***

XML (Extensible Markup Language)　popular data transmission format that has well-defined architectural rules but at the same time is flexible enough to handle a wide variety of data, including all of the data that cancer registries transmit.

X-ray　the common name for a roentgenogram or radiologic examination of an organ made by sending a beam of radiation through the organ to expose a special type of photographic film, which then provides an image of the organ for diagnosis; also called *radiographic study.*

y-axis　see ***axis.***

ZIP code　in the United States, a five-digit code designating a community or neighborhood postal delivery location. ZIP codes have no relation to political units or census divisions. Nine-digit ZIP codes are used to describe postal delivery locations more specifically.

index